Advances in Pain Research and Therapy
Volume 18

THE DESIGN OF ANALGESIC CLINICAL TRIALS

Advances in Pain Research and Therapy

Series Editor: John J. Bonica, M.D., D.Sc., F.F.A.R.C.S. (Hon.)

* Out of print in the original edition.

Advances in Pain Research and Therapy
Volume 18

The Design of Analgesic Clinical Trials

Editors

Mitchell B. Max, M.D.
Chief, Clinical Trials Unit
Neurobiology and Anesthesiology Branch
National Institute of Dental Research
National Institutes of Health
Bethesda, Maryland
Consultant, WHO Collaborating Center
for Research and Training
in Cancer Pain
New York, New York

Russell K. Portenoy, M.D.
Director of Analgesic Studies
Pain Service
Associate Attending Neurologist
Departments of Neurology and
Anesthesiology and
Critical Care Medicine
Memorial Sloan-Kettering Cancer Center
Assistant Professor of Neurology
Cornell University Medical College
Co-Director, WHO Collaborating Center
for Research and Training
in Cancer Pain
New York, New York

Eugene M. Laska, Ph.D.
Director, Statistical Sciences and Epidemiology Division
Nathan S. Kline Institute for Psychiatric Research
Director, WHO Collaborating Center for Training and Research
in Mental Health Program Management
Orangeburg, New York
Research Professor, Department of Psychiatry
New York University Medical Center
New York, New York

Raven Press 🦫 New York

Raven Press, 1185 Avenue of the Americas, New York, New York 10036

© 1991 by Raven Press, Ltd. All rights reserved. This book is protected by copyright. No part of it may be reproduced, stored in a retrieval system, or transmitted, in any form or by any means, electronic, mechanical, photocopying, recording, or otherwise, without the prior written permission of the publisher.

Made in the United States of America

Library of Congress Cataloging in Publication Data

The Design of analgesic clinical trials/editors, Mitchell B. Max,
  Russell K. Portenoy, Eugene M. Laska.
      p.   cm.—(Advances in pain research and therapy; v. 18)
    Includes bibliographical references and index.
    ISBN 0-88167-736-1
    1. Analgesics—Testing.   2. Pain—Chemotherapy.   3. Clinical
  trials—Design.   I. Max, Mitchell.   II. Portenoy, Russell K.
  III. Laska, Eugene M., 1939–   .   IV. Series.
    [DNLM: 1. Analgesics.   2. Clinical Trials—methods.   3. Pain—drug
  therapy.   W1 AD706 v. 18/QV 95 D457]
  RM319.D39   1991
  615'.783'0287—dc20
  DNLM/DLC
  for Library of Congress   90-9146
                                                                CIP

The material contained in this volume was submitted as previously unpublished material, except in the instances in which some of the illustrative material was derived.

Great care has been taken to maintain the accuracy of the information contained in the volume. However, neither Raven Press nor the editors can be held responsible for errors or for any consequences arising from the use of the information contained herein.

Materials appearing in this book prepared by individuals as part of their official duties as U.S. Government employees are not covered by the above-mentioned copyright.

987654321

FOREWORD

This book brings together an impressive group of experts in the area of analgesic trial design, to discuss the development and evaluation of new agents for pain control. I am pleased that a number of intramural scientists and extramural grantees of the National Institute of Dental Research (NIDR) are among the contributors. Pain research has been a long-standing interest of the NIDR. It was part of the institute's long-range plan for the 1970s and 1980s and has been a major component of its support of extramural and intramural research. The NIDR long-range plan for the 1990s has major sections devoted to the support of pain research.

In the intramural program at the NIDR, we have had a long-standing interest in pain mechanisms and the development of new methods of pain control. One of our major goals has been to facilitate the transfer of new knowledge gained in the neuroscience laboratory to the clinical situation. In 1973, when the Neurobiology and Anesthesiology Branch was first established, we were given the opportunity to develop a clinical arm of the program. I decided that an important first step was to develop improved methods for assessing pain that could be used to further our understanding of pain mechanisms in humans and to better evaluate the results of clinical trials. As this book indicates, progress has been made in both of these areas, but more needs to be done. I am pleased to see that extensive discussion of the design of repeat- and multiple-dose studies are included. The research in this area is meager. Very close to my own interests is the correlation of pain report and behavior with biochemical indices of pain. I believe advances in this area will lead to further understanding of the neurohumoral response to injury, as well as provide us with additional measures for assessing pain relief.

I hope that in the 1990s we can move to new approaches in the design and evaluation of clinical trials. We now have a variety of new pain assessment tools that have not yet been adopted by clinical pharmacologists. These tools provide more reliable and more valid measures of pain and pain relief. In addition, there is a real need for studies that not only evaluate drugs but also improve our understanding of their mechanisms of action. With such advances, we should be able to provide improved pain-control agents for acute and chronic pain conditions that plague our patients.

Ronald Dubner, D.D.S., Ph.D.
Neurobiology and Anesthesiology Branch
National Institute of Dental Research
National Institutes of Health
Bethesda, Maryland

PREFACE

> Imagination is the decisive function of the scholar. It serves the ability to expose real, productive questions, something in which, generally speaking, only he who masters all the methods of his science succeeds.
>
> H.–G. Gadamer

Recent developments in the clinic and the laboratory have made the study of pain a particularly promising area. In many medical specialties, groups of clinicians have emerged with a special interest in pain treatment. They are identifying new diagnostic categories of pain syndromes and defining the limitations of conventional analgesics. Scientific societies devoted to pain treatment and research and journals and meetings devoted to the subject have been rapidly expanding over the last decade. In a number of specialties, pain treatment and research is becoming established as a possible career track.

This interest in the clinical aspects of pain has been paralleled by a dramatic increase in knowledge about the neural basis of pain and analgesia. Stimulated by Melzack and Wall's "gate control theory of pain" in 1965 and the discovery of the opiate receptor in 1973, neuroscientists have generated a wealth of hypotheses about pain mechanisms in injured tissues and at synapses in spinal cord and brain. Few of these potential avenues for therapy have yet received clinical testing, but many investigational drugs suitable for probing these mechanisms are becoming available for use in humans.

There has also been considerable progress in a third area, clinical trials methodology and biostatistics. Current areas of advance include study designs for performing crossover studies in the presence of carryover effects; data collection methods, such as the patient's use of a stopwatch to directly measure onset and duration of subjective effects; and new statistical methods, such as survival and cure-rate models, that enable the researcher to better describe a clinical trial.

This book is intended as a resource for both the novice and the experienced analgesic investigator. The first of the book's three parts is intended for the investigator interested in studying the properties and potential clinical niche of a particular drug, where the researcher is free to choose from a variety of "pain models" and a range of single- or multiple-dose study designs. The second part, which is aimed at the clinical specialist interested in improving pain treatment for patients in a particular disease category, considers the crucial therapeutic questions in treating specific patient groups, the problems of performing analgesic trials in those diseases, and potential strategies for their solution. The third part addresses several other issues relevant to pain research, including innovations in pharmacokinetics and biostatistics, methods of evaluating interventions to improve clinicians' analgesic prescribing practices, the practice and training of analgesic research nurse observers, regulatory concerns, and issues in the study of nonpharmacological pain relief methods. Following many of the chapters are

vii

expert commentaries that highlight unresolved issues and ongoing controversies; these commentaries include excerpts of discussion from a January 1990 meeting at which preliminary versions of many of the chapters were presented to audiences of experts in analgesic research.

No single volume can cover all aspects of analgesic research. We have for the most part selected subjects related to randomized, controlled trials, although in many circumstances important information may be gathered by epidemiological surveys or observations of patients treated without randomization (1). The complex field of pain measurement has been summarized in several recent reviews (2–5) and is not explored in depth in this book, nor is the crucial clinical distinction between pain and suffering (6). Many of the chapters assume a familiarity with general principles of clinical trial design and elementary biostatistics, available in a number of standard texts (7–13). Although principles behind statistical approaches are discussed, few details are given; the reader is better served by consulting a biostatistician when planning, analyzing, and interpreting clinical trials.

Mitchell B. Max
Russell K. Portenoy
Eugene M. Laska

1. Feinstein AR. An additional basic science for clinical medicine: II. The limitations of randomized trials. *Ann Intern Med* 1983;99:544–550.
2. Chapman CR, Loeser JD, eds. *Issues in pain measurement.* New York: Raven Press, 1989.
3. Gracely RH. Pain psychophysics. *Adv Behav Med* 1985;1:199–231.
4. Price DD. *Psychological and neural mechanisms of pain.* New York: Raven Press, 1988;28–38.
5. Melzack R, ed. *Pain measurement and assessment.* New York: Raven Press, 1983.
6. Cassel EJ. The nature of suffering and the goals of medicine. *New Engl J Med* 1982;306:639–645.
7. Friedman LM, Furberg CD, DeMets DL. *Fundamentals of clinical trials,* 2nd ed. Littleton, Massachusetts: PSG Publishing Company, 1985.
8. Meinert CL. *Clinical trials: design, conduct, and analysis.* New York: Oxford University Press, 1986.
9. Pocock SJ. *Clinical trials: a practical approach.* Chichester, UK: John Wiley & Sons, 1983.
10. Shapiro S, Louis TA. *Clinical trials: issues and approaches.* New York: Marcel Dekker, 1983.
11. Bailar JC III, Mosteller F. *Medical uses of statistics.* Waltham, Massachusetts: NEJM Books, 1986.
12. Brown BW Jr, Hollander M. *Statistics: a biomedical introduction.* New York: John Wiley & Sons, 1977.
13. Ingelfinger JA, Mosteller F, Thibodeau LA, Ware JH. *Biostatistics in clinical medicine.* New York: Macmillan, 1983.

ACKNOWLEDGMENTS

The editors would like to thank a number of people for bringing this project to fruition. Many of the authors, in addition to writing their chapters, treated the entire project as their own, and their wealth of ideas considerably improved the organization and content of this book. An advisory committee consisting of William Beaver, Kathleen Foley, Raymond Houde, Louis Lasagna, and Abraham Sunshine provided invaluable counsel and encouragement. Carl Peck, John Harter, and their colleagues at the United States Food and Drug Administration (FDA), along with Abraham Sunshine and William Beaver, chairpersons of the Analgesic Guidelines Committee of the American Society for Clinical Pharmacology and Therapeutics, laid much of the groundwork for the book in the process of guiding the drafting of new FDA analgesic guidelines during 1989 and 1990. Members of the World Health Organization staff, most particularly Walter Gulbinat and Kenneth Stanley, offered valuable advice in shaping the project. We were fortunate to have the superb managerial support of Mary Callaway, who was ably assisted by Marilyn Herleth and Jean Itkin.

We are grateful for the sponsorship of the following organizations: International Association for the Study of Pain, American Pain Society, and United States Cancer Pain Relief Committee; the following corporate sponsors: E. I. du Pont de Nemours & Company, Janssen Pharmaceutica, McNeil Consumer Products Company/Robert Wood Johnson Pharmaceutical Research Institute, Pfizer, Inc., and The Procter & Gamble Company; and the following donors: Alza Corporation, Bristol-Myers Products, G. D. Searle & Company (Research and Development), Janssen Research Foundation, L.A.B., Inc., Lilly Research Laboratories, Merck Sharpe & Dohme Research Laboratories, Miles, Inc., Pharmaco Dynamics Research, Inc., The Purdue Frederick Company and Purdue Frederick Inc. of Canada, Roxane Laboratories, Inc., Wyeth Ayerst Research, and Zambon Corporation.

CONTENTS

III. Other Issues

CONTRIBUTORS

William T. Beaver, M.D. *Departments of Pharmacology and Anesthesia, Georgetown University School of Medicine, Washington, DC 20007*

Lennette J. Benjamin, M.D. *Comprehensive Sickle Cell Center, Montefiore Hospital Medical Center, Bronx, New York 10467; Department of Medicine, Albert Einstein College of Medicine, Bronx, New York 10467*

Charles B. Berde, M.D., Ph.D. *Pain Treatment Service, Children's Hospital, Boston, Massachusetts 02115; Departments of Anaesthesia and Pediatrics, Harvard Medical School, Boston, Massachusetts 02115*

Joseph R. Bianchine, M.D., Ph.D. *Medical Research Center, Adria Laboratories, Columbus, Ohio 43216*

Ralf Brueckner, M.D. *Division of Experimental Therapeutics, Walter Reed Army Institute of Research, Washington, DC 20307*

Eduardo Bruera *Palliative Care Unit, Edmonton General Hospital, Edmonton, Alberta, Canada T5K 0L4; Department of Medicine, University of Alberta, Edmonton, Alberta, Canada T5K 0L4*

Rocco L. Brunelle, M.S. *Lilly Research Laboratories, Eli Lilly and Company, Indianapolis, Indiana 46285*

Daniel B. Carr, M.D. *Analgesic Peptide Research Unit, Massachusetts General Hospital and Shriner Burns Institute, Boston, Massachusetts 02114; Departments of Anesthesiology and Medicine (Endocrinology), Harvard Medical School, Boston, Massachusetts 02115*

C. Richard Chapman, Ph.D. *Pain and Toxicity Program, Division of Clinical Research, Fred Hutchinson Cancer Research Center, Seattle, Washington 98104; Department of Anesthesiology, Department of Psychiatry and Behavioral Sciences, University of Washington School of Medicine, Seattle, Washington 98195*

Glenn T. Clark, D.D.S., M.S. *UCLA Dental Research Institute, School of Dentistry, University of California at Los Angeles, Los Angeles, California 90024-1762*

Charles S. Cleeland, Ph.D. *Pain Research Group, Department of Neurology, WHO Collaborating Center for Symptom Evaluation in Cancer Care, University of Wisconsin, Madison, Wisconsin 53706*

Barbara A. Coda, M.D. *Clinical Research Division, Pain and Toxicity Research Program, Fred Hutchinson Cancer Research Center, Seattle, Washington 98104; Multidisciplinary Pain Center, University of Washington, Seattle, Washington 98195*

Stephen Cooper, D.M.D., Ph.D. *Department of Pharmacology, University of Pennsylvania School of Dental Medicine, Philadelphia, Pennsylvania 19104*

Michael J. Cousins, M.D. *Department of Anaesthesia and Intensive Care, Flinders University of South Australia, Flinders Medical Centre, Bedford Park, South Australia 5042*

M. Yusoff Dawood, M.D. *Division of Reproductive Endocrinology, Department of Obstetrics, Gynecology, and Reproductive Sciences, University of Texas Health Science Center at Houston, Houston, Texas 77030*

Richard Deyo, M.D., M.P.H. *Back Pain Outcome Assessment Team, Northwest Health Services Research and Development Field Program, Seattle VA Medical Center, Seattle, Washington 98108; Departments of Medicine and Health Services, University of Washington, Seattle, Washington 98195*

Raymond A. Dionne, D.D.S., Ph.D. *Clinical Pharmacology Unit, Neurobiology and Anesthesiology Branch, National Institute of Dental Research, National Institutes of Health, Bethesda, Maryland 20892*

Gary W. Donaldson, Ph.D. *Pain and Toxicity Research Program, Fred Hutchinson Cancer Research Center, Seattle, Washington 98104*

Marilee I. Donovan, Ph.D., R.N. *Oregon Health Sciences University, Portland, Oregon 97201*

F. Michael Ferrante, M.D. *Pain Treatment Service, Department of Anaesthesia, Brigham and Women's Hospital, Harvard Medical School, Boston, Massachusetts 02115*

Kathleen M. Foley, M.D. *Pain Service, Department of Neurology, Memorial Sloan-Kettering Cancer Center, New York, New York 10021; Departments of Neurology and Pharmacology, Cornell University Medical College, New York, New York 10021*

James A. Forbes, M.S. *Department of Psychiatry, Johns Hopkins University School of Medicine, Baltimore, Maryland 21205*

James R. Fricton, D.D.S., M.S. *TMJ and Craniofacial Pain Clinic, Department of Diagnostic and Surgical Sciences, School of Dentistry, University of Minnesota, Minneapolis, Minnesota 55455*

Michael Friedman, Ph.D. *Statistical Services Department, Bristol-Myers Products, Hillside, New Jersey 07205*

Daniel Furst, M.D. *Department of Medicine/Rheumatology, University of Medicine and Dentistry of New Jersey, New Brunswick, New Jersey 08903; Ciba-Geigy Pharmaceuticals, Summit, New Jersey 07901*

David Goldstein, M.D., Ph.D. *Lilly Research Laboratories, Eli Lilly and Company, Indianapolis, Indiana 46285*

Richard H. Gracely, Ph.D. *Neurobiology and Anesthesiology Branch, National Institute of Dental Research, National Institutes of Health, Bethesda, Maryland 20892*

Kenneth M. Hargreaves, D.D.S., Ph.D. *Department of Restorative Sciences, University of Minnesota School of Dentistry, Minneapolis, Minnesota 55455*

John Harter, M.D. *Pilot Drug Evaluation Staff, Food and Drug Administration, Rockville, Maryland 20857*

Harlan F. Hill, Ph.D. *Clinical Research Division, Pain and Toxicity Research Program, Fred Hutchinson Cancer Research Center, Seattle, Washington 98104; Multidisciplinary Pain Center, University of Washington, Seattle, Washington 98195*

Raymond W. Houde, M.D. *Pain Service, Department of Neurology, Memorial Sloan-Kettering Cancer Center, New York, New York 10021*

Charles E. Inturrisi, Ph.D. *Department of Pharmacology, Cornell University Medical College, New York, New York 10021; Pain Research Program, Memorial Sloan-Kettering Cancer Center, New York, New York 10021*

Robert F. Kaiko, Ph.D. *Medical Department, The Purdue Frederick Company, Norwalk, Connecticut 06856*

Thomas G. Kantor, M.D. *Rheumatic Diseases Study Group, Department of Medicine, New York University Medical Center, New York, New York 10016*

Louis Lasagna, M.D. *Sackler School of Graduate Biomedical Sciences, Tufts University, Boston, Massachusetts 02111*

Eugene M. Laska, Ph.D. *Statistical Sciences and Epidemiology Division, Nathan S. Kline Institute for Psychiatric Research, WHO Collaborating Center for Training and Research in Mental Health Program Management, Orangeburg, New York 10962; Department of Psychiatry, New York University Medical Center, New York, New York 10016*

Klaus A. Lehmann, M.D. *Institute of Anesthesiology, University of Cologne Medical School, Cologne, Federal Republic of Germany*

Adam M. Mackie, M.D *Clinical Research Division, Pain and Toxicity Research Program, Fred Hutchinson Cancer Research Center, Seattle, Washington 98104; Multidisciplinary Pain Center, University of Washington, Seattle, Washington 98195*

Laurence E. Mather, Ph.D. *Department of Anaesthesia and Intensive Care, School of Medicine, Flinders University of South Australia, Bedford Park, SA 5042 Australia*

Mitchell B. Max, M.D. *Clinical Trials Unit, Neurobiology and Anesthesiology Branch, National Institute of Dental Research, National Institutes of Health, Bethesda, Maryland 20892*

Henry J. McQuay, M.D. *Oxford Regional Pain Relief Unit, Abingdon Hospital, OX14 1AG Abingdon, Oxon, United Kingdom*

Morris Meisner, Ph.D. *Statistical Sciences and Epidemiology Division, Nathan S. Kline Institute for Psychiatric Research, Orangeburg, New York 10962; Department of Psychiatry, New York University Medical Center, New York, New York 10016*

Joseph R. Migliardi, M.D. *Medical and Regulatory Affairs, Bristol-Myers Products, Hillside, New Jersey 07205*

Dwight Moulin, M.D. *Department of Clinical Neurological Sciences, Victoria Hospital, London, Ontario N6A 4G5*

David S. Muckle, M.D., F.R.C.S. (Eng), F.R.C.S. (Ed) *Department of Orthopedic Surgery, Middlesbrough General Hospital, Middlesbrough, Cleveland TS5 5AZ, England; Honorary Consultant, Football Association, England*

Prem K. Narang, Ph.D. *Pharmacokinetics/Dynamics Department, Adria Laboratories, Columbus, Ohio 43216*

Nancy Z. Olson, M.P.S., Abraham Sunshine, M.D., P.C., *New York, New York 10021*

Carl C. Peck, M.D. *Center for Drug Evaluation and Research, Food and Drug Administration, Rockville, Maryland 20857*

John L. Plummer, Ph.D. *Department of Anaesthesia and Intensive Care, Flinders University of South Australia, Flinders Medical Centre, Bedford Park, South Australia 5042*

Russell K. Portenoy, M.D. *Pain Service, Department of Neurology, Department of Anesthesiology and Critical Care Medicine, Memorial Sloan-Kettering Cancer Center, New York, New York 10021; Department of Neurology, Cornell University Medical College, New York, New York 10021*

Charles W. Prettyman, M.S. *Regulatory Affairs, The Purdue Frederick Company, Norwalk, Connecticut 06856*

Ada G. Rogers, R.N. *Pain Research Program, Pain Service, Department of Neurology, Memorial Sloan-Kettering Cancer Center, New York, New York 10021*

Bernard Schachtel, M.D.   *Medical Department, Whitehall Laboratories, Inc., New York, New York 10017; Clinical Epidemiology Unit, Yale University School of Medicine, New Haven, Connecticut 06510*

Carole Siegel, Ph.D.   *Statistical Sciences and Epidemiology Division, Nathan S. Kline Institute for Psychiatric Research, Orangeburg, New York 10962; Department of Psychiatry, New York University Medical Center, New York, New York 10016*

John E. Stambaugh, Jr., M.D., Ph.D.   *Oncology and Hematology Associates, P.A., Haddon Heights, New Jersey 08035; Department of Pharmacology, Thomas Jefferson University Medical College, Philadelphia, Pennsylvania 19107*

Patricia Stewart, M.D.   *Research and Development, McNeil Consumer Products, Fort Washington, Pennsylvania 19034*

Abraham Sunshine, M.D.   *Department of Medicine, New York University Medical Center, New York, New York 10016*

Howard T. Thaler, Ph.D.   *Department of Epidemiology and Biostatistics, Memorial Sloan-Kettering Cancer Center, New York, New York 10021*

Raja Velagapudi, Ph.D.   *Division of Biopharmaceutics, Center for Drug Evaluation and Research, Food and Drug Administration, Rockville, Maryland 20857*

Stanley L. Wallenstein, M.S.   *Analgesic Studies, Sloan-Kettering Institute (retired), New York, New York 10021*

T. Declan Walsh, M.Sc., M.R.C.P., F.A.C.P.   *Palliative Care Service, Department of Hematology and Medical Oncology, Cleveland Clinic Foundation, Cleveland, Ohio 44195-5236*

Richard I. H. Wang, M.D., Ph.D.   *Department of Pharmacology, The Medical College of Wisconsin, C.J.Z. VA Medical Center, 116E, Milwaukee, Wisconsin 53193*

C. Peter N. Watson, M.D., F.R.C.P.(C)   *Irene Eleanor Smythe Pain Clinic, Toronto General Hospital, Toronto, Ontario, Canada M5G 1L7; Department of Medicine, University of Toronto, Toronto, Ontario, Canada M5G 2C4*

Advances in Pain Research and Therapy, Vol. 18,
edited by M. Max, R. Portenoy, and E. Laska,
Raven Press, Ltd., New York © 1991.

1

Clinical Analgesic Research

A Historical Perspective

Louis Lasagna

*Sackler School of Graduate Biomedical Sciences, Tufts University,
Boston, Massachusetts 02111*

THE ERA BEFORE CONTROLLED CLINICAL TRIALS: ACHIEVEMENTS AND FAILURES

Enthusiasts for the modern controlled clinical trial would have one believe that prior to the advent of such methodology, very little in the way of useful scientific data was amassed. This overstates the case. For many years before clinical trials "established" their efficacy, drugs such as aspirin, phenacetin, acetaminophen, morphine, heroin, meperidine, and methadone were in clinical use in a number of countries, and subsequent controlled trials merely confirmed (at least in general qualitative terms) what traditional investigation and experience had uncovered. Even when failures occurred—such as the mistaken hope that heroin and meperidine were nonaddicting, or the inability to anticipate the syndrome of analgesic nephropathy—the truth was often ultimately discovered not by randomized, double-blind, placebo-controlled trials (RCCTs), but by what today would be called pharmacoepidemiologic data.

Recognition of the facts described above is important not only to instill humility in the hearts of hyperbolic RCCT enthusiasts, but to remind all of us that there will never be a time when all the information we should like to have about analgesics will derive from controlled trials. "Naturalistic" experience is important, and such experience must be efficiently tracked and reacted to, if we are to optimize medical care.

THE BEGINNINGS OF MODERN ANALGESIMETRIC TECHNIQUES

Major credit for the modern RCCT revolution in analgesic research must go to two groups, one at the Massachusetts General Hospital (MGH) and the other at Memorial Hospital in New York. In Boston, the leader was Henry K. Beecher, a charismatic and imaginative anesthetist—he detested the word "anesthesiologist"—who over the years recruited other anesthetists, internists, psychologists, statisticians, etc., to devise (and revise) techniques for measuring the safety and efficacy of analgesics. Beecher was taken with the impact of what he termed "the powerful placebo" (he always pronounced it play-see-boh) and with the quantification of "subjective" responses. Today's acceptance of our ability to measure pain, sedation, depression, cognitive impairment, anxiety, etc., by oral or written reports of "internal states" ignores the disdain with which science in general tended to treat such phenomena, despite the impressive track record of sensory psychologists interested in acoustic and visual research (1).

Beecher had at one time supported research in his laboratory on experimental pain in human subjects and had published on its ability to detect the analgesic effects of nitrous oxide and morphine. But with the passage of time, he became disenchanted with this approach because of its inconsistent results. For most of his career, Beecher denigrated experimental pain and praised what he called "pathological pain," i.e., pain arising as part of spontaneous disease or medical-surgical procedures, although with the arrival of Gene Smith in his laboratory, there was again a brief flirtation with experimental pain at the MGH laboratories.

The interest in placebo reactors was spurred by the paper of Lasagna et al. (2), which suggested that at the extremes of consistent placebo reactors and nonreactors, psychological and other variables were associated with placebo reactivity. Unfortunately for clinical trial design, placebo reactivity is not easy to predict and is not consistent, so the opportunity to "screen out" reactors and thus increase the sensitivity of clinical trials has never really materialized. Mosteller, Beecher's distinguished statistical consultant, did, however, suggest another way of maximizing the efficiency of drug studies with crossover designs. This consisted quite simply of ignoring subjects' responses where two drugs being compared gave identical results (e.g., analgesia or not, nausea or not) and focusing instead on those subjects who responded differently to two treatments. The technique was discussed in Beecher's book (1), with the credit for the original concept going to McNemar.

In New York, the two leaders were Raymond Houde and Stanley Wallenstein, one a physician-pharmacologist, the other a psychologist. Unlike Beecher, whose published research was voluminous, the work of the Memorial group was largely known, for many years, primarily to the aficionados who attended meetings of the Committee on Drug Addiction and Narcotics of the National Research Council, at which supported scientists like Beecher and Houde gave detailed annual progress reports. Sophisticated statistical analyses of their data marked the Memorial group's work from its beginning, and imaginative experimental designs (such as flexible, multilevel dose protocols) and the crossover technique were used to calculate potency ratios for standard and new drugs. Combinations of analgesics were also studied. Our debt to the MGH and Memorial groups is enormous.

EARLY CONTROVERSY

One bone of contention that surfaced early was the necessity of crossover designs for analgesic research. Proponents of such designs had theory on their side; it could reasonably be argued that because a person's internal standard for severity of pain was idiosyncratic, variance would be diminished by using each person as his own control. Both Beecher and Houde espoused this point of view, although Houde's patient population at that time—cancer patients with chronic pain—were much more likely to have stable pain and to return to baseline after a drug's effects had worn off than were Beecher's patients, whose postoperative pain was likely to be short-lived and was on average moving from severe to moderate, slight, and then none during the postoperative course. Also, Beecher's patients not infrequently failed to have severe pain long enough to allow the alternative therapy to be evaluated at the same predosing level as the first treatment.

Free and Peeters (3), however, showed that in certain populations, the order of administration of treatments was extremely important, suggesting that the benefits of crossover were possibly illusory. Although subsequent research has clearly confirmed the utility and efficiency of crossover in some situations, most analgesic assays today seem to be of the parallel-design variety.

One matter that never reached the point of actual research and controversy, but perhaps deserved such treatment, was the question of the variance contributed by different interviewers. At the MGH, Beecher had 24-hr coverage, with the technicians soliciting data from patient subjects at night being different from those who worked during the day. Houde, by contrast, used a talented and experienced nurse clinician, Ada Rogers, who only observed patients during the working day.

Although today randomization in its strict sense is routine, and is theoretically important in the estimation of statistical error, it is interesting to note that at least for a number of years the Beecher group simply alternated treatments (usually termed "A" and "B," rather than with different labels for each subject). Despite the theoretical disadvantages of Beecher's approach, in fact the potency estimates from his group and those of Houde's were generally in close agreement.

Another postulated effect of randomization—the equalization of baseline variables in the groups being compared—is in fact not as well achieved in small-size studies by pure randomization as it is by *stratified* randomization, wherein patients with severe pain at baseline are randomly allocated to the different treatments, as are those with moderate pain. Such an approach essentially guarantees that there will not be differences in baseline pain severity between treatment groups in parallel design studies.

For measuring pain, the earliest measures involved estimates, by patients, of the severity of pain, using such terms as "severe," "moderate," "slight," etc., with reevaluations of pain severity at various times after drug administration. The conversion of these shifts in pain levels to numerical values was based on the assumption that the increments from one level to another were of equal value and importance. (It certainly made the calculations easier.) Lasagna (4) tried to analyze this problem by research intended to assess the importance placed on these pain levels by subjects. His data suggested that although there was great individual variation in the importance attributed to these levels, in general a drop from "severe" to "moderate" was considered most important, with other single-level changes being deemed less so. The visual analogue scale approach (which in essence was used by Lasagna as one technique in his research) came into play later and in theory can serve to get around the nonhomogeneity of jumps from one quantal level to another (*vide infra*).

Keele (5) in the United Kingdom proposed that one should evaluate analgesic performance by scores that gave points for pain relief and subtracted points for adverse effects. Such an approach never achieved popularity among RCCT experts in the United States, in part at least because it was felt that such "salad scores" left the reader uncertain as to whether poor performance was owing to lack of efficacy or to unpleasant side effects. The use of "global satisfaction" ratings, however, has had a renaissance in recent years and will be discussed below.

Beecher's group did, for a short time, use quantitative judgments about "satisfactory" or "unsatisfactory" performance based on the achievement of pain relief within a certain period of time, and the providing of at least a certain degree of pain relief for a certain minimum of time to qualify as "satisfactory" (6). Such complex scores, although admittedly arbitrary, may serve better to transmit to prescribing physicians the likelihood of benefit from a drug than average pain or pain relief scores over time.

What to do with patients that fail on assigned treatments has always posed problems. Ethical principles demand that patients have the right to opt out of a trial at any time. If this occurs before a drug has had a chance to be absorbed, to be transported to the site of action, and to achieve its analgesic effect, there is no way of crediting the drug for benefit by interviews after the administration of the "rescue" medication.

Although all accept this inevitable truth, there has been disagreement as to what to do in the way of scoring. Suppose, for example, a patient gets *worse* after a medication. Should he be given only a zero for pain relief, or a negative score? And even if the rescue medication is demanded at a time when the pain is no worse than at baseline, what convention shall be adopted to assign scores for the interviews postrescue? Shall they arbitrarily be set at baseline? At whatever the pain level was at the time of rescue? At the worst possible pain level? There is no intuitively "correct" answer, so far as I can tell. These conventions differ in the degree to which they penalize failure, so that more "punitive" conventions pull apart good and poor drugs more than do less punitive conventions. There is one point of agreement, however: whatever convention is applied, it must be applied evenhandedly to all treatments before the code is broken.

The eliciting of adverse effects from analgesics has been attempted in various ways. One way has been to record the volunteered statements or responses to questions by patient subjects in clinical trials. Another has been to administer analgesics to healthy volunteers and then record the adverse effects reported by them, with the hope that although absolute percentages might differ between healthy volunteers and the sick (especially if healthy subjects were ambulatory during the study, to accentuate the ascertainment of nausea and vomiting liability), qualitatively the data would be comparable.

A similar situation obtains with the quantification of respiratory depressant effects of analgesics. Respiratory depression in the sick is not always easy to evaluate. Traditionally, therefore, studies have been performed in healthy young subjects, with sophisticated measurements of ventilation as well as blood and alveolar pCO_2. Again, the assumption has been that these studies are useful at least for comparative purposes in predicting clinical troubles. As in all studies of adverse effects, such research must involve equipotent doses of the drugs under study, if unfair and unwarranted conclusions are not to be drawn about relative side-effect liability.

The addiction potential of analgesics (at least of opioids) has long been studied in either "postaddicts" or drug-sophisticated volunteers as well as by behavioral pharmacologic techniques in animals.

MORE RECENT PROGRESS AND PROBLEMS

The accidental discovery that nalorphine was both an agonist and an antagonist (7) has led to the marketing of several agonist-antagonist analgesics and the study of many more. At an early point in the history of this category of analgesic research, Keats found that many of these drugs showed inverted U-shaped dose-response curves, rather than the traditional ones (8). Whatever may be the theoretical explanation for this fact, it has complicated the evaluation and marketing of a number of agonist-antagonist analgesics. Interestingly, naloxone—allegedly a pure antagonist—has been reported to show a similar U-shaped dose-response curve (9).

Postpartum pain at first was evaluated without reference to whether a patient suffered from steady episiotomy pain or crampy pain related to uterine contractions. In more recent years, Bloomfield et al. (10) have called attention to their own experience with such patients, indicating that drugs that inhibit prostaglandin production work better against crampy postpartum pain than do drugs of the opioid class, whereas both types of drugs work well against episiotomy pain.

A similar situation seems to exist with regard to pain related to third-molar extraction, where opioids work poorly but aspirin and newer nonsteroidal antiinflammatory drugs work well. (Acetaminophen, interestingly enough, also works well.)

Sriwatanakul et al. (11) at the University of Rochester have researched the semantics involved in the evaluation of pain and analgesics, showing how variable people are in their interpretation of descriptors. They also examined different modes of presentation of visual analogue scales (12), which have increased in popularity in the last decade or so. My own experience is that the various quantal and graded techniques now in use provide data that are always highly correlated (as one would expect) and that it is difficult to make a compelling case for any one technique usually being more discriminative than another in teasing apart different doses, or separating active drug from placebo.

On the other hand, I believe that we should pay more attention to describing the performance of analgesics in ways more readily comprehended by prescribing physicians than are SPID scores, or mean curves of pain intensity, pain relief, etc. For this purpose, asking patients to answer global evaluation questions as to degree of satisfaction with a drug's performance (which may include both efficacy and adverse-effects judgments) may be more to the point. In fact, such value judgments are often quite good at distinguishing between treatments.

CHALLENGES FOR THE FUTURE

Patient-administered analgesia has been demonstrated to be an effective way of providing "on-demand" pain relief, but this technology has thus far not seen much use in protocols intended to study analgesic potency and potency ratios. One hopes that it will be further explored for this purpose.

Unconventional analgesics are potential sources of scientific and therapeutic progress. One example is the utility of antidepressants (with or without a neuroleptic) for treating the refractory pain of postherpetic neuralgia and some other neurologic syndromes (13). Serendipitous leads of this sort should not be ignored.

Prescribing of analgesics continues to be suboptimal with regard to dosage, dosage interval, and drug selection (14). There is a great deal of patient benefit that could result from education of nurses and physicians. Hospice care and research in such settings have provided new insights into the optimal therapy of patients with chronic pain, stressing the difference in potency ratios for at least some opioids when given in single dose versus repeatedly, and the desirability of keeping patients pain-free throughout the entire day.

CONCLUSIONS

The progress in this field in the last four decades has been remarkable. Equally exciting is the prospect that much that is important remains to be done.

REFERENCES

1. Beecher HK. *Measurement of subjective responses. Quantitative effects of drugs.* New York: Oxford University Press, 1959.
2. Lasagna L, Mosteller F, von Felsinger JM, Beecher HK. A study of the placebo response. *Am J Med* 1954;16:770.

3. Free SM Jr, Peeters F. Statistical comparison of methods to evaluate analgesics. *J Chronic Dis* 1958;7:379.
4. Lasagna L. The clinical measurement of pain. *Ann NY Acad Sci* 1960;86:28.
5. Keele LA. The assay of analgesic drugs in man. *Analyst* 1952;77:111.
6. Denton JE, Beecher HK. New analgesics. I. Methods in the clinical evaluation of new analgesics. *JAMA* 1949;141:1051.
7. Lasagna L, Beecher HK. The analgesic effectiveness of nalorphine and nalorphine-morphine combinations in man. *J Pharm Exp Ther* 1954;112:3567.
8. Lasagna L. Benefit-risk ratio of agonist-antagonist analgesics. *Drug Alcohol Depend* 1987;20:385.
9. Lasagna L. Drug interaction in the field of analgesic drugs. *Proc R Soc Med* 1965;58:978.
10. Bloomfeld SS, Borden TP, Mitchell J. Aspirin and codeine in two postpartum pain models. *Clin Pharmacol Ther* 1976;20:499.
11. Sriwatanakul K, Kelvie W, Lasagna L. The quantification of pain: an analysis of words used to describe pain and analgesia in clinical trials. *Clin Pharmacol Ther* 1982;32–143.
12. Sriwatanakul K, Kelvie W, Lasagna L, Calimlim JF, Weis OF, Mehta G. Studies with different types of visual analog scales for measurement of pain. *Clin Pharmacol Ther* 1983;34:234.
13. Stimmel GL, Escobar JI. Antidepressants in chronic pain: a review of efficacy. *Pharmacotherapy* 1986;6:262.
14. Weis OF, Sriwatanakul K, Alloza JL, Weintraub M, Lasagna L. Attitudes of patients, housestaff, and nurses toward postoperative analgesic care. *Anesth Analg* 1983;62:70.

Advances in Pain Research and Therapy, Vol. 18,
edited by M. Max, R. Portenoy, and E. Laska,
Raven Press, Ltd., New York © 1991.

2

Phase I Studies

Initial Evaluation of Drug Toxicity, Dose Response, and Efficacy

Prem K. Narang and Joseph R. Bianchine

Adria Laboratories, Division of Erbamont, Columbus, Ohio 43216

After a therapeutic activity of a new chemical entity (NCE) has been identified using validated preclinical pharmacological models; and appropriate acute, subacute, and subchronic toxicological data have been gathered, preferably in a rodent and a nonrodent species; a sponsor seeks approval from its own governmental regulatory agency, e.g., the United States Food and Drug Administration (FDA), to initiate clinical studies in humans by submission of an Investigational New Drug Application (IND). The application includes a clinical protocol detailing the proposed initial investigations in humans, and an overview of the general clinical plan. These important initial studies are termed "Phase I studies."

The following review is limited to general aspects of Phase I investigations. Rules that govern these studies are basically similar for all classes of NCEs. It is not the intent of the authors to distinguish how Phase I studies for nonsteroidal analgesics, for example, ibuprofen, differ from those for a morphine-like analgesic. Clearly, Phase I studies for each of these drug types will differ; suffice it to say that most first-time-in-humans and other dose-ranging investigations are executed to assess safety and tolerance followed by an initial or pilot efficacy evaluation.

The primary objectives of Phase I clinical trials, according to the current FDA guidelines for drug development, can be classified as follows:

1. Initial assessment of safety and tolerance.
2. Initial assessment of efficacy.
3. Initial assessment of pharmacokinetics (PK)/pharmacodynamics (PD).

We will review the traditional approaches, where dosing is empirically based on preclinical safety data, and analysis is focused on mean rather than individual responses. Through the introduction of newer theories and study methods, the emphasis of current research is shifting to integrate pharmacokinetics in dose and dosing regimen selection, and to place greater emphasis on interindividual variation in response. We will discuss methods that make such analysis possible.

Phase I studies, except those for the drugs used in cancer chemotherapy and immunomodulation, are usually conducted in healthy normal volunteers. Depending on the pharmacological class of the NCE, one or more of the above goals can be addressed as a part of the dose-ranging studies. For example, a new morphine analogue may provide evidence of mood change, bowel motility change, or pupil diameter change, which will provide a clear pharmacologic endpoint. However, it is obvious that the efficacy of this new drug cannot be evaluated in Phase I if there is no pain present in the subject to be treated. In contrast, dose-ranging studies for an antihypertensive drug, even when conducted in healthy volunteers, provide "baseline" parameter estimates (unperturbed by the disease) for assessing safety, pharmacokinetics/dynamics, and therapeutic efficacy.

The approach to Phase I investigation is usually tempered by the researcher's philosophy, and by practical limitations that vary from one NCE to another. However, all Phase I studies involve careful, logical, ascending dose-ranging trials that attempt to estimate the so-called maximum tolerated dose (MTD), while assuring the safety of all subjects participating in the trial. This approach is intended to provide a quantitative relationship between the administered dose and the subjective and objective outcomes, first during single ascending dose and subsequently during multiple ascending dose studies. Objective endpoints may include vital sign measurements, special pharmacologic endpoints, and routine chemistry and/or hematological safety parameters. A dose versus response (toxicodynamic) curve may be constructed from some of these data. These curves tend to be S-shaped (Fig. 1), and are frequently used in preclinical toxicology and in general dose-ranging studies to estimate the maximally tolerated, safe, and/or therapeutic dose (1).

An alternative approach that is gaining popularity and scientific acceptance is based on obtaining systemic drug concentration versus time data, and thereby an estimate of systemic dose intensity or maximally tolerated systemic exposure (MTSE). This is also referred to as the concentration $\times$ time ($C \times T$) approach. In this approach, rather than developing quantitative dose-response relationships, rational dose selection decision making is based on the relationships developed between the pharmacokinetic parameters, e.g., area under the systemic drug concentration curve (AUC) as a function of time versus the response. Figure 2A shows a plot of the percent decrease in platelet count in patients treated with hexamethylene bisacetamide as a function of the AUC in individual cancer patients (2). It is apparent that parametric models, which can define such relationships, could be used in individualizing chemotherapy for a given patient. An oncologist can then aggressively treat the patient by providing the maximal systemic dose intensity while limiting the side effects to an acceptable level. For certain drugs, one may encounter a particular threshold of systemic drug concentration for response. Quinn et al. (3) successfully explains the variability in

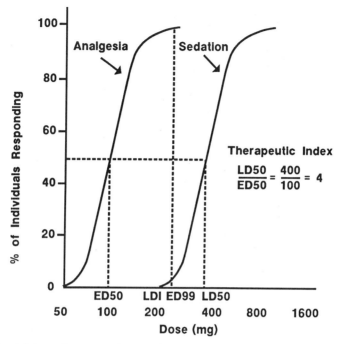

FIG. 1. Quantal dose-effect curves for an opioid analgesic. Dose required to produce a specific intensity of analgesia in 50% of individuals is called Median Effective Dose (ED_{50}). LD_{50} is the dose that causes sedation in 50% of individuals and LD_{50}/ED_{50} ratio gives the therapeutic index. (Adapted from ref. 1, with permission.)

the effectiveness (time to awakening) of hexobarbital in mice, rats, and rabbits by demonstrating that plasma hexobarbital concentration at awakening time was similar in all three species (Fig. 2B), although the disposition was greatly different. Figure 2B, based on their work, shows the threshold phenomenon (4).

The MTSE approach requires the availability of an adequate methodology to measure drug concentrations in biofluids, e.g., whole blood, plasma (serum), or urine. Traditionally, Phase I investigations have focused more heavily on the assessment of safety/tolerance issues, and therefore the need and the availability of adequate bioanalytical methods at the initiation of Phase I has lagged behind. However, in our opinion, it is imperative that a concerted effort be made to have a validated bioanalytical assay available early in the preclinical development, so that the pharmacodynamic profiles for the NCE can be determined during the acute, subacute, and subchronic toxicology studies.

Bioanalytical methods, if PK-PD approaches are applied, should not only be sensitive, but also must provide sufficient data at the lower end of the dynamic range to allow an assessment of precision and accuracy. Imprecise and biased methodologies alone can contribute errors of unknown magnitude in kinetic analysis, resulting in inaccurate estimates. MTSE or threshold-based approaches

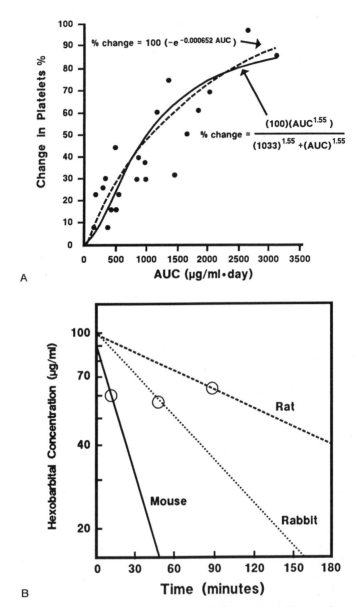

FIG. 2. A: Relationship of AUC of individual patients for the chemotherapeutic agent HMBA to percent decrease in platelet count observed in that same course. (From ref. 2, with permission.) **B:** Hexobarbital disposition in plasma following 50–100 mg/kg doses to mice, rats, and rabbits. Circles designate the concentration at which the animals awoke. AUC: Area under the plasma concentrations of the drug as a function of time curve; HMBA: Hexamethylene bisacetamide. (From ref. 4, with permission.)

that exploit integration of the pharmacokinetics, during single and multidose safety evaluation, can also provide a much better understanding of the drug pharmacology at early stages of preclinical development and assist in dose selection for the Phase I dose-ranging studies.

Plots of the dose versus a clinical response reveal two important features of the dose-response curve. The lowest dose level at which a subject elicits a response is called the threshold dose, whereas the lowest dose at which all subjects will respond at any dose is referred to as the plateau dose. Drug "resistance" or "nonresponders" can alter the slope of a dose-response plot and must be carefully assessed based on the preclinical or clinical drug disposition information. When a sensitive, specific, and validated bioanalytical methodology is available, the dose-ranging trials should evaluate both MTD and MTSE approaches by determining the drug's pharmacokinetics.

The advantage behind the concept of MTSE, depicted schematically in Fig. 3, is that it addresses the well recognized interpatient variability associated with drug absorption and disposition (Fig. 4A). As most drugs undergo biotransformation, drugs exhibiting low and high extraction (through liver) may show dispositional variability that depends on the intrinsic clearance of the drug (Fig. 4B). Models combining distribution and clearance concepts allow one to interpret

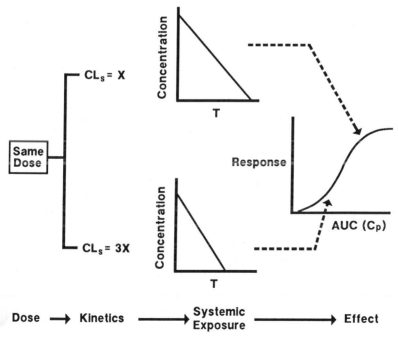

FIG. 3. Schematic of Maximally Tolerated Systemic Exposure (MTSE). AUC, area under the plasma drug concentration versus time curve (an estimate of exposure); CL_s, systemic clearance; C_p, the plasma concentration of a new chemical entity (NCE).

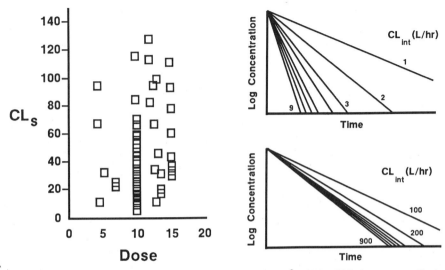

FIG. 4. **A:** Variability in the systemic clearance (CL_s; L/Hr/M²) of idarubicin in cancer patients following IV administration of 5–15 mg/M²/day doses. **B:** Expected plasma drug concentration-time profiles following an intravenous bolus dose with changes in intrinsic clearance for drugs of low-extraction ratio (*top*) and high-extraction ratio (*bottom*). Intrinsic clearance was varied over a ninefold range in both cases, from 1 to 9 liters/hr for the poorly extracted drug and from 100 to 900 liters/hr for the highly extracted drug. This simulation was based on the well-stirred model of hepatic elimination assuming hepatic elimination only, a hepatic blood flow of 90 liters/hr, and a volume of distribution greater than 30 liters. (From ref. 6, with permission.)

such dispositional variability. Variabilities associated with the amount of a given liver enzyme responsible for metabolism, drug binding to plasma or tissue constituents, hepatic blood flow, and hepatic extraction ratio need to be isolated for each new candidate and the contribution of these kinetic variables defined. The variability associated with drug disposition can be significantly greater and hence more important than the small test dose variations in a dose-ranging trial. This is especially true for those drugs that are subject to extensive hepatic metabolism. Many drugs exhibit highly variable disposition in humans, even within small populations of patients with clinically normal renal and hepatic function. For example, systemic clearance of doxorubicin and cyclophosphamide has been shown by Crom et al. (7) to differ by a factor of 3 to 10 among children with cancer; significant distributional and clearance variability has been recognized within adult leukemia patients being treated with idarubicin (5,8); and large variability has also been observed in kinetic parameters pertaining to the absorption for 6-mercaptopurine (9) in humans.

Therefore, selection of an optimal dose to conduct efficacy studies becomes a major challenge for an investigator in face of wide (at times tenfold) intersubject variability. As is evident from the foregoing discussion, it is often quite difficult to select a rational dose from dose-response Phase I studies for use in Phase II studies.

DOSE-RESPONSE AND BIOLOGIC VARIABILITY

The selection of the size of an initial dose for a first-time-in-humans Phase I trial is usually based on extrapolation from animal toxicology data and experience with other structurally (pharmacologically) similar chemical entities. However, the traditional approaches to a dose-ranging trial to find a MTD (for assessment of safety/tolerance) and/or an estimate of the size of the initial dose (for assessment of efficacy) do not characterize the inter- and intrasubject variations in response (Fig. 5). It can be seen that a range of doses can produce the same response (intensity of effect), or varying responses could be observed from the same dose in different patients (intersubject) or in the same patient (intrasubject). This is a likely scenario for all study designs in which a subject receives more than one dose.

In an excellent recent article, Sheiner et al. (10) have addressed the issues of inter- and intrasubject variability, mentioned above, by proposing that one additional goal of a dose-ranging trial should be to assess and estimate these components of variability. Implementing appropriate design characteristics during the early development phases, as discussed later (Common Study Designs), can usually provide estimates of population characteristics of patient-specific dose-response relationships.

ASSESSMENT OF PHARMACOKINETICS/PHARMACODYNAMICS

Phase I investigations provide a rich environment to obtain vital information on drug absorption, distribution, metabolism, and excretion. A carefully thought

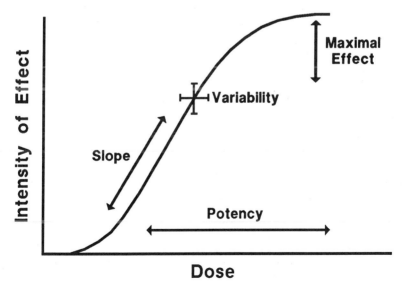

FIG. 5. The log dose-effect relationship with its four characterizing variables.

out plasma and urine sampling strategy, followed by quantitation of drug and/or metabolite concentrations using validated methodology, and a detailed kinetic/dynamic analysis can reveal information pertaining to the relative contributions of organs of drug clearance, possible influences of disease states, role of tissue binding, and major organ blood flow (11,12). Peck and Collins (13) have expressed strong encouragement of the FDA for incorporation of pharmacokinetic and pharmacodynamic investigations as a routine part of Phase I studies. Peck (14) proposes that early derivation of kinetic/dynamic intelligence in drug development may lead to compressed drug development times, while improving the ability to provide physicians with dosing instructions for individualizing therapy for their patients.

Pharmacokinetics

The study of the metabolic disposition of xenobiotics in humans is an essential element of early Phase I investigation. The findings from such a study can provide valuable information in the design of future clinical/preclinical protocols.

Single-Dose Studies

The first single-dose study in humans can provide vital kinetic information pertaining to drug distribution, excretion, and elimination. Early estimates of plasma protein binding, elimination half-life, distribution volumes, and metabolic patterns also help define kinetic features of the NCE.

Single-rising dose-ranging trials provide information on proportionality (system linearity) over the tested range. Deviations from a linear system, e.g., a curvilinear relationship between the drug dose and AUC or a unidirectional change in systemic clearance, suggest changes in drug disposition with dose. For example, an increase in AUC with increasing doses of an intravenously administered drug may indicate metabolic saturation or saturation of an active secretory process contributing to the overall excretion. Understanding dose dependency in disposition is extremely important in the correct interpretation of response. Quantitation of metabolites, in addition to the parent drug in plasma and urine, may provide insights that would otherwise be reflected in the dose-response relationships as unexplained intersubject variability. Characterization of active metabolites is also crucial for valid application of MTSE with tolerance and efficacy.

Multiple-Dose Studies

Most therapeutic agents are administered more than once. To understand the effects of repeat administration of an agent, pharmacokinetic studies are undertaken, usually in concert with safety/tolerance evaluation. Multiple dosing dose-ranging trials not only provide safety/tolerance data, but also elucidate metabolic inhibition, saturation, stimulation, or autoinduction in humans that may not have been apparent from single-dose studies. Drug accumulation and changes in the drug disposition patterns can thus be isolated. Pharmacokinetic analysis using mathematical modeling approaches (especially for regimens with varying dosing interval) can help elucidate properties of the drug under a steady state or clinically relevant environment.

Pharmacodynamics

Extensive progress has been made in the last two decades in collecting, analyzing, and modeling the plasma drug concentration versus time data to describe drug pharmacokinetics. However, the time course of drug concentration cannot in itself predict the time course or the magnitude of the elicited effect. When drug concentrations at the effect site are in equilibrium with systemic levels, the concentration versus effect relationship is termed pharmacodynamics. Dynamic studies are designed to elucidate or demonstrate the nature of drug action and its dependence on time, dose, and concentration of the drug in body fluids. Our brief presentation of these concepts does not allow us to provide, in detail, the various types of dynamic models that have been proposed and tested. Interested readers should review the work of Sheiner and Holford (15) and Chapter 24 of this book.

Pharmacokinetics/Pharmacodynamics

Figure 6 is a simplistic schematic representation of a pharmacokinetic (PK) and pharmacodynamic (PD) model that can describe a dose-effect relationship

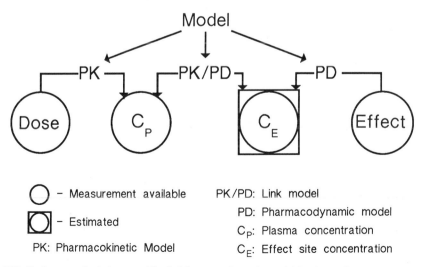

FIG. 6. A conceptual pharmacokinetic/pharmacodynamic model for dose-effect relationship.

by using drug concentration (C) measurements (15). The application of pharmacodynamics to the study of drug action *in vivo* requires linking of pharmacokinetics and pharmacodynamics to first predict the dose concentration and then the concentration-effect relationship, followed by linking the two with a PK/PD link model. However, delays in drug equilibration with the receptor site, presence of metabolites with varying potencies, or use of indirect or surrogate measures of drug effect often necessitate formulation and testing of more complex models (15). As drug effects are often mediated by the unbound drug, kinetic issues pertaining to drug binding must be considered when developing dose versus effect relationships.

Efficacy or toxicity-response measurements and their relationships to the dose or systemic concentration are evaluated by pharmacodynamic models that are based on the Hill equation (16). The equations describing these models are similar to those used for enzyme (Michaelis-Menton) and protein-binding kinetics. Although their use in pharmacodynamics can be justified on theoretical grounds alone (17,18), they are useful empirically because of two important features: (a) prediction of a maximal drug effect (E_{max}), and (b) no effect in the absence of the drug. A simple model (shown below) based on a hyperbolic relationship correlates effect (E) to the plasma drug concentration (C), where EC_{50} is the concentration producing 50% of E_{max} response.

$$E = \frac{E_{max}\,C}{EC_{50} + C}$$

The use of this and other minor variants of the parametric model has grown over the past five years as more efforts are targeted at defining the concentration-response, rather than the dose-response, relationships.

The study of pharmacokinetics/pharmacodynamics and simultaneous modeling of kinetic and dynamic data for parent drug and active metabolites have raised several other important issues. Some issues that all investigators dealing with Phase I clinical pharmacology must keep in mind during the design, analysis, and review of the published data pertain to drug dosing route, disposition, and data analysis.

Route of Administration

In general, most portal routes of drug entry into systemic circulation are prone to potentially erratic absorption and bioavailability (especially for poorly soluble and slowly absorbed drugs). There is also a higher propensity for enhanced first-pass metabolism of those drugs that are administered by the oral, rectal, and subcutaneous routes. Influence of lipophilicity, protein binding, pH, and other physicochemical factors is discussed elsewhere in this volume. Some opioids, e.g., morphine, lose a significant proportion of their potency when administered orally because of large first-pass metabolism. However, when given intravenously, a small dose of morphine can produce the same response.

The route of administration can affect the shape of the time-effect curves by influencing distribution, metabolism, and bioavailability, and can also alter the duration of drug action. Therefore, attention should be given to route of administration when developing kinetic-dynamic relationships.

Active Metabolism

Biotransformation of drugs usually results in metabolites that are more polar, less lipid soluble, distribute less extensively in tissues, and undergo faster elimination than the parent. Drug metabolism, therefore, fosters elimination and often results in inactivation of the compound. However, many metabolites have pharmacodynamic activity and hence contribute to the overall pharmacodynamic response of the parent, or may at times have a totally different effect of their own, therapeutic or toxic, until they are excreted or further metabolized. In developing an understanding of the dose-effect or systemic exposure-effect relationships, an up-to-date understanding of the available information on active metabolites and their dispositional features is extremely important.

Heroin, for example, is rapidly metabolized to monoacetylmorphine (MAM), which, in turn, is hydrolyzed to morphine. Both MAM and heroin are more lipid soluble and hence enter the brain more readily than morphine. In contrast, most of the analgesic activity is associated with MAM and morphine. As would be expected, persistence of dynamic effect is more closely related to the presence of these metabolites than to heroin itself.

Meperidine is metabolized to an active metabolite, normeperidine, by N-demethylation in the liver. In patients with underlying disease, e.g., cirrhosis and/ or renal disease, the bioavailability of the parent and the half-lives of both the parent and the active metabolite are significantly increased. Therefore, the total systemic exposure owing to the parent and an active metabolite varies significantly from subject to subject. Hence, for compounds being evaluated as analgesic agents, kinetic-dynamic evaluations should simultaneously assess the contribution of active metabolites to the response of the parent molecule.

Parameter Estimation

As PK/PD data bases develop based on systemic dose intensity versus effect concepts, the use of models will play an important role in understanding drug disposition, effects, and mechanisms. Modeling and discriminating the correct structural model among several alternatives can usually yield valuable insights into pharmacokinetic-pharmacodynamic mechanisms. An important goal of data analysis is estimating model parameters for drug response and population variability. Optimal sampling schemes that minimize the number of blood samples to be drawn can be applied once the pharmacostatistical models have been developed and tested. Such approaches are useful in gathering information from Phase I studies in special populations, e.g., pediatric and geriatric.

DATA ANALYSIS: MEAN PARAMETERS OR MEAN RESPONSES (PARAMETRIC VS. ANOVA DOSE RESPONSE MODELS)

The traditional approach to safety or efficacy data analysis, over the studied dose range, has employed the analysis of variance (ANOVA) models. This approach, based on the estimation of mean response, has a major drawback in that it does not provide a good way to estimate dose increments for a specific patient. Recently Sheiner et al. (10) have shown that with knowledge of the population parameters, including an assessment of the magnitude of intraindividual observational variability, not only can the mean responses of a typical patient at any dose be computed, but the mean and standard deviation (SD) of the responses in the population at any dose can also be approximated. Parametric PK-PD models can therefore be used to describe both subject-specific response and mean response curves. ANOVA models, on the other hand, include a different parameter for the mean response at each distinct dose. As has been pointed out previously, three major differences apparent between these two models are (a) the response depends on the magnitude of dose in the parametric but not in the ANOVA model, (b) there are few parameters in the parametric model, but as many as there are doses in the ANOVA models, and (c) whereas the parametric models are global (carry information about doses not yet tested), the ANOVA models tend to be local and provide information only about the dose level tested.

TABLE 1. *Performance of various design/analysis approaches to estimating population mean parameters*

Design/analysis	Estimation error (%)[a]			
	E_{max}	D_{50}	$\omega(E_{max})$	$\omega(D_{50})$
Parallel-dose/WLS				
Bias (ME)	3.9	39[b]	—	—
Precision (MAE)	22	100	—	—
Crossover/WLS				
Bias (ME)	−4.5	4.4	—	—
Precision (MAE)	6.5	19	—	—
Crossover/FO				
Bias (ME)	−1.1	−2.9	−7	−13
Precision (MAE)	5.3	18	32	77
Dose-escalation/WLS				
Bias (ME)	−33	−75	—	—
Precision (MAE)	33	91	—	—
Dose-escalation/FO				
Bias (ME)	−.3	−4.0	−15	−20
Precision (MAE)	6.4	20	35	77

WLS, weighted least-squares analysis; ME, mean error; MAE, mean absolute error; FO, first-order method.

[a] Expressed as a percentage of true parameter value.

[b] The estimated bias is surprisingly large. This is, in part, because of Monte Carlo sampling error. Another run used 200 replications and obtained a bias of 21.7 ± 6.4 (SEM), still a large bias.

(From ref. 10, with permission.)

It should, however, be kept in perspective that parametric models are dependent on numerous assumptions.

Using Monte Carlo simulations, Sheiner et al. (10) have tested the ability of several different data analysis methods, e.g., weighted least-squares, extended least-squares, and first-order, to estimate population parameters from different study designs commonly employed for dose-ranging efficacy study. The efficiency of each method for a given study design, weighted least-squares or first-order, was assessed with separate simulation of 50 data sets for a hypothetical antihypertensive drug. Table 1 shows precision and accuracy in parameter estimates of the E_{max} model, with interindividual standard deviations denoted $\omega(E_{max})$ and $\omega(D_{50})$ (parameter similar to EC_{50} discussed earlier), respectively. If the validity of the assumptions underlying the PK-PD model is verified, the analysis demonstrates the potential utility of the patient specific dose-response parametric model to provide a proper basis for dose selection.

Simulation of pharmacokinetic/pharmacodynamic models provides a tool to evaluate drug input paradigms *a priori* for other Phase I studies. A proper dose and a regimen can then be proposed for the Phase II program that will provide a certain exposure (systemic dose intensity) or drug concentration above a certain "threshold level" that is consistent with the understanding of both the pharmacokinetics and pharmacodynamics of the NCE.

DOSE-RANGING TRIALS

Selection of Initial Starting Dose

The starting dose for human trials, as mentioned earlier, is usually extrapolated from animal toxicology data or human experience with pharmacologically similar analogs. Traditionally, the initial starting dose has been selected from early acute and subacute toxicological evaluations, based on a highest no effect (toxicity) dose with a safety factor of 1:10 in a rodent and 1:6 in a nonrodent species. Species susceptibility to a class of similar pharmacological agents should be kept in perspective during such selection and decision making. It is widely known that the dog, for example, is extremely sensitive to drugs belonging to the anthracycline class. Therefore, dose selection for the Phase I study in humans must not be based on the standard $\frac{1}{6}$ of the LD_{10} in this species. The National Cancer Institute (NCI) has devised a protocol that allows investigators to estimate toxic doses in mice, dogs, and monkeys (19) for chemotherapeutic agents. The MTD is defined as the highest dose that kills none of the animals; the toxic dose low (TDL) is defined as the minimum dose at which any toxicity is seen; and the lethal dose 10 (LD_{10}) is defined as the dose at which 10% of the animals deaths are considered drug induced. In any case, the primary goal of such recommendations and safety committees is to avoid starting at a dose either too toxic to humans or so low as to require many dose escalations before any pharmacologic effect is seen.

Dose-Escalation Schemes

If the assignment of doses in a dose-ranging study is fixed without prior human experience, then there is no way of knowing where the preselected doses lie relative to the dose-response curve (Fig. 1). If they happen to cluster to the left or the right, then too few or too many responses will be observed and information regarding the plateau or threshold doses, respectively, will not be obtained. A Phase I study should not require more than six to eight escalations (20) if animal toxicology data can to some extent be accurately extrapolated to man. Unfortunately, extrapolation of animal data does not always provide the dose-range in man, because of species related dispositional variability.

The process of dose escalation must balance two conflicting considerations: an ethical need to escalate slowly, so as to avoid going from no observable toxicity to lethality, counterbalanced by the need to escalate rapidly so as not to expose a large number of healthy subjects to a new drug or patients to ineffective doses. Another important effect of slow escalation in safety dose-ranging studies is that the overall drug development process slows down.

A reasonable compromise between the need to escalate slowly to be safe and fast enough to be efficient is the modified Fibonacci scheme. A commonly used dose-escalation scheme is based on the Fibonacci sequence (21), demonstrated to be an optimal strategy for the sequential search for the maximum of a unimodal function that begins with the integers 1, 1, 2, 3, 5, . . . , each following number being the sum of its two predecessors. In the modified Fibonacci scheme of dose escalation, successive groups of patients receive n (starting dose), 2n, 3.3n, 5n, 7n, 9n, 12n; then doses increase by a third of the previous dose. This scheme, also shown in Fig. 7, is slower than the Fibonacci sequence so that a greater percent of increase in dose escalation occurs earlier in the trial. A retrospective analysis of 30 Phase I chemotherapeutic trials, designed according to the modified Fibonacci scheme, showed favorable evidence in that only 3 of 30 trials required more than ten steps while 8 of 30 required no more than six steps to reach the human MTD (22). Although this scheme is not always ideal, no dose-escalation model has been proposed that is both safe and efficient for all drugs. Therefore, each Phase I dose-escalation protocol should be devised based on the steepness of preclinical toxicity versus dose or exposure curves.

Two other escalation schemes have been proposed (4) for chemotherapeutic agents that are based on the pharmacokinetic principles of MTSE (or the $C \times T$ approach). They require determination of the LD_{10} dose and $C \times T$ at that dose in mice, initially starting the first-time-in-humans testing at a safe dose (1/10 LD_{10}), obtaining a $C \times T$ estimate by integrating pharmacokinetics, and choosing escalation based on a comparison of the $C \times T$ in humans and in mice. Table 2 shows dose ratio (mg/m^2 basis) and the $C \times T$ data for five chemotherapeutic agents, where pharmacokinetic exposure was estimated in both humans and mice, and supports the ability of systemic exposure as a useful predictor of the relative toxicity in mice and humans.

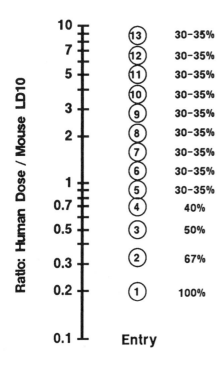

FIG. 7. Modified Fibonacci dose escalation scheme for Phase I trials (semilogarithmic plot). The starting dose in humans is $\frac{1}{10}$ of the LD_{10} in mice (normalized to body weight or surface area). The first escalation step doubles the dose. Each subsequent escalation step is a decreasing percentage of the previous dose. Escalations continue at 30–35% of the previous dose until limiting toxicity (maximum tolerated dose) is reached. (From ref. 4, with permission.)

As brisk early escalation steps are important for efficiency, the alternatives to modified Fibonacci escalation schemes shown in Table 3 are often a good compromise between the desired caution and boldness. These are based on the underlying assumption that the MTSE approach may provide better relationships with response than the MTD approach. These have been tested in the area of chemotherapy (Table 4) and have demonstrated significant savings in both time and money, but are still not widely applied. The authors feel that the applicability of these schemes and MTSE (or C × T, or simply concentration vs. response) approach should be tested in other therapeutic areas to better understand their utility and predictability in studying drug dynamics and pharmacology.

TABLE 2. *Mouse as a quantitative predictor of human toxicity: comparison of dose ratio (mg/m² basis) and C × T ratio for human MTD to mouse LD_{10}*

Drug	Dose ratio	C × T ratio
Doxorubicin	5.0	0.8
Diaziquone	1.0	1.0
Amsacrine	0.8	1.3
Pentostatin	0.7	1.1
Indicine *N*-oxide	0.9	0.6

(From ref. 4, with permission.)

TABLE 3. *Pharmacologically guided escalation schemes*

Proposal A:	Square root (or geometric mean) method
	First escalation step is equal to the square root of the ratio of the C $\times$ T at the mouse LD_{10} to the C $\times$ T for initial (entry) human dose. Subsequent escalations follow Fibonacci modified scheme.
Proposal B:	Extended factor of 2 method
	Maximum escalation step size assumed to be a factor of 2 until the human C $\times$ T is 40% of the mouse C $\times$ T at LD_{10}. Then escalation steps are reduced according to modified Fibonacci scheme.

(From ref. 4, with permission.)

Common Study Designs for Dose-Ranging Studies

Dose-ranging studies are designed to explore the range of doses that may be safely tested in human studies. These studies estimate the lowest active and maximally tolerated dose. We will briefly discuss various dose-ranging designs below.

Ascending-Descending Dose Design

In an attempt to choose doses that migrate toward the desired therapeutic dose range, especially if a response can be predefined, an ascending-descending or up-and-down approach has been employed in dose-ranging studies. This approach, first introduced by Bliss (23), basically involves assigning each subject's dose based on the previous observation. If the previous observation was a nonresponse, then the dose is increased to the next higher level for the next administration and if it produced a response, the dose is decreased to the next lower level. Use of this method in estimating the "median effective dose" has been described by Dixon and Mood (24). These methods can be useful in estimating threshold and plateau doses.

TABLE 4. *Escalation steps required from entry dose ($\frac{1}{10}$ LD_{10}) to maximum tolerated dose for various strategies*

	No. of escalation steps required		
Drug name	Modified Fibonacci	Proposal A (square root)	Proposal B (extended 2s)
Doxorubicin	11	5	6
AMSA	4	2	3
Pentostatin	4	3	3
Indicine *N*-oxide	5	3	3

(From ref. 4, with permission.)

Bolognese (25) has presented three up-and-down designs for maximum dose-ranging information that are meant for use in early, small-sample, clinical pharmacology studies. These designs encompass dosing of the test drug to each of the n subjects and some of the designs allow for repeated observations to be made in the same subject. In principle, decision making leads to an increase or decrease in dose by one predefined level depending on whether the meaningful predefined response is achieved or not. The use of these designs is evident from the two dose-ranging efficacy studies with lisinopril (26) and felodipine (27). It should be kept in perspective, however, that the doses given in this design are not really independent of the responses obtained; each dose except the first depends on the preceding response of the subject. The cumulative dose-response plot in such cases will have carryover effects that may bias the analysis of response. Hence, these studies may only serve as a helpful tool in the design of other statistically robust dose-ranging trials.

Parallel-Dose Design

Traditionally, significant effort is devoted to the design and analysis of efficacy studies, but minimal effort is directed toward the dose-ranging trials. According to Temple (28), of the FDA and current clinical practices, a parallel-dose design comparing several doses with a placebo is a preferred methodology for defining the dose-response relationship. In a parallel-dose design each subject is randomized to receive either a placebo or just one of the doses of active drug. Therefore, if there are m dose levels including the placebo and n subjects are studied at each dose, then the total number of subjects (N) for the study is mn. The desirable qualities that favor this design during Phase I studies are a single exposure of subjects to a new NCE, and therefore a lack of carryover or period effects. If one chooses a parametric PK-PD approach for data analysis, the major problem with this design (10) is that it provides poor estimates of variability and biased parameter estimates (Table 1). Unfortunately, parameter estimation problems associated with this design cannot be solved by adopting alternative methods of data analysis (see Table 1). Another disadvantage is the requirement of a large number of subjects and increased costs. Table 5, abstracted from a recent article by Sheiner et al. (10), well documents the potential advantages and pitfalls associated with various designs for dose-ranging studies, based on parametric modeling approach.

Crossover-Dose Design

As each subject is studied only once in the parallel-dose design, there is relatively poor information on intrasubject variability in the population parameters in dose-response curves. The rationale behind the crossover design is to have more than one point on each subject's dose-response curve. Each of n subjects receive

TABLE 5. *Potential problems for various dose-ranging study designs*

Problem	Parallel dose	Crossover	Dose escalation
Ethical	++	+++	0
Problems in study execution			
Need for many centers	++	+	+
Complexity of protocol	0	++	+/+++
Problems in study analysis			
Reliance on modeling assumptions	0	+	+++
Carryover effects	0	++	+
Period effects	0	++	++
Center effects	++	+	+
Few doses examined	++	++	0
Biased parameter estimates	+++	0	+
Poor/no estimates of variability	+++	+	+
Problems in extrapolation			
Not representative of individual response	+++	0	0
Not representative of clinical practice	++	+++	0
Not representative of patient group	+	+++	0

0, Absence of problem; +, problem minor; ++, problem moderate; +++, problem major.
(From ref. 10, with permission.)

all *a priori* selected m doses (m − 1 active doses, plus placebo) over m periods. So as not to confound the period or carryover effects with dose effects, m doses are given to groups in chosen sequence to which subjects are previously randomized. Since all subjects receive all doses, n needs to be a multiple of m, e.g., for a total of 5 doses (4 active and 1 placebo), the number of subjects need to be 5, 10, 15, 20 . . . , mx, where x is the number of subjects receiving a dose in each period. (Alternatively, one may use a partially balanced design in which each patient gets only some of the doses.)

A major ethical concern with this design during early Phase I dose-ranging safety studies is the exposure of all, rather than a few, subjects to potentially toxic higher doses of the new NCE. Conversely, for dose-ranging efficacy studies, the concern is the use of low and ineffective doses throughout the study. It is apparent that unlike the parallel-dose design, m − 1 additional dose periods increase the duration of the study. Potential concerns and advantages of the crossover-dose design are summarized in Table 5, and the performance of various analysis procedures in estimating population mean parameters of a parametric model, used by Sheiner et al. (10) in evaluating an antihypertensive, is shown in Table 1. As is evident from Table 1, assuming no carryover (which is a major assumption), the parameter estimation bias is much less than that seen with the parallel design because the interindividual component of the random variability in the data is smaller. For Phase 1 safety and efficacy data analysis, both discrete (ANOVA and repeated measures ANOVA) and parametric approaches have been used. As Table 1 shows, traditional methods employing ANOVA, assuming parallel response curves for all participating subjects, do not provide correct interindividual estimates of variability (10). However, the parametric approach (10) in concert with the first-order method, which recognizes correlation among the repeated measures in the same subject (29), has been demonstrated to be an effective and flexible methodology that provides estimates of mean parameters and their interindividual variability.

Dose-Escalation Design

A dose-escalation design allows one to gather significantly more data than other designs at several dose levels and does not suffer from the ethical concerns of the crossover design. These designs vary for safety and efficacy assessments. Basically, doses are slowly increased (in a predetermined manner) and the response is measured. An attempt is usually made to obtain several responses in the same individual at various doses. A typical design includes administration of a placebo dose to all subjects and measurement of the response. After a predetermined period of time, the lowest active dose is given and the response monitored. If the response does not meet predefined criteria of a clinical endpoint and no unacceptable toxicity is seen, the dose is increased to the next highest of $m - 1$ active doses. Figure 8 shows one variant of the dose-escalation design for a dose-ranging efficacy study of an antihypertensive (10).

If a response is seen at any dose, the dose is maintained at that level for the study duration and measurement of the response continues. The data from these studies consist of all responses from all subjects. As doses are always escalated, never decreased, the carryover effects associated with the crossover design are reduced. Each level of increasing dose is expected to overwhelm any pharmacological carryover from the previous dose, although the design remains vulnerable to other factors that can produce carryover effects (e.g., patient expectation and other psychological effects).

A minor variant of this design, particularly useful in Phase I safety studies, is the randomized block dose-escalation scheme that may allow examination of more than one dose in each subject. A total of N subjects are randomly divided into two or three blocks, and the subjects are then escalated through the preselected doses. For example, subjects in each block could be studied at placebo and three to four additional but different escalating-dose levels. Sheiner et al. (10) have suggested that the analysis of data from studies employing a dose-escalation design and a parametric patient-specific dose-response model, although based on modeling assumptions, may allow one to better assess the results of dose-ranging studies than does the traditional ANOVA approach. This can potentially provide both patient-specific and population estimates for individualizing drug therapy.

One of the problems with the dose-escalation design is that period effects can be confounded with dose effects and also period-by-dose interactions, e.g., dependence of response on time. In analgesic studies, the fact that patients know

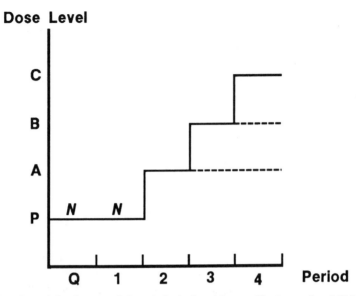

FIG. 8. A variant of the dose-escalation study design. After qualification and an initial placebo period, as in the parallel-dose design, all subjects are advanced to the lowest active dose (A). At the end of period 2, if response (BP for an antihypertensive) has not fallen below the escalation threshold, dose is increased (*solid line*) to the next highest level (B). If BP is below the threshold, dose A is continued (*broken line*) for all subsequent periods. The same procedure is repeated at the end of the next two periods for those who were escalated at the end of the current period. (From ref. 10, with permission.)

that they will receive progressively higher doses is of particular concern; their expectations that relief should increase with rising doses can produce a strong placebo effect.

Other Statistical Concepts

This section briefly addresses some of the other important statistical concepts that must be incorporated into a Phase I dose-ranging protocol.

Randomization/Blinding

Randomization is a fundamental requirement for safety and efficacy evaluation during Phase I. In these studies, randomization enhances validity of statistical testing, improves balance between the various treatments with respect to known or unknown prognostic factors, and significantly eliminates bias from the overall investigation. Most statistical books and computer software (e.g., SAS, BMDP, SPSS) provide tables or programs to generate randomization sequences. Some alternative schemes, e.g., adaptive randomization, can be employed in Phase I efficacy studies. Adaptive randomization increases the likelihood of comparability of the various treatment groups at baseline. In this process, an eligible patient's prognostic and baseline variables are first compared with similar information on all patients already entered in the study. The patient assignment to a treatment group is adopted in a way so as to minimize group heterogeneity and ensure maximum balance among groups.

When feasible, the initial Phase I trials should also be double blinded. During Phase I safety studies, it is customary to have a physician and statistician unblinded: a physician to provide advice to the investigator treating subjects in cases of medical emergency, and a statistician for unbiased interim data analysis. It has also been suggested (30) that the adequacy of the blinding procedures should be checked by asking patients what drug they think they are taking, and how they made the guess. The requirement that treatment drugs be indistinguishable in appearance, taste, and other respects from placebo can necessitate special formulation work at an early stage of the drug development.

Sample Size

If the results of experimental investigations are to be convincing and statistically sound, consideration must be given to the size of the sample chosen to represent the population. Sample size is influenced by patient availability, expected dropout rate, definition of a meaningful response and, of course, by the basic study design and the chosen method of data analysis. Table 5 shows the relative requirements for the number of patients for various designs.

Early Phase I investigations rely more on in-depth clinical observations than on conventional statistical conclusions. Phase I dose-ranging studies customarily employ at least six to eight subjects per treatment group, randomized with a 1: 2 ratio of placebos to active drug. Other constraints, e.g., not exposing a large number of subjects to a new drug, along with the resources that may be available, can also play a role in determining the sample size. Once the safety component for a NCE has been properly defined, attempts should be made in Phase I/II efficacy trials to achieve a respectable power for the study. At this juncture it is usually informative to compute adequate sample size based on different values of α, β error, estimates of variability, and effect size.

Use of Placebo

The use of placebo in early Phase I safety studies is also crucial. As these studies are normally conducted in healthy volunteers, a placebo arm or some placebo controls assist in delineating responses that may be related to the drug or any apprehension that the subjects feel in taking an NCE. It is important, as mentioned earlier, that a double-blind trial with placebo controls will require that the drugs and the dosage form be matched by color, shape, and taste.

SUMMARY

Phase I studies comprise the initial investigations of an NCEs safety, tolerance, and pharmacokinetics/pharmacodynamics. We have reviewed the traditional approaches for conducting these studies, empirically based on the findings from animal studies, that focus on group mean response evaluation. Newer, alternative methodologies have been proposed that may increase the value of information learned from the Phase I studies. These methodologies specifically address inter- and intraindividual variability components that are important in optimally characterizing the use of the drug in the target population. Proper Phase I work focuses on questions to be answered during early Phase II evaluation, providing estimates of optimal dose and regimens for Phase III.

The development of more powerful analgesics requires that not only an attempt be made to understand and quantitate the pain, but also effective tools and methodologies be developed for Phase I studies. PK/PD approaches, interindividual variability estimates for kinetics and dynamics, evaluation of maximally tolerated systemic exposure, and use of alternative study designs for dose-ranging studies are new methods that may better characterize the efficacy and toxicity of the NCE.

REFERENCES

1. Gilman AG, Goodman LS, Rall TW, Murad F, eds. *The pharmacological basis for therapeutics,* 7th ed. New York: Macmillan, 1980.
2. Egorin MJ, Sigman LM, Van Echo DA, et al. Phase I clinical pharmacokinetic study of hexamethylene bisacetamide (NSC95580) administered as a five-day infusion. *Cancer Res* 1987;47: 617–623.
3. Quinn GP, Axelrod J, Brodie BB. Species, strain and sex differences in metabolism of hexobarbital, amidopyrine, antipyrine, and aniline. *Biochem Pharmacol* 1958;1:152–159.
4. Collins JM, Zaharko DS, Dedrick RL, Chabner BA. Potential roles of preclinical pharmacology in phase I clinical trials. *Cancer Treat Rep* 1986;70:73–80.
5. Narang PK, Gerber M. Is disposition of idarubicin dose dependent? International union of pharmacology (IUPHAR), IV World Conference on Clinical Pharmacology and Therapeutics. *Eur J Clin Pharmacol* 1989;36:A308.
6. Rowland M, Sheiner LB, Steimer JL, eds. *Variability in drug therapy: description, estimation, and control.* New York: Raven Press, 1985.
7. Crom WR, Glynn-Barnhart AM, Rodman JH, et al. Pharmacokinetics of anticancer drugs in children. *Clin Pharmacokinet* 1987;12:168–213.
8. Berman E, Raymond V, Daghestani A, Arlin A, et al. 4-demethoxy daunorubicin (idarubicin) in combination with 1-β-D-arabino furanosylcytosine in the treatment of relapsed or refractory acute leukemia. *Cancer Res* 1989;49:477–481.
9. Zimm S, Collins JM, Riccardi R, et al. Variable bioavailability of oral mercaptopurine: is maintenance chemotherapy in acute lymphoblastic leukemia being optimally administered? *New Engl J Med* 1983;308:1005–1009.
10. Sheiner LB, Beal SL, Sambol NC. Study designs for dose ranging. *Clin Pharmacol Ther* 1989;46: 63–77.
11. Rowland M, Tozer TN, eds. *Clinical pharmacokinetics: concepts and applications.* Philadelphia: Lea and Febiger, 1980;138.
12. Gibaldi M, Perrier D, eds. *Pharmacokinetics,* 2nd ed. New York: Marcel Dekker, Inc., 1982.
13. Peck CC, Collins JM. First time in man studies: a regulatory perspective—art and science of phase I trials. *J Clin Pharmacol* 1990;30:218–222.

14. Peck CC. The randomized concentration-controlled clinical trial (CCT); an information-rich alternative to the randomized placebo-controlled trial. *Clin Pharmacol Ther* 1990;47:148.
15. Holford NHG, Sheiner LB. Understanding the dose-effect relationship: clinical application of pharmacokinetic-pharmacodynamic models. *Clin Pharmacokinet* 1981;6:429–453.
16. Hill AV. The possible effects of the aggregation of the molecules of haemoglobin on its dissociation curves. *J Physiol (Lond)* 1910;40:iv–vii.
17. Ariens EJ, Simonis AM. A molecular basis for drug action. *J Pharm Pharmacol* 1964a;27:137–257.
18. Ariens EJ, Simonis AM. A molecular basis for drug action. The interaction of one or more drugs with different receptors. *J Pharm Pharmacol* 1964b;16:289–312.
19. Priem DJ, Young DM, Davis RD, et al. Procedures for preclinical toxicologic evaluation of cancer therapeutic agents: Protocols of the laboratory of toxicology. *Cancer Chemother Rep* 1973;4:1–30.
20. Penta JS, Rozenscweig M, Guarino AM, et al. Mouse and large animal toxicology studies of twelve antitumor agents: relevance to starting dose for phase I clinical trials. *Cancer Chemother Pharmacol* 1979;3:97–101.
21. Forsythe GE, Malcolm MA, Moler CB. *Computer methods for mathematical computations.* Englewood Cliffs, New Jersey: Prentice Hall, 1977;178–182.
22. Goldsmith MA, Slavik M, Carter SK. Quantitative prediction of drug toxicity in humans from toxicology in small and large animals. *Cancer Res* 1975;35:1354–1364.
23. Bliss CI. The calculation of the dosage-mortality curve. *Ann Appl Biol* 1935;22:134–167.
24. Dixon WJ, Mood AM. A method for obtaining and analyzing sensitivity data. *J Am Statist Assoc* 1948;43:109–126
25. Bolognese JA. A Monte-Carlo comparison of three up-and-down designs for dose ranging. *Controlled Clin Trials* 1983;4:187–196.
26. Dickstein K. Hemodynamic, hormonal, and pharmacokinetic aspects of treatment with lisinopril in congestive heart failure. *J Cardiovasc Pharmacol* 1987;9(suppl 3):S73–S81.
27. Frecling P, Harvard-Davis R, Goves JR, Burton RH, Orme-Smith EA. Control of hypertension in elderly patients with felodipine and metoprolol: a double blind, placebo-controlled clinical trial. *Br J Clin Pharmacol* 1987;24:459–464.
28. Temple R. Government viewpoint of clinical trials. *Drug Info J* 1982;16:10–17.
29. Beal SL, Sheiner LB. NONMEM users guides. NONMEM project group, UCSF, 1989, San Francisco, CA.
30. Moscucci M, Byrne L, Weintraub M, Cox C. Blinding, unblinding and placebo effect: an analysis of patients' guesses of treatment assignment in a double-blind clinical trial. *Clin Pharmacol Ther* 1987;41:259–265.

DISCUSSION

Dr. Carl Peck: I agree with almost all of the theses put forth by Drs. Narang and Bianchine, and congratulate them on a superb manuscript. I would, however, like to make an alternative interpretation of a fundamental goal in drug development. Narang and Bianchine suggest that in addition to safety and efficacy, dose response is an important matter in drug development. Certainly we have been promoting dose-response studies in recent years as a method to prove effectiveness, and as a basis for physicians' treatment of their patients.

I would like to go a step further. Our goal ought to be to develop a knowledge base that would allow physicians to individualize therapy for patients. In that way, therapy could be optimized for the individual, not for the population. That is where the emphasis of Narang and Bianchine on kinetics and dynamics is right on target, because I think that is a valuable framework for such dosing strategies.

Advances in Pain Research and Therapy, Vol. 18,
edited by M. Max, R. Portenoy, and E. Laska,
Raven Press, Ltd., New York 1991.

3

Experimental Pain Models

Richard H. Gracely

*Clinical Pain Section, Neurobiology and Anesthesiology Branch, National Institute of
Dental Research, National Institutes of Health, Bethesda, Maryland 20892*

EVOLUTION OF EXPERIMENTAL ANALGESIA: SUCCESS, FAILURE, SUCCESS, REINTERPRETATION

Over 40 years ago, experimental methods were used successfully to evaluate analgesic agents. Using predominantly the pain sensation threshold evoked by a radiant heat source, analgesic potency and dose-response curves were routinely demonstrated (1–3). The validity of these results, however, was quickly challenged. In a paper that set standards for present clinical analgesic trials, Denton and Beecher (4) instituted double-blind placebo controls and found no effect of a 15 mg dose of morphine using the radiant heat threshold technique. This failure was replicated by many other investigators during the next 15 years (2). Experimental methods were deemed useless for analgesic assessment, and investigators were left with a puzzle. Why did narcotics modify pain associated with injury or disease and not pain produced experimentally?

In 1966, this puzzle was apparently solved. Beecher (2) described a study by Smith and coworkers (5) in which a continuously increasing pain was produced by exercising an arm rendered ischemic by a tourniquet. The time required for this pain to reach distressing or unbearable levels was reliably increased by morphine as compared to a double-blind placebo. The effect at less intense levels was not statistically significant. These investigators concluded that morphine analgesia resulted from the reduction of an emotional "reaction component." This component was assumed to accompany clinical pain conditions and to be evoked by especially severe experimental pain stimulation. According to this model no morphine effect is observed for less intense stimulation because little reaction component is associated with the "brief flickering jabs" (5) of discrete, threshold-level pain perceptions.

This interpretation profoundly influenced medical and scientific thought. Until recently standard medical texts (6) explained that opiates produce analgesia by reducing pain reaction with little effect on pain sensation, e.g., "I still feel it but it does not bother me any more." Recent findings have modified this interpretation. There is general agreement that previous negative results reflected the use of pain threshold as a dependent measure, focusing on the very bottom of the pain range. For many stimuli, opiate analgesia is demonstrated with difficulty at these levels but routinely at more intense levels. There is also general acknowledgment that pain can be divided into sensory and emotional components, that it is a particular sensory experience accompanied by immediate feelings of discomfort and distress. However, increasing evidence indicates that the unpleasant reaction component is not necessary for the demonstration of experimental analgesia. In the past decade, opiate analgesia has been demonstrated routinely using brief electrical (7–23) and thermal (14,24–34) stimuli, including dose-response relationships (28,30,31). Experimental analgesia has been demonstrated also with less potent agents, detailed below. In addition, converging anatomical, physiological, and behavioral evidence strongly suggests that opiate analgesia includes a significant reduction in the magnitude of pain sensation independent of alteration of the aversive or emotional qualities associated with the sensation (35–38).

Thus, previous failures to demonstrate experimental analgesia resulted from use of threshold, rather than suprathreshold, methodology. The emotional "reaction component" associated with clinical pain conditions is not a necessary prerequisite for the experimental demonstration of opiate analgesia. The "reaction component," however, remains an important concept in pain assessment and treatment, one that can be evaluated by experimental methods. Both simple (18,39) and complex (40,41) verbal scales have separately evaluated the intensity and unpleasantness of pain sensations evoked by experimental stimuli. Visual analogue scales also have been used (42,43), with discriminatory power approaching that of the verbal methods (44,45). Scales of the intensity and unpleasantness of pain sensations evoked by brief stimuli have been dissociated by both pharmacological (18,31,39,46,47) and nonpharmacological (42,48–51) interventions. In addition, the amount of unpleasantness associated with a specific pain intensity has been shown to systematically vary among different types of experimental pain stimuli (52–54) and with age (55).

UTILITY OF EXPERIMENTAL PAIN MODELS

The present advantages of experimental methods for the evaluation of analgesic efficacy include those described 30 years ago. These methods can provide fast, efficient evaluations in normal populations under controlled conditions. They also are less expensive than clinical trials, statistically more powerful, and permit toxicity testing in healthy individuals.

Previous criticisms also are still valid. Experimental pain sensations cannot duplicate the experience of clinical pain syndromes. Experimental stimulation also may not activate higher-level processes present in clinical syndromes, processes ranging from spinal summation to the experience of anxiety, concern, and affective distress. Experimental stimulation may not duplicate crucial sensory characteristics of a syndrome, such as pain associated with inflammation or with injury to neural systems mediating pain sensation. Thus, experimental pain stimuli may neither provide an adequate stimulus nor duplicate the sensory, affective, and cognitive consequences of clinical pain.

However, several lines of evidence indicate that human psychophysical pain methods can provide considerable utility in the face of these limitations. First, many of the paradigms used in analgesic development possess these limitations to a much greater degree. The rat tail flick, hot plate, and advanced animal models do not duplicate the afferent characteristics or psychological gestalt of human syndromes. These methods are useful for their correlative power; agents that appear potent in a tail flick paradigm will likely result in human analgesia. On a continuum from actual clinical pain to the rat tail flick, the human psychophysical models may compare more favorably to clinical pain than accepted animal models. Second, psychophysical methods have already been shown to reliably respond to at least one class of agents used in clinical pain control. The experimental demonstrations of opiate analgesia, and recent investigations of nonopiate agents, are discussed below. Third, recently acquired knowledge of pain mechanisms and the afferent effects of experimental stimulation combine to increase the information resulting from the outcome of an experimental pain evaluation. Fourth, experimental methods may serve as an adjunct to clinical pain assessment, either by direct comparisons to clinical pain sensation (56–59), or by methods that evaluate the influence of clinical pain on experimental pain perception (60–67). Finally, experimental methods can provide direct information about the subject's ability to perform a rating task. Stimulus control allows measures of sensitivity and scaling performance (27,28,68–72). This information can be used to evaluate the quality of experimental data. If the goal is evaluation of potency or analgesic mechanisms, use of high-quality data improves sensitivity. Use of performance measures in designs that compare experimental and clinical pain also may allow inferences about clinical scaling ability (56–59).

Thus, experimental methods can serve as a correlative analogue of clinical syndromes. Specific classes of drugs shown to exert experimental analgesia will also generally show an effect in the clinical situation. Regardless of outcome, experimental tests will provide information on side effects and toxicity in healthy individuals skilled in describing subjective sensations. Positive results will demonstrate at least part of the analgesic action of a test drug. Negative results will provide information on toxicity, and will demonstrate mechanisms not activated by the agent.

MODALITIES AND METHODS

Discrete pain sensations are most often evoked either by application of electrical stimuli to the skin or teeth, or by application of thermal stimuli to the skin by a contact probe or by a radiant lamp or laser source. Continuous pain sensations are usually evoked by the cold pressor method or by the tourniquet ischemia method. The cold pressor procedure involves immersion of a limb (usually the hand) in ice water. Tourniquet ischemic pain is produced by exercising a hand to which circulation has been occluded by a blood pressure cuff. Pressure pain is now being used more frequently. It is usually applied by continuously increasing the pressure of a small probe applied to the finger or other bony location. A recent application squeezes the finger web. Stimuli can be administered in discrete brief presentations of varying intensities. The choice of a particular method may be based on several factors, such as naturalness, repeatability, severity, selective stimulation of primary afferents, and sensitivity to specific analgesic interventions (73).

Psychophysical pain methods have been detailed in several reviews (56,57,73–78). These methods can be divided into three simple classes:

1. *Continuous stimulation, growing in intensity or severity (intolerability) over time, or use of discrete stimuli to mimic such stimulation.* This class includes most pain threshold procedures and methods that evaluate the elapsed time (or number or intensity of discrete stimuli) to reach suprathreshold subjective criteria such as distressing or intolerable. Judgments of pain magnitude also may be requested at specific time points.

2. *Random presentations of a fixed set of discrete stimuli.* This class includes a majority of the psychophysical scaling procedures such as category scaling, magnitude estimation, cross-modality matching, and Sensory Decision Theory (SDT) methods. Results can be analyzed in terms of pain magnitude by determining a specific response magnitude to each stimulus. The ability to discriminate between stimuli also can be used to construct a response scale (79). SDT analysis, which separately measures discrimination and response behavior, has been applied extensively to pain judgments (9–12,24–26,29,34,67–71). The classical threshold "Method of Constant Stimuli" is also in this class. It presents stimuli near pain threshold and evaluates probability of a threshold response at each stimulus level. A modification of a fixed stimulus set method, little used in pain research, requires a single response to an integrated impression (average, sum, difference) of two or more stimuli (72,80,81).

3. *Interactive or adaptive methods.* These procedures do not present a fixed stimulus set but rather adjust the stimulation based on previous responses. The classical threshold "Method of Adjustment" is related to this class. The staircase modification of the "Method of Limits" is another threshold procedure in which stimulus intensity is increased by negative reports and decreased by positive ones. The result is a series of stimulus intensities that track pain threshold (82). This method is considered most efficient because most of the stimuli contribute to the analysis. It has been applied recently to scaling of suprathreshold pain sensation by randomly switching between several independent staircases, each tracking at a different subjective level (27).

WHAT METHODS ARE SENSITIVE TO WHICH ANALGESICS?

Most studies of experimental analgesia have evaluated the effects of powerful opiates. Morphine has long been the standard in analgesic assays, and the use of a powerful agent maximizes the chance of a positive result. Thus, the few and often conflicting demonstrations of sensitivity to nonopiate agents may reflect either the general paucity of these studies or insufficient experimental sensitivity.

Opiates

Results with opiates are numerous and unequivocal. Morphine has reduced pain sensations produced by brief electrical (8,14,20,22), thermal (14,31–34), or pressure (14) stimuli, and by the continuous pains evoked by cold pressor (83) and tourniquet ischemia (5). Experimental analgesia has been demonstrated with similar opiates such as oxycodone by electrical tooth-pulp stimulation (R. H. Gracely, unpublished observations), meperidine by tourniquet ischemia (84), and dipipanone by the cold pressor method (85). One study showed that the synthetic enkephalin analog FK33-824 increased pain tolerance to an ascending series of electrical stimuli applied to the earlobe (21). The short-acting opiate fentanyl and its derivatives have been used widely, showing analgesia to electrical tooth pulp stimulation (17–19) and heat applied to skin by a contact thermode (27,30,86). Recent studies using fixed stimulus sets or interactive methods have demonstrated opiate dose-response relationships (28,30,31), antagonism (87,88), and effects of infusion rate, multiple infusions, and simulated or real potentiation (87,89,90). Analgesia to weak opiates has been assessed less frequently. Codeine analgesia has been demonstrated by electrical skin stimulation (23,91), cold pressor (90), and tourniquet ischemia (93).

Antiinflammatory Agents

Results with nonsteroidal antiinflammatory drugs (NSAIDs) appear equivocal. Aspirin has reduced pain associated with pressure applied to the finger web (94), while aspirin, indomethacin, and ibuprofen failed to show a response in cold pressor tests (83,92,95). Studies using tourniquet ischemia have shown both analgesia (96) and negative results (93). Electrical skin stimulation also has resulted in analgesia in one case (8) but not in another (22), whereas subjective ratings of electrical tooth pulp stimulation, as well as cortical evoked potentials, have been reduced by aspirin (97,98).

This variability across and within stimulation modalities may reflect both the relatively weak potency of this class of medications, and their selective peripheral action. Specific stimulus modalities may provide a more "adequate stimulus" amenable to NSAID attenuation. For example, the above results suggest that pressure pain may activate peripheral processes affected by NSAIDs whereas cold pressor pain does not. The lack of an effect on electrical stimulation is consistent with the fact that electrical stimuli activate primary afferent fibers directly. This stimulation bypasses the receptor and therefore the consequence of the stimulation is not influenced by change in receptor sensitivity. The positive reports with electrical stimulation are somewhat puzzling, since NSAIDs are assumed to reduce pain at the receptor level. However, the effects of NSAIDs on late evoked potentials and the finding that ketoprofen alters the nociceptive reflex evoked by electrical skin stimulation in normals but not in paraplegic patients suggest a central mechanism of NSAID action (97–99).

Thus, there is indication of NSAID effects with specific stimuli, and with conflicting results with others. Additional evidence is needed to clarify results with the tourniquet and electrical methods, to replicate the positive results found with pressure pain, to specify the characteristics of an adequate stimulus, and to determine site(s) of NSAID action.

Antidepressants

Doxepin was indistinguishable from placebo using the electrical tooth pulp model (9), while imipramine reduced pain sensations produced by electrical stimuli applied to the skin (100). Amitriptyline did not alter pain sensations produced by contact heat stimuli in patients suffering from diabetic neuropathy (101) or facial pain (102). Thus, preliminary results suggest that thermal stimuli are not sensitive to antidepressants, and the sensitivity to electrical stimulation may be drug or stimulus dependent. Again, insufficient data are available to draw firm conclusions.

Benzodiazepines

Discrimination of thermal pain sensations have been reduced by diazepam, indicating possible analgesia (34). However, another study found no such reduction (24). In addition, results of a stimulus integration task suggest that diazepam-produced changes in discrimination may represent a disruption of psychophysical performance and not a reduction in pain sensitivity (103). Stimulus integration tasks [functional measurement (72,80,81,103), conjoint measurement (104)] require a single integrated impression to two stimuli, providing more information than that available from a response to a single stimulus. This increased power may clarify changes in pain discrimination such as those found · with diazepam. The critical issue is whether pain sensation or rating consistency is affected by the drug (70).

Additional studies have shown that diazepam reduced the unpleasantness but not the intensity of sensations produced by electrical skin stimulation (39) and did not alter judgments of electrical tooth pulp stimulation (18). Diazepam has been shown to increase tolerance to tourniquet ischemia (24) but did not alter continuous ratings of pain intensity to the same stimulus (93). These results are consistent with clinical anecdotal results that minor tranquilizers alter emotional factors but do not provide analgesia.

Anesthetics

Thirty or more years ago, 25 to 50% nitrous oxide, 0.35 to 0.5% trichloroethylene, and 1 to 2% ether, but not 0.5% halothane, had been shown to reduce pain produce by pressure to the tibia (105), and 20% nitrous oxide had been shown to reduce pain from radiant heat and tourniquet ischemia (106). More recent studies have shown that ketamine reduces pain from tourniquet ischemia (84), and nitrous oxide in concentrations between 15 and 50% reduces pain sensations evoked by heat applied to the skin (107), and by electrical stimulation of the tooth pulp (10,11,108–112). A series of studies using an ascending series of electrical tooth pulp stimuli have shown that the information presented to subjects about the expected effects and potency of nitrous oxide can result in changes in pain ratings indicative of either increased analgesia or hyperalgesia (110–111). These results are consistent with the hypothesis that particular pain rating paradigms may be more open to modification by conscious or unconscious factors (see below). In addition, the findings that the experimental context can be arranged to result in nitrous oxide hyperalgesia is consistent with the moderate potency demonstrated in experimental studies and observed in clinical practice. A recent study which minimized the opportunity for biased responding found a rapid and significant analgesic effect of 50% nitrous oxide to contact heat stimuli that was about one-half to one-third the magnitude of analgesia produced by 1.1 μg/kg fentanyl using the same method (Kaufman, Chastain, Gaughan, and Gracely, *unpublished observations*).

COMMON EXPERIMENTAL PAIN PARADIGMS AND THEIR PITFALLS

Ascending and/or Continuous Stimulation: The Simulation Pitfall

All psychophysical methods of pain evaluation require subjects to form judgments of perceived sensation. Many methods share a common major weakness: they allow manipulation of the results independent of perceived sensation. This pitfall takes different forms, depending on the method. In methods in which a continuous pain is increasing over time (cold pressor, tourniquet ischemia), judgments are confounded with time and possibly with number of response trials. For example, a common cold pressor method (immersion of hand in ice water) requires pain ratings on a numerical scale at 15-sec intervals for 1 min. Subjects give four numbers in increasing order. After a manipulation, it is very easy to give another four numbers that indicate a desired effect, such as lowered numbers if the subject assumes an analgesic was administered. Rather than request responses at specific time points, variants of the method measure the elapsed time to endpoints such as pain threshold, pain tolerance, or intermediate levels such as uncomfortable or distressing. Subjects may use estimates of elapsed time to provide "appropriate" data. This pitfall is also present in methods that simulate continuous stimuli by presenting a train of continuously increasing discrete stimuli (20).

This pitfall is also present in paradigms in which brief stimuli of varying intensity are presented in random sequence. Ideally, stimulus intensities should be spaced close enough together for sufficient "confusion"; subjects are unaware of how many different stimuli are used and of which one is presented on each trial. If stimuli are spaced widely apart each specific intensity can be recognized, e.g., "that is the bottom one," or "that one is the second from the top." This identification allows the same manipulation of the result possible with continuous measures.

This problem could be labeled the "simulation pitfall." Regardless of the method, subjects can easily manipulate the result without attending to and independently judging the pain sensation. The degree to which subjects actually manipulate results is not known. The importance of this classification is that methods vulnerable to this conscious manipulation also are vulnerable to unconscious bias (82); the outcome may be subtly altered in response to internal expectations or external demands.

The type, character, and direction of the alteration or simulation depends more on details of experimental design than of method. Subject expectations may be shaped by real or perceived goals of the experiment, and uncontrolled events may cue them to emit an appropriate response. For example, a psychometric examination of repeat reliability requires assessment on more than one occasion. Subjects may perceive an implicit goal of stable responding, and "look good" by giving the same responses to identified stimuli or response trials, or at specific times. In another example, subjects may perceive side effects in an analgesic assessment, assume they received the active medication, and "look good" by lowering their responses or lengthening their response times.

Random Presentation of a Fixed Set of Discrete Stimuli: The Pitfall of Perceptual Bias

The simulation pitfall discussed above can be classified as a bias that occurs "outside of the psychophysical process" (OPP) of applying responses to perceived sensations. It is an OPP bias because orderly data and appropriate effects can be generated without judging the magnitude of (or even feeling) the stimulus-evoked sensations. Results can be biased without attending to stimulation-evoked sensations, or by identifying which stimulus is presented. Other biases, in contrast, occur "within the psychophysical process" (WPP). These WPP biases influence or modulate the judgments of a perceived sensation, and occur in all psychophysical paradigms, including those with random stimulation that cannot be easily simulated. The effects are often directional, amplifying or attenuating the entire function. These effects may be caused by expectations (received an analgesic), by personality or cultural traits (stoicism), or by situational factors (male subject impressing female experimenter, anxious subject). They may be unconscious, or represent a conscious desire to modify pain responses. Like the simulation pitfall, they allow subjects to give a specific result. Unlike the simulation pitfall, this effect must occur within the context of perceiving and labeling sensation.

Perceptual biases may also be nondirectional. There is considerable evidence that subjects in a psychophysical task engage in consistent rating behaviors that systematically influence results. The sensitivity of methods to stimulus range, spacing, and frequency and to a constricted response range all stem from a single tendency (45,56,113,114). When subjects are required to make repeated judgments of varying stimuli on a defined scale, they tend to spread their responses over the scale. Their response distribution remains relatively constant regardless of the composition of the stimulus ensemble.

This tendency to produce a constant response distribution is related to the response scale used, and thus can be termed a "response behavior pitfall." This pitfall can distort psychophysical functions and reduce the sensitivity of analgesic assessments. It may also result in response centering effects, in which extreme scores tend to normalize independent of any manipulation. This effect is known by several names, such as "regression to the mean," "Law of Initial Values," or "floor-ceiling effects." The influence of response behavior can be minimized by administration of uniform stimulus distributions and use of responses with a large possible range such as magnitude estimation or line production. There is evidence that specific subject instruction (45) or the use of randomized descriptors (39,44,45) can minimize this effect. The use of interactive methods in which the response distribution remains relatively constant should also reduce the influence of response behaviors (27,28).

Detection of Analgesia from Side Effects or from the Rating Task

Detection of perceived side effects may influence pain judgments (47,115), presumably because these effects indicate that an analgesic has been administered. The influence of side effects is a design issue discussed below. The pain assessment method also can provide feedback to the subject that analgesia has occurred. The time or number of trials to endpoints may be increased in the continuous methods, or the range of sensation experienced from a fixed stimulus set may be lowered. This detection may mediate conscious or unconscious behaviors that distort the results, leading to incorrect inferences about analgesic mechanisms or dose-response relationships. The interactive methods continuously adjust the stimuli to produce the same responses (and assumed sensations) before and after an analgesic administration. Thus, cues of analgesia such as reduced sensory range are minimized in comparison to other methods (27,28).

Perceptual biases are a nuisance variable present to some degree in all subjective judgments. Sophisticated psychophysical methods and analyses have been used to reduce bias effects. However, because pain is an experience with both sensory and affective components, it may not be assessed adequately by methods that focus exclusively on sensory characteristics. The clinically significant component of pain sensation, its associated feelings of aversion, distress, and suffering, may be most appropriately evaluated by methods used to assess other conceptual variables such as opinion or attitude. Measurement biases with these methods are most effectively minimized by careful experimental design and control. In the case of pain assessment, instructions should specify a uniform set of expectations. Cues signaling analgesic administration should be minimized, and "active" placebos should be employed to mimic unavoidable side effects. For example, Max et al.'s (47) crossover studies in neuropathic pain mimic the sedation and cholinergic side effects of amitriptyline by use of an active placebo containing diazepam and benztropine. If side effects of a test drug are unique and hard to duplicate, they could be masked (a) by administering an active placebo with strong subjective effects to all groups (18), (b) by administering the test drug to all groups and then assessing incremental analgesia produced by either an increased dose or a second administration (28,90), or (c) by assessing the effects of an antagonist (87,88).

CONCLUSION

It is acknowledged that pain sensations evoked by experimental stimulation cannot precisely duplicate the pain of an acute clinical condition or chronic syndrome. However, recent findings indicate that these procedures can provide significant information. Experimental pain methods have evolved from simple threshold tests of analgesia. Increasingly sophisticated methods evaluate and control for human reporting behavior. These methods embrace the complexity of pain experience, and serve as tools that can facilitate evaluation of analgesic efficacy, and investigations of the mechanisms of pain and analgesia.

The design and use of these tools can be improved further. It is all too easy to use an inappropriate measure, design a confounded study, or produce a biased result. It is hoped that future evolution will bring both improved methods and increased appreciation of what experimental methods can do, and a critical appreciation of when they do it properly or poorly.

REFERENCES

1. Beecher HK. *Measurement of subjective responses.* New York: Oxford University Press, 1959.
2. Beecher HK. Pain: one mystery solved. *Science* 1966;151:840–841.

3. Hardy JD, Wolff HG, Goodell HS. *Pain sensations and reactions.* New York: Hafner, 1952.
4. Denton JE, Beecher HK. New analgesics I. Methods in the clinical evaluation of new analgesics. *JAMA* 1949;141:1051–1057.
5. Smith GM, Egbert LD, Markowitz RA, Mosteller F, Beecher HK. An experimental pain method sensitive to morphine in man: the submaximum effort tourniquet technique. *J Pharmacol Exp Ther* 1966;154:324–332.
6. Jaffe JH, Martin WR. Opioid analgesics and antagonists. In: Gilman AG, Goodman L, Gilman I, eds. *The pharmacological basis of therapeutics,* 6th ed. New York: Macmillan, 1980;494–543.
7. Bromm B, Seide K. The influence of tilidine and prazepam on withdrawal reflex, skin resistance reaction and pain ratings in man. *Pain* 1982;12:247–258.
8. Buchsbaum MS, Davis GC, Coppola R, Naber D. Opiate pharmacology and individual differences I: Psychophysical pain measurements. *Pain* 1981;10:357–366.
9. Chapman CR, Butler SH. Effects of Doxepin on perception of laboratory-induced pain in man. *Pain* 1978;5:253–262.
10. Chapman CR, Gehrig JD, Wilson ME. Acupuncture compared with 33 percent nitrous oxide for dental analgesia: a sensory decision theory evaluation. *Anesthesiology* 1975;42:532–537.
11. Chapman CR, Murphy TM, Butler SH. Analgesic strength of 33 percent nitrous oxide: A signal detection evaluation. *Science* 1973;179:1246–1248.
12. Chapman CR, Wilson ME, Gehrig JD. Comparative effects of acupuncture and transcutaneous stimulation on the perception of painful dental stimuli. *Pain* 1976;2:265–283.
13. Chatrian GE, Fernandes de Lima VM, Lettich E, Canfield RC, Miller RC, Soso MJ. Electrical stimulation of tooth pulp in humans II: Qualities of sensations. *Pain* 1982;14:233–246.
14. Cooper BY, Vierck CJ Jr, Yeomans DC. Selective reduction of second pain sensation by systemic morphine in humans. *Pain* 1986;24:93–116.
15. Craig KD, Coren S. Signal detection analyses of social modelling influences on pain expressions. *J Psychosom Res* 1975;19:105–112.
16. Fernandes de Lima VM, Chatrian GE, Lettich E, Canfield RC, Miller RC, Soso MJ. Electrical stimulation of tooth pulp in humans. I. Relationships among physical stimulus intensities, psychological magnitude estimates, and cerebral evoked potentials. *Pain* 1982;14:207–232.
17. Gracely RH, Dubner R, McGrath PA. Narcotic analgesia: fentanyl reduces the intensity but not the unpleasantness of painful tooth pulp stimulation. *Science* 1979;203:1261–1263.
18. Gracely RH, Dubner R, McGrath PA. Fentanyl reduces the intensity of painful tooth pulp sensations: controlling for detection of active drugs. *Anesth Analg* 1982;61:751–755.
19. McGrath PA, Sharav Y, Dubner R, Gracely RH. Masseter inhibitory periods and sensations evoked by electrical tooth pulp stimulation. *Pain* 1981;10:1–17.
20. Parry WL, Smith GM, Denton JE. An electric-shock method of inducing pain responsive to morphine in man. *Anesth Analg* 1972;51:573–578.
21. Stacher G, Bauer P, Steinringer H, Schreiber E, Schmierer G. Effects of the synthetic enkephalin analog FK33-824 on pain threshold and pain tolerance in man. *Pain* 1979;7:159–172.
22. Wolf BB, Kantor TG, Jarvik ME, Laska E. Response of experimental pain to analgesic drugs. I. Morphine, aspirin and placebo. *Clin Pharmacol Ther* 1966;7:224–238.
23. Wolf BB, Kantor TG, Jarvik ME, Laska E. Response of experimental pain to analgesic drugs. II. Codeine and placebo. *Clin Pharmacol Ther* 1966;7:323–331.
24. Chapman CR, Feather BW. Effects of diazepam on human pain tolerance and sensitivity. *Psychosom Med* 1973;35:330–340.
25. Clark WC, Yang JC. Acupunctural analgesia? Evaluation by signal detection theory. *Science* 1974;184:1096–1098.
26. Feather BW, Chapman CR, Fisher SB. The effect of placebo on the perception of painful radiant heat stimuli. *Psychosom Med* 1972;34:290–294.
27. Gracely RH, Lota L, Walther DJ, Dubner R. A multiple random staircase method of psychophysical pain assessment. *Pain* 1988;32:55–63.
28. Gracely RH. Multiple random staircase assessment of thermal pain perception. In: Dubner R, Bond M, Gebbart G, eds. *Proceedings of the Fifth World Congress on Pain.* Amsterdam: Elsevier, 1988;391–394.
29. Lloyd MA, Wagner MK. Acupuncture analgesia and radiant-heat pain: a signal detection analysis. *Anesthesiology* 1976;44:147–150.

30. Price DD, Harkins SW, Baker C. A simultaneous comparison of fentanyl's analgesic effects on experimental and clinical pain. *Pain* 1986;24:197–203.
31. Price DD, von der Gruen A, Miller J, Rafii A, Price C. A psychophysical analysis of morphine analgesia. *Pain* 1985;22:261–269.
32. Wolskee PJ, Gracely RH, Sayer MJ, Dubner R. Effect of morphine on experimental pain and measures of clinical pain in chronic pain patients. *Pain* 1981;(Suppl 1):155.
33. Wolskee PJ, Gracely RH. The effects of morphine on experimental pain response in chronic pain patients. *Soc Neurosci Abstr* 1980;6:246.
34. Yang JC, Clark WC, Ngai SH, Berkowitz BA, Spector S. Analgesic action and pharmaco-kinetics of morphine and diazepam in man: an evaluation by sensory decision theory. *Anesthesiology* 1979;51:495–502.
35. Dubner R, Bennett GJ. Spinal and trigeminal mechanisms of nociception. *Annu Rev Neurosci* 1983;6:381–418.
36. Leibeskind JC, Paul LA. Psychological and physiological mechanisms of pain. *Annu Rev Psychol* 1977;28:41–60.
37. Mayer DJ, Price DD. Central nervous system mechanisms of analgesia. *Pain* 1976;2:379–404.
38. Price DD, Dubner R. Neurons that subserve the sensory-discriminative aspects of pain. *Pain* 1977;3:307–338.
39. Gracely RH, McGrath PA, Dubner R. Validity and sensitivity of ratio scales of sensory and affective verbal pain descriptors. *Pain* 1978;5:19–29.
40. Chen ACN, Treede RD. The McGill Pain Questionnaire in the assessment of phasic and tonic experimental pain: behavioral evaluation of the "pain inhibiting pain" effect. *Pain* 1985;22:67–79.
41. Klepac RK, Dowling J, Hauge G. Sensitivity of the McGill Pain Questionnaire to intensity and quality of laboratory pain. *Pain* 1981;10:199–207.
42. Price DD, Barrell JJ, Gracely RH. A psychophysical analysis of experiential factors that selectively influence the affective dimension of pain. *Pain* 1980;8:137–149.
43. Price DD, McGrath PA, Rafii A, Buckingham B. The validation of visual analogue scales as ratio scale measures in for chronic and experimental pain. *Pain* 1983;17:45–56.
44. Duncan GH, Bushnell MC, Lavigne GJ. Comparison of verbal and visual analogue scales for measuring the intensity and unpleasantness of experimental pain. *Pain* 1989;37:295–303.
45. Price DD. *Psychological and neural mechanisms of pain.* New York: Raven Press, 1988.
46. Heft MW, Gracely RH, Dubner R. Nitrous oxide analgesia: a psychophysical evaluation using verbal descriptor scaling. *J Dent Res* 1984;63:129–132.
47. Max MB, Schafer SC, Culnane M, Dubner R, Gracely RH. Association of pain relief with drug side-effects in postherpetic neuralgia: a single dose study of clonidine, codeine, ibuprofen and placebo. *Clin Pharmacol Ther* 1988;43:363–371.
48. Hargreaves KM, Dionne RA, Meuller GP, Goldstein DS, Dubner R. Naloxone, fentanyl and diazepam modify plasma beta-endorphin levels during surgery. *Clin Pharmacol Ther* 1986;40:165–171.
49. Johnson JE. Effects of accurate expectations about sensations on the sensory and distress components of pain. *J Pers Soc Psychol* 1973;27:261–275.
50. Malone MD, Kurts RM, Strube MJ. The effects of hypnotic suggestion on pain report. *Am J Clin Hypn* 1989;31:221–230.
51. Price DD, Barber J. An analysis of the factors that contribute to the efficacy of hypnotic analgesia. *J Abnorm Psychol* 1987;96:46–51.
52. Heft MW, Gracely RH, McGrath PA, Brown FJ. Assessment of pain produced by electrical and natural stimulation of teeth. *J Dent Res* 1977;56(Special Issue B):194.
53. Price DD, Harkins SW, Baker C. Sensory-affective relationships among different types of clinical pain and experimental pain. *Pain* 1987;28:297–307.
54. Rainville P, Feine JS, Saulnier C, Rivard C, Duncan GH, Bushnell MC. Perceived intensity and unpleasantness of four modalities of experimental pain. *Am Pain Soc Abstr* 1989;8:64.
55. Harkins SW, Price DD, Martelli M. Effects of age on pain perception—thermonociception. *J Gerontol* 1986;41:58–63.
56. Gracely RH. Psychophysical assessment of human pain. In: Bonica JJ, Liebeskind JC, Albe-Fessard D, eds. *Advances in pain research and therapy, vol. 3.* New York: Raven Press, 1979;805–824.
57. Gracely RH. Subjective quantification of pain perception. In: Bromm B, ed. *Neurophysiological correlates of pain.* Amsterdam: Elsevier Press, 1984.

58. Heft MW, Gracely RH, Dubner R, McGrath PA. A validation model for verbal descriptor scaling of human clinical pain. *Pain* 1980;9:363–373.
59. Price DD, Harkins SW. The combined use of visual analogue scales and experimental pain in proving standardized assessment of clinical pain. *Clin J Pain* 1987;3:1–8.
60. Brands AEF, Schmidt AJM. Learning processes in the persistence behavior of chronic low back pain patients with repeated acute pain stimulation. *Pain* 1987;30:329–337.
61. Cohen MJ, Naliboff BD, Schandler SL, Heinrich RL. Signal detection and threshold measurement to loud tones and radiant heat in chronic low back pain patients and cohort controls. *Pain* 1983;6:245–252.
62. Lipman JJ, Blumenkopf B, Parris WCV. Chronic pain assessment using heat beam dolorimetry. *Pain* 1987;30:59–67.
63. Malow RM, Olson RE. Changes in pain perception after treatment for chronic pain. *Pain* 1981;11:65–72.
64. Naliboff BD, Cohen MJ, Schandler SL, Heinrich RL. Signal detection and threshold measurement for chronic back pain patients, chronic illness patients and cohort controls to radiant heat stimuli. *J Abnorm Psychol* 1981;90:271–274.
65. Schmidt AJM, Brands AEF. Performance level of chronic low back pain patients in an acute pain situation. *J Psychosom Res* 1985;30:339–346.
66. Wolskee PJ, Gracely RH. Effect of chronic pain on experimental pain response. *Am Pain Soc Abstr* 1980;2:4.
67. Yang JC, Richlin D, Brand L, Wagner J, Clark C. Thermal sensory decision theory indices and pain threshold in chronic pain patients and healthy volunteers. *Psychosom Med* 1985;47:461–468.
68. Chapman CR. Sensory decision theory methods in pain research: a reply to Rollman. *Pain* 1977;3:295–305.
69. Clark WC, Yang JC. Applications of Sensory Decision Theory to problems in laboratory and clinical pain. In: Melzack R, ed. *Pain measurement and assessment.* New York: Raven Press, 1983.
70. Coppola R, Gracely RH. Where is the noise in SDT pain assessment? *Pain* 1983;17:257–266.
71. Rollman GB. Signal detection theory measurement of pain: a review and critique. *Pain* 1977;3:187–211.
72. Gracely RH, Wolskee PJ. Semantic functional measurement of pain: integrating perception and language. *Pain* 1983;15:389–398.
73. Gracely RH. Methods of testing pain mechanisms in normal man. In: Wall PD, Melzack R, eds. *Textbook of pain.* London: Churchill Livingstone, 1989;257–268.
74. Chapman CR, Casey KL, Dubner R, Foley KM, Gracely RH, Reading AE. Pain measurement: an overview. *Pain* 1985;22:1–31.
75. Gracely RH. Pain measurement in man. In: Ng L, Bonica JJ, eds. *Pain, discomfort and humanitarian care.* New York: Elsevier, 1980;111–137.
76. Gracely RH. Pain psychophysics. In: Manuk S, ed. *Advances in behavioral medicine,* vol 1. New York: JAI Press, 1985.
77. Procacci P, Zoppi M, Maresca M. Experimental pain in man. *Pain* 1979;6:123–140.
78. Wolff BB. Methods of testing pain mechanisms in normal man. In: Wall PD, Melzack R, eds. *Textbook of pain.* London: Churchill Livingstone, 1984.
79. Thurstone LI. *The measurement of values.* Chicago: University of Chicago Press, 1959.
80. Algolm D, Raphaeli N, Cohen-Raz L. Integration of noxious stimulation across separate somatosensory systems: a functional theory of pain. *J Exp Psychol [Hum Percept]* 1986;12:92–102.
81. Jones B. Algebraic models for integration of painful and nonpainful electric shocks. *Percept Psychophys* 1980;28:572–576.
82. Cornsweet TN. The staircase-method in psychophysics. *Am J Psychol* 1962;75:485–491.
83. Jones SF, McQuay HJ, Noore RA, Hand CW. Morphine and ibuprofen compared using the cold pressor test. *Pain* 1988;34:117–122.
84. Maurset A, Skoglund LA, Hustveit O, Oye I. Comparison of ketamine and pethidine in experimental and postoperative pain. *Pain* 1989;36:37–41.
85. Posner J, Telekes A, Crowley D, Phillipson R, Peck AW. Effects of an opiate on cold-induced pain and the CNS in healthy volunteers. *Pain* 1985;23:73–82.
86. Wolskee PJ, Gracely RH, Dorros CM, Schilling RM, Taylor F. Fentanyl reduces thermal pain

intensity: effect of stimulus range on response method. *Am Pain Soc Abstr* 1983;4:74.
87. Gracely RH, Gaughan AM, Meister BM, Dionne RA, Hargreaves KM, Dubner R. Staircase assessment of opiate analgesia time-course: effect of infusion rate and naloxone antagonism. *Abstr Am Canad Pain Soc* 1988;SS-5d.
88. Wolskee PJ, Gracely RH, Greenberg RP, Dubner R, Lees D. Comparison of effects of morphine and deep brain stimulation on chronic pain. *Am Pain Soc Abstr* 1982;3:36.
89. Price DD, von der Gruen A, Miller J, Rafii A, Price C. Potentiation of systemic morphine analgesia in humans by proglumide, a cholecystokinin antagonist. *Anesth Analg* 1985;64:801–806.
90. Gracely RH, Gaughan AM. Staircase assessment of simulated opiate potentiation. *Pain* 1990;(Suppl 5):S482.
91. Wolf BB, Kantor TG, Jarvik ME, Laska E. Response of experimental pain to analgesic drugs. III. Codeine, aspirin, secobarbital and placebo. *Clin Pharmacol Ther* 1969;10:217–228.
92. Garcia de Jalon PD, Harrison FJJ, Johnson KI, Kozma C, Schnelle K. A modified cold stimulation technique for the evaluation of analgesic activity in human volunteers. *Pain* 1985;22:183–189.
93. Posner J. A modified submaximal effort tourniquet test for evaluation of analgesics in healthy volunteers. *Pain* 1984;19:143–151.
94. Forster C, Anton F, Reeh PW, Weber E, Handwerker HO. Measurement of the analgesic effects of aspirin with a new experimental algesimetric procedure. *Pain* 1988;32:215–222.
95. Telekes A, Holland RL, Peck AW. Indomethacin: effects on cold-induced pain and the nervous system in healthy volunteers. *Pain* 1987;30:321–328.
96. Smith GM, Beecher HK. Experimental production of pain in man sensitivity of a new method to 600 mg of aspirin. *Clin Pharmacol Ther* 1969;10:213–216.
97. Chen ACN, Chapman CR. Aspirin analgesia evaluated by event-related potentials in man: possible central action in brain. *Exp Brain Res* 1980;39:359–364.
98. Rohdewald P, Derendorf H, Drehsen G, Elgar CE, Knoll O. Changes in cortical evoked potentials as correlates of the efficacy of weak analgesics. *Pain* 1982;12:329–341.
99. Willer JC, De Borucker T, Bussel B, Roby-Brami A, Harrewyn JM. Central analgesic effect of ketoprofen in humans: electrophysiological evidence for a supraspinal mechanism in a double-blind cross-over study. *Pain* 1989;38:1–7.
100. Bromm B, Meier W, Scharein E. Imipramine reduces experimental pain. *Pain* 1986;25:245–257.
101. Max MB, Culnane M, Schafer SC, Gracely RH, Walther DJ, Smoller B, Dubner R. Amitriptyline relieves diabetic neuropathy pain in patients with normal or depressed mood. *Neurology* 1987;37:589–596.
102. Sharav Y, Singer E, Schmidt E, Dionne RA, Dubner R. The analgesic effect of amitriptyline on chronic facial pain. *Pain* 1987;31:199–209.
103. Gracely RH, Wolskee PJ, Deeter WR, Dubner R. Differential effects of fentanyl and diazepam on pain sensation and psychophysical performance. *Soc Neurosci Abstr* 1981;7:340.
104. Heft MW, Parker SR. An experimental basis for revising the graphic rating scale. *Pain* 1984;19:153–161.
105. Dundee JW, Moore J. Alteration in response to somatic pain associated with anaesthesia. IV: The effect of sub-anaesthetic concentrations of inhalation agents. *Br J Anaesth* 1960;32:453–459.
106. Chapman WP, Arrowood JG, Beecher HK. The analgetic effects of low concentrations of nitrous oxide compared in man with morphine sulfate. *J Clin Invest* 1943;22:871–875.
107. Yang JC, Clark WC, Ngai SH. Antagonism of nitrous oxide analgesia by naloxone in man. *Anesthesiology* 1980;52:414–417.
108. Benedetti C, Chapman CR, Colpitts YH, Chen AC. Effect of nitrous oxide concentration on event-related potentials during painful tooth stimulation. *Anesthesiology* 1982;56:360–364.
109. Chapman CR, Benedetti C. Nitrous oxide effects on cerebral evoked potentials to pain. *Anesthesiology* 1979;51:135–138.
110. Dworkin SF, Chen ACN, Schubert MM, Clark DW. Cognitive modification of pain: information in combination with N_2O. *Pain* 1984;19:339–351.
111. Dworkin SF, Chen ACN, LeResche L, Clark DW. Cognitive reversal of expected nitrous oxide analgesia for acute pain. *Anesth Analg* 1983;62:1073–1077.

112. Heft MW, Gracely RH, Dubner R. Nitrous oxide analgesia: a psychophysical evaluation using verbal descriptor scaling. *J Dent Res* 1984;63:129–132.
113. Parducci A. Contextual effects: a range-frequency analysis. In: Carterette EC, Friedman MP, eds. *Handbook of perception,* vol 2. New York: Academic Press, 1974;127–141.
114. Poulton EC. Models for biases in judging sensory magnitude. *Psychol Bull* 1979;86:777–803.
115. Gracely RH, Dubner R. Reliability and validity of verbal descriptor scales of painfulness. *Pain* 1987;29:175–185.

Advances in Pain Research and Therapy, Vol. 18,
edited by M. Max, R. Portenoy, and E. Laska,
Raven Press, Ltd., New York © 1991.

Commentary

Experimental Pain Models and Analgesic Efficacy

C. Richard Chapman

*Pain and Toxicity Program, Division of Clinical Research, Fred Hutchinson Cancer
Research Center, Seattle, Washington 98104; and Department of Anesthesiology,
Department of Psychiatry and Behavioral Sciences, University of Washington
School of Medicine, Seattle, Washington 98195*

Richard H. Gracely briefly described the history of experimental pain models
and discussed several issues that surround their use in the evaluation of analgesic
efficacy. He also addressed the seemingly poor fit of human laboratory research
using experimental pain models to clinical analgesia and explained why these
difficulties have occurred. Finally, Dr. Gracely explored the utility of experimental
pain models and provided an overview of current experimental pain paradigms.
I comment here on two aspects of his discourse: (a) Why human studies of
experimental analgesia have proven difficult historically; and (b) The nature and
potential value of such models for future research.

ON THE APPARENT LIMITATIONS
OF EXPERIMENTAL ANALGESIA

Dr. Gracely has accurately described the difficult evolution of human models
for experimental research on analgesic states. He identified a methodologic
shortcoming in early research as the principal reason for the failure of early
studies to match clinical observations of analgesic states: investigators used
threshold rather than suprathreshold stimulus intensities. I agree that the problem
has been methodologic and that the use of the pain threshold as an effect variable
has impaired progress, but I would emphasize the importance of weak pharmacologic control in early human laboratory research. Early investigators and
many contemporary researchers have failed to appreciate the complex nature
of pharmacologic analgesic states and to control them rigorously.

Opioid analgesia research provides an excellent example because we have a
good understanding of opioid analgesic mechanisms. Opioids modulate the centripedal transmission of nociception when they bind to selective receptors in the

central nervous system and initiate inhibitory processes. We can introduce carefully controlled doses of these drugs to systemic circulation, but their effects on the brain are not always straightforward. The physiochemical characteristics of a given drug determine the rate and extent to which the drug crosses the blood-brain barrier, binds to opioid receptors, and the rate at which it washes out of the brain. Speaking broadly, many lipophilic drugs tend to enter and leave the central nervous system readily, and apart from the occulting effects of hysteresis, one can typically demonstrate a relationship between plasma concentration and the effect on the brain. Hydrophilic opioids, however, show a weak apparent relationship between rapidly changing plasma concentration following intravenous bolus administration and the drug's effects on the brain.

There are also marked pharmacokinetic differences between experimental subjects. People differ in how they distribute and eliminate drugs introduced to systemic circulation. The practical effect of such differences in experimental analgesia studies of opioids is a confounding of the experimenter's control over standardized drug dosage. When drugs are administered in fixed amounts on the basis of body weight alone, pharmacokinetic variability will ensure that some subjects receive much more drug at central nervous system sites than others. This adds variability to estimates of dose-effect relationships.

One can see the value of pharmacokinetic control over drug administration from data that Hill et al. (1,2) previously published. I limit my description to morphine, since most of the early research on experimental analgesia involved this drug.

We gave human subjects intravenous boluses of morphine so that we could assess them pharmacokinetically. From plasma samples obtained after the morphine bolus, we estimated the pharmacokinetic parameters of each individual. Using this information, we designed a morphine infusion test session so that we might evaluate analgesic states when pharmacokinetic differences were removed. We initiated morphine administration by giving a loading bolus of drug and sustained a stable plasma concentration by subsequent infusion at an exponentially declining rate. Loading bolus size and rate of infusion were individually derived from each subject's pharmacokinetics.

With this procedure, we successfully predicted and achieved a steady state plasma concentration of drug during the laboratory infusion session. Moreover, we could increase plasma concentrations and hold them by repeating the process. This control allowed us to minimize variability in concentration of morphine in the brain over time. The effects of individual pharmacokinetic differences on analgesic states were largely removed.

In a study of 15 volunteers (2), we investigated the analgesic effects of morphine at four plasma concentrations: 0, 25, 50, and 100 ng/ml. In these nontolerant subjects, the effects associated with these plasma concentrations ranged from minimal analgesic effect to slight depression of ventilatory drive. We used electrical stimulation of tooth pulp to induce experimental pain and measured both the subjective report of pain intensity and the brain evoked potential.

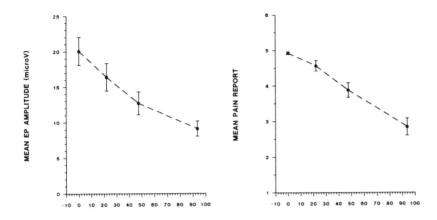

FIG. 1. A: Mean changes in the amplitude of the dental evoked potential (EP) during individually fitted, stepwise, steady-state infusions of morphine in 15 subjects. *Vertical bars* indicate standard errors of the means. **B:** Mean changes in pain report (±SE) obtained at the same time. These findings were previously reported by Hill et al. (2).

Figure 1 depicts the mean results. Both evoked potential and pain report showed unequivocal mean concentration–effect relationships. We included a sham increase in plasma concentration as a control (not shown), but no placebo effects occurred. These findings demonstrate clearly that strong control of pharmacologic parameters yields unambiguous analgesic results in the human studies laboratory. Moreover, the degree of analgesia we observed with morphine in laboratory volunteers accords well with the results we obtain in the clinic with bone marrow transplant patients who require morphine for the control of severe oral mucositis pain (3).

Clearly, the assessment of analgesic states in the human studies laboratory is not a simple undertaking. Precise control over drug action is time consuming, costly, and technically demanding. In return for our trouble, however, we are able to attain far greater control and precision than one observes in conventional animal laboratory or human clinical research.

THE ROLE OF HUMAN EXPERIMENTATION IN FUTURE RESEARCH ON ANALGESIC STATES

Dr. Gracely has argued that experimental methods offer a "correlative analogue" of clinical pain syndromes. I think it is important to further clarify the nature of the analogy between the experimental context and clinical intervention for pain.

As Dr. Gracely has noted, experimental methodology falls short of providing us with a miniaturization of clinical pain. Indeed, there are many manifestations of clinical pain, and experimental paradigms could never hope to represent all or even most clinical pain states.

The value of experimental methodology depends, I believe, entirely upon theory. Our experimental efforts are meaningful only so long as strong, clearly articulated theory permits us to make definitive predictions about the effects of analgesic interventions. Theory provides the bridge between clinical phenomena and patient care; without it, the laboratory researcher is simply fishing for parallel outcomes that may or may not be a clue to some relationship between the two arenas of research. In the case of opioid analgesia, we have a strong theoretical understanding of how opioids work within the central nervous system to modulate the centripedal transmission of nociceptive information. On the basis of this information and pharmacokinetic theory that accounts for the distribution and elimination of such drugs, we can predict experimental phenomena rather well. Moreover, we can draw upon theory confirming or extending data from animal research arenas and validate the clinical potential of such findings via work in the human environment.

It follows that two important roles of the human subjects laboratory are (a) the validation or refinement of theoretical principles, and (b) the replication of findings obtained in basic research with animals. The latter is important because some phenomena are species-specific, and dose ranges may vary markedly between animal and human subjects. The human studies laboratory provides a staging environment in which new developments in basic research can be translated and refined for human clinical testing.

Furthermore, the human studies laboratory provides an opportunity for technologic development and refinement. For example, our research team has conceptualized, constructed, and evaluated a computer-based system for the delivery of pharmacokinetically tailored opioid infusions. After demonstrating a high degree of control and accuracy in human subject experimentation, we were able to take this immediately to clinical trial (see Chapter 23). Drug delivery technology as well as specific drugs and dosing schedules can thus be tested in a human subjects environment, facilitating clinical application and minimizing the research burden of trial and error work with patients.

Figure 2 depicts an idealized relationship between animal laboratory, human laboratory, and human clinical research. The animal research environment introduces new phenomena and provides a theoretical framework to the human studies laboratory. Human laboratory researchers, however, are also influenced by the clinical arena. Clinical problems define and prioritize the research goals of the human laboratory investigator and give both direction and focus to his or her work. In turn, human laboratory work feeds backward to the animal research environment, providing feedback about the applicability of phenomena and theoretical refinements to human pain control. It feeds forward to the human clinical environment through its validation and refinement of phenomena from basic research, its definition of dose ranges and analgesia to side effect ratios, and its technical innovation.

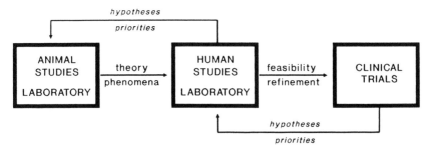

FIG. 2. Relationship of the human studies laboratory to the basic science laboratory and clinical research.

CONCLUSIONS

The future for experimental human laboratory research on analgesic states is bright. Technologic advances have provided us with greater control over experimental parameters than earlier researchers could achieve. More importantly, theory on analgesic mechanisms has matured sufficiently to provide us with clear guidelines for research in pharmacologic areas. The issue of whether experimental pain really represents clinical syndromes is no longer relevant.

There are still significant areas of difficulty for human researchers. As Gary W. Donaldson and I have emphasized in Chapter 32, nonpharmacologic interventions are extremely difficult to investigate in either clinical or laboratory settings. We are unable to achieve control overdosing and, in most cases, even to conceptualize what gradation of treatment means. In some cases, we lack sufficient theory to make strong predictions about experimental outcomes. In these areas, human laboratory investigators must await further technical and theoretical development before they can project major contributions.

REFERENCES

1. Hill HF, Saeger L, Bjurstrom R, et al. Steady-state infusions of opioids in human: I. Pharmacokinetic tailoring. *Pain,* in press.
2. Hill HF, Chapman CR, Saeger LS, Bjurstrom R, Walter MH, Kippes M. Steady-state infusions of opioids in human: II. Concentration-effect relationships and therapeutic margins. *Pain,* in press.
3. Hill HF, Chapman CR, Kornell J, Sullivan K, Saeger L, Benedetti C. Self-administration of morphine in bone marrow transplant patients reduces drug requirement. *Pain* 1990;40:121–129.

Advances in Pain Research and Therapy, Vol. 18,
edited by M. Max, R. Portenoy, and E. Laska,
Raven Press, Ltd., New York © 1991.

4

Single-Dose Analgesic Comparisons

Mitchell B. Max* and Eugene M. Laska**

*Clinical Trials Unit, Neurobiology and Anesthesiology Branch, National Institute of
Dental Research, National Institutes of Health, Bethesda, Maryland 20892;
**Statistical Sciences and Epidemiology Division, Nathan S. Kline Institute for
Psychiatric Research, Orangeburg, New York 10962; and Department of Psychiatry,
New York University Medical Center, New York, New York 10016

Single-dose analgesic comparisons are the most common designs used in the investigation of new analgesics and have provided much of our knowledge about the drugs used in practice. In these approaches, patients rate pain or relief for several hours following a randomly assigned dose of test drug, standard analgesic, or placebo. Although single-dose comparisons have obvious limitations in guiding chronic treatment, they do indicate if a test medication is active and can reveal many of the clinical properties of a new analgesic in comparison to a standard.

This chapter reviews general issues in designing and analyzing a single-dose analgesic comparison that an investigator should consider and address in the study protocol. These include (a) the purpose of the study, (b) the type of patients to be studied, (c) the primary measures of efficacy and safety, (d) the mechanics of study execution, (e) the choice of treatments and doses, (f) the experimental design, and (g) some comments on analyzing the data.

For further reading on these topics, the reader is referred to classic reviews of analgesic clinical trials methods written by Houde, Wallenstein, Beaver, and Lasagna (1–5), and to several excellent reviews (6,7) and multiauthor volumes (8,9) that elucidate the conceptual foundations of pain assessment and the variety of assessment methods. Texts on clinical trial design (10–13) and statistical methods (14–16) are also recommended.

PURPOSE OF STUDY

In the discussion that follows, it is assumed that the compound to be studied has completed Phase I toxicity studies and single-blind dose-ranging observations for analgesic efficacy (Chapter 2) that have established the doses likely to produce analgesia and toxicity, the nature of the common side effects, and the profiles of absorption, distribution, and elimination.

Naturally, a design should be tailored to the specific question being addressed and the audience that will assess the results. Studies intended to satisfy regulatory authorities may focus on demonstrating that the drug is safe and unequivocally effective relative to a placebo or standard. Other studies may be intended to guide the prescribing clinician in a particular clinical situation, and may provide comparisons with the common clinical alternatives. A full program of research should attempt to elucidate the range of response among individuals: Which patients will respond and with what probability? Among those who respond, how long will it take to obtain pain relief, and how much time will elapse before they require remediation? It will be useful to have an estimate of the drug's efficacy relative to a standard. A clinician would like to know the conditions under which there are advantages or disadvantages in efficacy or toxicity compared to optimal doses of the standard. Still other studies (see Chapter 25) may be primarily designed to address a more basic scientific principle and audience, e.g., "Can the pharmacological release of pituitary beta-endorphin relieve pain?"

TYPE OF PATIENTS TO BE STUDIED

Type of Pain

In the evaluation of new analgesics, a variety of patient populations have been studied. Patients with acute pain following major surgery and those with chronic cancer pain are appropriate for evaluating the higher dose ranges of potent analgesics. Patients with pain following minor surgery, oral surgery, mild trauma, sore throat, and childbirth are suitable for evaluating weaker agents, although in each of these groups there may be a considerable range of pain severity. Selection of the appropriate groups for study will be narrowed by the route of administration of the test drug, and by patient availability. Specific advantages and limitations of particular patient populations are discussed in detail in Part II of this volume.

In the 30 years since Beecher asserted that in assessing analgesics in man, "neither source of pain nor type (acute or chronic) are important considerations" (17), research has revealed distinctions among types of pain with differing sensitivities to different analgesics. Pain caused by peripheral nerve damage or infiltration, for example, often responds poorly to opiates or aspirin-like compounds (18,19), whereas dysmenorrhea, acute inflammatory pain, and malignant bony pain respond particularly well to the nonsteroidal antiinflammatory drugs (NSAIDs). Therefore, the pathophysiology of the patient's pain must be considered in defining study entry criteria.

In choosing whether to limit enrollment to a narrow group of patients (for example, patients undergoing hysterectomy), or a wider variety of patients (any postoperative inpatient with severe pain), the investigator faces some tradeoffs. In a narrowly defined patient group, the variation in factors that can influence the patient's pain and relief is reduced. A more homogeneous population has the potential for reducing the error variance and the sample size needed to detect treatment differences. For example, in a study limited to hysterectomy patients, patients will have less variation in age and medical condition, anesthetic techniques and drugs, associated discomforts such as nausea or distention, and adjunctive treatments for these symptoms. Patients are also likely to be in the same wards, with less variety in the daily care routines that can exacerbate pain. Moreover, when the investigators interact repeatedly with a relatively small group of clinicians caring for the patients, the primary caregivers will usually assist to further standardize these variables. A narrowly defined patient group is particularly important when the purpose of the study is to address a particular biological principle of pain relief (20). For example, if one wished to determine whether kappa-receptor opiate agonists interact with visceral afferent input, one might limit a study to patients with tumor involving intraperitoneal structures, ruling out those with uncertain or mixed origin of pain.

On the other hand, in some investigations it may be more appropriate to include a broader range of patients, for example, patients with pain following a mixed group of surgical procedures. If the variance is not greatly increased by such a strategy, it may be possible to complete studies more rapidly. Studies using a wider pool of patients have several other potential advantages. New analgesic agents may affect one type of pain better than others, and inclusion of a broader spectrum of patients may allow a retrospective exploration of which classes of pain tend to respond more favorably. For application to clinical practice, a conclusion based on experience with a broad range of patients may be more convincing than one based on a single homogeneous subset of patients.

MEASURES OF EFFICACY AND TOXICITY

Measures of Efficacy

Desirable qualities for pain measures used in clinical analgesic trials include the following:

1. *Ease in use by ill patients.* Simplicity and speed of completion are crucial in the patient with acute postoperative pain, for example, who may be distracted by pain, fatigue, anxiety, or nausea. If asked to complete a pain assessment measure that takes several minutes of concentration, the patient may become upset or not attend to the measure, increasing the variability in the study and the likelihood that the patient will drop out.

2. *Sensitivity sufficient to detect differences among treatments.* Sensitivity relates to the ability of the scale to distinguish, with reasonable probability for

reasonable sample sizes, treatments known to be different, e.g., a standard analgesic from placebo, or a high from a low dose of a standard analgesic.

3. *Clarity for the clinicians who will use the analgesic.* The scales used should permit the ascertainment of practical dimensions of analgesia such as speed of onset and duration, and global patient satisfaction.

Most investigators agree that standard subjective measures based on category and visual analogue scales (VAS) meet the above criteria reasonably well (21). Examples of these measures are illustrated in Fig. 1. Many more complex pain measures have been developed for use in psychophysical studies and chronic pain diagnosis and management (6–9), but are infrequently used in acute pain studies.

Pain Intensity Category Scale

The oldest of the standard measures is the four-point pain intensity category scale. Although this measure is still the most widely used scale, it has been criticized on several counts. Patients have indicated that a four-point pain intensity scale does not have enough levels to allow them to accurately describe their pain level. For example, a patient in whom an analgesic reduces pain from "greater than severe" to "below severe, but well above moderate" must choose

Pain Intensity Category Scale (4-point)		Pain Relief Category Scale (5-point)	
Severe	3	Complete	4
Moderate	2	Lots	3
Mild	1	Moderate	2
None	0	Slight	1
		None	0

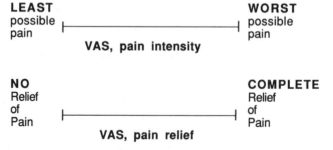

FIG. 1. Examples of standard category and visual analogue scales (VAS) used to assess pain and pain relief in analgesic studies. (Adapted from ref. 21, with permission.)

"severe" each time, an approximation that might greatly reduce the measure's sensitivity in detecting an effective analgesic.

A second common criticism has been that numerical scores for the categories are arbitrarily set to equal step integers, without evidence that the levels of pain to which they correspond are spaced apart an equal number of "discernible difference units." Lasagna (22) suggests that there is a greater difference for patients between severe and moderate pain than between moderate and slight, or slight and none. Such inaccurate assignment of numerical equivalent scores could reduce the sensitivity of an analgesic assay, he argued. In efforts to remedy the two purported shortcomings of the four-point pain intensity category scale, Gracely et al. (23) and Tursky (24) have developed longer lists of pain descriptors, with numerical equivalents determined by cross-modality matching techniques, but there are as yet no data showing either of these scales superior to the four-point scale in detecting analgesia. Wallenstein et al. (25) compared the ratings of 257 patients using the category pain scale to the VAS pain scale (see below) and found that the four categories were not far from equal spacing (Fig. 2). Laska et al. (26,27) have developed two techniques for assigning scores to categorical values on the basis of the dose-response curve, which are briefly described in Chapter 29.

Relief Category Scale

Unlike pain intensity measures, which focus on the present experience, relief scales rely on the patient's memory of pain at the baseline period. This rarely

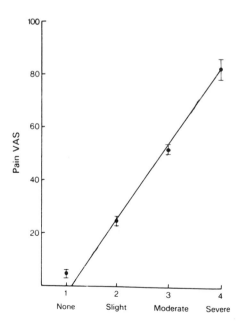

FIG. 2. Relationship of pain category scale to VAS pain ratings made by 264 patients in analgesic studies. The four categories are spaced in a roughly even manner, although the spacing between "none" and "slight" pain is somewhat smaller than the other two intervals. (From ref. 25, with permission.)

presents difficulty in a 4 to 6 hr single-dose study, but may reduce reliability of relief data in longer or more complex studies. Compared to the pain intensity category scale, relief category scales have been reported to be more sensitive to small reductions in pain. Littman et al. (28) examined reports of over one thousand patients at baseline and 1 hr after receiving the opiate dezocine or a control. In 31% of 157 patients whose pain intensity category remained unchanged at "moderate," the relief category scale detected a change: "a little" relief in 19%, "moderate" relief in 11%, and "a lot" of relief in 1%. As with the pain intensity category scale, Wallenstein (29) has found the relief categories to be rather evenly spaced, relative to their equivalent VAS ratings (Fig. 3).

Fifty Percent Relief Measure

Following Beecher's lead, early analgesic investigators asked patients whether pain was "at least 50% relieved," and used the number of hours during which they reported such relief as an indicator of analgesia. This measure, which is highly correlated with other standard measures (Chapter 15) but reduces the available information for no valid reason, is falling out of use.

Visual Analogue Scale (VAS) Pain

A visual analogue scale is a line whose ends are labeled with descriptors of the extremes of a subjective category, e.g. "least possible pain" and "worst possible pain" (Fig. 1). The patient is asked to mark the line at a point corresponding to his present pain level. Visual analogue pain scales, introduced into pain mea-

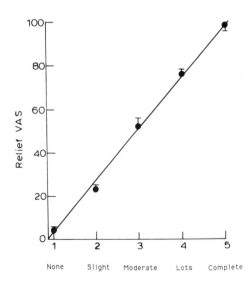

FIG. 3. Relationship of pain relief category scale to pain relief VAS ratings. (From ref. 29, with permission.)

surement in the 1970s (30,31), share the simplicity and brevity offered by category scales, and offer several potential advantages. Because visual analogue scales are continuous, they may avoid the serious boundary error of category scales. Based on a series of studies in subjects with experimentally induced and chronic pain (32), Price (7) suggested that visual analogue scales are relatively free of some of the biases that may complicate category scales, e.g., the tendency of patients to try to use as much of the range of words as possible. It has been suggested that the most "bias-free" VAS scales may be those that are between 10 and 15 cm in length (7), and are anchored by words delineating extremes (e.g., the least possible pain, the worst possible pain). Horizontal lines may produce more reliable results than vertical lines (33). Several authors have mentioned that occasionally, patients have more difficulty understanding VAS scales than category scales (28,34), but this can usually be prevented by careful instructions by the nurse observer.

Visual Analogue Scale, Relief

VAS measures have also been used to assess relief, but only a minority of investigators use them routinely (35). Like the category relief scale, the relief VAS serves to expand the part of the scale corresponding to slight relief, potentially increasing the sensitivity over that offered by the pain VAS. (See also Commentary by Wallenstein following this chapter.)

Using Serial Pain Measures to Approximate an Analgesic's Time-Effect Curve

In order to compare analgesics, investigators use serial measures of pain and relief, as described above, to estimate the time course and magnitude of analgesia. Figure 4 (top) shows the hypothetical time course of pain relief that a patient might describe if relief could somehow be continuously assessed. The actual interview points and relief readings on a visual analogue scale are represented by the open circles; in most analgesic studies, measurements are taken hourly, and more frequently in the first hour, e.g., an initial reading at 30 min. In this example, the patient experienced "meaningful relief" well before the first observation. Data collected at only the scheduled interview points might not distinguish a drug of rapid onset from one of slower onset, an important distinction for the patient. Some patients never have onset of relief with a particular drug and dose.

Laska et al. (36) and Siegel et al. (37) have suggested that in order to characterize the effects of a specified dose of an analgesic, the following information is needed: (a) the probability of relief occurring at all; (b) in those patients that have meaningful relief, the distribution of times of onset; (c) the magnitude of relief while the drug is working, including the peak relief obtained; (d) the probability that

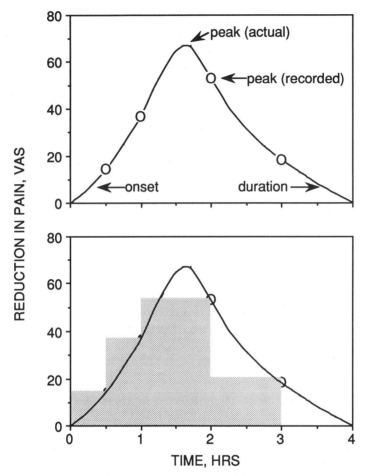

FIG. 4. Approximating the analgesic time-effect curve with intermittent pain and relief measures. Reduction in pain is plotted against time elapsed since administration of study medication. *Open circles* correspond to the patient's pain assessment at scheduled interviews. Onset and duration of meaningful analgesia are indicated by *arrows* (*top panel*); in this example, onset occurs well before the first scheduled interview. The area under this hypothetical curve (*bottom panel, shaded*) is often approximated by the sum of the products of each pain relief reading at a scheduled interview and the time since the previous interview.

pain relief will end, often defined by request for remedication, before the end of the observation period; and (e) the distribution of times of offset of analgesic effect. (We will use the term "duration of effect" to mean the time from onset of meaningful relief to the time of offset; that is, the moment at which the patient no longer experiences meaningful relief [36–38]).

Measures Derived From Category and VAS Scales

Historically, analgesic investigators have focused on the third of the above dimensions, the magnitude of analgesia, using several measures calculated from scores obtained using category and VAS scales. To account for differences in baseline pain intensity among patients in the study, pain intensity category scores and VAS scores are converted into "pain intensity difference (PID)" scores by subtracting them from the pain score taken at baseline. Positive scores indicate reduction in pain, making the PID scores analogous to relief scores. (An alternative method is to use analysis of covariance.) PID or relief scores are commonly summed over the observation period, weighted for the time between observations, and the summed scores respectively termed SPID (summed pain intensity differences) or TOTPAR (total pain relief). These summary variables are estimates of the area under the time-effect curve (AUC), as illustrated in Fig. 4 (bottom). Let P_t denote the pain intensity and R_t the relief at time t. Expressed algebraically:

$$PID_t = P_t - P_0;$$

$$SPID = \sum PID_t \times [\text{time (hrs) elapsed since previous observation}]$$

$$TOTPAR = \sum R_t \times [\text{time (hrs) elapsed since previous observation}]$$

Some investigators compute "% SPID," defined as SPID/maximum possible SPID. The latter is the value of SPID that would be obtained if the patient was pain-free for the total period of observation. This adjustment may partly correct for the tendency for SPID scores to be higher in patients with greater initial pain (39,40).

In comparing treatment effects, investigators use:

1. *Hourly scores.* A graph of the primary pain or relief measure over time is a standard part of an analgesic study report. It is also useful to display the actual number of subjects that are available for the comparison, because dropout rates can affect the interpretation of the estimates. For patients who drop out before a trial is over, many investigators carry the last observation forward or assign the baseline level of pain intensity and no pain relief to the rest of the observations (see p. 88). This approach should be used with caution, as erroneous inferences can result if the dropout rate is high.

2. *Peak PID or relief scores for each patient.* This is a particularly relevant measure if one is focusing on treating severe pain in the "resistant" patient. Demonstrating differences between drugs using peak scores has often required a large sample size, however (41).

3. *SPID or TOTPAR scores.* These AUC measures have been widely used because they are relatively sensitive, often showing statistically significant differences between graded doses of an analgesic when peak scores or a scores from a single hour do not (35). However, SPID and TOTPAR scores, like any AUC measures, confound onset and duration of analgesic effect with magnitude. A

short-acting, highly effective drug cannot be distinguished from a long-acting, marginally effective drug.

Comparison of Various Measures Derived from Category and VAS Scales

Littman et al. (28) compared the pain intensity category, relief category, and pain intensity VAS scales in 20 clinical trials in 1,497 patients receiving the opiate agonist-antagonist dezocine, standard opiate analgesics, and placebo. For AUC scores as well as scores 1 hr after drug (usually corresponding to peak relief), the relief category scale was consistently the most sensitive to treatment differences, the VAS pain scale of intermediate sensitivity, and the pain category scale the least sensitive. These differences were not marked, however; the three scales gave the same overall conclusions in 17 of 20 studies.

The relief category scale was also favored in a survey of experienced analgesic researchers in which 9 of 13 ranked the summed relief category score (TOTPAR) as the "most important derived variable" in assessing analgesic effect (35). Wallenstein et al. (25, and Commentary following this chapter) suggested that the VAS relief scale was yet more sensitive than the category relief scale, but consensus has not been reached regarding whether this scale should be more widely used.

Other Measurements that Guide Clinicians in Using Treatments

Measures of Pain Onset and Duration

In order to prescribe a drug effectively, the clinician must be aware of several of the other "dimensions of analgesia" listed above—the distribution of times of onset and duration of analgesia among individual patients. In older studies, where onset measures were not directly taken, onset may have been missed because the first postdrug observation was usually 30 to 60 min after administration. Information on duration of analgesia has rarely been obtained for the shorter-acting drugs, although some investigators have reported "time to remedication" as a surrogate indicator. The latter measure may exaggerate duration of effective analgesia because the patient may feel that he should "hold out" as long as possible before asking for remedication, and even after the patient decides to request remedication, the nurse may not be immediately available.

Siegel et al. (37) and Laska et al. (38) have introduced two methods to directly measure onset and offset of analgesia. Initially they asked patients who reported relief at a regularly scheduled observation to estimate how long ago relief began. More recently they have given each patient two stopwatches that are started at the time of medication. The patient is instructed to stop the "onset" stopwatch as soon as he feels "meaningful pain relief," and to stop the "offset" watch as soon as "the medication is not giving meaningful relief." These data may be used to provide estimates of the probability of obtaining an effect and, for patients who obtain an effect, the distribution of time to onset and the probability of needing remediation, and if so, the distribution of time to remediation. Methods for analyzing onset and duration data are discussed in Chapter 32.

Global Ratings

Many investigators ask patients for global reports of satisfaction with the analgesic, e.g., poor, fair, good, excellent (42). In a crossover study, patients may be asked which drug they preferred, and why. In the case of drugs that are powerful analgesics but produce unpleasant side effects, the patient's global assessment regarding the balance of effects may be a valuable guide for choosing treatments in a clinical setting.

The Multiple-Scale Problem

In their focus on assessing magnitude of analgesia, investigators have traditionally used a number of different scales looking at this dimension in each study. A typical trial may report data from the pain intensity category and VAS relief category, and perhaps several additional scales of interest to the investigator. These are looking at the same dimension of analgesia, and have been shown by all reviewers to be highly correlated with one another (2,28,29, and Chapter 15). Such use of redundant scales may needlessly introduce problems, particularly when the resulting statistical conclusions differ to some degree among the scales.

One solution commonly advocated in textbooks on clinical trials is to choose primary measures for the outcomes in question before the experiment starts (13,43), designating the others as secondary outcome measures. For analgesic studies, one might select one primary measure for each of the dimensions of pain relief discussed above—probability and time of onset, magnitude of relief (peak or summed scores), and probability and time of remediation. In view of the limited amount of data comparing the scales, investigators accustomed to using a number of measures of relief magnitude might feel uncomfortable with the arbitrary choice of one measure. An alternative solution is to continue to use multiple scales that measure more or less the same dimension of analgesia, and incorporate the data in multivariate analyses such as multivariate analyses of variance and multivariate bioassay methods to determine relative potency (44,45, and Chapter 30).

It is necessary to add that although univariate statistical comparisons of each hourly score are commonly performed, one must be leery of the so-called multiplicity problem; that is, performing many statistical tests, some of which will be significant merely by chance. Also, if there are many treatments or many measures of effect in the trial, the multivariate nature of the multiple comparisons must be considered. This can make finding true differences difficult.

Measures of Adverse Effects

The quantitative assessment of common adverse effects during single-dose studies in patients is likely to become an important area for innovation during the next decade. This is because common analgesic side effects, particularly those of the opiates, often prevent effective analgesic dosing, may increase morbidity, and limit patients' activities. As more is learned about the receptors, neurotransmitters, and other physiological mechanisms responsible for these effects, many novel analgesics or adjuvants that may increase the analgesia/ toxicity ratio will become available for clinical trials. A direct demonstration of such an improved therapeutic ratio in the target population will provide the most convincing evidence for adopting a new treatment.

In most of the single-dose analgesic comparisons to date, however, there has been little effort to quantitatively define adverse effects of the agents studied. The usual practice is to ask the patient at each observation time, "Have you noticed any other effects of the medication?" or "How do you feel?" The patient grades any volunteered symptoms as mild, moderate, or severe, and the observer inquires about those symptoms, and elicits new complaints at subsequent observation times (46).

Single-dose comparisons are inadequate, by themselves, to characterize drug toxicity for several reasons:

1. Customary sample sizes of 30 to 50 patients per treatment are insufficient to detect uncommon side effects with any certainty; it takes 228 patients, for example, to have a probability of .9 of observing in at least one patient a side effect whose frequency in the treated population is 1% (46).

2. Toxicity may be underestimated in the controlled clinical setting of a single-dose trial. Some side effects may only occur with repeated dosing and drug accumulation. Activity-related side effects, e.g., ataxia, nausea, or subtle changes in mental acuity, may not be revealed in acutely ill, bedridden subjects of inpatient analgesic studies (3).

3. Methods used to assess side effects are often cumbersome and impractical in acutely ill patients, or might distract from assessment of pain. Examples include respiratory responses to CO_2 and subtle tests of motor skills and cognitive function (47).

Because of the potential difficulties described in points 2 and 3, a number of investigators have carried out complementary studies examining analgesic effects of a drug in patients with pain, and side effects in normals (48–52). One large cooperative research program, however, has demonstrated that it is feasible to quantify side effects and analgesia in the clinical setting. In the Veterans Administration Cooperative Analgesic Study, Belville et al. (46) used side effects spontaneously reported by postoperative patients, rated as slight, moderate, or severe, to calculate relative potencies, using bioassay methods to be discussed below. For intramuscular pentazocine and morphine, the relative potencies for sedation and analgesia were similar.

As one would expect, a higher proportion of patients report a given side effect when they are specifically asked about its presence than when only spontaneous reports are recorded. This may occur in placebo-treated patients as well as in those given active drug. The few studies to date in which spontaneous reports were compared to those elicited with a checklist have not proven that standardized elicitation of side effects increases the power with which treatments can be distinguished (13). The analyses presented used present-or-absent criteria, however, not category, VAS, or AUC measures. By analogy with pain assessment methodology, it is plausible that in clinical settings where one or two common drug side effects are of particular interest, prospective examination at each observation using sensitive measures may prove superior to waiting for volunteered reports.

As described in the above section on pain measures, a none/mild/moderate/severe category scale may be suboptimal because patients can often make more subtle distinctions for sensory experiences (53). In an effort to increase sensitivity, some investigators are using more extensive descriptor scales (54), or visual analogue scales for common side effects such as sedation (55) and nausea (56). As with the pain VAS, the use of horizontal lines of 10 to 15 cm, with the two anchor phrases clearly delineating extremes, may be a more sensitive measure than a four-point category scale (7). Side effect scores might be analyzed using similar methods to those described above for analgesic efficacy scores.

It is difficult to compare the reported side effect rates across studies because of the variations in methods used to elicit information as well as the clinical setting in which the side effect is rated. For example, opiate-induced nausea might be slight and not significantly different from placebo-associated nausea unless the patient ambulates, and sedation may be affected by the patient's activity. For some adverse reactions such as sedation and cognitive impairment, performance measures may prove valuable in evaluating potentially less toxic therapeutic alternatives (57–59).

THE MECHANICS OF STUDY EXECUTION

Interacting with the Patient

The nurse-observer plays a crucial role, communicating with the patient and striving to maintain uniformity in study methods. Specific issues related to preparing the patient, obtaining informed consent, and interview technique are discussed at length in Chapter 26.

Timing of Study

A study begins when the patient has pain requiring medication and can effectively communicate subjective assessments to the study's personnel. Patients undergoing minor surgical procedures such as oral surgery, or those having regional or local anesthesia, such as many obstetric patients, are well suited for study on the day of surgery. For major surgery requiring general anesthesia, the more usual practice is to defer study until the morning of the first postoperative day. When patients are studied within several hours of general anesthesia, they may be too groggy to respond to questions reliably and frequently have nausea and vomiting. It is often difficult to assure that anesthetists who are not co-investigators will use uniform methods for patients in the study and this variability may reduce the sensitivity of studies on the day of surgery.

Prior Medication

Policies about prior and concomitant medications need to be specified in the study protocol. Patients with chronic pain or those studied a day or more after their surgery or trauma will obviously need analgesics before the study begins. The customary practice is to allow any standard analgesic with relatively short duration, e.g., morphine, hydromorphone, codeine, oxycodone, acetaminophen, aspirin, ibuprofen. Analgesic antagonists or potentiators, and long-acting agents such as methadone, levorphanol, sustained-release opiate preparations, or piroxicam are not desirable. One research group prefers to avoid any opiate that will be used during the study itself, because of their impression that chronic treatment with a particular opiate induces more tolerance to that analgesic than to other opiates (1).

For studies that begin on postoperative day one, orders for the preceding evening must ensure that the patient will get adequate medication to maintain analgesia until the customary 8 or 9 AM starting time, but not receive long-acting agents that will prevent or interfere with the study. One common approach is to ask the floor nurse to offer the patient an analgesic at 5 or 6 AM, making it likely that remedication will be needed at the appropriate time for study. After the nurse-observer arrives, the patient's pain level is monitored frequently until the patient reports moderate or severe pain and requests medication. Some groups use reports of pain at rest, whereas others claim that studies are more sensitive when pain is measured after a maneuver that intensifies baseline pain, such as having a patient turn or cough. A specified time, depending on the patient's maintenance analgesic and route of administration, must have elapsed since the previous standard analgesic was given (2).

With the growth of interest in postoperative pain management, many alternatives to the traditional intramuscular (IM) opiate are being employed, including patient-controlled analgesic infusions, and epidural infusions of opiates or local anesthetics. Although the researcher might prefer a uniform prestudy analgesic method, this may not be acceptable to anesthesiology staff or patients. One compromise solution is to require the use of relatively short-acting opiates or anesthetics, and to either stratify the randomization of treatments based on the anesthetic technique or retrospectively analyze and control for the effect of pretreatment on the results.

Concomitant Medications

Other medications that may be required for intercurrent clinical problems could cause problems of interpretation. Typically, it is assumed that, unless they are known to potentiate or antagonize analgesia, they do not affect the outcome of the trial. For example, nausea may be treated with phenothiazine injections or suppositories. With the exception of methotrimeprazine (60), it is believed that these agents do not potentiate opiate analgesia (61,62). Drugs thought to enhance analgesic action such as caffeine and antihistamines should be avoided.

Blinding and Placebos

The pain relief that follows any treatment is to some extent a product of the expectations and interactions of patient and clinicians (63); such so-called placebo effects underlie much of the analgesia observed with potent drug and sugar pill alike (63,64). During the early years of analgesic trials, some investigators sought to identify and exclude "placebo reactors" (65), but it soon became clear that with repeated challenges, the large majority of patients at least occasionally report relief after placebo (2). The likelihood and intensity of placebo analgesia vary with the patient's pain intensity, prior treatments, expectations, and other clinical circumstances (64,66). "Reverse placebo effects" have been documented as well: When investigators mistakenly believed that subjects would be given only placebo or opiate antagonist, the patients' pain tended to increase, suggesting that patients were responding to the investigators' nonverbal cues (67).

For these reasons, investigators now accept the necessity of blinding themselves and patients to the identity of treatments whenever possible. This requires that drugs be identical in color, pill shape, taste, and if possible, have similar side effects. The last is often difficult to achieve because many analgesics, particularly the opiates, have side effects that permit the sophisticated patient to distinguish them from an inert placebo. Similar "unmasking" may also occur when one drug causes pain on injection, becomes effervescent when given in solution, or has a recognizable odor. Side effects of a new compound may spuriously indicate modest analgesic efficacy by suggesting to patients that they have received a potent analgesic, which in itself may alter their pain experience (19). Such potential difficulties can be addressed in the experimental design, for example, by using a standard analgesic or a nonanalgesic ("active placebo") that mimics the side effects of the test compound, or by using multiple doses of the test compound. It has been suggested that investigators routinely check the adequacy of the blinding procedures by asking patients what drug they think they are taking and how they make that guess (68,69), but this has not been described to date in acute analgesic studies.

When different routes of administration are compared, each patient must receive a treatment by each route. In a placebo-controlled comparison of an intrathecal (IT) to an intramuscular (IM) opiate, for example, the patient might receive simultaneous injections of opiate IT and saline IM, saline IT and opiate IM, or saline IT and saline IM.

Randomization and Stratification

In most studies, patients are randomly assigned to treatments. Randomization methods are well discussed in general texts on clinical trials (12). In the simplest method, a list of patient numbers is prepared, grouped into blocks; the block size is the number of possible treatments or a multiple of that number. Within each block, the treatment order is either individually randomized or assigned according to the requirement of a specific design, such as a Latin square.

Approximate equivalence of patients in the treatment groups is a crucial issue in parallel group studies (70). There is a risk of obtaining a spurious result if the treatment groups are imbalanced for some prognostic variable that strongly predicts treatment response. Although an imbalance for any particular factor becomes less likely as the sample size in a study increases, the overall risk of at least one imbalance rises with the number of factors. In general, analgesic studies may benefit from measures to assure balancing the treatment groups during the trial. Such efforts depend upon a clear understanding of the factors influencing response, and the practical ease of implementing measures to maintain balance. If prospective efforts to balance the groups are not used, however, post hoc adjustments during the analysis of the study may be possible.

One of the most important variables that may affect analgesic response is initial pain severity. Patients who begin a study with severe pain have the possibility of higher PID scores, by definition, than patients who begin with moderate pain, and studies have confirmed this occurs (40). It has also been demonstrated that the relief scores of patients with severe starting pain tend to be lower than those of patients with moderate pain (40), i.e., it is harder to completely relieve severe pain than moderate pain.

Kaiko and coworkers (71,72) have done the most extensive analysis of other variables that predict response in analgesic assays. In studies in 715 patients who received intramuscular morphine for chronic cancer pain, TOTPAR scores were significantly greater in the elderly compared to the young, in blacks compared to whites, in patients with dull pain compared to sharp pain, and in patients with abdominal pain compared to arm or chest pain (Fig. 5). The same workers found that in postoperative patients, the higher AUC scores in the elderly reflected an increased duration of analgesia, probably related to their slower rates of metabolizing morphine (72,73); peak analgesia was affected little by age. Belville et al. (74) have also reported a greater response to morphine in elderly patients. If the effects of race, pain site, and pain quality are confirmed by others, they might be important variables to balance among groups.

In order to assure equal distribution of the critical prognostic variables among

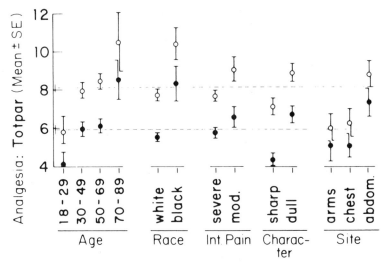

FIG. 5. Variables that may predict response to morphine. TOTPAR scores in relation to age, race, initial pain intensity, pain character, and pain site following 8 mg (*filled circles*) and 16 mg (*open circles*) doses of intramuscular morphine sulfate in cancer patients with pain. TOTPAR is the sum of the hourly pain relief scores. Upper and lower *dashed lines* indicate mean scores for all patients following the 16 mg and 8 mg doses, respectively. (From ref. 72, with permission.)

treatments, some investigators choose to stratify patients, that is, to assign patients to separate blocked randomizations depending on their initial pain level (35), type of surgical procedure, or other variables. Note that it is easier to assign treatments and prepare medications based on prognostic variables if they are known ahead of time—e.g., sex, race, surgical site—than if the variable can be assessed only at the moment the study begins, as in the case of pain severity or quality. For example, suppose that one wished to stratify on surgical procedure and initial pain level. Before the study began, one might assign numbers 1 to 80 to orthopedic procedures, 101 to 180 for thoracic cases, and 201 to 280 for gynecological cases. For the first thoracic case, the nurse must obtain medications 101 *and* 180 from pharmacy and bring them to the bedside, administering 101 if starting pain is moderate or 180 if pain is severe. The complexity increases if there is need to stratify for additional variables.

A larger number of prognostic variables can be kept in balance by using various computer-assisted methods of "adaptive randomization," i.e., adapting the probabilities of allocation of treatment to the characteristics and the prognostic features of the current patient, based on those patients who have already completed the study (13,75). Although use of these methods is increasing in a number of medical specialities, they have been little used in acute analgesic studies. At present the limited knowledge about prognostic variables for analgesia and the cumbersome requirement of bringing multiple medications to the bedside may discourage their use.

CHOICE OF TREATMENTS AND DOSES

Simple Efficacy Study: Test Drug, Placebo, Positive Control

Although the simplest of the classic single-dose designs consists of two treatments—the test medication and a placebo—most modern trials also include a standard analgesic "positive control," such as morphine, aspirin, or ibuprofen. In order to demonstrate the value of each of the two types of controls, and the potential consequences of their omission, a number of possible outcomes are illustrated in Fig. 6.

Figure 6A shows data from a hypothetical study comparing Drug X, an investigational analgesic, with a morphine positive control and a placebo. According to the primary outcome measure chosen for this study, summed relief category scores (TOTPAR), Drug X tended to be slightly but not statistically significantly more effective than morphine, and both were statistically superior to placebo. The conclusions are straightforward: Drug X is an effective analgesic, and the study methods were sufficiently sensitive to distinguish morphine-level analgesics from placebo.

The omission of a positive control does not fatally flaw the study if Drug X is superior to placebo (Fig. 6B), although one cannot be certain about the strength of the effect. The positive control serves as a yardstick against which to compare the magnitude of Drug X's ability to produce analgesia. In pain syndromes for which there is no known "positive control"—e.g., neuropathic pain—the comparison of test drug to placebo must suffice. Should Drug X fail to outperform placebo, however, the omission of the positive control will render the study uninterpretable (Fig. 6C). One cannot reliably conclude that Drug X is ineffective in this condition. Perhaps the drug usually relieves pain in patients with this condition, but the study failed. This could happen because patients were too stressed by the clinical setting to respond to medication, the pain questionnaires were insensitive, the procedures of the nurse-observer were variable or confusing (see Chapter 26), or merely because of random variation. With a positive control included, one might find that this standard analgesic, at a dose well known to be effective in the target condition, is superior to Drug X and placebo (Fig. 6D). That would demonstrate that the methods in this study were sufficiently sensitive, and it is probable that Drug X is inactive in this population. Alternatively, one might find Drug X and the standard analgesic equivalent to placebo (Fig. 6E). In this case, it is probable that the study methods were ineffective.

What are the consequences of omitting the placebo and comparing Drug X only to a standard analgesic? As in the previous case, this omission is less damaging when the assay shows a difference between the two treatments. The data in Fig. 6F suggest that Drug X is an effective analgesic in this population, although one cannot be sure how much of the Drug X and morphine analgesia are owing to placebo effects. If the responses to Drug X and standard analgesic were similar, however (Fig. 6G), interpretation would be troublesome. The data might reflect either that Drug X and morphine were both effective analgesics, or that neither was effective and there was a large placebo effect.

If the use of a placebo group is difficult, an alternative approach is to use a second dose level of the standard analgesic. Figure 6H shows that morphine 12 mg surpassed morphine 6 mg, demonstrating the sensitivity of the study methods, and implying that the effects of both Drug X and morphine 12 mg were not merely placebo effects.

In addition to the test-standard-placebo triad explored above, most analgesic studies include additional treatment groups, chosen to address the major question to be answered in the study. To test the soundness of various alternative designs for the intended purpose, the investigator may wish to graph the various possible outcomes as in Fig. 6 to ensure that whatever the outcome, light will be shed on the issue.

Determining the Dose-Response Curve of an Analgesic

To fully characterize an analgesic, the drug's dose-response curve for analgesia and side effects should be determined. Dose-response relationships are usually described on a logarithmic dose scale, as schematized in Fig. 7. Important features of the curves, which may differ among individuals and among pain syndromes with different pharmacological mechanisms, are the threshold for analgesia, the slope of the linear portion of the curve, the presence of a "ceiling" for analgesia, and the limits to dosage imposed by side effects. The new drug may resemble the aspirin-like drugs, with a shallow slope and a ceiling effect (76); the morphine-like opiate agonists, with a steep slope and no ceiling for analgesia, dosage being limited only by side effects (2); or some of the opiate agonist-antagonists, with a steep slope and an analgesic ceiling.

It is highly recommended that early in the development of a new analgesic, the dose-response curve be explored in one or several models whose assay sensitivity is well known (77; United States Food and Drug Administration Draft Analgesic Guidelines, 1990). Along with Phase I and II pharmacokinetic and pharmacodynamic data, this will help to guide selection of several specific doses for testing in a wide variety of patient populations during Phase III, compared to standard medications used in treating these conditions.

Most analgesic studies have used fixed doses, regardless of the patients' weight or body surface area. This has mainly been an issue of convenience—it is more cumbersome to have a pharmacist or one of the nonblinded investigators make up individual dosing units. Also, several early investigations failed to find a clear relationship between pain relief and body weight following a fixed dose of analgesic (78,79); further investigations of this point may be in order using more sensitive modern methods and drugs with steep dose-response slopes.

The exploration of an analgesic's dose-response relationship will generally require studies in several different patient populations with differing levels of

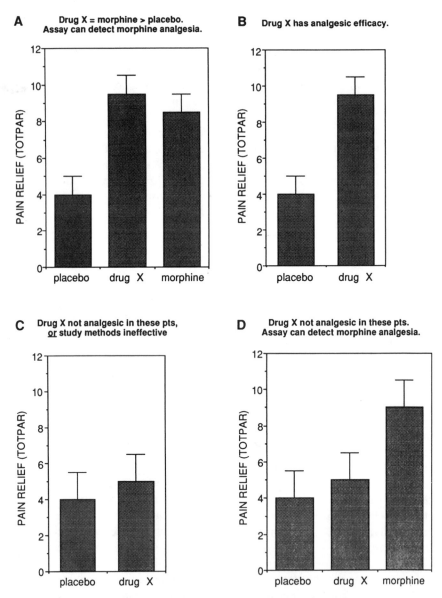

FIG. 6. A–D: Placebo and standard analgesic in the interpretation of analgesic trials (see text). **E–H:** Placebo and standard analgesic in the interpretation of analgesic trials (see text). The symbol > denotes "statistically significantly greater than," and = denotes "not significantly different from."

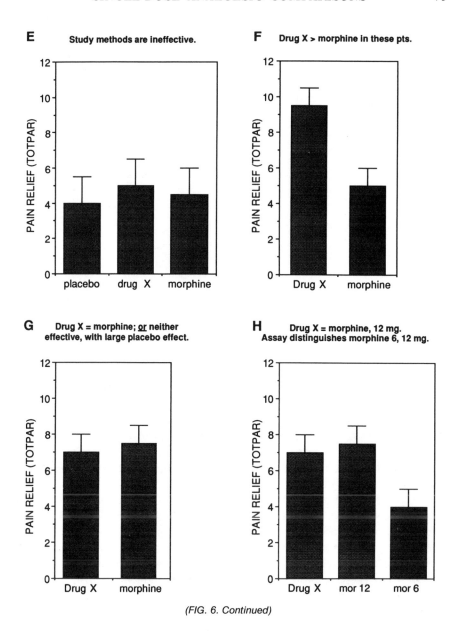

(FIG. 6. Continued)

pain severity and sensitivity to analgesics, e.g., patients requiring potent analgesics for major surgical procedures or cancer pain as well as the models commonly used to evaluate weaker agents—oral surgery, postpartum pain, lesser surgical procedures, and mild trauma. The dose-response curves may be different in these two groups. If patients in the latter groups were used, they might get nearly

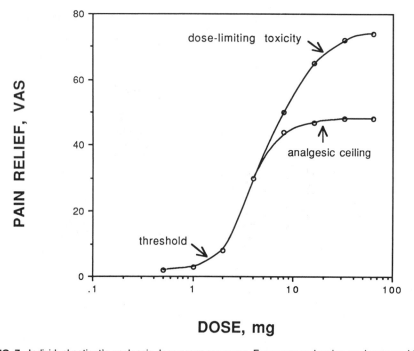

DOSE, mg

FIG. 7. Individual patient's analgesic dose-response curve. For some analgesics, such as morphine and other mu-receptor opioid agonists, the upper dose is limited only by side effects, but short of complete relief of pain, no "analgesic ceiling" is reached (*upper curve*). Other analgesics, including the aspirin-like drugs and the mixed agonist-antagonist opioids, have an analgesic ceiling (*lower curve*). Clinical trials will be the most efficient in distinguishing between treatments when the doses tested are on the steep part of the dose-response curve.

complete relief with low doses of test drug, whereas those in the former groups might get little or no relief from the same dose.

This point is illustrated by Fig. 1 of Chapter 29, a summary of data on aspirin dose-response from eight studies by Laska et al. (27). The curves represent the percent of patients obtaining complete relief from placebo or aspirin, 325 mg, 650 mg, or 1,300 mg in five patient groups: postpartum uterine cramp with either moderate (labeled U_2) or severe (U_3) baseline pain intensity; moderate (E_2) or severe (E_3) episiotomy pain; or severe pain following cesarean section or other gynecological surgery (S_3). The data suggest that patients with uterine cramp might be an excellent choice to demonstrate efficacy of low doses of an aspirin-like drug, as the 325 mg dose is widely spaced from placebo. However, it is difficult to differentiate higher aspirin doses in this model because the lowest dose already gives more than 50% of the patients complete relief. Likewise, except at minimal doses, it would be unproductive to study any stronger analgesics in this model. In contrast, the episiotomy and surgical populations are better able to distinguish the lowest from the higher aspirin doses, and are likely to be better models for assessing analgesics stronger than aspirin, 1,300 mg.

When one tests more than one dose of a study drug, hoping to learn whether higher doses yield additional analgesia, additional controls may be needed besides the placebo and the single dose of standard analgesic illustrated in Fig. 6. If the two doses of Drug X differ in effect, a dose of standard analgesic whose effect is in the range of that of the high dose of Drug X is not crucial to the conclusion, although it will improve the ability to make clinical comparisons. If, however, the two doses of Drug X are not statistically distinguishable and there is no standard analgesic with greater effect than the higher dose of Drug X (Fig. 8, top), one cannot tell whether the results reflect a ceiling effect for Drug X, or alternatively, that the pain model chosen cannot demonstrate the effect of any analgesic more powerful than the lower dose of Drug X. The inclusion of a

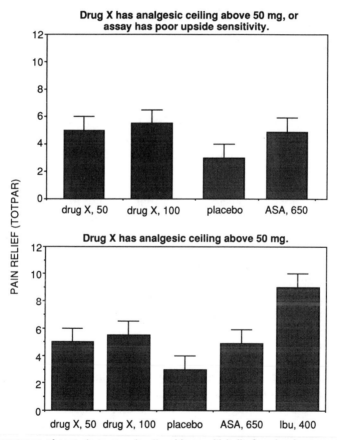

FIG. 8. Importance of controls to examine "upside sensitivity" of analgesic assay. *Top:* If the assay does not distinguish graded doses of Drug X, and there is no standard control more powerful than the Drug X doses, one cannot distinguish whether these results reflect a true analgesic ceiling effect or insensitivity of the model to more potent analgesics. *Bottom:* The addition of a more effective control (here, ibuprofen, 400 mg) establishes that Drug X reaches an analgesic ceiling near the 50 mg dose.

higher dose of standard, or a different standard of a more powerful class would resolve this issue (Fig. 8, bottom). If the higher standard were more effective than Drug X, one could conclude that the model has "upside sensitivity," i.e., the ability to detect additional analgesia on the upper side of the Drug X dose in question, but that Drug X has a ceiling for analgesia above 50 mg. On the other hand, the failure of an accepted standard in the model, e.g., ibuprofen 400 mg in moderate surgical pain, to surpass Drug X or a weaker standard analgesic would have suggested that this particular study lacked the upside assay sensitivity to evaluate the higher dose of Drug X.

The above comments are predicated on analytic methods of data analysis that are limited to consideration of a single study. However, it may be more appropriate to consider statistical models that incorporate known relationships among drugs and doses that have been determined from previous studies. A discussion of such methods is beyond the scope of this chapter, but is discussed in papers by Ramsey (80) and Kuo (81,82).

Relative Potency Studies

The relative potency of a test drug to a standard drug is the dose of the standard drug necessary to obtain an equivalent effect to that achieved by a unit dose of the test drug. Relative potency bioassays consist of a comparison of doses of a test drug with doses of a standard (Figure 9A). A common design is the "four-point relative potency assay," consisting of two doses each of test and standard. A placebo may not be necessary in such trials because the demonstration of a statistically significant positive slope for the dose-response curves establishes assay sensitivity. A placebo is necessary, however, if one wishes to estimate the lowest dose at which analgesic efficacy might be detected.

Historically, the extensive use of four-point relative potency assays by a number of groups in the 1950s and 1960s provided the most impressive evidence that analgesics can be scientifically assessed (Table 1). Although the absolute level of analgesia observed with a particular drug varied from center to center, the relative potencies of various drugs to morphine tended to be quite uniform (2). Relative potency estimates have also been made for one drug given by several routes (Fig. 10) (83).

Relative potency studies are most informative when the test compound and standard are similar enough that they can be treated as different dilutions of a single agent—that is, having a similar time-course of onset and duration and a similar slope of the dose-response curve—and when the ranges of analgesic effects produced by the chosen doses of test and standard drugs overlap (4). As mentioned above, the relative potency of the test drug to the standard can be calculated for analgesia as well as for common side effects. The analgesic calculation has usually been based on a specific measure of analgesia, such as peak relief or an AUC measure (SPID, TOTPAR). Alternatively, multivariate techniques are now available to combine multiple measures in the estimate (44; Chapter 30).

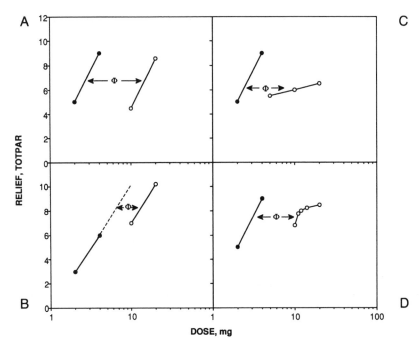

FIG. 9. Assumptions of relative potency bioassay. The relative potency (Φ) determined by this assay will apply for any doses in the range tested, provided the effects of the drug doses chosen are in a similar range, the dose-response curves are parallel and linear [all true in panel (**A**)] and the time-course of effects are similar. Dosing predictions based on the relative potency may be incorrect in at least part of the dose range if the effect range tested in the assays differs for the treatments (**B**), if the dose-response curves are not parallel (**C**) or linear (**D**), or if the time-courses of effects differ greatly (see Fig. 10).

There are several advantages in expressing the outcome of a study or group of studies (84) in terms of relative potency. First, such estimates allow clinicians to tailor the dosing of a new drug to the individual patient, based on the specific dose of the standard usually used by that patient. Second, this method obviates the problem of expressing a drug's effect in units on an arbitrary analgesic scale, measurements whose absolute size is difficult to interpret and which vary with the patient population, study methods, and placebo effect. Finally, relative potency studies may be a valuable tool in developing safer analgesics. As knowledge of neural mechanisms of the therapeutic and toxic effects of analgesics grows, a number of agents may be developed with milder side effects than standard agents. If the doses of test drug are compared only to single doses of one or more controls, a direct comparison of side effects at equianalgesic doses will not be possible unless a dose of test drug and standard fortuitously produce the same amount of analgesia. If a relative potency design is used, however, the side effects and analgesia at any dose in the range tested can be estimated and compared for test drug and standard. In this way, an advantage in "therapeutic ratio" of a new compound may be more convincingly demonstrated.

TABLE 1. *Relative potency estimates of several narcotic analgetics adapted from the results of a number of investigators in different institutions*

Drug	Patient population	Investigator	Potency relative to morphine
Oxymorphone	Cancer	Wallenstein and Houde	9.8
	Cancer	Eddy and Lee	9.9
	Postoperative	DeKornfeld	10.0
Phenazocine	Cancer	Houde et al.	3.2
	Postoperative	DeKornfeld and Lasagna	3.3
Dextromoramide	Cancer	Bauer et al.	2.0
	Postoperative	Keats et al.	1.9
	Cancer	Houde and Wallenstein	1.3
Dipipanone	Cancer	Houde and Wallenstein	0.49
	Cancer	Seed	0.47
	Cancer	Cochin	0.88
Normorphine	Cancer	Houde and Wallenstein	0.40
	Postoperative	Lasagna	0.25
Dihydrocodeine	Cancer	Seed et al.	0.15
	Postoperative	Beecher	0.17
	Postoperative	Keats et al.	0.17

From ref. 2, with permission.

The investigator considering relative potency designs must also be aware of their pitfalls. If the dose-response curves of the test and standard drugs are not linear, not parallel, or the doses chosen are not in the same analgesic range, requiring extrapolation of the curves, the calculated relative potency may be incorrect or meaningless (Fig. 9B–D). For discussion of the value of relative potency even when the lines are not parallel, see Cornfield (85). When a drug is compared to itself, the estimated relative potency should be one whether peak analgesia, hourly PID, or AUC scores are used. If the drugs to be compared have different kinetics, however, peak, hourly, and AUC scores may produce very different relative potency values. For example, AUC scores will favor the drug with longer duration (Fig. 10A). The meaning of relative potency in these circumstances must be carefully considered.

In the early stages of the study of a new drug, the doses may be erroneously chosen so that there is little overlap of analgesic ranges (Fig. 9B and Fig. 10B). To guard against that, Beaver and Feise (86) have conducted relative potency studies using several different dose pairs of test drug. After each complete block of patients complete the study, the data are examined and the test drug doses for the next block chosen according to the results of that block, to ensure that equianalgesic dose ranges are used. Formal statistical methods to explore dose range and use of all of the data generated to obtain an estimate of relative potency are relatively crude at present, but there is current research to address the design issues (87–89).

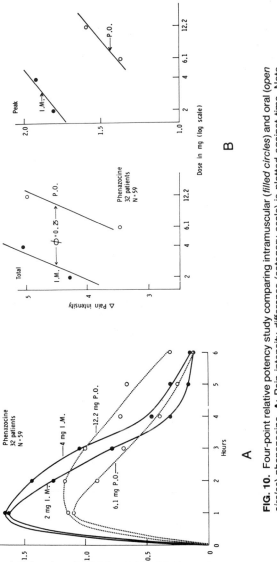

FIG. 10. Four-point relative potency study comparing intramuscular (*filled circles*) and oral (*open circles*) phenazocine. **A:** Pain intensity difference (category scale) is plotted against time. Note the difference between the time-course of analgesia for the two routes. **B:** Total (*left*) or peak (*right*) change in pain intensity are plotted against dose. For total scores, oral phenazocine is one-fourth as potent as intramuscular drug. For peak scores, no relative potency can be calculated because there was no overlap between the level of response seen with the two routes. Because the time-course of response differs between the routes, note that the relative potency calculated for total scores will change according to the length of the study; e.g., if only the first three hours were considered, the IM/PO disparity would have appeared even greater. (From ref. 83, with permission.)

Analgesic Combinations

The United States Food and Drug Administration's general policy regarding fixed-combination prescription drugs, 21 CFR, 300.50 (a), is:

> Two or more drugs may be combined in a single dosage form when each component makes a contribution to the claimed effects and the dosage of each component (amount, frequency, duration) is such that the combination is safe and effective for a significant patient population requiring such concurrent therapy . . .

There are a number of rationales for treating pain with drug combinations (90). The most common strategy is to combine two analgesics with different mechanisms of action, in order to enhance analgesic effects and reduce side effects. In addition, nonanalgesics are sometimes added to analgesics if the non-analgesic potentiates analgesic action, counteracts a side effect of the analgesic, treats another symptom of the disease for which the drug is intended, alters the absorption of the analgesic, or prevents diversion and abuse. The specific rationale and claims for the combination determine the research design issues; different rationales may call for different experimental designs. In this section, we comment only on studies of drug combinations intended to enhance analgesia.

Historically, the most common design used to evaluate analgesic combinations has been the 2×2 factorial design, in which the treatments are the two individual ingredients, the combination, and a placebo. The comparison of each ingredient to the placebo shows whether the ingredient is effective alone, and a favorable comparison of the combination to each ingredient satisfies the FDA requirement that "each component makes a contribution to the claimed effects."

If it is already known that one of the ingredients is not an analgesic alone but potentiates the analgesic in the combination, many believe that it can be considered as a placebo, and a fully inert placebo can be omitted. The combination must be shown to be superior to the nonanalgesic and analgesic ingredients alone, and for consistency, the analgesic ingredient must be superior to the nonanalgesic ingredient or placebo (U.S. Food and Drug Administration Draft Analgesic Guidelines, 1990).

The 2×2 factorial design combination study has usually been analyzed using analysis of variance techniques. To demonstrate at the 0.05 level of significance that "each component makes a contribution to the claimed effects," it is sufficient to show that the contrast between the combination and each component (using, for example, t-tests or rank tests) are statistically significant, each at the .05 level (91,92). Although it has been claimed that the size and sign of the interaction term in a factorial analysis of variance may suggest whether the ingredients work at similar or different sites of action (90), such inferences are not warranted, because the size of the interaction term, I, will vary according to (a) the size of the placebo effect, and (b) the steepness of the individual dose-response curves, neither of which directly depend on the analgesic mechanism.

To see this, recall that the interaction term is defined by:

$$I = (AB - P) - (A - P) - (B - P)$$
$$= AB + P - A - B$$

where A, B, AB, and P denote the mean effect of treatments A, B, the combination of A and B, and placebo, respectively. Thus the sign and size of I can be substantially affected, indeed determined, by the magnitude of P. As for the effect of the steepness of the dose-response curves, suppose that A and B are the same drug, say A, given at the same dose. Then the combination is just A given at twice the dose, say A_2. Then $I = A_2 + P - 2A$. Then I is positive, negative, or zero according to whether the slope of the dose-response curve is steep or flat. For example, if P is zero, then the sign of I depends on whether the dose-response line of A is above, on, or below the 45° line.

Another criticism of the 2×2 factorial design is that it does not give the clinician enough information to decide whether the combination treatment is clinically advantageous. From the prescriber's viewpoint, it is a trivial result that a combination of component A and component B gives more analgesia than either alone. The clinically interesting question is whether the physician should prescribe the combination or merely raise the dose of A or B. This point is moot, of course, if conventional doses of drug A or B are already at the maximum effective or tolerated dose levels, as is often the case for aspirin and the nonsteroidal antiinflammatory drugs.

To answer the question of whether the combination is clinically desirable, one needs to use a more complex design. For the case where both components are analgesic when given alone, a complete analysis would include multiple doses of each component and the combination (93), with careful attention to side effects as well as pain relief. Loewe (94) describes the use of isobolograms to fully characterize this situation, but the large number of treatment groups required has discouraged the use of this approach in clinical studies. Several groups (95–97; Commentary by Goldstein and Brunelle following this chapter) are developing modeling approaches that may prove more practical in the clinical setting.

If it has been established that one component of the combination has little or no analgesic effects by itself, one might choose to do a relative potency comparison of the analgesic and the analgesic-potentiator combination (98); such studies provided the most convincing published evidence of enhanced analgesia resulting from the addition of caffeine to aspirin or acetaminophen (84) and ibuprofen (99).

SAMPLE SIZE

How many patients should be included in the trial? Many texts on clinical trial design and statistical methods discuss sample size selection (13). The specific computation technique to decide on the number of patients depends in general on the underlying assumption about the distribution of the random variables, the power desired for a particular effect size difference, and upon the particular experimental design used. Recall that a type I error is the rejection of the null hypothesis of equal effects of two drugs, when in truth they are equal (a so-called false-positive result). A type II error is the failure to reject the null hypothesis of equality of drug effects, when in truth the effects are unequal. For a given test, the probability of a type I error is called the size of the test, or the α-level, whereas power is the probability of rejecting the null hypothesis when it should be rejected (commonly denoted by $1 - \beta$, where β is the probability of a type II error). For a fixed probability of a type I error under certain statistical assumptions in a parallel design, the required sample size to achieve a given level of power for a fixed treatment effect size is proportional to the variance of the outcome measure, and inversely proportional to the square of the treatment effect magnitude one wishes to detect. For example, to halve the amount of pain relief that a study can detect at the same size and power, one must either quadruple the sample size, or reduce the variance by a factor of four.

It is difficult to calculate with any certainty the required sample size for a given α, effect magnitude, and power because the variance is generally unknown. However, estimates of the variance may be obtained from previous similar studies, when available. There are many studies in the literature that report on statistically significant differences between a standard analgesic and a placebo using 30 to 50 patients per group in parallel single-dose designs, and 15 to 25 patients in a crossover design. For small differences and heterogeneous samples, larger sample sizes may be required. On the other hand, the use of rather homogeneous groups, e.g., standardized surgical trauma, together with meticulous technique may allow the sample size in a parallel single-dose design to be as small as 12 to 20 patients per treatment (Chapter 25). As data accumulates, continuing review of methodology used in previous studies together with analysis of patient subgroups facilitates rational planning for future studies, and may reduce the sample size requirements.

EXPERIMENTAL DESIGN: PARALLEL GROUP VERSUS CROSSOVER STUDIES

In a parallel group (also termed "completely randomized") design, each patient receives a single treatment. In a crossover design, each patient receives some (incomplete block) or all (complete block) of the treatments being studied.

Single-dose analgesic studies often require large sample sizes because detection of a drug effect must compete with so many other causes of variation in pain report: the subject's painful lesion, psychological makeup, previous pain experience, age, race, weight (78,79), interaction with the nurse observer, tolerance to opiate medications, etc. Much of this variation can be eliminated when the study treatments are compared in the same patient (100–102), resulting in more power because "each patient is his own control." However, there may be other problems with the use of crossover designs that must be carefully considered before they are used.

Carryover Effects

A major concern with crossover studies is the possibility that conclusions drawn from them may be biased by unequal "carryover effects." These are changes in the efficacy of treatments resulting from treatments given in earlier periods.

Figure 11 shows a hypothetical comparison of a new opiate agonist-antagonist to morphine, and assumes that the test drug has antagonist activity at tissue

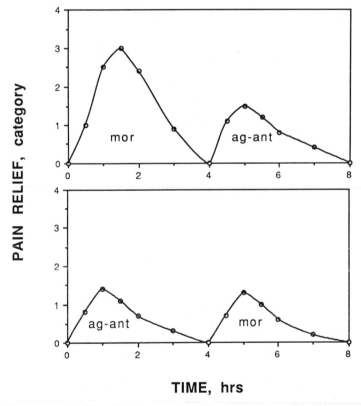

TIME, hrs

FIG. 11. Drug carryover effect. A new opiate agonist-antagonist (ag-ant) is being compared to morphine (mor). The true level of efficacy of the agonist-antagonist is about one-half that of morphine, as evidenced by a comparison of first dose data (*left side, top and bottom*). If enough antagonist activity persists from the first dose of test drug to inhibit morphine analgesia (*bottom*), while residual analgesic effects are negligible, the test drug's relative potency will be spuriously increased by inclusion of second dose data. In order to lessen pharmacological carryover effects, some investigators study only one dose every 24 hr.

levels well below those required for analgesia. A parallel-group comparison, using first-dose data only, would show that the antagonist is about half as effective as morphine (Fig. 11, left side of both panels). If we also assume there is little residual analgesic effect of morphine, the effect would be similar if the mixed agonist were given after morphine (Fig. 11, top) but when morphine followed the mixed agonist, the residual antagonist activity might largely prevent morphine analgesia (Fig. 11, bottom). Because of this, the averaged results for the crossover study would exaggerate the mixed agonist's efficacy relative to morphine. Conversely, a crossover comparison between morphine and an agent that potentiates morphine might show the potentiator to be relatively less effective than would be found in a parallel study.

In addition to direct pharmacological interactions of the two drugs in tissue, carryover effects may be mediated by drug-induced changes in neurotransmitters, drug metabolism, behavior, or psychological factors. In an example of a psychological carryover effect, Laska and Sunshine (66) found that the ratings of analgesia in patients treated with placebo were closely correlated with the dose of active analgesic they had previously received. Higher previous doses of the analgesic produced higher mean analgesia with the subsequent placebo treatment.

Some have suggested that when carryover effects are found in a study, then the first-dose data alone can be used. Brown (103) has pointed out, however, that carryover effects can be difficult to detect because the statistical test for carryover, which depends on a between-patient comparison, has very low power. He has concluded that if differential carryover effects are suspected to be substantial in a two-treatment, two-period study, then a parallel-group design should be used instead.

Dropouts

In crossover studies of postoperative pain and other acute spontaneously resolving pain syndromes, many patients may never request subsequent doses, resulting in a high dropout rate. Apart from the costs of lost time and data, a high dropout rate would prompt some reviewers to doubt the general applicability of the results, as they only reflect the subset of patients with prolonged pain.

Although data from several small studies are often cited to document the dangers of crossover studies (104,105), a more recent series of 59 four-dose crossover studies involving thousands of postoperative patients—the Veterans Administration Cooperative Analgesic Study—suggests that crossover studies can be advantageous even if pain steadily decreases over time. In this series, patients could receive a second dose of study analgesic within the same day if it fit into the nurse-observer's 8 to 10 hr shift; otherwise patients resumed their standard analgesic care until the next morning. [Some investigators (1) give only one dose of study medication per day, potentially reducing the carryover effect because of the long washout period, but increasing the chance that pain resolves before the patients receive all assigned treatments.] Although in the Veterans Administration study, only 40% of patients required all four study medications (101), the authors reported that they still achieved greater power utilizing that subgroup's four-dose crossover, as opposed to all of the patients' first-dose data. To achieve similar power, a one-dose parallel design would have had to enroll 2.4 times the number of patients that entered the original study, or 6 times the number that completed all four doses. Differential residual effects of the drugs on subsequent treatment periods were negligible whether pain (SPID) or pain relief (TOTPAR) scores were considered (106).

Because most single-dose comparison studies involve three or more treatments, it may be unrealistic to expect that most patients with acute pain will complete the entire series in the usual case where a nurse observer is available for a single daily shift and the patient has had a procedure that causes severe pain for only a day or two. In this setting, one can employ various incomplete block designs, in which each patient gets several, but not all, of the treatments. The "twin crossover" (107,108) is an incomplete block design in which patients receive either (a) the high dose of test drug and low dose of standard, or (b) the low dose of test drug and hi*p*h dose of standard, in either order, to make four possible treatment assignmc. .s. However, because certain combinations of treatments are excluded in this design, it has statistical weaknesses for bioassay studies. For example, one cannot test whether the two dose-response curves are parallel. Without any loss of efficiency, one may use many other incomplete block designs to overcome this difficulty (109).

Newer Crossover Designs

New designs and statistical methods make it possible to estimate the true treatment effects, even if there are carryover effects. To consider two simple examples, suppose one is comparing treatments A and B. If patients can receive three treatments, only two treatment sequences are needed, A-B-B and B-A-A. If only two treatment periods are possible, the four treatment sequences A-B, B-A, A-A, and B-B are used. These designs allow the carryover effect of each treatment to be estimated using a within-patient analysis (109–111). In addition to removing a source of bias, direct measurement of carryover effects may give additional information about the clinical effects of the analgesic to be expected with repeated dosing. More complex designs that incorporate measures of carryover effects are discussed by Jones and Kenward (109) and in Cochran and Cox (112).

ANALYSIS OF DATA

Review of Each Day's Data

After completing each patient interview, the researchers should review the data to assure that there are no gross inconsistencies or missing information. On occasion, data may be excluded from an analysis if it is clear, for example, that the patient misunderstood the scales, the patient required rescue medication before the expected peak activity of the study drugs, or an intercurrent medical event made it unlikely that the data would reflect analgesia of the study drugs. Such events might include the patient vomiting the study pills or developing a probable pulmonary embolism in midstudy. Decision rules regarding exclusion of data should be specified in advance in the written protocol and exclusions made prior to unblinding the randomization, with care that the procedures not bias the analysis in favor of one or another of the treatments. Patients whose data are excluded from the main analysis should still be included in an analysis of toxicity and, when appropriate, in so-called intent-to-treat analyses (13).

Rescue Medication

When patients require rescue medication after the time study drugs should have taken effect but before the end of the observation time, scores for unobserved subsequent pain and pain relief have historically been assigned values according to predetermined rules. Common conventions have included (a) pain and relief scores are set to the scores at the time of rescue; (b) pain scores are set to baseline pain level, and relief to zero; and (c) pain scores are set to the highest possible rating, and relief to zero. The first method appears to adhere most closely to actual patient observations. Sriwatanakul et al. (35) found that all of these methods led to similar statistical conclusions in four analgesic studies in which they were compared, but naturally these results depend on such factors as the size of the differences between treatments, the sample size, and the frequency and timing of required rescue medication. Today, however, wholesale imputation of data values is frowned upon, particularly for comparison of hourly PID or relief scores. In the latter case, misleading conclusions can be reached, especially if the treatments differ greatly in duration. For example, if the majority of patients are remedicated and set to a single conventional value, this can result in a spuriously low variance and make similar drugs appear to differ statistically. Moreover, there may be very few real observations used in the comparison. As noted above, presentations of data should indicate how many patients remained in the study and how remedicated patients were handled. Also, the use of duration parameters (Chapter 32), e.g., the probability of needing rescue medication and the survival distribution time of analgesic offset, is a more appropriate way to handle the data in the late hours of the trial.

When to Conduct Analyses, Early Stopping

Investigators who conduct long-term medical and surgical clinical trials frequently plan a number of analyses using sequential or group sequential methods (113–115) and are prepared to stop the trial early if a therapeutic or toxic effect is seen. By allowing "multiple looks" at the data, group sequential methods enable the early stopping of a study if treatments differ, but at a cost of stricter requirements for concluding that a significant treatment difference exists. Such methods are often used in clinical trials with a single outcome variable, e.g., survival or death, but have rarely been employed in analgesic studies, where there are multiple outcomes and measures. As the correlational structure of analgesic measures become better understood (Chapter 30), sequential methods may be more frequently applied in future studies. At present, it is more common to continue an analgesic study until a predetermined sample size has been reached. Investigators may find it useful to do interim analyses after one-third or one-half of subjects have completed, to verify that study methods are working and to help plan future studies. This can be done without changing the probability of a type I error, provided that one renounces the right to stop the study and declare a statistically significant difference.

Some Comments on Statistical Analysis of Analgesic Data

The approach to the analysis of data from an analgesic clinical trial depends naturally on the design of the experiment, the purpose of the analysis, and the assumptions about the underlying measures or random variables. Although there are some special features of analgesic trials that raise particular statistical issues, the general considerations in the analysis of data from any clinical trials are relevant and apply here as well. Several advanced statistical issues that have been the subject of recent research and are particularly relevant to clinical trials of analgesics are discussed in Chapters 29 and 30. A few comments on the traditional methods of data analysis applied in analgesic trials are given below.

Adjustments for Imbalance

A well-designed randomized experiment attempts to allocate patients to treatment groups in such a way that known influential variables are approximately equally distributed. Strategies such as stratification and adaptive randomization methods mentioned above may be used. Nonetheless, if there are a sufficiently large number of prognostic variables, it is almost certain that there will be imbalance among groups. As a first step in data analysis, an assessment of the degree of imbalance among groups is typically performed. Although tests of hypotheses about the equivalence of treatment groups with respect to a variable such as age, sex, and disease class are commonly done, mere lack of statistical significance does not necessarily guarantee that the groups are, in fact, equivalent. For example, if a prognostic variable has a large variance there may be considerable imbalance, but a statistical test may not have sufficient power to uncover it. An examination of the sample probability distribution of the prognostic variable is therefore quite useful. Evidence of imbalance in the data set suggests that in subsequent analyses of efficacy parameters, adjustments be made to overcome the implications on inference. In extreme cases of imbalance, e.g., all males in one group and all females in the other, it may be that no post hoc adjustment is possible. In most cases, it is possible to adjust by introducing the prognostic variables into the model, e.g., the analysis of covariance, or by performing analyses within strata and pooling across the strata.

Analysis of Efficacy Measures

In the statistical analysis of efficacy measures, the commonly used approaches are: analysis of variance (ANOVA) techniques based on normality assumptions or nonparametric techniques based on ranks, contingency table methods designed generally for categorical variables, and survival methods used for time measures such as onset or duration. The majority of published studies of analgesic clinical trials analyze the data by contrasting mean treatment effects using analysis of variance methods. Such analyses are based on assumptions of a linear sum of effects such as treatment, subject, investigator, site, and interactions among them. In the simplest case of comparing two treatments, the ANOVA approach reduces to the computation of a student's *t*-test.

For many outcome measures in analgesic trials, particularly data collected as categorical variables, the underlying assumption of normality may need to be reviewed. This can be done by examining the residuals. Sometimes the data may be transformed to make this assumption more tenable. Alternatively, nonparametric procedures may be used to contrast treatments. Tests such as the Wilcoxon and the normal scores test are analogous to the pairwise *t*-test mentioned above. The analogue of the parametric analysis of variance is the Friedman analysis of variance. Instead of being based on the actual magnitude of the variables, these nonparametric statistical methods are based on the *ranks* of the variables in the pooled samples. Such methods are often quite efficient, and may yield hypothesis tests with validity (accurate α level) that are considerably more certain than is possible under the assumptions of the usual normal theory-based ANOVA.

Typically, in analgesic trials there are multiple contrasts among the treatments—for example, all treatments in the trial are compared to placebo, to the standard, and often to each other. Because of this multiplicity of testing, the experimentwise error rate needs to be considered so that incorrect rejections of pairwise null hypotheses concerning equality of treatment means do not occur with high probability. To accomplish this objective, adjustments to the analyses are sometimes made by techniques such as Bonferroni, Tukey, Scheffé, and others. However, there are times when use of such adjustments are inappropriate and lead to excessively conservative analyses. For example, in testing whether a combination treatment is superior to both of its ingredients, no adjustment need be made.

For data that are categorical, a natural layout for summarizing the observations is a contingency table, possibly of high dimension. Analyses of such tables generally are based on either log linear models or tests such as the generalized Mantel-

Haenszel. In the special case where the contingency table is two-dimensional, the log linear model corresponds to the familiar chi square test of independence.

The use of survival time methods in the analysis of time-related data from clinical trials has increased dramatically in the last decade. Their great strength is that they can be used when the results contain observations that are censored, that is, either the observation or only a lower bound of the value of the observation is observed. For example, in the collection of duration data, if the patient continues to receive relief at the end of the clinical trial, the observation on the length of effect of the treatment is censored (Chapter 32). The principal nonparametric technique for estimating the distribution function of a survival random variable in the presence of censoring was introduced by Kaplan and Meier (116). Subsequent methods have been developed, most notably the Cox proportional hazards model (117), which includes techniques for handling covariates and enable comparisons to be made across treatments.

In dose-response studies, the typical analytical approach is based on regression methods. The general shape of the curve, usually linear in some dose range, is assumed. The parameters that characterize the curve, e.g., slope and intercept, are then fit by least squares. Studies in which the dose-response of a test drug is compared to the dose-response of a standard treatment are often performed to obtain an estimate of the relative potency, as discussed earlier. The estimate of relative potency depends on the measure of analgesia used, the mathematical model selected to represent the dose-response curve, and the relationship between the test and the standard. The theory that is most widely used assumes linearity and parallelism of the two dose-response lines. The linearity assumption can be on any scale for which a transformation of the analgesic measure produces a straight line in the dose range in which the model holds. Statistical tests are generally applied to obtain some level of assurance as to the validity of the underlying assumptions. Unfortunately, these tests may have relatively low power to detect departures from the assumptions unless sample sizes are relatively large, so one cannot be completely sure of their veracity. However, even when one cannot be certain that all of the underlying assumptions are valid, the relative potency is a useful summary measure for relating two drugs. As to which variable to use, a recent advance in relative potency assay methodology permits an analysis based on many variables, as long as all satisfy the underlying assumptions (Chapter 30). Similar techniques may be applied to the problem of analysis of side effects or laboratory values.

ACKNOWLEDGMENTS

We would like to thank Kenneth Hargreaves, Richard Gracely, David Goldstein, and Bernard Schachtel for their review of the manuscript.

REFERENCES

1. Houde RW, Wallenstein SL, Beaver WT. Evaluation of analgesics in patients with cancer pain. In: Lasagna L, ed. *Clinical pharmacology, section 6, International encyclopedia of pharmacology and therapeutics.* New York: Pergamon Press, 1966;59–97.

2. Houde RW, Wallenstein SL, Beaver WT. Clinical measurement of pain. In: de Stevens G, ed. *Analgetics.* New York: Academic Press, 1965;75–122.
3. Lasagna L. The evaluation of analgesic compounds in patients suffering from postoperative pain. In: Lasagna L, ed. *Clinical pharmacology, section 6, International encyclopedia of pharmacology and therapeutics.* New York: Pergamon Press, 1966;51–58.
4. Wallenstein SL, Houde RW. The clinical evaluation of analgesic effectiveness. In: Ehrenpreis S, Neidle A, eds. *Methods in narcotics research.* New York: Marcel Dekker, 1975;127–145.
5. Beaver WT. Measurement of analgesic efficacy in man. In: Bonica JJ, Lindblom U, Iggo A, eds. *Advances in pain research and therapy,* vol 5. New York: Raven Press, 1983;411–434.
6. Gracely RH. Pain psychophysics. *Adv Behav Med* 1985;1:199–231.
7. Price DD. Psychological and neural mechanisms of pain. New York: Raven Press, 1988;28–38.
8. Melzack R, ed. *Pain measurement and assessment.* New York: Raven Press, 1983.
9. Chapman CR, Loeser JD, eds. *Issues in pain measurement.* New York: Raven Press, 1989.
10. Pocock SJ. *Clinical trials: a practical approach.* Chichester, UK: John Wiley & Sons, 1983.
11. Shapiro S, Louis TA. *Clinical trials: issues and approaches.* New York: Marcel Dekker, 1983.
12. Meinert CL. *Clinical trials: design, conduct, and analysis.* New York: Oxford University Press, 1986;71–89.
13. Friedman LM, Furberg CD, DeMets DL. *Fundamentals of clinical trials,* 2nd ed. Littleton, Massachusetts: PSG Publishing Company, 1985.
14. Bailar JC III, Mosteller F. *Medical uses of statistics.* Waltham, Massachusetts: NEJM Books, 1986.
15. Brown BW Jr, Hollander M. *Statistics: a biomedical introduction.* New York: John Wiley & Sons, 1977.
16. Ingelfinger JA, Mosteller F, Thibodeau LA, Ware JH. *Biostatistics in clinical medicine.* New York: Macmillan, 1983.
17. Beecher HK. *Measurement of subjective responses.* New York: Oxford University Press, 1959;51.
18. Glynn C, Dawson D, Sanders R. Double-blind comparison between epidural morphine and epidural clonidine in patients with chronic non-cancer pain. *Pain* 1988;34:123–128.
19. Max MB, Schafer SC, Culnane M, Dubner R, Gracely RH. Association of pain relief with drug side effects in postherpetic neuralgia: a single-dose study of clonidine, codeine, ibuprofen, and placebo. *Clin Pharmacol Ther* 1988;43:363–371.
20. Schwartz D, Lellouch J. Explanatory and pragmatic attitudes in therapeutic trials. *J Chronic Dis* 1967;20:637–648.
21. Fishman B, Pasternak S, Wallenstein SL, Houde RW, Holland J, Foley KM. The Memorial pain assessment card: a valid instrument for the evaluation of cancer pain. *Cancer* 1987;60:1151–1158.
22. Lasagna L. The clinical measurement of pain. *Ann NY Acad Sci* 1960;86:28–37.
23. Gracely RH, McGrath P, Dubner R. Validity and sensitivity of ratio scales of sensory and affective verbal pain descriptors: manipulation of affect by diazepam. *Pain* 1978;5:19–29.
24. Tursky B. The development of a pain perception profile: a psychophysical approach. In: Weisenberg M, Tursky B, eds. *Pain: new perspectives in therapy and research.* New York: Plenum Press, 1976;171–194.
25. Wallenstein SL, Heidrich G, Kaiko R, Houde RW. Clinical evaluation of mild analgesics: the measurement of clinical pain. *Br J Clin Pharmacol* 1980;10:319S–327S.
26. Laska EM, Meisner M, Takeuchi K, Wanderling JA, Siegel C, Sunshine A. An analytic approach to quantifying pain scores. *Pharmacotherapy* 1986;6:276–282.
27. Laska EM, Sunshine A, Wanderling JA, Meisner MJ. Quantitative differences in aspirin analgesia in three models of clinical pain. *J Clin Pharmacol* 1982;22:531–542.
28. Littman GS, Walker BR, Schneider BE. Reassessment of verbal and visual analog ratings in analgesic studies. *Clin Pharmacol Ther* 1985;38:16–23.
29. Wallenstein SL. Scaling clinical pain and pain relief. In: Bromm B, ed. *Pain measurement in man: neurophysiological correlates of pain.* Amsterdam: Elsevier, 1984;389–396.
30. Scott J, Huskisson EC. Graphic representation of pain. *Pain* 1976;2:175–184.
31. Huskisson EC. Visual analogue scales. In: Melzack R, ed. *Pain measurement and assessment.* New York: Raven Press, 1983;33–37.
32. Price DD, McGrath PA, Rafii A, Buckingham B. The validation of visual analogue scales as ratio scale measures for chronic and experimental pain. *Pain* 1983;17:45–56.

33. Sriwatanakul K, Kelvie W, Lasagna L, Calimlim JF, Weis OF, Mehta G. Studies with different types of visual analog scales for measurement of pain. *Clin Pharmacol Ther* 1983;34:234–239.
34. Kremer E, Atkinson JH, Ignelzi RJ. Measurement of pain: patient preference does not confound pain measurement. *Pain* 1981;10:241–248.
35. Sriwatanakul K, Lasagna L, Cox C. Evaluation of current clinical trial methodology in analgesimetry based on experts' opinions and analysis of several analgesic studies. *Clin Pharmacol Ther* 1983;34:277–283.
36. Laska E, Gormley M, Sunshine A, et al. A bioassay computer program for analgesic clinical trials. *Clin Pharmacol Ther* 1967;8:658–669.
37. Siegel C, Sunshine A, Richman H, et al. Meptazinol and morphine in postoperative pain assessed with a new method for onset and duration. *J Clin Pharmacol* 1989;29:1017–1025.
38. Laska E, Siegel C, Sunshine A. Onset and duration: measurement and analysis. *Clin Pharmacol Ther* 1991; in press.
39. Laska EM, Sunshine A, Zighelboim I, et al. Effect of caffeine on acetaminophen analgesia. *Clin Pharmacol Ther* 1983;33:498–509.
40. Lasagna L. The psychophysics of clinical pain. *Lancet* 1962;2:572–575.
41. Belville JW, Forrest WH, Brown BW. Clinical and statistical methodology for cooperative clinical assays of analgesics. *Clin Pharmacol Ther* 1968;9:290–302.
42. Calimlim JF, Wardell WM, Davis HT, Lasagna L, Gillies AJ. Analgesic efficacy of an orally administered combination of pentazocine and aspirin, with observations on the use and statistical efficiency of GLOBAL subjective efficacy ratings. *Clin Pharmacol Ther* 1977;21:34–43.
43. Pocock SJ, Hughes MD, Lee RJ. Statistical problems in the reporting of clinical trials: a survey of three medical journals. *New Engl J Med* 1987;317:426–432.
44. Laska EM, Meisner MJ. Statistical methods and applications of bioassay. *Annu Rev Pharmacol Toxicol* 1987;27:385–397.
45. Sunshine A, Laska EM, Olson NZ. Analgesic effects of oral oxycodone and codeine in the treatment of patients with postoperative, postfracture, or somatic pain. In: Foley KM, Inturrisi CE, eds. *Opioid analgesics in the management of clinical pain.* New York: Raven Press, 1986;225–234.
46. Belville JW, Forrest WH, Elashoff J, Laska E. Evaluating side effects of analgesics in a cooperative clinical study. *Clin Pharmacol Ther* 1968;9:303–313.
47. Hindmarch I, Stonier ID, eds. *Human psychopharmacology: measures and methods,* vol 1. Chichester, U.K.: John Wiley & Sons, 1987.
48. Denton JE, Beecher HK. New analgesics. I. Methods in the clinical evaluation of new analgesics. *JAMA* 1949;141:1051–1057.
49. Belville J, Escarraga L, Wallenstein SL, Houde RW, Howland W. Relative respiratory depressant effects of oxymorphone (numorphan) and morphine. *Anesthesiology* 1960;21:397–400.
50. Houde RW, Wallenstein SL, Belville JW, Escarraga LA. The relative analgesic and respiratory effects of phenazocine and morphine. *J Pharmacol* 1964;144:337–345.
51. Keats AS, Telford J. Studies of analgesic drugs. VIII. A narcotic antagonist analgesic without psychotomimetic effects. *J Pharmacol* 1964;143:157–164.
52. Brown CR, Forrest WH, Hayden J, James KE. Respiratory effects of hydromorphone in man. *Clin Pharmacol Ther* 1973;14:331–337.
53. Gescheider GA. *Psychophysics: method, theory, and application,* 2nd ed. Hillsdale, New Jersey: Lawrence Erlbaum Associates, 1985.
54. Melzack R, Rosberger Z, Hollingsworth ML, Thirlwell M. New approaches to measuring nausea. *Can Med Assoc J* 1985;133:755–761.
55. Inturrisi CE, Colburn WA, Kaiko RF, Houde RW, Foley KM. Pharmacokinetics and pharmacodynamics of methadone in patients with chronic pain. *Clin Pharmacol Ther* 1987;41:392–401.
56. Morrow GR. The assessment of nausea and vomiting. *Cancer* 1984;53:2267–2280.
57. Bruera E, Macmillan K, Hanson J, MacDonald RN. The cognitive effects of the administration of narcotic analgesics in patients with cancer pain. *Pain* 1989;39:13–16.
58. Sjogren P, Banning A. Pain, sedation and reaction time during long-term treatment of cancer patients with oral and epidural opioids. *Pain* 1989;39:5–12.
59. Wood MM, Cousins MJ. Iatrogenic neurotoxicity in cancer patients. *Pain* 1989;39:1–4.
60. Beaver WT, Wallenstein SL, Houde RW. A comparison of the analgesic effects of methotrimeprazine and morphine in patients with cancer. *Clin Pharmacol Ther* 1966;7:436–446.

61. Keats AS, Telford J, Kurosu Y. "Potentiation" of meperidine by promethazine. *Anesthesiology* 1961;22:31–41.
62. Houde RW. On assaying analgesics in man. In: Knighton RS, Dumke PR, eds. *Pain.* Boston: Little, Brown, 1966;183–196.
63. White L, Tursky B, Schwartz GE, eds. *Placebo: theory, research, and mechanisms.* New York: Guilford Press, 1985.
64. Spiro HM. *Doctors, patients, and placebos.* New Haven: Yale University Press, 1986.
65. Beecher HK, Keats AS, Mosteller F, Lasagna L. The effectiveness of oral analgesics (morphine, codeine, acetylsalicylic acid) and the problem of placebo "reactors" and "non-reactors." *J Pharmacol Exp Ther* 1953;109:393–400.
66. Laska E, Sunshine A. Anticipation of analgesia: a placebo effect. *Headache* 1973;13:1–11.
67. Gracely RH, Dubner R, Deeter WR, Wolskee PJ. Clinicians' expectations influence placebo analgesia (letter). *Lancet* 1985;1:43.
68. Karlowski TR, Chalmers TC, Frenkel LD, et al. Ascorbic acid for the common cold. A prophylactic and therapeutic trial. *JAMA* 1975;231:1038–1042.
69. Moscucci M, Byrne L, Weintraub M, Cox C. Blinding, unblinding, and the placebo effect: an analysis of patients' guesses of treatment assignment in a double-blind clinical trial. *Clin Pharmacol Ther* 1987;41:259–265.
70. Lavori PW, Louis TA, Bailar JC, Polansky M. Designs for experiments—parallel comparisons of treatment. *New Engl J Med* 1983;309:1291–1298.
71. Kaiko RF, Wallenstein SL, Rogers AG, Houde RW. Sources of variation in analgesic responses in cancer patients with chronic pain receiving morphine. *Pain* 1983;15:191–200.
72. Kaiko RF, Wallenstein SL, Rogers AG, Grabinski PY, Houde RW. Clinical analgesic studies and sources of variation in analgesic responses to morphine. In: Foley KM, Inturrisi CE, eds. *Opioid analgesics in the management of clinical pain. Advances in Pain Research and Therapy, vol 8.* New York: Raven Press, 1986;13–24.
73. Kaiko RF. Age and morphine analgesia in cancer patients with postoperative pain. *Clin Pharmacol Ther* 1980;28:823–826.
74. Belville JW, Forrest WH, Miller E, et al. Influence of age on pain relief from analgesics. *JAMA* 1971;217:1835–1841.
75. Taves DR. Minimization: a new method of assigning patients to treatment and control groups. *Clin Pharmacol Ther* 1974;15:443–453.
76. Beaver WT. Mild analgesics: a review of their clinical pharmacology. *Am J Med Sci* 1965;577–599.
77. U.S. Food and Drug Administration. *Guidelines for the clinical evaluation of analgesic drugs.* Washington, D.C.: U.S. Government Printing Office, 1979.
78. Jackson GL, Smith DA. Analgesic properties of mixtures of chlorpromazine with morphine and meperidine. *Ann Intern Med* 1956;45:640–652.
79. Sunshine A, Laska E, Meisner M, Morgan S. Analgesic studies of indomethacin as analyzed by computer techniques. *Clin Pharmacol Ther* 1964;5:699–707.
80. Ramsey FL. A Bayesian approach to bioassay. *Biometrics* 1972;28:841–858.
81. Kuo L. Bayesian bioassay design. *Ann Statistics* 1983;11:886–895.
82. Kuo L. Linear Bayes' estimators of the potency curve in bioassay. *Biometrika* 1988;75:91–96.
83. Beaver WT, Wallenstein SL, Houde RW, Rogers A. A clinical comparison of the effects of oral and intramuscular administration of analgesics: pentazocine and phenazocine. *Clin Pharmacol Ther* 1966;9:582–597.
84. Laska EM, Sunshine A, Mueller F, Elvers WB, Siegel C, Rubin A. Caffeine as an analgesic adjuvant. *JAMA* 1984;251:1711–1718.
85. Cornfield J. Comparative bioassays and the role of parallelism. *J Pharmacol Exp Ther* 1964;144:143–149.
86. Beaver WT, Feise GA. Twin crossover relative potency analgesic assays in man. I. Morphine vs. morphine. *J Clin Pharmacol* 1977;17:461–479.
87. Dixon WJ, Mood AM. A method for obtaining and analyzing sensitivity data. *J Am Statist Assoc* 1948;43:109–126.
88. Bolognese JA. A Monte Carlo comparison of three up-and-down designs for dose ranging. *Controlled Clin Trials* 1983;4:187–196.
89. Sheiner LB, Beal SL, Sambol NC. Study designs for dose-ranging. *Clin Pharmacol Ther* 1989;46:63–77.

90. Beaver WT. Combination analgesics. *Am J Med* 1984; (September 10 Suppl. 3A):38–53.
91. Laska EM, Meisner MJ. Hypothesis testing for combination treatments. In: Peace K, ed. *Statistical issues in drug research and development.* New York: Marcel Dekker, 1989.
92. Laska EM, Meisner MJ. Testing whether an identified treatment is best. *Biometrics* 1989;45: 1139–1151.
93. Levine JD, Gordon NC. Synergism between the analgesic actions of morphine and pentazocine. *Pain* 1988;33:369–372.
94. Loewe S. The problem of synergism and antagonism of combined drugs. *Arzneimittelforschung* 1953;3:285–290.
95. Carter WH Jr, Carchman RA. Mathematical and biostatistical methods for designing and analyzing complex chemical interactions. *Fundam Appl Toxicol* 1988;10:590–595.
96. Plummer JL, Short TG. Statistical modelling of the effects of drug combinations. *J Pharmacol Methods* 1990;23:297–309.
97. Brunden MN, Vidmar TJ, McKean JW. *Drug interactions and lethality analysis.* Boca Raton, Florida: CRC Press, 1988.
98. Lavigne GJ, Hargreaves KM, Schmidt EA, Dionne RA. Proglumide potentiates morphine analgesia for acute surgical pain. *Clin Pharmacol Ther* 1989;45:666–673.
99. Forbes JA, Beaver WT, Jones KF, Kehm CK. An evaluation of ibuprofen and ibuprofen-caffeine combinations in postoperative oral surgery pain. *Clin Pharmacol Ther* 1990, in press.
100. Houde RW, Wallenstein SL, Rogers A. Clinical pharmacology of analgesics. 1. A method of assaying analgesic effect. *Clin Pharmacol Ther* 1960;1:163–174.
101. James KE, Forrest WH, Rose RL. Crossover and noncrossover designs in four-point parallel line analgesic assays. *Clin Pharmacol Ther* 1985;37:242–252.
102. Louis TA, Lavori PW, Bailar JC, Polansky M. Crossover and self-controlled designs in clinical research. *New Engl J Med* 1984;310:24–31.
103. Brown BW Jr. The crossover experiment for clinical trials. *Biometrics* 1980;36:69–79.
104. Meier P, Free SM, Jackson GL. Reconsideration of methodology in studies of pain relief. *Biometrics* 1958;14:330–342.
105. Free SM, Peeters F. Statistical comparison of methods to evaluate analgetics. *J Chronic Dis* 1958;7:379–384.
106. Forrest WH, James KE, Ho TY. Residual analgesic effects of morphine in 55 four-period crossover analgesic studies. *Clin Pharmacol Ther* 1988;44:383–388.
107. Beaver WT, Feise GA. Twin crossover relative potency analgesic assays in man. I. Morphine vs. morphine. *J Clin Pharmacol* 1977;17:461–479.
108. Beaver WT, Feise GA. Twin crossover relative potency analgesic assays in man. II. Morphine vs. 8-methoxycyclazocine. *J Clin Pharmacol* 1977;17:480–489.
109. Jones B, Kenward MG. *Design and analysis of cross-over trials.* London: Chapman and Hall, 1989.
110. Laska EM, Meisner M, Kushner HB. Optimal crossover designs in the presence of carryover effects. *Biometrics* 1983;39:1087–1091.
111. Laska EM, Meisner M. A variational approach to optimal two-treatment crossover designs: applications to carryover-effects models. *J Am Statist Assoc* 1985;80:704–710.
112. Cochran WG, Cox GM. *Experimental designs,* 2nd ed. New York: John Wiley & Sons, 1957.
113. Lan KKG, DeMets DL. Discrete sequential boundaries for clinical trials. *Biometrika* 1983;70: 649–653.
114. O'Brien PC, Fleming TR. A multiple testing procedure for clinical trials. *Biometrics* 1979;35: 549–556.
115. Pocock SJ. Group sequential methods in the design and analysis of clinical trials. *Biometrika* 1977;64:191–199.
116. Kaplan EL, Meier P. Non-parametric estimation from incomplete observations. *J Am Statist Assoc* 1958;53:457–481.
117. Cox DR, Hinckley DV. *Theoretical statistics.* London: Chapman and Hall, 1974.

Advances in Pain Research and Therapy, Vol. 18,
edited by M. Max, R. Portenoy, and E. Laska,
Raven Press, Ltd., New York © 1991.

Commentary

The VAS Relief Scale
and Other Analgesic Measures

Carryover Effect in Parallel and Crossover Studies

Stanley L. Wallenstein

Analgesic Studies, Sloan-Kettering Institute (retired), New York, New York 10021

I would like to present some new perspectives on two relatively unrelated but significant issues as a supplement to the excellent discussion of the state of the art in the large and complex area of clinical analgesic research, and illustrate them with examples from our own work at the Memorial Sloan-Kettering Cancer Center. First I will discuss the relative merits of a variety of analgesic measurement tools, with special emphasis on the Visual Analogue Scale for relief. Second, I will present some relatively unconventional thoughts on carryover effects, and how they relate to crossover and parallel-group analgesic studies.

ANALGESIC SCALES

The categorical scale for relief consists of two absolute categories at polar ends of the scale, "no relief" and "complete relief," and usually three categories in between, "slight," "moderate," and "lots" of relief. The sensitivity of the scale is a function of these categories. The visual analogue relief scale (VAS relief), which we use, is a 10-cm line bounded on the left by "no relief of pain" and on the right by "complete relief of pain." Patients are free to evaluate their relief and mark the scale at any point along the line, or indeed at the boundaries. Measurements are customarily made in terms of millimeters from the "no relief" boundary, providing, in effect, a 100-point relief scale (Chapter 4, Fig. 1). Responses on the categorical and VAS relief scales bear a linear relationship to one another, demonstrating that arithmetic increments on one scale are proportional to arithmetic increments on the other.

This relationship contrasts with the relationship that exists between the VAS and the categorical pain intensity difference (PID) scales when the VAS PID

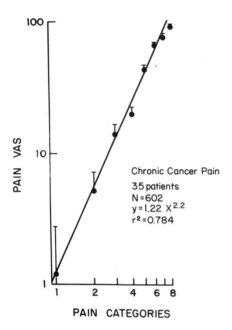

Chronic Cancer Pain

35 patients
N = 602
$y = 1.22 \ X^{2.2}$
$r^2 = 0.784$

FIG. 1. Power function of VAS pain intensity and the categorical scale for extended pain score. The pain categories are, in order: no pain, just noticeable, weak, mild, moderate, strong, severe, and excruciating. (From ref. 2, with permission.)

scale and an eight-point extended categorical PID scale are compared. The following pain categories are employed in the extended scale: no pain, just noticeable, weak, mild, moderate, strong, severe, and excruciating. The scale is derived from an experimental model employed by Tursky (1) in which the eight selected pain categories were found to be related as a power function (log-log) to an electric shock stimulus. We employed this scale in clinical analgesic studies in an attempt to better define the meaning to the patient of responses along the VAS pain scale, and also to determine if the terms employed bore a similar relationship in patients with clinical pain to what Tursky found in volunteers in an experimental pain situation. We found that the relationship between the extended pain scale and the VAS pain scale in cancer patients is also best defined in terms of a power function (Fig. 1) (2). These results suggest some consistency in the way patients and volunteers in experimental situations employ words to define pain. They also suggest that the discrete categories of pain used in clinical analgesic studies may not bear a linear relationship to one another. This is in contrast to the linear relationship we found to exist between categorical and VAS pain relief scales. There is some evidence that the log conversion of the extended pain scale provided analgesic measures equal or superior to other peak or total, categorical or VAS analgesic, measures in terms of assay sensitivity in a relative potency assay (3).

The VAS relief scale has been employed in a variety of analgesic studies in different pain populations both in the United States and in England, including a variety of postoperative pains and chronic cancer pain. Table 1 summarizes

TABLE 1. *Relative potencies, 95% confidence limits, and lambdas[a] for studies employing a variety of categorical and visual analogue parameters of analgesia*

Study	Design	Parameter[b]	N	Lambda	R	95%	Limits
Morphine,	Twin[c] 6 dose	Peak VAS relief	337	1.45	5.45	0.45	12.20
buprenorphine	postop	Peak relief	339	1.78	3.57	Infinite	
(6)		Peak VAS PID	334	1.95	6.20	Infinite	
		Peak PID	339	2.35	4.02	Infinite	
Morphine,	Twin 6 dose	Peak VAS relief	231	0.90	0.06	0.03	0.11
meptazinol (7)	postop	Peak relief	240	0.86	0.07	0.04	0.11
		Peak VAS PID	231	0.92	0.08	0.04	0.15
		Peak PID	240	0.72	0.09	0.06	0.15
Morphine,	Twin 6 dose +	Peak VAS relief	287	1.21	0.09	0.04	0.25
fenaprofen,	ASA postop	Peak relief	288	1.22	0.07	0.03	0.16
aspirin (8)		Peak VAS PID	287	2.00	0.07	0.00	2.36
		Peak PID	288	1.60	0.06	0.01	0.22
Morphine IM,	Twin 4 dose	Peak VAS relief	40	0.36	0.15	0.05	0.35
zomepirac PO	postop	Peak relief	40	0.56	0.12	Infinite	
(9)							
Morphine 8 & 16	Twin 4 dose	Peak VAS relief	56	0.36	3.27	1.21	4.66
IM, heroin, 2 &	postop	Peak relief	69	0.53	3.30	0.53	6.56
4 IM (10)		Peak VAS PID	54	0.33	4.25	0.23	6.54
		Peak PID		0.65	3.13	Infinite	
Morphine, 8 & 16	Twin 4 dose	Peak VAS relief	65	0.53	2.60	1.10	3.77
IM, heroin, 4 &	postop	Peak relief	65	0.68	2.22	Infinite	
8 IM (10)		Peak VAS PID	64	0.70	2.30	Infinite	
		Peak PID	78	0.76	1.85	Infinite	
Methadone IM,	Twin 4 dose	Peak VAS relief	148	1.52	0.10	Infinite	
LAAM IM	postop	Peak relief	149	1.37	0.14	0.03	0.44
		Peak VAS PID	148	1.17	0.23	Infinite	
		Peak PID	149	1.31	0.26	Infinite	
Morphine,	Twin 4 dose	Peak VAS relief	150	0.82	0.10	0.00	0.17
meperidine	postop	Peak relief	152	0.86	0.09	0.00	0.17
		Peak VAS PID	150	2.11	0.03	Infinite	
		Peak PID	152	1.19	0.04	Infinite	
Heroin,	Parallel group 4	Peak VAS relief	161	0.63	4.30	1.92	5.22
hydromorphone	dose postop	Peak relief	161	0.60	3.65	1.44	5.09
(3)		Peak VAS PID	161	0.59	5.85	2.41	6.36
		Peak PID	161	0.58	4.99	2.89	5.28
Morphine, 8 & 16	Complete	Peak VAS relief	263	2.18	2.27	Infinite	
IM, heroin, 4 &	crossover 4	Peak relief	263	3.55	6.69	Infinite	
8 IM (11)	dose chronic	Peak VAS PID	263	3.77	1.08	Infinite	
	cancer	Peak PID	263	6.78	13.73	Infinite	
Morphine, IM, PO	Complete	Peak VAS relief	84	1.25	0.07	Infinite	
	crossover 4	Peak relief	84	1.34	0.05	Infinite	
	dose chronic	Peak VAS PID	84	0.87	0.06	Infinite	
	cancer	Peak PID	84	2.87	0.04	Infinite	

[a] Lambda is the ratio of common slope to the standard error. In general, the smaller the value of lambda, the more sensitive the assay.

[b] "Peak relief" and "Peak PID" scores were based on standard categorical scales of relief.

[c] "Twin" refers to twin crossover, a particular incomplete block design.

our experiences with this and the other major analgesic parameters for measuring peak drug effects in 11 studies and over 1,800 comparisons. Study designs include parallel group and complete and incomplete (twin) crossover relative potency assays in patients with chronic cancer pain or postoperative pain. The value lambda, calculated as the standard error divided by the common slope for the test drugs in a parallel-line bioassay, represents a measure of assay efficiency independent of the parameter employed (4). The lower the value of lambda, the more sensitive the assay. By this measure, in 8 of the 11 assays in the table, the VAS peak relief scales were more sensitive measures of drug and dose differences than the corresponding categorical scales, and in five instances, VAS peak relief provided valid relative potency assays with finite confidence limits whereas other parameters failed to do so. In contrast, the categorical scale for peak relief produced a valid assay in only one instance when the VAS scale failed to do so.

The ability of the analogue scales to measure smaller changes in effect than can be observed with ordinal scales having a limited number of categories may also contribute to the increased sensitivity of the VAS scales in terms of peak effect. Analysis of total effects produce similar results; however, the differences between VAS and categorical total pain relief (TOTPAR) are not as striking as those obtained in terms of peak effects. In our experience, total scores on all scales are more sensitive measures of drug effects than are corresponding peak scores. Thus, differences between VAS and categorical measures of total effect are not as critical for assay sensitivity as corresponding differences among peak measures. This is particularly true in studies where relatively large numbers of patients contribute to the stability of the results.

There are other inherent advantages to VAS relief scales that, although theoretical rather than statistical, are nevertheless meaningful. Pain intensity difference scores are calculated and derived, and are numerically dependent on the pain level at 0 hour. In an attempt to free the PID scores from the mathematical limitations of dependence on initial pain, some investigators have calculated intensity difference scores based on percent of maximum possible effect (5), and this appears to lend some stability to analgesic scores based on the PID scales. Relief scales, on the other hand, being direct measures of effect, offer certain practical and theoretical advantages over pain intensity scales. The interpretation of the meaning of the VAS relief scale is simplified and straightforward as a result of its linear relationship to the usually employed categorical relief scales, and the 100 mm VAS relief scale provides a direct reading of analgesia which, in effect, is equivalent to the percent of maximal effect as calculated for PID. It avoids the problems in interpretation of PID scores when patients start at different pain-intensity levels. This can be most important in some special situations, such as in pharmacokinetic studies correlating analgesic effect with blood level, where the VAS relief scale is the parameter of choice.

CARRYOVER EFFECTS IN PARALLEL-GROUP AND CROSSOVER STUDIES

Carryover effects can involve anything from direct or indirect drug interactions to psychological carryover, and when present in a clinical analgesic study, may influence reported treatment effects. The possibility of carryover is often presented as a justification for the preference of parallel group over crossover design as the methodology of choice for clinical analgesic studies, with the implication that the problem of carryover is unique to crossover studies. Carryover may indeed occur among treatments in a crossover study, and may be temporal, pharmacological, or psychological. The possibility of their influencing results should be taken into account in the study design and analysis. However, interactions need not be limited to treatments specified within the study design, nor need they be limited to crossover studies. The potential for carryover exists in any clinical analgesic study, regardless of design.

With the possible exception of some special pain models, it is common for patients on analgesic studies to have received other analgesics, or drugs that may influence analgesic response, prior to being placed on study. This is the case for patients in postoperative studies who will have received other drugs in surgery or in the recovery room, and it is obviously applicable for patients with chronic pain. The problem of the influence of prior treatments external to the study will exist whether the study design is crossover or parallel group, but it is rarely examined, as it is not usually a routine part of analgesic study design and analysis to examine the effects of treatments prior to the time when patients enter the study. In an attempt to define some of the dimensions of this problem, we evaluated a variety of demographic factors, including aspects of prior drug experience, as part of our analgesic assay of heroin and hydromorphone. The study was a parallel group assay in cancer patients with postoperative pain after a variety of surgical procedures including abdominal procedures, thoracotomies, orthopedic procedures, and excisions of soft tissue cancers. Some of the patients had had preoperative pain owing to cancer, which had been treated with opiates. All patients received analgesics for pain as needed after surgery prior to being placed on study on the second postoperative day. The statistical evaluation included covariate analysis for time since last analgesic, amount of narcotic taken in the prior 48 hrs (in terms of morphine equivalents), and the length of time the patients were on narcotics prior to surgery (Table 2) (3).

TABLE 2. *Analysis of variance for VAS TOTPAR by treatments with covariates, and relative potency estimate for VAS TOTPAR and VAS peak relief for heroin and hydromorphone*

Source of variation	df	Mean square	F	Level of significance
Covariates	5	270390.437	16.124	<.001
Age	1	51214.212	3.054	.083
Last analgesic	1	132205.452	7.884	.006
Opioid history				
48 hrs	1	216606.690	12.917	<.001
Duration	1	5592.996	0.334	>.1
VAS PI 0 hr	1	24390.767	1.454	>.1
Treatments	3	90594.341	5.402	.001
Pooled regression	1	252408.337	15.011	<.001
Parallelism	1	1623.292	0.097	>.1
Preparations	1	10910.176	0.649	>.1
Error	152	16769.425		
Relative potency	VAS TOTPAR 5.630 (3.844–5.325)		VAS peak relief 4.301 (1.918–5.218)	

df, degrees of freedom; F, the ratio of the mean square for each individual source of variation to the mean square for the study error; PI, pain intensity.
From ref. 3, with permission.

Both time since last analgesic and amount of narcotic consumed in the prior 48 hrs proved to be highly significant covariance factors influencing analgesic response in this study. The analgesic score (VAS TOTPAR) was negatively correlated with the amount of narcotic consumed in the prior 48 hrs and was positively correlated with time since the prior analgesic. Whether these findings resulted from more frequent narcotic consumption owing to increased narcotic tolerance, or from increased levels of pain, or a combination of these factors, is a matter of speculation. In any event they can be looked on as measures of pain behavior, and taking them into account result in a considerable increase in assay sensitivity, even in a parallel group assay such as this.

These results clearly demonstrate that carryover is not limited to crossover studies. If one assumes no carryover in this type of parallel-group study, one is adopting an unrealistic "out of sight, out of mind" approach. Parallel-group studies can hide but not cure the problem of prior drug interaction in analgesic studies. In this sense they offer no advantage over crossover studies. It is our conviction that wherever feasible crossover studies of analgesics should be carried out. The crossover design can not only provide increased precision over parallel-group studies, but also offers the capability, not found in parallel-group studies, of evaluating for potential interaction among the study drugs. The statistical evaluation of the extent and significance of carryover resulting from treatments within the study can only be carried out in appropriately designed crossover studies, and this can indeed be worthwhile and important clinical information in treating patients with pain. Parallel-group studies by their very nature cannot provide this potentially useful information and merely leave the problem of carryover to speculation about a potential unknown.

REFERENCES

1. Tursky B. The development of a pain perception profile: a psychological approach. In: Weisenberg W, Tursky B, eds. *Pain: new perspectives in therapy and research.* New York: Plenum Press, 1976;171–194.
2. Wallenstein SL. Scaling clinical pain and pain relief. In: Bromm B, ed. *Pain measurement in man: neurophysiological correlates of pain.* Amsterdam: Elsevier, 1984;389.
3. Wallenstein SL, Houde RW, Portenoy R, Lapin J, Rogers A, Foley KM. Clinical analgesic assay of repeated and single doses of heroin and hydromorphone. *Pain* 1990;41:5–13.
4. Gaddum JH. Bioassays and mathematics. *Pharmacol Rev* 1953;5:87–134.
5. Laska EM, Sunshine A, Zighelboim I, Roure C, Marrero I, Wanderling J, Olsen N. Effects of caffeine on acetaminophen analgesia. *Clin Pharmacol Ther* 1983;33:498–509.
6. Wallenstein SL, Kaiko RF, Rogers AG, Houde RW. Crossover trials in clinical analgesic assays: studies of buprenorphine and morphine. *Pharmacotherapy* 1986;6(5):228–235.
7. Kaiko RF, Wallenstein SL, Rogers AG, Canel A, Jacobs B, Houde RW. Intramuscular meptazinol and morphine in postoperative pain. *Clin Pharmacol Ther* 1985;37:589–596.
8. Kaiko RF, Wallenstein SL, Lapin J, Houde RW. Oral fenoprofen compared to intramuscular morphine and oral aspirin in cancer patients with postoperative pain: relative analgesic potency, effectiveness, side effects, mood and age. In: Harris LS, ed. *National Institute on Drug Abuse Monograph Series: Problems of drug dependence, 1983.* Washington, DC: U.S. Government Printing Office, 1984;205–211.

9. Wallenstein SL, Rogers AG, Kaiko RF, Heidrich G, Houde RW. Relative analgesic potency of oral zomepirac and intramuscular morphine in cancer patients with postoperative pain. *J Clin Pharmac* 1980;20(No 4, Part 2):250–258.

10. Kaiko RF, Wallenstein SL, Rogers AG, Grabinski PY, Houde RW. Analgesic potency, mood and side effects of heroin and morphine in cancer patients with postoperative pain. *N Engl J Med* 1981;304:1501–1505.

11. Kaiko RF, Wallenstein SL, Rogers AG, Grabinski PY, Houde RW. Clinical analgesic studies of intramuscular heroin and morphine in postoperative and chronic pain. In: Foley KM, Inturrisi CE, eds. *Opioid analgesics in the management of clinical pain. Advances in pain research and therapy, vol 8.* New York: Raven Press, 1986;107–116.

Advances in Pain Research and Therapy, Vol. 18,
edited by M. Max, R. Portenoy, and E. Laska,
Raven Press, Ltd., New York © 1991.

Commentary

Outcome Measures
and the Effect of Covariates

Howard T. Thaler

*Department of Epidemiology and Biostatistics, Memorial Sloan-Kettering
Cancer Center, New York, New York 10021*

Single dose, controlled clinical trials have been used extensively to evaluate efficacy of analgesics in a hospital setting. Design and analysis considerations for such trials are discussed at length and amply referenced by Max and Laska in Chapter 4. Here we elaborate on particular approaches to two aspects: choice of outcome measures and incorporation of information on prognostic factors. Patients in these trials were asked to rate pain intensity and relief at regular intervals by marking visual analogue scales (VAS) or selecting from a set of verbal descriptors. The sequences of measurements recorded following each administration of a test dose to a patient need to be summarized and studied not only in relation to the current drug and dose, but also in relation to other quantitative and qualitative information available on the patient, called covariates, that may be determinants of analgesic response.

Traditional analyses taking the area under the time-effect curve as a single outcome measure were, and still are, very useful. It became apparent, however, that the analgesic response may be multifaceted. Appropriate choice of two or more summary values can facilitate study of the temporal pattern of analgesia. Furthermore, identification of statistically significant covariates can lead to improved accuracy of drug effect estimates and aid in the design of more efficient future trials. Since definitive results pertaining to either of these goals require larger samples than would usually be available in a single trial, data from several trials run under similar conditions need to be combined.

This chapter considers a combination of simple summary values that correlate with duration of relief and peak effect, namely, time to remedication (remed time) and maximum VAS pain relief score (maxVPR), respectively. Multiple linear regression is used to establish the relation between these two outcome variables and a set of covariates describing demographic, clinical, and prior treatment factors in a large data base.

DESCRIPTION OF DATA SOURCE

A data base comprising results of over 2,600 administrations of test drugs from a series of clinical trials conducted at Memorial Sloan-Kettering Cancer Center between 1976 and 1987 provided a basis for studying data summaries and covariate effects with statistical power not otherwise attainable. The trials were either parallel group or crossover designs intended to evaluate the relative potency and efficacy of opioids, both investigative drugs and standard treatment, in chronic cancer and postoperative pain models.

To achieve greater homogeneity of the study sample, analyses were limited to postoperative patients only and to the drug most frequently used in these trials: 4, 8, or 16 mg doses of intramuscular morphine, yielding a total of 614 observations in 8 trials. Although heterogeneity still remains with respect to such factors as sequencing of morphine doses relative to other study and nonstudy drugs, type of cancer, and type of surgery, limiting the sample strengthens the results establishing the importance of evaluating covariates vis-à-vis different summary values in a particular clinical setting. The analyses need to be repeated for other drugs and patient groups.

Patients rated their pain immediately prior to the test dose, and rated pain intensity and relief at hourly intervals thereafter, until they required remedication (generally, when pain returned to, or exceeded, the initial level) or to a maximum of 6 hrs. VAS scores ranged from 0 to 100 according to the positions marked on the pain evaluation cards.

Relevant information for each patient could be classified as demographic (age, sex, race, height, weight), clinical (initial pain intensity, site, and character, and time since surgery) and treatment-related (length of prior opioid exposure, total morphine-equivalent dosage in past 48 hrs, time since last previous dose, and test dose). These formed the basis of the analysis of prognostic factors. Data on other potentially important covariates, such as type and extent of surgery, biochemical profile, concomitant medication, or presence of pertinent medical conditions, were not readily available. Kaiko et al. (1) conducted an analysis of sources of variation in analgesic responses based on an earlier series of trials limited to two doses of morphine in chronic cancer pain. They used total pain relief (TOTPAR) as a single outcome based on categorical rather than VAS scores and did not have access to detailed prior treatment data. Wallenstein (pp. 101–102) refers to a more limited covariate analysis in a single trial of hydromorphone versus heroin.

SUMMARIZING TWO DIMENSIONS OF ANALGESIA

The shapes of time-effect curves that are the basis of summary values such as total pain relief (TOTPAR) and sum of pain intensity difference (SPID) depend on several components, such as time of onset of meaningful relief, peak effect, time to peak effect, and duration of meaningful relief. These components tend to be interrelated. For example, earlier onset may correlate with greater peak relief. Nevertheless, curve shapes can vary substantially between patient characteristics or between drugs that differentially affect the components of response. A change in TOTPAR or SPID may be attributable to a change in any or all of the components.

It is useful, therefore, to consider multiple summary values as they relate to prognostic factors and treatment. The analyses in this commentary focus on two such summaries: remed time as a behavioral correlate of duration of analgesia and maxVPR as an approximation to peak effect. These two outcomes had a correlation of 0.531 in the data under study. Although they may not be an optimal choice, they are simple and useful in demonstrating several points.

TIME-EFFECT CURVES

Observations can be grouped according to remed time in order to explore the temporal pattern of analgesia. Table 1 shows the overall distribution of remed times in the study sample. When mean VAS pain relief (VPR) is plotted versus time for each group, assuming zero initial relief, several patterns are seen (Fig. 1). Patients who remedicated later tended to have more rapid onset, and greater, later, and more prolonged peak effect. Note that patients remedicated with near-zero relief except at 6 hrs, suggesting that the latter group included patients remedicating simply because the study ended.

A similar plot for mean VAS pain intensity shows the complementary pattern (2), with the peak of pain relief corresponding to the "trough" of pain intensity. However, another aspect emerges that bears on an assumption made in computing SPID, namely, that pain intensity difference never goes below zero and remains at zero from remed time (or other stopping time) until the "projected" end of the study. Patients remedicating before 6 hrs tend to do so at a higher

TABLE 1. *Distribution of remedication times*[a]

Hours after test dose	Number remedicating	Percent	Cumulative percent
1	4	0.7	0.7
2	82	13.4	14.0
3	183	29.8	43.8
4	127	20.7	64.5
5	68	11.1	75.6
6	61	9.9	85.5
>6	89	14.5	100.0
	Total 614		

[a] Nearly 76% of patients remedicated before the projected end of the observation period. Patients in "6 hr" and ">6 hr" groups were combined for subsequent covariate analyses but only "6 hr" patients were included in Figs. 1 and 2.

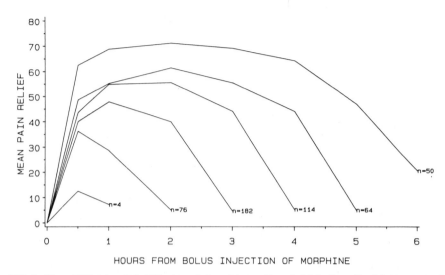

FIG. 1. Mean VAS pain relief at 30 min and at each hour after administration of test dose, grouped by remedication time in order to more precisely display time-effect curves. Only patients with full VAS data are included.

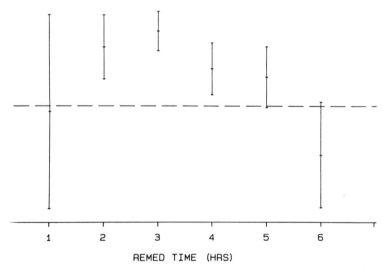

FIG. 2. Means of final VAS pain intensity minus initial VAS pain intensity (mean $\pm$ 2 SEM) grouped by remedication time. Only four patients remedicated at 1 hr. "Overshoot" decreases from 2 and 3 hrs to 4 and 5 hrs. Some patients remedicating at 6 hrs did so only because the study ended.

level of pain than they had initially and this difference is greater at 2 or 3 hrs than at 4 or 5 hrs remed time (Fig. 2).

COVARIATE RESULTS

All of the covariates enumerated above that were statistically significant when tested univariately for their relationship to either outcome variable were included in an analysis of covariance. Any that were no longer significant when adjusted for the other covariates were eliminated, leaving seven in the final model that are coded in Table 2. The direction of the correlation with both outcome measures was the same for each covariate, but in some instances the strength of relationship differed markedly. Notably, older age was a strong predictor of longer remed time ($p < 0.001$) but not significantly related to maxVPR. Kaiko (3) found similar results. Conversely, low initial level of pain was a very strong predictor of high maxVPR ($p < 0.0001$) but only marginally related to remed time. The existence of differences in prognostic factors supports the hypothesis that these two outcomes represent different components of the analgesic responses, although the correlation between them after adjusting for covariates and treatment remains at a level of 0.434.

THE IMPORTANCE OF COVARIATES

Knowledge of covariate effects may give clues to the study of factors influencing both pain and analgesic effectiveness and can be used in determining dosage requirements for individual patients. In terms of the technical aspects of study design, incorporation of covariates into the statistical model for evaluating a

TABLE 2. *Results of covariate analyses showing coding used, direction of factors favorable for better response, and regression coefficients for both outcome measures*

Covariate	Coding units	Favorable direction	Regression coefficients[a] Remed time	Max VPR
Age	years/10	Older	0.127^2	—
Sex	1 = male, −1 = female	Female	-0.150^2	3.52^2
Initial pain[b]		Lower	-0.102^1	5.55^3
Time since surgery	1, 2, 3⁺ days	Longer	0.355^3	5.74^2
Time since last analgesic	≤3, 4, . . . , 7⁺ hr	Longer	0.161^3	1.31^1
Prior time on opioids[c]		Shorter	-0.068^1	-2.09^2
Prior exposure (48 hrs)	mg. equiv. morph./10	Less	-0.486^2	-5.33^1
Log test dose	4, 8, 16 mg = 0, 1, 2	More	0.423^3	8.42^3

[a] Statistical significance for the test that the regression coefficient for each covariate is zero, adjusted for all other covariates in the model: 1, $0.05 < p < 0.09$; 2, $0.0001 < p < 0.001$; 3, $p < 0.0001$.

[b] Tursky scale responses were used for initial pain in order to include remed time data for which VAS was unavailable.

[c] Prior time on opioids was scored as follows: 0, none; 1, <1 day; 2, 1–3 days; 3, 4–7 days; 4, 8–14 days; 5, 15–31 days; 6, 2 months; 7, 2–6 months; 8, >6 months.

particular treatment will reduce the unexplained, experimental variation in the data and thereby increase the accuracy of estimates of efficacy and relative potency. This will improve the chances for statistically significant conclusions or, conversely, reduce the required sample size when planning a trial.

For the data described in this commentary, adjusting for the covariates in the analysis reduced the error variance for measuring the slope of the linear regression on log dose by 17% for remed time and by 11% for maxVPR. Although even the unadjusted estimates of dose-response slopes were accurate and highly significant in this large data base, the same percent improvement owing to covariate analysis could make the difference between significant and nonsignificant results in a single, smaller trial.

POOLING DATA FROM DIFFERENT STUDIES

In the results described thus far, we have implicitly assumed that the clinical trials from which the data were drawn were similar enough in terms of patient populations and the way in which they were conducted that their results could be pooled. The trials covered a span of 10 years during which changes could have occurred in the patient population and in concomitant medication. There were variations in study design, in the order in which morphine was administered, and in the drug(s) being compared with morphine. Nevertheless, "poolability" is partially a statistically testable hypothesis using analysis of covariance with "study" as a classification variable and including the significant covariates as well as test dose of morphine. In fact, differences in overall levels of response between studies were at most marginally significant when adjusted for covariates, and the slope of the log dose versus response regression line was not different between studies for either outcome. Nevertheless, one should exercise caution when pooling data and look for factors that explain any apparent differences between studies.

SUMMARY

In this commentary we have used a large data base of clinical trials to illustrate an approach to two issues in the analysis of the results of single-dose analgesic clinical such trials: the use of more than one summary outcome measure and the importance of incorporating information on prognostic factors, or covariates, in statistical analyses. Time to remediation and maximum VAS pain relief were chosen as two simple summary values that correlate with duration of analgesia and peak effect, respectively. Although not independent of each other, they in part represent two dimensions of response, and grouping by remed time was useful in depicting the temporal pattern of analgesia. Analysis of covariance was used to evaluate the statistical significance of prognostic factors vis-à-vis each outcome measure and was shown to improve the accuracy with which drug effects could be estimated. The importance of incorporating covariate information in study design and analysis has been demonstrated and differences in significance of covariates for the two outcome measures studied suggest that the analgesic response is more than one-dimensional. The following topics are suggested for further study:

1. Other measures of the components of analgesic response such as (a) direct "stopwatch" recording of onset and duration of relief and (b) use of more efficient weighted averages of currently available, repeated measurements of pain intensity and relief ratings to replace or amplify TOTPAR and SPID.

2. Parametric statistical modeling of time-effect curves, including multivariate analysis that considers the inherent correlation between outcome measures with respect to drug and covariate effects.

3. Expansion of the list of potentially relevant prognostic factors and replication of the analyses on other patient groups and for other drugs, where the covariate effects may in fact differ.

ACKNOWLEDGMENT

I would like to thank Dr. Raymond W. Houde, Stanley L. Wallenstein, and Ada G. Rodgers, whose years of devoted research developed the data base on which these analyses were based.

REFERENCES

1. Kaiko RF, Wallenstein SL, Rogers AG, Houde RW. Sources of variation in analgesic responses in cancer patients with chronic pain receiving morphine. *Pain* 1983;15:191–200.
2. Thaler HT, Friedlander-Klar H, Cirrincione C, Portenoy RK, Wallenstein SL, Foley KM, Houde RW. A statistical approach to measuring analgesic response. In Bond MR, Charlton J, Woolf C, eds. *Proceedings of the VIth World Congress on Pain.* Amsterdam: Elsevier, 1991, in press.
3. Kaiko RF. Age and morphine analgesia in cancer patients with postoperative pain. *Clin Pharmacol Ther* 1980;28:823–826.

Advances in Pain Research and Therapy, Vol. 18,
edited by M. Max, R. Portenoy, and E. Laska,
Raven Press, Ltd., New York © 1991.

Commentary

Pain Measurement Scales in Single-Dose Comparisons

Bernard P. Schachtel

*Medical Department, Whitehall Laboratories, Inc., New York, New York 10017;
and Clinical Epidemiology Unit, Yale University
School of Medicine, New Haven, Connecticut 06510*

Assay sensitivity, the ability to demonstrate the statistically significant activity of an analgesic agent compared to placebo or to another agent, represents a noteworthy achievement for any analgesic trial. It is particularly praiseworthy when one considers the minimal sample size that is employed in most analgesic trials, in contrast to the much larger sizes of other therapeutic trials. Indeed, even known active agents, our so-called positive controls, cannot be distinguished from placebo in every clinical study.

Beyond this feat, often expected as ordinary, lies the ultimate challenge to the clinical investigator—upside assay sensitivity, the comparison of one active drug with another or comparison between doses of an active drug. Besides those mentioned by Max and Laska (Chapter 4), there are other features of the "successful" study that should be heeded to enhance the sensitivity of a pain model. In their discussion of the type of patient to be evaluated, for example, Max and Laska cite the condition being evaluated as a determination of the homogeneous status of patients before treatment. Within each diagnosis, however, lie several cogent clinical features that may distinguish one patient with a diagnosed condition from another patient with the same condition. For example, as Bloomfield et al. (1) and Kantor et al. (2) have shown in their work, the postpartum patient with severe postepisiotomy pain *and* severe uterine cramps differs from the patient with predominantly severe postepisiotomy pain. These and other clinical features may have prognostic import: the primiparous woman suffering postepisotomy pain may have a different reaction to pain than the multiparous woman, as may the constipated postpartum patient, or the extremely anxious patient, etc. The clinical features that can influence patient response to an analgesic agent should be taken into account, if possible, to assure baseline homogeneity. Unless specified *a priori,* these factors can reduce the sensitivity of an assay considerably.

In our research on patients with sore throat (3,4) for example, we were able to distinguish another feature of the general condition being evaluated as a potentially confounding variable. Just as the postepisiotomy condition does not exclusively classify the state of a postpartum patient, the patient with a sore throat will have other expressions of upper respiratory infection, too. If nasal congestion coexists with a sore throat, as it often does, the patient may be forced to mouth-breathe, causing dryness in the throat, thus confounding his/her assessment of throat pain. If this clinical hunch had not been identified, we would not have been able to show the efficacy of aspirin or acetaminophen in relieving throat pain (Chapter 17, Fig. 4). However, when patients without severe nasal congestion and mouth-breathing are examined, both agents were readily distinguished from placebo (Chapter 17, Fig. 5).

The precision used to define the clinical condition associated with sore throat pain (3,4), in fact, is primarily responsible for the sensitivity of the sore throat pain model (see Chapter 17). In several clinical trials, its sensitivity has been consistently observed. Similar to Cooper's dental impaction model (p. 117), the sore throat pain model has a reproducibly low placebo response, leaving much "room" for the detection of analgesia by positive controls, such as aspirin 650 mg, and to evaluate stronger analgesics. In general, specification of cogent clinical features is necessary both to obtain baseline homogeneity and to discern treatment effects.

Equally important as attention to the pretreatment status of patients, the construction of rating scales for use *after* treatment is critical to the success or failure of a clinical trial. The visual analogue scale, for example, has drawn much attention as a relatively new, sensitive device for measuring pain intensity or relief (5). However, a word of caution is in order concerning the anchor words for this scale. As can be appreciated from our experience during a pilot study we were conducting on a musculoskeletal pain model (6), the words themselves can influence a subject's response on the scale. At the last assessment of pain from an acute sprained ankle, a divinity school graduate student completed a 10-cm visual analogue pain intensity scale (with "no pain" on the left extreme and "severe pain" on the right) by placing a mark corresponding to approximately 8 cm. Having just finished the study, with all rating scales collected, he agreed to complete another scale, identical to the other but having "worst pain possible" at the right extreme. On this scale, in response to the same question, "Place a line on the scale that best describes your pain now," his mark corresponded to approximately 3 cm. I asked him if his ankle pain had changed in the intervening 5 minutes or so, and he told me that the pain was the same. Showing him both scales, I asked him to explain the difference. The first represented how he felt, he said (and was certainly in accord with the trend of his ratings over the assessment period). But, he said, pointing to his pregnant wife and toddler, "She has the worst pain possible (during childbirth). I don't. That's why I gave my pain a lower score."

This vignette, though unconfirmed in a controlled trial, illustrates what is intuitively true: the choice of the anchor words for a visual analogue scale is key. To be useful, the words on this scale should be appropriate to the condition and meaningful to the patient.

There is another kind of visual analogue rating scale, the "quality-of-pain" rating scale. Rather than employ words of pain intensity or relief, these scales directly address a quality of pain that is specific to the pain condition being evaluated. We have pursued this line of investigation in different acute pain conditions by asking subjects to describe their pain using their own words. As Melzack and Torgerson (7) reported from their research, patients with acute pain tend to describe it with sensory terms (frequently those found in the clusters of sensory words in the McGill Pain Questionnaire). However, rather than administer the entire questionnaire repeatedly throughout a trial, as Heidrich et al. (8) and others have done, we have used the one or two words that are frequently selected by the subjects themselves and adapted these words to new visual analogue rating scales.

To be consistent, I will again cite an example from our sore throat research. In hundreds of interviews, patients with sore throat repeatedly described their difficulty swallowing, tantamount to the symptom of dysphagia which a clinician elicits from a patient. For the investigator, difficulty swallowing confers not only a sensory quality of the pain state but also a change over time as a result of therapy. Therefore, we designed a visual analogue rating scale for the patient with difficulty swallowing (9). When used to study ibuprofen 400 mg, acetaminophen 1,000 mg, and placebo, this scale indicated definite therapeutic effects (Chapter 17, Fig. 13). Although these results confirmed those from conventional rating scales (pain intensity and relief), it is noteworthy that they were obtained on patients with relatively mild baseline scores, lower than the baseline pain intensity scores. Furthermore, when we applied the conventional criterion of a relatively severe level to this new scale, though used by one-quarter fewer patients, the difficulty swallowing scale yielded the same statistically significant results. Now confirmed in other studies, these results suggest that this quality-of-pain scale is quite sensitive.

Concerning the categorical relief scale, one can speculate why it may be a more sensitive indicator of therapeutic effect than the categorical pain intensity scale, as several investigators have reported. One reason is that the relief scale relies on a *direct* assessment by the patient, in contrast to the pain intensity difference derived by the investigator. A similar scale that also permits the subject to make a direct assessment is the transitional change-in-pain scale (Chapter 17, Fig. 1). At one end of this visual analogue scale are the words "much worse"; at the other end "much better"; and in the middle, the word "same." The patient is asked to use this scale at each posttreatment time-point in response to the following question: "How does your pain compare now to the last time I asked you?" Thus the patient is making a direct comparison to how he felt half an hour or an hour ago. Just as the clinician in the office asks the patient, "How are you now (compared to the last time we spoke)?," the investigator can use this scale so that the patient can directly relate *change in pain,* with familiar terms as anchor words on the scale, yielding meaningful results (Chapter 17, Fig. 6). When properly explained to the patient, this change-in-pain scale complements and occasionally augments the pain intensity and relief rating scales.

In sum, as Max and Laska have succinctly summarized, the seminal efforts and achievements of Beecher, Lasagna, Houde, and Beaver have created the fundamental scientific tools of analgesiology, which they developed in single-dose pain models. The continued evaluation and refinement of these tools should facilitate future innovations and improvements in the study of analgesic agents.

REFERENCES

1. Bloomfield SS, Mitchell S, Cissell G, Barden TP. Analgesic sensitivity of two post-partum pain models. *Pain* 1986;27:171–179.
2. Kantor T, Sunshine A, Laska E, Meisner M. Different dose response curves for aspirin in two types of postpartum pains (abstract). *Fed Proc* 1966;25:501.
3. Schachtel BP, Fillingim JM, Beiter DJ, Lane AC, Schwartz LA. Subjective and objective features of sore throat. *Arch Intern Med* 1984;144:497–500.
4. Schachtel BP, Fillingim JM, Beiter DJ, Lane AC, Schwartz LA. Rating scales for analgesics in sore throat. *Clin Pharmacol Ther* 1984;36:151–156.
5. Sriwatanakul K, Lasagna L, Cox C. Evaluation of current clinical trial methodology in analgesimetry based on experts' opinions and analysis of several analgesic studies. *Clin Pharmacol Ther* 1983;34:277–283.
6. Schachtel BP, Sorrentino JV, Wooley BH, Davis B, Brown J. Qualities of pain rated as indicators of therapeutic response (abstract). *Clin Pharmacol Ther* 1985;37:226.
7. Melzack R, Torgerson WS. On the language of pain. *Anesthesiology* 1971;34:50–59.
8. Heidrich BG, Slavic-Svircen V, Kaiko RF. Efficacy and quality of ibuprofen and acetaminophen plus codeine analgesia. *Pain* 1985;22:385–397.
9. Schachtel BP, Fillingim JM, Thoden WR, Lane AC, Baybutt RI. Sore throat pain in the evaluation of mild analgesics. *Clin Pharmacol Ther* 1988;44:707–711.

Advances in Pain Research and Therapy, Vol. 18,
edited by M. Max, R. Portenoy, and E. Laska,
Raven Press, Ltd., New York © 1991.

Commentary

Single-Dose Analgesic Studies: The Upside and Downside of Assay Sensitivity

Stephen A. Cooper

*Division of Advanced Education, Temple University School of Dentistry,
Philadelphia, Pennsylvania 19140*

There are different pain models and varying methods for studying analgesic agents. The term "pain model" is being used to describe the type of pain being studied, e.g., orthopedic surgery, general postsurgical, postpartum, dental impaction, etc. Early in the clinical development of a drug, single-dose efficacy studies in a variety of pain models are used to determine the optimal analgesic dosage and time-effect of that drug as well as its relative efficacy to known standards. If an investigational drug is not efficacious in these early studies, the drug that looked so promising in the laboratory usually receives an early burial.

Single-dose studies could be faulted for not measuring the cumulative effects of a drug over several doses or days. However, there is some rationale for quickly eliminating an agent for use in *acute pain* that, on the very first dose, does not have some advantage over the standard treatments. The fact is that single-dose studies have been excellent predictors of efficacy for analgesics (1–3).

As was discussed in the preceding chapter, the ability of a study to establish statistically significant differences between treatments depends on several factors: the mean differences in effect between the treatments, the variance, and the sample size. This commentary will restrict itself to the first of these factors, proposing a method for comparing the spacing of effect levels among placebo, standard analgesics, and more powerful active agents that are commonly used pain models. In doing this, it is assumed that differences in cross-study variances are small and similar sample sizes are used. Special emphasis is placed on separating the aspirin-like standards from placebo (downside sensitivity) and the test treatments from these standards (upside sensitivity). In fact, separating active drug from placebo turns out to be rather easy in most pain models. The more difficult challenge is to select models that have adequate upside assay sensitivity. This issue revolves around both the amount of the efficacy scale that is being used by the standards and how much of the remaining scale is actually available for use by the test drugs. Theoretically, if aspirin uses 50% of the given analgesic efficacy scale, then 50% should be left. However, what seems intuitively obvious is clearly not a clinical reality.

This commentary illustrates a method for comparing levels of response to analgesics among commonly used pain models. If this information were available before initiating a study, then the model could be matched to the most appropriate standards and the study results might better distinguish the efficacy of the medications, instead of the results being manipulated by the limitations of the model. For example, in a very unfavorable model the placebo might consistently use 60% of the total pain relief (TOTPAR) scale, whereas the best any drug could achieve would be 80% of the scale. This leaves a mere 20% of the TOTPAR scale to statistically separate drugs, which, in most instances, would be a difficult task. In this situation, the variance would have to be quite small and the sample size large to separate treatment effects. A more ideal situation would be one in which the placebo uses only 15%, a typical standard 40 to 50%, and the best possible achiever 80%.

The data presented in this commentary explore the effect of placebo and aspirin and the practical limits of separating mean treatment effects in different pain models. The results are based on a survey of over 70 studies. The approach used to address this component of assay sensitivity centered around obtaining data from several established investigators that used similar methods in a variety of pain models. The literature was of some value; but many investigators do not publish whereas others published results with insufficient data. The majority of data used in this paper was obtained by direct written request to investigators. The data base suffers the inherent weaknesses of any retrospective study that sets specific inclusion criteria and then attempts to collect representative data. The studies had to be single dose, parallel group, double-blind, randomized, placebo controlled, six or more hourly observations, and use one or more orally administered nonsteroidal antiinflammatory drugs (NSAIDs). Any study found in the literature or submitted to us by an investigator that met these criteria was included in the data base.

With respect to the etiology of the pain, the postpartum and dental models were homogeneous, whereas the postsurgical studies represented a variety of general surgery procedures. No attempt was made to block the postsurgical studies by type of procedure. The dental pain studies were drawn mostly from dental impaction pain; but the model was further subdivided to compare dental impaction, dental extraction (nonimpaction), and periodontal postsurgical pain. Also, a comparison was made with the dental impaction studies between retaining patients for observations versus the use of take-home diaries. To the best of our knowledge, the studies from all models evaluated the first oral dose of pain medication taken by patients.

A derived measure known as "percentage *t*heoretical *m*aximum *T*OTPAR" (%TMT) was used for comparing pain models. The %TMT attempts to standardize across studies the scores derived from relief categorical scales using varying gradations. The formula is

$$\%TMT = \frac{\text{6-hr TOTPAR}}{\text{Theoretical Maximum TOTPAR}} \times 100$$

By comparing the same treatments both within a given pain model and then across pain models, it is possible to estimate both the consistency and one aspect of assay sensitivity of these models. With this information, it would then be possible to estimate the potential of a model for testing analgesics of different strengths. The 6-hr TOTPAR was chosen because TOTPAR has been recognized as a sensitive measure of efficacy and 6 hrs is a common time for drug evaluation. One could always argue the choice of efficacy measure, length of measured observation interval, criteria for study inclusion, and final choice of studies, but we feel that the method as well as the results fairly represent this important aspect of assay sensitivity. The concept of using percent scores to compare across study results was previously presented by Laska et al. (4).

In a 6-hr study using a five-point categorical scale (0–4) such as none (0), a little (1), some (2), a lot (3), or complete (4), the TMT is 24 (complete relief: $6 \times 4 = 24$). Since even the best drugs take some time to be effective and since pain can vary from patient to patient, it is logical that no drug can achieve the perfect mean score of 24. Another important issue relates to the percentage of the scale used by placebo. One way to look at assay sensitivity is as the difference between the portion of the scale used by placebo and the practical (not theoretical) maximum of that scale (Fig. 1). Of course, other variables not being discussed in detail such as variance and sample size also influence assay sensitivity. Using our own dental impaction studies as a reference, in a typical 6-hr study using a sample size of 40 per treatment group, it takes approximately 10% of the TOT-PAR scale (2.4 units) to demonstrate a statistically significant difference. Pain models with greater standard errors due to more variability or smaller sample sizes would require a greater percentage of the scale to demonstrate statistical significance, whereas models with smaller standard errors would require a correspondingly smaller percentage of the TMT to demonstrate statistical superiority.

Table 1 summarizes the %TMT for several studies in postpartum, postsurgical, and dental pain models.[a] These data suggest that in the particular studies selected, there are some clinically relevant differences among the models.

The dental impaction model achieved the lowest %TMT for placebo which, assuming equal variance across models, would permit the greatest opportunity for upside scale sensitivity. When the results for other investigators using the dental impaction model were compared to our own data set, the results were very similar. The other dental pain models—nonimpaction and periodontal—had a somewhat higher %TMT for placebo as did the postsurgical model, but all were under 25%. The postpartum model had the extremely high %TMT of over 40% for placebo. The range was from 27.9 to 50.4% (Table 1).

---

[a] All the published papers used in the tables are alphabetically referenced in Appendix A. All other data were submitted by the investigators and complete references were not available.

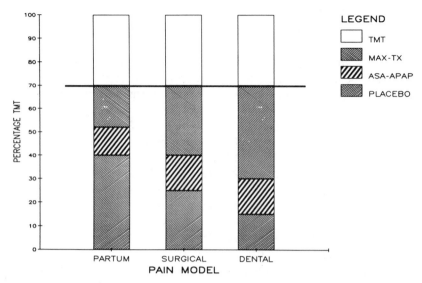

FIG. 1. The %TMT (percentage of total maximum TOTPAR) is used to demonstrate assay sensitivity and the ceiling effect in postpartum, postsurgical, and dental impaction pain models. The data in this figure are hypothetical and the *horizontal bar* at 70% represents an estimate of the maximum effect any drug could achieve. MAX-TMT denotes the effect of a powerful analgesic and ASA-APAP the effect of a standard dose of aspirin or acetaminophen in the respective pain models. The *horizontal bar* at 70% TMT indicates the approximate ceiling effect of a typical pain study.

TABLE 1. *Summary of percentage TMT data for postsurgical, postpartum, and dental impaction pain models*

Model	Treatment[a]		
	Placebo	Aspirin 650 mg	Standard treatment
Postsurgical	24.8 ± 2.0[c]	46.4 ± 9.1	39.8 ± 2.8
(n)	(16)	(3)	(15)
range	14.1–39.3	32.9–63.8	
Postpartum	41.9 ± 2.6	52.9 ± 3.5	—
(n)	(7)	(6)	
range	27.9–50.4	38.8–64.5	
Impaction	16.7 ± 2.4	27.1 ± 2.2	29.6 ± 2.9
(n)	(11)	(7)	(9)
range	8.7–35.1	17.4–35.3	
Impaction-C[b]	15.1 ± 0.8	28.1 ± 3.0	27.7 ± 2.3
(n)	(29)	(13)	(23)
range	7.1–24.8	11.8–47.3	

[a] Standards were either aspirin 600 to 650 mg, acetaminophen 500 to 1,000 mg, or codeine 60 mg. All medications were orally administered.

[b] C, Cooper studies.

[c] Means are the study means ± SE of study means.

Using aspirin 600 to 650 mg as the common standard, the models followed the same pattern as for placebo. The dental impaction model had the lowest %TMT (<30%) and the postpartum model the highest with 52% (Table 1). The postsurgical model demonstrated the largest separation between placebo and aspirin with over 22%, whereas the postpartum and dental impaction were closer to 10%.

The mean %TMT scores for test treatments are not included in Table 1. This was done intentionally to avoid presenting potentially misleading information on a potpourri of agents that, in many instances, actually may not have been any more efficacious than the standards. Nevertheless, it was interesting to observe that the best treatments in the entire data base were 78.9% (dental impaction), 75.8% (postpartum), and 69.2% (postsurgical). Only 13 of the surveyed studies had test treatments with a %TMT over 60%. It may be a reasonable assumption that 80% is a relative ceiling %TMT for any pain model. Overall, the differential between test treatments and placebo was greatest for the dental impaction model and smallest for the postpartum model. In the opinion of the author, the ceiling effect of most models evaluating oral analgesics will fall well below 80%. This has important implications when estimating the potential for upside assay sensitivity.

Using only our own data base of dental studies, the dental impaction model appeared potentially more sensitive than either the periodontal or nonimpaction dental models (Table 2). This was most evident with the lower %TMT for placebo. When the impaction studies were blocked for inpatient observations versus take-home diaries, the mean placebo response was lower with the inpatient technique; but the differences were small and both had placebo %TMTs under 20% (Table 3). In the 29 studies, none had a placebo %TMT over 25%, but the four that were over 20% all used the take-home diary. In looking at the response to aspirin 650 mg, there was only a 2% difference between the inpatient observations versus the take-home diary techniques.

TABLE 2. *Summary of percentage TMT data for dental pain models: Cooper data base*

	Treatment			
Model	Placebo	Standard treatment[a]	Aspirin 650 mg	Test treatment[b]
Impaction	15.1 ± 0.8[c]	27.7 ± 2.3	28.1 ± 3.0	43.6 ± 2.3
(n)	(29)	(23)	(13)	(25)
Nonimpaction	24.5 ± 5.0	47.9 ± 3.0	—	51.9 ± 4.2
(n)	(5)	(3)		(4)
Periodontal	23.0 ± 2.8	39.8 ± 3.8	39.3 ± 7.4	58.1 ± 2.8
(n)	(6)	(6)	(3)	(6)

[a] Standards were either aspirin 600 to 650 mg, acetaminophen 500 to 1,000 mg, or codeine 60 mg. All medications were orally administered.
[b] Test treatment represents the best performance of a treatment in the study.
[c] Means are the study means ± SE of study means.

In the studies surveyed, the dental impaction model had a very low placebo response (n = 40) and the postpartum model had a high placebo response (n = 7). A placebo response in excess of 30% might limit assay sensitivity, assuming similar variances and sample sizes across pain models; if the ceiling remains relatively stationary, then the available scale for separating drugs becomes smaller. The postpartum model also was the only pain model to have a mean aspirin response of over 50%, reinforcing the possibility that the maximum ceiling limit might occur even with the evaluation of mild analgesic agents. The postsurgical, periodontal, and nonimpaction models all had placebo %TMTs under 25%, consistent with reasonable potential for upside assay sensitivity.

Based on the studies in this survey, the maximum %TMT that any drug can achieve appears to be up to 80%, but the vast majority of studies were in the 50 to 60% range. It should be noted that this survey only evaluated oral analgesics, and possibly injectable drugs could do better because of their faster onset of action. Another interesting finding was that there was only a small difference in mean effect level between the inpatient observation and take-home diary techniques.

This commentary represents a preliminary survey since the data base is too small to draw any definitive conclusions; however, the results do indicate that there is a rational basis to further explore the use of %TMT as a tool to predict a component of model sensitivity. A much larger data base needs to be collected that includes more studies from each of the commonly used pain models. Once this is available, more extensive model and individual site analysis can be performed. It also may be feasible to evaluate the performance of specific standard and test drugs across the various pain models. For example, it may be possible to evaluate if certain models are more advantageous for NSAID drugs or narcotic analgesics.

Since the identity of investigators and investigational drugs are not necessary, possibly the Food and Drug Administration (FDA) could provide access to such data. I believe the effort would prove worthwhile because it may contribute to

TABLE 3. *Summary of percentage TMT data for dental impaction model: inpatient observations versus take-home diary*

Model	Treatment			
	Placebo	Standard treatment[a]	Aspirin 650 mg	Test treatment[b]
Inpatient observations	11.2 ± 0.7[c]	25.4 ± 3.7	27.2 ± 4.3	41.6 ± 3.6
(n)	(11)	(11)	(7)	(10)
Take-home diaries	17.6 ± 0.9	29.8 ± 2.8	29.2 ± 4.4	45.0 ± 3.0
(n)	(18)	(12)	(6)	(15)

[a] Standards were either aspirin 600 to 650 mg, acetaminophen 500 to 1,000 mg, or codeine 60 mg. All medications were orally administered.
[b] Test treatment represents the best performance of a treatment in the study.
[c] Means are the study means ± SE of study means.

a rational basis for choosing the most appropriate pain models and standard treatments when evaluating investigational drugs. Equally important, new clinical sites will have a method and existing data base to evaluate the utility of their models.

ACKNOWLEDGMENT

The author acknowledges the assistance of Ms. Laurie Strow in the preparation of this commentary.

REFERENCES

1. Beaver WT. Mild analgesics: a review of their clinical pharmacology. Part I. *Am J Med Sci* 1966;250: 577–604.
2. Beaver WT. Mild analgesics: A review of their clinical pharmacology. Part II. *Amer J Med Sci* 1966;251:576–599.
3. Cooper SA. New peripherally acting oral analgesic agents. *Annu Rev Pharmacol Toxicol* 1983;23: 617–647.
4. Laska LM, Sunshine A, et al. Effect of caffeine on acetaminophen analgesia. *Clin Pharmacol Ther* 1983;33:498–509.

APPENDIX A: REFERENCES USED IN DATABASE[b]

1. Baird WM, et al. Comparison of zomepirac, APC with codeine, codeine and placebo in the treatment of moderate and severe postoperative pain. *J Clin Pharmacol* 1980;20:243–249.
2. Beaver WT, et al. Analgesic effect of intramuscular and oral nalbuphine in postoperative pain. *Clin Pharmacol Ther* 1981;29:174–180.
3. Bloomfield SS, et al. Ketorolac versus aspirin for postpartum uterine pain. *Pharmacotherapy* 1986;6:247–252.
4. Brunelle RL, et al. Analgesic effect of picenadol, codeine and placebo in patients with postoperative pain. *Clin Pharmacol Ther* 1988;43:663–667.
5. Cooper SA, et al. The relative efficacy of ibuprofen in dental pain. *Comp Contin Educ Dent* 1986;7:578–597.
6. Cooper SA, et al. The analgesic efficacy of ketoprofen compared to ibuprofen and placebo. *Adv Ther* 1988;5:43–53.
7. Cooper SA, et al. Double-blind comparison of meclofenamate sodium (Meclomen) with acetaminophen with codeine, and placebo for relief of postsurgical dental pain. *J Clin Dent* 1988;1:31–34.
8. Cooper SA, et al. Ibuprofen and acetaminophen in the relief of acute pain: a randomized, double-blind, placebo-controlled study. *J Clin Pharmacol* 1989;29:1026–1030.
9. Desjardins PJ, Cooper SA, et al. The relative analgesic efficacy of propiram fumarate, codeine, aspirin and placebo in post-impaction dental pain. *J Clin Pharmacol* 1984;24:35–42.
10. Forbes JA, et al. A 12-hour evaluation of the analgesic efficacy of diflunisal, acetaminophen, an acetaminophen codeine combination, and placebo in postoperative pain. *Pharmacotherapy* 1983;3: 47S–54S.
11. Forbes JA, et al. A 12-hour evaluation of the analgesic efficacy of diflunisal, zomepirac sodium, aspirin and placebo in postoperative oral surgery pain. *Pharmacotherapy* 1983;3:38S–46S.
12. Forbes JA, et al. Analgesic effect of acetaminophen, phenyltoloxamine and their combination in postoperative oral surgery pain. *Pharmacotherapy* 1984;4:221–226.
13. Forbes JA, et al. Analgesic effect of fendosal, ibuprofen and aspirin in postoperative oral surgery pain. *Pharmacotherapy* 1984;4:385–391.

14. Forbes JA, et al. Nalbuphine, acetaminophen and their combination in postoperative pain. *Clin Pharmacol Ther* 1984;35:843–851.
15. Forbes JA, et al. Analgesic effect of naproxen sodium, codeine, a naproxen codeine combination and aspirin on the postoperative pain of oral surgery. *Pharmacotherapy* 1986;6:211–218.
16. Forbes JA, et al. Analgesic effects of an aspirin-codeine-butalbital-caffeine combination and an acetaminophen-codeine combination in postoperative oral surgery pain. *Pharmacotherapy* 1986;6: 240–246.
17. Jain AK, et al. Comparison of oral nalbuphine, acetaminophen, and their combination in postoperative pain. *Clin Pharmacol Ther* 1986;39:295–299.
18. Mahler DL, et al. Assay of aspirin and naproxen analgesia. *Clin Pharmacol Ther* 1976;19:18–23.
19. Markowitz RN, et al. Comparison of meclofenamate sodium with buffered aspirin and placebo in the treatment of postsurgical dental pain. *J Oral Surg* 1985;43:517–522.
20. Rowe NH, et al. Control of pain with meclofenamate sodium following removal of an impacted molar. *Oral Surg* 1985;59:446–448.
21. Sunshine A, et al. Analgesic effects of oral propiram fumarate, codeine sulfate and placebo in postoperative pain. *Pharmacotherapy* 1983;3:299–303.
22. Sunshine A, et al. A comparative oral analgesic study of indoprofen, aspirin and placebo in postpartum pain. *J Clin Pharmacol* 1985;25:374–380.
23. Sunshine A, et al. A double-blind, parallel comparison of ketoprofen, aspirin and placebo in patients with postpartum pain. *J Clin Pharmacol* 1986;26:706–711.
24. Sunshine A, et al. Comparative study of flurbiprofen, zomepirac sodium, acetaminophen plus codeine and acetaminophen for the relief of postsurgical dental pain. *Am J Med* 1986;80(3A): 50–54.
25. Sunshine A, et al. Analgesic efficacy of piroxicam in the treatment of postoperative pain. *Am J Med* 1988;84(5A):16–22.

[b] Studies are all included in the database. Several other studies in the database were provided by the investigators and are not listed.

Advances in Pain Research and Therapy, Vol. 18,
edited by M. Max, R. Portenoy, and E. Laska,
Raven Press, Ltd., New York © 1991.

Commentary

Dose-Response Model for Combination Analgesic Drugs

David J. Goldstein and Rocco L. Brunelle

Lilly Research Laboratories, Eli Lilly and Company, Indianapolis, Indiana 46285

Combinations of analgesics with different mechanisms of action can reduce the adverse event profile that a single agent could produce at a comparable level of analgesia. Additionally, combinations can simplify treatment and compliance. However, the determination of optimal levels of the components tends to be haphazard. The optimal safe and effective dose for each component of a combination drug should be obtained with the same care and precision as the optimal safe and effective dose for a single agent. The dose and frequency of administration for an analgesic should be determined early in the clinical phase of the drug research process. Similarly, the optimal dose of each combination should be determined early in the research of a combination drug.

This commentary briefly reviews the issues involved with obtaining the dose of a single analgesic agent and gives a simple additive model for testing the effectiveness of a combination analgesic drug. Both of these techniques are combined into a factorial design that can be used for a response surface model that will aid the researcher in choosing an optimal combination dose that is both safe and effective.

DOSE-RESPONSE MODEL FOR A SINGLE AGENT

An optimal safe and effective dose should be established early in the development of a new analgesic therapy. Although this can be obtained by conducting a moderate size dose-response study, a series of studies using a single dosage level of the experimental drug are often done instead. These studies are attractive in their simplicity, lower cost, and fewer patients exposed to the drug; however, they provide very little information on the clinically optimum dose (a dose that has sufficient analgesic efficacy with a low incidence of acceptable adverse events). Even after conducting many of these single-dosage studies, one may not have an accurate estimate of the optimum safe and effective dose.

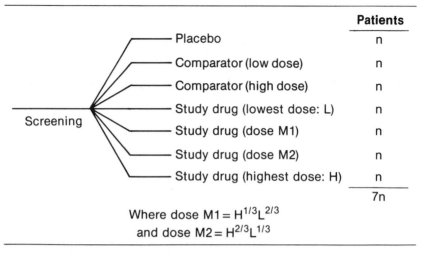

	Patients
Placebo	n
Comparator (low dose)	n
Comparator (high dose)	n
Study drug (lowest dose: L)	n
Study drug (dose M1)	n
Study drug (dose M2)	n
Study drug (highest dose: H)	n
	7n

Where dose $M1 = H^{1/3}L^{2/3}$
and dose $M2 = H^{2/3}L^{1/3}$

FIG. 1. Study design for a dose-response study.

Dose-response studies for analgesic drugs are often reported in the literature. Recent examples are Forbes et al. (1) and Desjardins (2). Typically, dose-response studies are randomized, double-blind, placebo and analgesic comparator controlled studies. They should have a minimum of three dosage levels of the study drug in order to fit various models. We recommend at least four carefully selected dosage levels of the study drug in order to evaluate different dose-response models.

The first dose-response study should cover the entire range of possible doses (Table 1). The highest dose should be the largest dose recommended by the basic pharmacology studies and the lowest dose should be below the expected level of efficacy. At least two more doses should be chosen between these two levels. We recommend that the doses be picked using a log scale since this scale usually parallels the biological dose response relationship.

A typical design for a dose-response study is presented in Fig. 1 and the summary of the analysis[a] in graphical form[b] is presented in Fig. 2. After completing a dose-response study, the researcher usually has an accurate estimate of the appropriate dose to use in extended efficacy and safety studies.

---

[a] After the experiment is completed the mean analgesic scores among the treatments can be compared using a one-way analysis of variance (ANOVA) model. A dose-response model for the study drug can also be estimated from this data.

Table 1 shows the analysis of variance table for a dose-response study.

[b] The multiple comparison intervals are a graphical presentation of the Protected Least Significant Difference multiple comparison technique (11). These intervals are obtained by adding and subtracting one-half of the Least Significant Difference value to each of the treatment means and then using these upper and lower bounds as the multiple comparison intervals. This graphical presentation obviates the need for large, complex pairwise comparison tables, since treatments that have comparison intervals that do not overlap are significantly different from one another at the 0.05 level of significance.

TABLE 1. *Analysis of variance for a dose-response study*[a]

Source of variation	df	Mean squares	F value	p value
Treatment	6	MST	MST/MSR	
Study drug				
Linear	1	MSL	MSL/MSR	
Lack of Fit	2	MSN	MSN/MSR	
Residual	7 (n − 1)	MSR		

[a] The linear and lack-of-fit components were obtained by using only the data from the patients receiving the study drug. The doses were transformed to logs and then a regression model was fit to this data using linear, quadratic, and cubic terms in the model. The quadratic and cubic terms were combined for the lack-of-fit component. The residual mean squares for the entire model was used to test both the overall treatment effect and the study drug model fits. If appropriate, the placebo dose can also be used in determining the dose-response model.

df, degrees of freedom; MST, mean squares treatment; MSR, mean squares residual; MSL, mean squares linear; MSN, mean squares nonlinear.

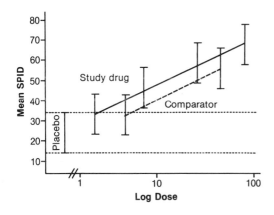

FIG. 2. Example results from a dose-response study. Means and multiple comparison intervals—sum of pain intensity difference (SPID).

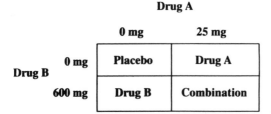

Drug A

		0 mg	25 mg
Drug B	**0 mg**	**Placebo**	**Drug A**
	600 mg	**Drug B**	**Combination**

FIG. 3. Example of a 2 by 2 factorial design.

ADDITIVE MODEL FOR A COMBINATION DRUG

A basic study that is often used to evaluate the combination of two known analgesics is the 2 by 2 factorial design (3–5) (Fig. 3). A factorial design requires that each level of a factor is combined with the level of every other factor. Thus a 2 by 2 factorial design has four categories. A detailed discussion of this model can be found in Winer (6).

The 2 by 2 factorial design facilitates evaluating the effectiveness of each of the individual drugs and of the combination compound (Table 2). However, the optimum dose must be approximated using multiple experiments and thus has the same limitations as one-dose studies. The combination drug is deemed additive if the combination response is equal to the sum of the individual components minus the contribution of the placebo. A departure from additivity indicates two possible alternatives: the combination effect is more than additive or it is less than additive. This can be determined by examinations of the mean plots. Figure 4 presents examples of results in the graphical form of a 2 by 2 factorial design study.

DOSE-RESPONSE MODEL FOR A COMBINATION DRUG

An obvious problem with the 2 by 2 factorial model in evaluating the efficacy of a combination drug is the assumption that the optimum effective dose is the same as the optimum dose of each of the components. A response surface design

TABLE 2. *Analysis of variance for a 2 by 2 factorial model*

Source of variation	df	Mean squares	F value	p value
Drug A	1	MSA	MSA/MSR	
Drug B	1	MSB	MSB/MSR	
Nonadditivity	1	MSNA	MSNA/MSR	
Residual	4 (n − 1)	MSR		

df, degrees of freedom; MSA, mean squares Drug A; MSB, mean squares Drug B; MSNA, mean squares nonadditivity; MSR, mean squares residual.

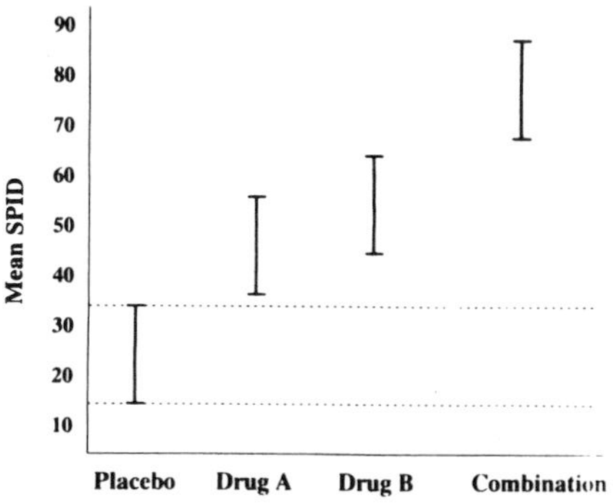

FIG. 4. Example of results from a 2 by 2 factorial design study. Means and multiple comparison intervals—sum of pain intensity difference (SPID).

permits evaluation of the relationship between the two components in different concentration ratios over a wide range of dosages and estimation of the optimum safe and effective combination dose (7,8).

There are many types of response surface designs that can be used (9). One such design is the central composite design which is an optimum design for examining the relationship between the combination doses and the response variable. This design has been used extensively in studies optimizing the manufacture of chemicals and for the reduction of pollutants.

Another response surface design uses an expanded factorial design with more than two levels of each of the components. The expanded factorial design can be used to evaluate the relationship between the combination doses and the response in order to estimate the optimum safe and effective combination dose. The factorial design model is a simpler design than the central composite design. However, this design loses the ability to estimate over a larger surface when compared to the central composite design (i.e., a larger range of possible doses of both components). This wide range of assessments is not required for most drug studies and may not be possible because of limitations owing to the adverse event profile. An example of the expanded factorial design is presented in Fig. 5. The results of this study can be evaluated using an analysis of variance technique (Table 3).

		Drug A			
		0 mg	20 mg	45 mg	100 mg
Drug B	0 mg	Placebo			
	250 mg				
	500 mg				
	1000 mg				

FIG. 5. Combination dose-response study using a 4 by 4 factorial design.

TABLE 3. *Analysis of variance for a 4 by 4 factorial model[a]*

Source of variation	df	Mean squares	F value	p value
Drug A	3	MSA	MSA/MSR	
Drug B	3	MSB	MSB/MSR	
Interaction	9	MSI	MSI/MSR	
Residual	16 (n − 1)	MSR		

[a] This ANOVA model tests for the main effects of each therapy and the interaction of the two therapies. Further analysis of the dose-response relationship for each drug independently is also possible. This model also permits one to assess the departure from linearity or from parallelism of the combination of the two drugs. This is similar to the test for nonadditivity in the 2 by 2 factorial model. However, this effect does not explain the relationship of the interaction.

df, degrees of freedom; MSA, mean squares Drug A; MSB, mean squares Drug B; MSI, mean squares interaction; MSR, mean squares residual.

A dose-response model for the combination therapy can be fit to the results from this factorial design.[c] After evaluating the adequacy and goodness of fit of this model, it is advantageous to show the results with a three-dimensional plot (Fig. 6). Computer packages that produce three-dimensional plots as in Fig. 6 can also show the model in various positions (10). One can rotate both the ordinate and abscissa to aid in examining the entire dose-response surface (Fig. 7).

Just as the single treatment dose-response study permits visualization over a range of doses of an individual component, the response surface analysis permits visualization of various combinations of the test medications, which aids the researcher in choosing the optimal clinical combination dose. In addition, one can make accurate estimates about the effects of any dosage combination on the surface even though the specific doses were not used.

Safety data (i.e., incidence of adverse events) can be analyzed using a similar technique: categorical analysis and logistic regression for the dose-response surface. Also, simple coloration of the efficacy dose-response surface to reflect various levels of adverse events can provide another dimension of information on the dose-response surface plot. This gives a four-dimensional plot!

Repeat doses at fixed intervals can be analyzed similarly. This results in a series of surfaces and permits an evaluation of the analgesic efficacy at steady-state concentrations. The dose picked from such studies can then be used in pivotal 2 by 2 factorial design efficacy and safety studies. The sample sizes for these studies can be estimated from the results of the response surface study to permit demonstration of efficacy.

[c] The following quadratic regression model was used to fit a three-dimensional dose-response surface for the analgesia scores:

$$Y = b_1 + b_2A + b_3B + b_4AB + b_5A^2 + b_6B^2$$

where Y = sum of pain intensity differences (SPID) score, A, B = log of the levels of Drugs A and B, and b_is = model parameters.

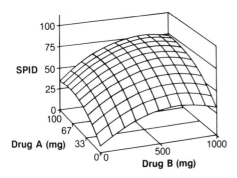

FIG. 6. Example of a response surface model obtained from the 4 by 4 factorial design.

Finally, if there is some prior evidence of the optimum combination dose, one can weight certain key cells in the expanded factorial design (i.e., increase the number of patients in these cells) to produce a 2 by 2 factorial design within the expanded factorial design. This imbedded design increases the power of showing a treatment effect for certain comparisons. The analysis of the response surface design should include the same number of patients in each cell so that each cell contributes equally to the response surface model. For such cases a

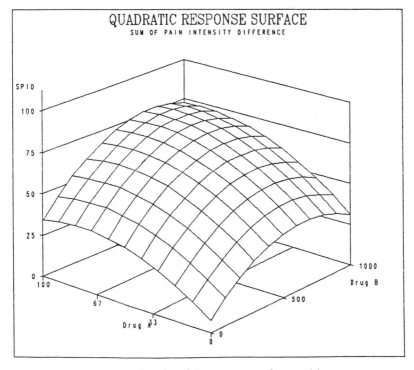

FIG. 7. Rotation of the response surface model.

proportion of the individuals in these weighted cells can be randomly selected to balance the factorial design.

Thus, despite the more complicated and more expensive initial effort using the response surface analysis, the potential benefits—more ideal selection of doses, lack of necessity for doing a series of 2 by 2 factorial design studies to approximate the optimum dose, and the potential to do efficacy and safety studies in parallel—outweigh these deficits.

REFERENCES

1. Forbes JA, Yorio CC, Selinger LR, Rosenmertz SK, Beaver WT. An evaluation of flurbiprofen, aspirin, and placebo in postoperative oral surgery pain. *Pharmacotherapy* 1989;9(2):66–73.
2. Desjardins PJ. Analgesic efficacy of piroxicam in postoperative dental pain. *Am J Med* 1988;84(5A): 35–41.
3. Forbes JA, Kolodny AL, Chachich BM, Beaver WT. Nalbuphine, acetaminophen, and their combination in postoperative pain. *Clin Pharmacol Ther* 1984;35:843–851.
4. Bently KC, Head TW. The additive analgesic efficacy of acetaminophen, 1000 mg, and codeine, 60 mg, in dental pain. *Clin Pharmacol Ther* 1987;42:634–640.
5. Forbes JA, Barkaszi AB, Ragland RN, Hankle JJ. Analgesic effect of acetaminophen, phenyl-toloxamine and their combination in postoperative oral surgery pain. *Pharmacotherapy* 1984;4: 221–226.
6. Winer BJ. *Statistical principles in experimental design,* 2nd ed. New York: McGraw-Hill, 1971;394–397.
7. Box GEP, Hunter WG, Hunter JS. *Statistics for experimenters—an introduction to design, data analysis, and model building.* New York: John Wiley & Sons, 1978.
8. Solana RP, Chinchilli VM, Carter WH Jr, Wilson JD, Carchamn RA. The evaluation of biological interactions using response surface methodology. *Cell Biol Toxicol* 1987;3:263–277.
9. Goldberg MR, Offen WW, Rockhold FW. Factorial design. An approach to the assessment of therapeutic drug interactions in clinical trials. *J Clin Res Drug Dev* 1988;2(4):215–225.
10. SAS Institute, Inc. *SAS user's guide: statistics,* version 5 ed. Cary, North Carolina: SAS Institute Inc., 1985.
11. Andrews HP, Snee RD, Sarner MH. Graphical display of means. *Am Statist* 1980;34(4):195–199.

DISCUSSION: SINGLE-DOSE COMPARISON (Chapters 4 and 5)

Dr. John Harter: At the FDA, we are not very enamored with the area under the curve measures such as SPID, TOTPAR, or TMT. We look at onset, duration, and peak effect as distinct aspects of analgesic performance, and we will be conveying this information to physicians in the new package inserts we are developing.

We are quite concerned about dropouts, particularly since different treatments have different dropout rates. In a typical postoperative pain study of 50 patients initially given placebo, for example, by 6 hrs all but one or two may have already received a rescue dose of analgesic, whereas a considerable number of patients given the test drug may have avoided remedication. We are concerned with how you analyze patients for times after they remedicate. In the time-effect curves presented in this volume, the points in the later hours of the study largely reflect assigned scores for dropouts. If you did not include those scores, the curves would change substantially. For example, the placebo curve, instead of going up and coming down, would go right up to the end of the trial because the placebo patients who remain in the trial are doing as well as anybody.

We are also interested in the potential gains to be made by measuring drug levels along with pain relief scores. Among patients who do poorly, for instance, you will find more people with low serum drug levels than among the patients who do well. There is some additional power to discriminate among treatments that can be gained by adjusting for serum levels. An early demonstration of that was a study by Laska and Sunshine (1) where their pain relief data and blood levels showed a bioequivalency problem with a particular formulation of ibuprofen.

The choice of dose is very important. In many of the applications the FDA reviews, people have studied too narrow a dose range. Our studies of the pharmacokinetic variability of drugs has demonstrated that if you are not going to do sophisticated pharmacokinetic-pharmacodynamic analyses, you should at least pick doses far enough apart that there is a good separation between the resulting blood levels. In the case of ketorolac, we were able to select a recommended dosage level that had not been studied, in part because the sponsor had studied a ninefold range of dose levels. Sponsors who study just a threefold dose range may be left with insufficient information to adequately guide prescribing.

A final topic I'd like to comment on is that a number of investigators have mentioned that it is more difficult today than a decade ago to recruit patients for studies, partly because of the increased requirements of informed consent. This may have some impact on the study results. For example, it is more difficult for standard doses of standard drugs such as aspirin to beat placebo than it was 10 years ago. In some cases, I think I understand how such a bias is introduced; in repeated dose studies of NSAIDs in arthritis, for example, the only patients you can recruit are those that haven't responded to the standard NSAIDs used in practice. But it is more complicated than that, and it would behoove us to think about this phenomenon, and how we are going to adjust to it.

REFERENCE

1. Laska EM, Sunshine A, Marrero I, et al. The correlation between blood levels of ibuprofen and clinical response. *Clin Pharmacol Ther* 1986;40:1–7.

DISCUSSION

Dr. Raymond Houde: Drs. Max and Laska criticized the use of assigned scores for times after patients receive a rescue analgesic. I do not agree with them that the conventional methods of defining the area under the time-effect curve use "fictitious numbers." Beyond the point where the patient no longer has pain relief, and requires a rescue analgesic, it is reasonable to say that he has zero pain relief. It makes clinical sense.

Dr. Saul Bloomfield: I'd like to comment about differences among pain models. The preceding chapter points out that different types of pain have differing severity and sensitivity to various analgesics. Our group in Cincinnati is studying another area of possible distinction among pain models. In several studies, we have compared time-effect relationships of NSAIDs for pain following major surgery, oral surgery, and childbirth (postpartum uterine cramping), and determined onset, time to peak, and duration. Preliminary results suggest that in the postoperative pain model one could readily delineate differences in onset, time to peak, and duration among the various NSAIDs; in oral surgery pain we could distinguish differences in onset and duration; and in postpartum cramping we could distinguish duration. We are analyzing additional studies to see whether these are consistent features of the three models.

Dr. Lawrence Mather: I have a concern with the data presented comparing various pain models in assessing drugs. How can one compare these results without taking into account the many factors that affect the physiology of drug absorption and distribution? For example, the type of anesthesia and premedication may have profound effects on gastric emptying and drug absorption. Although the randomization may cancel out some of this variation, such factors may muddy the situation enormously.

Dr. Abraham Sunshine: As you point out, there are a whole host of factors that can impact on a study. One can still tell if the clinical trial retains the sensitivity that you need, though, by including graded doses of a standard analgesic in the study. If you can distinguish 100 mg, 200 mg, and 400 mg ibuprofen and there is a positive slope of the dose-response curve, you know that you have overcome these variable factors in the assay. Dr. Bloomfield adequately demonstrated dose-response relationships in the studies to which he referred.

Dr. Robert Kaiko: Before Drs. Laska, Siegel, and Sunshine began to measure onset and duration directly with a stopwatch, these variables were estimated from the data from the scheduled interview times. What method of deriving onset and duration from these data comes reasonably close to the direct stopwatch measure?

Dr. Eugene Laska: We have spent an enormous amount of time looking at that question, but I would have to say that none of the indirect measures is very good. With a very large number of measurements with a crude instrument, one can get closer to an accurate estimate, but the measure remains crude nonetheless. Dr. Sunshine has used a "recall method," for example. At the first scheduled interview where the patient reports relief, the nurse asked the patient to estimate how long ago it began. Almost always, the estimate was a number divisible by 5 or 10. If one needs to characterize a drug with onset at 6 min after injection, this isn't any way to do business.

Dr. Bloomfield: I have some reservations about the stopwatch method for measuring drug onset. For one thing, the placebo response tends to be a very early effect and is included in the onset of whatever agent is administered. Second, for some types of pain, such as intermittent or cramping pain, the whole idea of onset measured by a stopwatch is not going to be meaningful at all. We have tried it, and it makes no sense in those types of pain.

Dr. Laska: Perhaps I have not been clear. There are two phenomena, I think, that are being mixed up in your objection. One has to do with measurement and the second has to do with inference about the measurement. I think it is fair to say that when the patient says he has onset—however that is defined—that is the time of onset, whatever it was that caused it.

There are lots of things that went into that decision by the patient to report onset. Some of the relief may be a placebo effect, and some of it is the drug. Whatever the cause, that observation of the patient is the phenomenon that we are interested in studying. So to reject the stopwatch as a measurement device for that reason is to say that you are not interested in the phenomenon of onset time for that patient.

Now regarding attribution of effects to the drug, the placebo effect, or to anything else, the issues are the same whether one is considering onset or any other measure of efficacy. Perhaps you would wish to argue that the difference between onset time for a drug and placebo is the real difference in onset time, but I wouldn't. The most important feature in the data I have looked at is the probability of getting onset, not the time to onset or the placebo issue.

I had an interesting debate with Chuck Inturrisi a long time ago about whether it is possible to have an onset time that differs as you go up the scale in doses. As I recall, Chuck said that couldn't be the case because of the pharmacokinetic models and the way the equations look. But that isn't consistent with data we have, which support the notion that as you raise the dose, the onset time shortens.

Dr. Donald Jasinski: In our studies of opiate abuse potential, we recently had some findings to confirm Dr. Laska's suggestion that higher doses give earlier onset. We asked addicts to rate subjective effects every 60 sec following doses of transnasal butorphanol. In a double-blind crossover study, subjects could discriminate onset of a 4-mg dose much earlier than a 1-mg dose.

Dr. Laska: I think it would be difficult in an analgesic trial to ask the patient every few seconds, "Do you still have your headache?" That isn't necessary with the stopwatch method.

Dr. Russell Portenoy: I'd like to point out that fine measurements of onset are important only for certain drugs—particularly those targeted for intermittent use in acute pain. For drugs with a very slow onset, or for those to be used for chronic dosing only, I'm not sure the stopwatch technique is critical.

Dr. Abraham Sunshine: With Dr. Laska, we have proposed a method to measure onset, but we by no means say that it is the only method to measure onset. We report our work and encourage others to look at it differently.

In our initial pilot study, we asked patients to tell us when they had the onset of effect from parenteral morphine or meptazinol. Within minutes, patients would say "I feel something," usually before we left the room. We realized that that question would not give us the information we were looking for. We then made the question a bit more rigorous by asking patients to tell us when they had onset of "meaningful" relief, each patient defining this for himself. Others may come up with a different methodology, but this approach has helped us to differentiate time-effect curves for onset and duration quite well.

When other investigators studied meptazinol, many used AUC variables such as SPID and TOTPAR and missed the fact that meptazinol is a very short-acting drug. Its relative potency at 30 min and 1 hr are very high compared to morphine, and then it falls off precipitously.

Dr. Thomas Kantor: In any analgesic trial, there are people who don't respond at all to the drug—they never have onset. The proportion of nonresponders at each dose is an important outcome measure that should be analyzed; it is something that a clinician really wants to know. This feature is included in the methods that Dr. Laska has described.

Dr. Richard Gracely: Dr. Laska has presented some new designs for crossover studies, and has criticized the two-treatment, two-period crossover design. I recognize that the possibility of carryover effects limits the ability of this design to accurately estimate relative potency, but in several of our studies it has served us well in determining whether a drug is efficacious compared to placebo. The most common carryover effect is that of a drug in the first period carrying over into the second period. That will reduce the mean effect and if anything, is conservative. The lower variance of the within-patient crossover tends to preserve the sensitivity of the crossover relative to a parallel comparison. Are the more complex designs such as AB, BA, AA, BB or ABB, BAA always preferable?

Dr. Laska: Whatever the nature of the carryover effect, you can disentangle it from the true treatment effects if you use the designs I presented. When you don't use such designs, you can't tell what is going on. Another question that is more relevant, I think, is whether you do better with these newer crossover designs or with a parallel-group design. W. B. Brown has written about this at length, pointing out that in addition to purely statistical issues, one must consider the cost of recruiting a subject, the comparative costs of various numbers of treatment periods, and the possibility of dropout along the way.

Dr. John Harter: With regard to Dr. Laska's recommended crossover designs, how important is the consistency of the condition to your assumptions? Does your design take care of the possibility that the patient's disease has gotten worse or gone away during the trial? That is the problem that bothers the FDA statisticians and ourselves the most—the possibility that we may not be dealing with the same disease process at different points in the study.

Dr. Laska: The requirement of a stable baseline remains a problem in the new crossover designs we presented, just as it does in the two-treatment, two-period crossover.

I'd also like to comment on the argument Drs. Wallenstein and Houde have made in support of crossover studies. They seek to counter the common criticism of crossover studies—that there may be carryover effects from one study drug to the next—by pointing out that even in parallel-group studies, patients will have carryover effects from the standard treatment they received just before the study began. The argument, as I understand it, says that as long as we are in big trouble anyway on the first dose, we might as well be in big trouble on the second dose.

Despite my being an enthusiastic supporter of crossover designs, I find that argument a bit unpersuasive. I would prefer to focus on specific measures to handle such carryover effects, such as taking previous treatments into account as covariates (as Dr. Wallenstein has done), and using designs such as ABB, BAA to directly measure the carryover effect.

Dr. Dwight Moulin: In comparing new treatment methods, for example, Patient Controlled Analgesia versus continuous opioid infusion, I have difficulty determining what is an appropriate sample size. I'm familiar with the standard formulae for parallel dose and crossover study sample size calculations, but could you offer some guidelines for using them?

Dr. Laska: Regrettably, I can't give you guidelines, but I can give you philosophy, which may be more helpful. If you are beginning a new experimental procedure and really don't know anything, you have to act in a way described by statisticians as "Bayesian." You are accumulating information to try and model phenomena, getting background information about parameters to be estimated later. Many journal editors will not publish an early study without formal calculations of sample size, but this is unfortunate; it frequently results in an uninformative mechanical massage of the data. By the time you are ready to do a more formal clinical trial and know a lot about the procedure, there are tables and formulae that can answer your question precisely.

Advances in Pain Research and Therapy, Vol. 18,
edited by M. Max, R. Portenoy, and E. Laska,
Raven Press, Ltd., New York © 1991.

5

Multidose Short-Term Analgesic Studies

Patricia E. Stewart

*Research and Development, McNeil Consumer Products,
Fort Washington, Pennsylvania 19034*

Definitive evidence of the efficacy of a new analgesic compound has traditionally come from single-dose comparisons with placebo or an acceptable reference standard. The methodology for these single-dose comparative studies has been well established and is outlined in the *Guidelines for the Clinical Evaluation of Analgesic Drugs* published in 1979 by the Food and Drug Administration (FDA) (1). The methods described in these guidelines, along with several modifications and enhancements made since their publication, still serve as the cornerstone for evaluating efficacy of new analgesics. The methodology for these single-dose analgesic studies is extensively reviewed in Chapter 4 by Max and Laska.

Over the last decade, there has been a growing recognition of the importance of augmenting the traditional approach of single-dose analgesic studies with multidose efficacy trials. In fact, clinical development of analgesic compounds has now evolved to the point that short-term multidose clinical trials will likely be a requirement for United States marketing approval. A consensus on the methodology for these multidose studies has not yet been developed. The 1979 FDA Guidelines noted that "In certain important areas (e.g., the evaluation of repeated dose regimens of analgesics), currently existing methodology is relatively primitive . . ." In his review of analgesic clinical trial methodology, Beaver (2) noted that "The need to put repeat-dose studies of analgesics on a quantitative footing as firm as currently exists for single-dose studies constitutes the most important current challenge facing clinical analgesimetry." (pp. 432–433). Thus, although there is currently an established "requirement" that multidose studies be conducted, no recognized consensus exists regarding the specifics of acceptable study designs.

RATIONALE FOR SHORT-TERM MULTIDOSE STUDIES

The rationale for the inclusion of short-term, multidose clinical studies in the development program for new analgesic compounds is multifaceted. The primary reason for their inclusion is that these studies—in contrast to single-dose trials—

closely approximate the "real-life" clinical setting. Patients with pathologic pain typically require more than one dose of medication to alleviate their pain. A second reason for conducting multidose analgesic studies is that information concerning the optimal dosing frequency in various pain states can best be obtained from a formal evaluation of repeat dosing schedules. Yet another reason for conducting multidose studies is that some analgesics have demonstrated an augmentation of efficacy with repeated dosing; thus, data on the drug's efficacy following the second or third dose could provide useful prescribing information.

Finally, multidose studies are crucial to the evaluation of a drug's side effect profile. Single-dose studies have repeatedly been shown to be unreliable predictors of a drug's side effect liability. It is not uncommon in single-dose studies for the frequency of side effects to be greater among placebo-treated patients than among drug-treated patients. Multidose studies more accurately approximate known side effect profiles of reference drugs and are more reliable predictors of the side effect liability of a new drug. Despite the usefulness of short-term multidose studies, the definitive study design for establishing the safety profile of any new analgesic compound involves long-term studies in appropriate chronic pain models such as osteoarthritis or cancer pain.

REVIEW OF REPRESENTATIVE PUBLISHED LITERATURE ON SHORT-TERM MULTIDOSE STUDIES

For all of the reasons outlined in the preceding section, there is a general consensus that the efficacy and safety of a new analgesic should be evaluated in multidose studies in patients with acute pain requiring short-term therapy. There is no consensus, however, concerning the design features of such studies. A review of the published literature on short-term multidose analgesic studies reveals a variety of approaches. Table 1 summarizes the design features of representative short-term, multidose analgesic studies published in the literature. As with single-dose analgesic studies, various clinical pain models have been evaluated in multidose studies. Notably, short-term multidose evaluations in pain arising from surgery (3–9), dental procedures (10–16), cancer pain (17–19), headache (20), or orthopedic pain (21) have been published.

Because no accepted methodology has yet emerged, existing analgesic development programs will need to rely on investigator experience and expertise as well as currently available models in designing short-term multidose clinical studies. Scientists at the FDA should not be overlooked as a source of information concerning the appropriateness of a particular study design since they have broad access to studies conducted for analgesics under Investigational New Drug (IND) Applications or New Drug Applications (NDAs).

DESIGN AND METHODOLOGY ISSUES IN SHORT-TERM MULTIDOSE STUDIES

Several issues need to be resolved when designing a short-term, multidose analgesic study. Among these issues are: choice of a pain model and duration of treatment period; choice of a control agent(s); dosage regimen; efficacy measurement scales; safety assessments; and statistical analysis. Previous FDA guidelines for analgesic drugs (1) have been silent on these issues as they relate to repeat-dose studies. Since there is no standardized methodology, each study will need to address these issues within the framework of existing scientific data and clinical judgment.

A discussion of the various design issues relevant to short-term multidose analgesic studies follows.

Choice of a Pain Model and Duration of Treatment

Obviously the pain model selected for study in a multidose trial should be one that typically requires more than 1 day of therapy. It seems reasonable that the type of pain evaluated in short-term multidose studies should be anticipated to persist for 3 to 10 days. In evaluating efficacy with repeated dosing, it also seems reasonable that at least three doses of the study drug be given. Several days of multiple dosing would be ideal, particularly in conditions where the pain persists at a somewhat constant level for that length of time.

Table 2 presents information on the percent of patients who were medicated at least once on days 2 through 7 in each of five multidose studies involving zomepirac sodium. Each of these studies was 1 week in duration and their design was essentially similar. Two doses of the test drug (zomepirac sodium) were compared in a double-blind manner to a standard reference analgesic; patients were allowed to administer study medication on a prn basis. Focusing on day 4 in Table 2 as a marker, it is obvious that a reasonable percentage of patients are still remedicating in the cancer, oral surgical, and acute orthopedic pain models, but that the mixed postoperative and postpartum pain models have few remaining patients at this time.

Postoperative Pain Model

The postoperative pain model seems an obvious candidate for evaluation of short-term multidose therapy. There are many types of surgery, some of which may be more appropriate for evaluation of a particular drug than others. Although there is a good correlation between the extent of the surgery and the duration of pain, extensive major surgery is typically complicated by the need for parenteral analgesic therapy. For this reason, major surgical models are precluded in the study of oral analgesics. Ouellette and his colleagues (7,8), however, did use a major surgery model successfully for short-term, multidose evaluations of the parenteral analgesic, buprenorphine, in comparison to other parenteral narcotic agents.

More moderate surgical procedures, particularly overnight and outpatient procedures, often result in a significant variability with respect to the extent and duration of pain. Furthermore, with more moderate surgical procedures, a decision

TABLE 1. *Summary of representative published studies of short-term multidose analgesic evaluations*

Ref.	Pain model	Drugs evaluated	Dosing regimen	Study duration	Evaluation intervals	Efficacy measurements[a]
3	Postoperative pain (mixed)	Zomepirac, pentazocine	PRN up to 6 doses	24 hours	Predose, 4 hr postdose	Pain intensity (predose); pain relief; pt. & inv. global ratings (poststudy)
4	Postoperative pain (plastic surgery)	Zomepirac, clometacin, placebo	PRN up to 4 doses/day	4 days	Predose, 4 hr postdose	Pain intensity (predose); pain relief; pt. & inv. global ratings (poststudy)
5	Postpartum pain	Zomepirac, APC[b]	PRN q 4 hr up to 6 doses/day	5 days	Predose, 4 hr postdose	Pain intensity (predose); pain relief; pt. & inv. global ratings (poststudy)
6[b]	Postoperative pain (mixed)	Zomepirac, dihydrocodeine	PRN up to 30 doses	5 days	Daily	Pain intensity, adequacy of sleep; best pain relief; pt. global ratings (poststudy)
7	Postoperative pain (abdominal)	Buprenorphine, meperidine	PRN q 30 min up to 10 doses	48 hours	0.5–8 hr postdose 1st injection (hourly)	Pain intensity; pain relief; inv. global ratings (poststudy); no. pts. ≥4 hr btn inj.; time to remedicate
8	Postoperative pain (mixed)	Buprenorphine, morphine	PRN q 3 hr	3 days	0.5–8 hr postdose 1st injection/ day (hourly)	Pain intensity; pain relief; inv. global ratings (poststudy); time to remedicate; time to return to baseline pain
9	Postoperative pain (mixed)	Buprenorphine, morphine	PRN up to 12 doses/day	3 days	0.5–8 hr postdose 1st injection/ day (hourly)	Pain intensity; pain relief; inv. global ratings (poststudy); time to remedicate
10	3rd molar extraction	Acetaminophen + codeine	1st dose imm. postop; 2nd dose PRN	12 hours	0–12 hr postdose (hourly)	Pain intensity; time to remedicate
11	Oral surgery (mixed)	Zomepirac APC[b]	PRN q 4 hr up to 42 doses/wk	7 days	Predose; 4 hr postdose	Pain intensity (predose); pain relief; pt. & inv. globals (poststudy)

12	3rd molar extraction	Ibuprofen, ibuprofen/codeine	PRN up to 3 doses/day	6 days	0–6 hr postdose (1st 2 doses) (hourly)	Pain intensity; pain relief; pt. global ratings (daily)
13	3rd molar extraction	Acetaminophen, diflunisal	PRN q 2 hr up to 2 doses	10 hr	0–10 hr postdose (hourly)	Pain intensity; no. pts. needed rescue med.
14	3rd molar extraction	Codeine, propoxyphene, acetaminophen	PRN q 2 hr	Approx. 10–12 hr	Hourly until study end	Pain intensity; time to remedicate
15	3rd molar extraction	Acetaminophen, codeine	PRN q 2 hr	10 hr	0–10 hr postdose (hourly)	Pain intensity; time to remedicate
16	3rd molar extraction	Acetaminophen, acetaminophen + codeine	PRN q 2 hr up to 5 doses	Approx. 10–12 hr	Hourly until study end	Pain intensity; time to remedicate
17	Cancer pain	Ibuprofen,[c] placebo	PRN up to 4 doses/day	7 days	Daily	Pain intensity; pain relief; narcotic drug use; pt. & inv. global ratings (poststudy)
18[c]	Cancer pain	Dezocine, butorphanol	PRN	7 days	Daily	Pt. global ratings; inv. overall global ratings
19[c]	Cancer pain	Zomepirac, percodan	PRN q 4 hr up to 6 doses/day	7 days	After each dose	Analgesic acceptability per dose; pt. overall global ratings
20	Headache	Zomepirac, placebo	PRN q 4 hr up to 3 doses/episode	4 episodes per 2 mos	Predose; 4 hr postdose	Pain intensity (predose); analgesic acceptability; inv. & pt. global ratings (poststudy)
21	Orthopedic pain	Zomepirac, APC[b]	PRN q 4 hr	7 days	Predose; 4 hr postdose	Pain intensity (predose); pain relief; inv. & pt. global ratings (poststudy)

[a] Key: pt., patient; inv., investigator; btn, between.
[b] APC, aspirin + codeine (30 or 60 mg).
[c] Study also had single-dose component; information presented from multidose component only.
[d] All patients on oxycodone/acetaminophen throughout study.

TABLE 2. *Percentage of patients remedicating on days 2 to 7 in multidose studies of zomepirac sodium and reference analgesics in various pain models*

Pain model (reference)	Percent of patients remedicating					
	Day 2	Day 3	Day 4	Day 5	Day 6	Day 7
Oral surgical (11)	92	59	49	36	24	13
Acute orthopedic (21)	80	74	63	49	39	27
Cancer (19)	78	59	59	53	45	38
Mixed postoperative (3)	49	24	13	6	5	3
Postpartum (5)	46	25	6	—	—	—

must be made to evaluate the subjects on an inpatient or outpatient basis. With continuing pressures on hospitals and clinics to discharge patients as soon as possible postoperatively, it seems prudent to design multidose studies in postoperative pain with both an inpatient and an outpatient component.

Ideally, in designing an analgesic trial, one should select a postoperative procedure with a relatively homogeneous patient group. Such homogeneity limits intersubject variability and should provide more consistent results. Thus, instead of evaluating an analgesic compound in a general postoperative model, it may be more desirable to consider evaluations in specific types of surgery, such as orthopedic procedures (e.g., joint replacements), cesarean sections, and podiatry procedures. Experience with the impacted third molar extraction model discussed below is an example of a pain model that has more homogeneity than most. To date, however, almost all of the published reports of short-term, multidose analgesic studies in postoperative pain have not limited patient selection to a particular surgical procedure (3,6–8).

Postpartum cramping and/or postepisiotomy pain have been extensively evaluated in single-dose analgesic studies. The sensitivity of this model relative to other available models is poor, however. Particularly problematic for repeat dose studies is that pain duration in these models is often limited and historically, many patients have required only a single dose of analgesic medication (see Table 2).

Musculoskeletal Pain Models

Acute musculoskeletal injuries can also be considered for short-term multidose studies since these conditions typically require several days of outpatient therapy. As Honig (22) has outlined, there are several problems with using this model in clinical trials. Identifying study sites that have access to adequate numbers of patients with homogeneous conditions is difficult and developing objective parameters with which to assess improvement is problematic, particularly since many of the injuries involve more than one anatomical site. In this pain model, Honig recommends evaluation of sports-related injuries and the use of global pain relief scores along with other more traditional pain assessment scales. Another type of acute orthopedic pain, that arising from a fracture, can also be considered for evaluation of a new analgesic compound; however, this pain model is limited because of the rapid reduction in pain following casting.

Dental Pain Models

Oral surgical and other dental models have been used extensively in single-dose analgesic studies with good model sensitivity. The impacted third molar extraction model has been the most successful of the dental models, probably because of the homogeneity of the procedure and the relative homogeneity of the patient population (see Chapter 15 by Forbes). The model has proven successful in both inpatient and outpatient settings. Because pain arising from this surgical procedure usually persists for 3 to 4 days, the impacted third molar extraction model lends itself well to short-term multidose evaluations. The usefulness of this model in repeat dose studies is underscored by the number of studies listed in Table 1 that have employed the model. Another dental model that may be appropriate for short-term multidose analgesic evaluations is periodontal pain, although the duration of this pain is less consistent than that arising from third molar extraction.

Intermittent Pain Models

Intermittent pain models, such as headache or dysmenorrhea, might also be considered for short-term multidose trials. In nonvascular headache pain, the doses may be spaced over a period of several weeks or months and more than one dose may be required for each headache episode. In Diamond's (20) study of zomepirac sodium and placebo in patients with recurrent muscle contraction headache, patients were instructed to take medication prn for up to four episodes of headache within a 2 month period. Dysmenorrhea pain lends itself well to short-term, multidose study designs provided that patient selection is limited to those patients with a history of a sufficient need for analgesics each month. In this patient group, repeat doses of medication over several cycles can be evaluated.

Other Pain Models

Chronic pain models such as cancer pain and pain arising from osteoarthritis can also be considered for study on a short-term basis. Stambaugh has been successful in evaluating several analgesic medications using a short-term multidose design in the cancer pain model (17–19).

Another model that has recently emerged for consideration in analgesic studies is that of sore throat pain (see Chapter 17). Although the duration of this type of pain is not well characterized, it often persists for several days, making it a candidate for evaluation in repeat-dose studies. Other acute, infectious, or other disease-related pain models have not been adequately described. Some longer-term pain models, such as burn pain, rheumatoid arthritis pain, low back pain with muscle spasm, and migraine headache pain, have a plethora of complicating factors and therefore, short-term evaluation of analgesic compounds in these models is likely to be beset with many problems.

Choice of Control Groups

Like their single-dose counterparts, multidose, short-term analgesic trials should be double-blind and well-controlled. The choice of controls for multidose studies should be appropriate to the known pharmacokinetic properties of the test compound and to the pain model selected for evaluation. Comparative results of the test drug with control agents will help to position the new drug within the spectrum of marketed analgesics. Typical analgesic benchmark standards are as appropriate for multidose studies as they are for single-dose trials. These standards include aspirin, acetaminophen, ibuprofen, codeine, and aspirin (acetaminophen)/codeine combinations. The choice of control agents for multidose studies, however, need not be limited to these standards.

A placebo control group is essential in most single-dose study designs and the use of rescue medication is standard. In multidose analgesic studies, however, the use of a placebo control is problematic. It is certainly of questionable ethics to withhold analgesic therapy from patients in pain and it is unlikely that any institutional review board will approve a repeat-dose study with a placebo control in the absence of provisions for rescue medication. Nevertheless, in repeat-dose trials the use of rescue medication among patients assigned to a placebo control group introduces an active "placebo" and makes data interpretation almost impossible. On the other hand, if placebo patients are allowed to discontinue the study after use of a rescue medication, the analysis of the study is severely compromised owing to the large dropout rate.

An alternative approach for repeat-dose designs is to include a placebo control for the first dose of medication with subsequent randomization to either the test drug or an active control agent. McQuay et al. (6) used this approach in their evaluation of zomepirac sodium and dihydrocodeine in patients with postoperative pain. In essence this type of design is a single-dose evaluation followed by a rerandomization for subsequent doses. In McQuay et al.'s study, rerandomization following the initial dose was done only for patients who received placebo as the first dose; those who received one of the active drugs were maintained on the same drug during the multidose study phase.

There may be certain situations where the use of a placebo control throughout the multidose study is appropriate. For example, in his evaluation of the efficacy of ibuprofen as add-on therapy in cancer patients, Stambaugh randomized patients receiving an oxycodone/acetaminophen combination to either prn ibuprofen or placebo treatment for 7 days (17; Chapter 6). One of the efficacy measurements evaluated in this study was the use of the oxycodone/acetamin-ophen combination in each group during the study period. In this study, the use of the combination was significantly less in patients receiving add-on ibuprofen treatment than in those receiving add-on placebo.

Dosage Regimen

Pharmacokinetic and pharmacodynamic evaluations of an analgesic agent typically guide selection of the dose-to-dose interval for administration of the agent. In repeat-dose evaluations, study medication can either be administered on a fixed dose regimen or prn. Prn dosing with a recommended dose-to-dose interval is the standard dosage recommendation for analgesic drugs. It seems reasonable, therefore, to design multidose studies that incorporate this dosing pattern. Such trials should assess the actual dosing interval necessary for the drug in a given pain condition. Inherent in a study design incorporating prn dosing is an established pain level prior to each dose; this greatly aids meaningful interpretations of efficacy results.

Multidose studies that use a fixed dosing schedule should include an assessment of pain prior to each dose along with assessments of pain relief. An obvious problem with fixed dose schedules is that patients may be treated in the absence of baseline pain, thus making interpretation of pain relief scales difficult. In pain models where there is a declining pain level over time, the use of fixed dosage regimens may preclude meaningful assessments of the drug's efficacy. Fixed dose study designs are most appropriate in pain models that do not have naturally decreasing pain, such as cancer pain or pain of osteoarthritis.

Efficacy Measurement Scales

Multidose, short-term analgesic studies can use the same efficacy measurements scales developed for single-dose studies. Both verbal and visual analogue pain intensity and pain relief scales can be used successfully in multidose studies. The actual frequency of use of these scales, however, needs to be carefully considered in multidose studies. In single-dose studies, efficacy measurements are typically made at hourly intervals for some period of time postdose. Continued hourly assessments are not feasible over a period of several days, so alternatives need to be considered.

One approach in multidose studies is to use hourly assessments made after the first dose followed by dose-to-dose relief and/or global assessments thereafter. This approach capitalizes on the more careful hourly assessments collected with single-dose studies and thus increases model sensitivity. This particular type of approach has been used by Forbes, as described in Chapter 15 on the oral surgery postoperative pain model. Another approach would be to use a single assessment of relief and/or global efficacy measures after each dose.

Efficacy measures can also be assessed at set intervals, such as once or twice daily (e.g., morning/evening). Although this approach provides a less detailed assessment of pain relief given by a particular dose, it typically has greater overall clinical acceptability. In addition, it will tend to reduce any bias favoring short-acting drugs that provide more immediate pain relief but less overall effectiveness.

It may be possible to obtain hourly efficacy measurements following the first two doses, thus increasing the probability of reliably evaluating potential differential efficacy with repeat doses. Quiding and his colleagues have used this approach with some success in their multidose assessments of analgesic drugs in the impacted third molar extraction model (10,13–16). In their studies, patients completed hourly assessments of pain relief and intensity from the time of surgery (performed usually before noon) until midnight; multiple doses of the study drugs can be administered throughout this interval, provided at least 2 hrs separated each dose. Yet another option in multidose studies is to include additional hourly pain measurement assessments at designated time points within the study.

It should be noted that the validity of relief scales in multidose studies has been questioned, specifically the pain level the patient is evaluating relief against. If the patient is evaluating relief with respect to the level of baseline pain, there is concern that recall of this pain may be poor, particularly as the interval between baseline and subsequent efficacy measurements increases. Thus, the patient should be instructed to measure relief against the pain present prior to each dose.

There is no established consensus as to the best efficacy measurement scale to employ. Furthermore, there has yet to be a published report of a study in which multiple-dose data distinguish the efficacy of various treatments better than single-dose data. Additional insights into this issue will surely emerge as more multidose analgesic studies are completed and published.

Safety Assessments

Valuable safety information can be obtained from short-term multidose studies since these studies closely approximate the manner in which the analgesic drug will ultimately be used. Adverse experience profiles observed in these studies are relatively predictive of future marketed experience. In contrast, single-dose studies do not provide reliable information concerning the safety of a specific drug, although these studies can provide a "red flag" if a product has a relatively unique safety concern. This particular point was illustrated in a study by McQuay et al. (6) which included both a single-dose and a multidose component. Following administration of the single dose, very few side effects were noted; however, approximately 50% of patients in the active treatment groups reported at least one side effect following multidose administration for 5 days. Although short-term multidose studies provide useful information concerning the safety of a new drug, chronic studies provide the definitive safety profile.

Adverse experience information is typically elicited through use of a patient diary or through reports to the investigator or study nurse at scheduled visits. In certain situations, it may be desirable to ask the patient to answer questions relating to the occurrence of specific side effects. Such questions should be used judiciously since they can artificially inflate the natural incidence of the side effect.

It is also possible to collect vital-sign data in multidose studies; however, unless the pharmacologic profile of the drug suggests an effect on a specific vital sign parameter, the usefulness of such information is questionable. Routine measurement of clinical laboratory parameters, electrocardiograms, or pulmonary function tests have not typically been done in short-term, multidose analgesic studies, but they may be considered in special situations where a question has arisen concerning the effect of the test drug on a specific parameter.

Statistical Analysis

Obviously, the statistical techniques used to analyze data from multidose studies need to be appropriate to the design options selected for a particular study. The choice of parametric versus nonparametric statistical tests needs to be made based on the assumptions concerning the data collected. This issue is addressed in Chapter 4 on single-dose study designs.

Two interesting theoretical questions arise concerning analysis of multidose studies. One concerns the need to adjust for differences in the number of doses a patient has taken. One possibility is to weight patients' data based on the number of doses taken; an alternate approach is to ignore differences in the number of doses taken and evaluate each patient equally. In many of the published studies to date, the only adjustment made for differing number of doses was to divide the pain reduction summary measures by the number of doses.

A typical approach has been to average all measurements of a particular efficacy parameter for each patient and then for all patients in a particular treatment group before evaluating intergroup differences. This approach has provided statistical separation of treatment groups. Information about individual patient response to repeat doses of analgesics can be masked with this approach; therefore, it is important to analyze not only the efficacy parameter(s) but the number of doses and the interval between doses. Such dosage interval data can be useful in drafting labeling information for the product.

New methods are emerging for modeling, estimating, and testing longitudinal data (23–27). Undoubtedly, as short-term multidose analgesic study designs become better characterized, corresponding statistical methods will also be established.

SUMMARY

It seems clear that short-term multidose studies evaluating both efficacy and safety will be required in new development programs for analgesic compounds.

These studies will generally be considered late Phase II or Phase III studies for NDA submissions and their intent is to evaluate pain types and dosage regimens that are appropriate to the intended clinical use of the drug.

After reviewing available short-term multidose studies of analgesic drugs it is apparent that no standardized methodology exists for conducting these studies. Until such a methodology is developed, investigators and sponsors will need to rely on current scientific data and clinical judgment in designing short-term multidose studies. Certain guidelines can be recommended for these studies. Entrance criteria (including pain state) and dosage regimen should be based on the anticipated use of the drug. Except under special situations the use of a placebo control should be avoided. Efficacy measurements can include pain relief and intensity scales developed for single-dose studies and safety assessments should include adverse experience monitoring.

Although short-term multidose analgesics may not provide the degree of assay sensitivity achievable with single-dose studies, they do offer a more reliable assessment of the drug under circumstances more closely resembling the intended clinical use.

REFERENCES

1. U.S. Dept. of Health, Education and Welfare. Guidelines for the clinical evaluation of analgesic drugs. FDA 80-3093. Washington, DC: U.S. Government Printing Office, November, 1979.
2. Beaver WT. Measurement of analgesic efficacy in man. In: Bonica JJ, ed. *Advances in pain research and therapy.* New York: Raven Press, 1983;411–434.
3. DeAndrade JR, Honig S, Ciccone WJ, Leffall L. Clinical comparison of zomepirac with pentazocine in the treatment of postoperative pain. *J Clin Pharmacol* 1980;20:292–297.
4. Elbaz JS, Bernard A. A controlled repeat-dose comparison of zomepirac and clometacin in pain after plastic surgery. *J Clin Pharmacol* 1980;20:303–308.
5. Messer RH, Vaughn T, Harbert G. Clinical evaluation of zomepirac and APC with codeine in the treatment of postpartum episiotomy pain. *J Clin Pharmacol* 1980;20:279–284.
6. McQuay HJ, Bullingham RES, Moore RA, et al. Zomepirac, dihydrocodeine and placebo compared in postoperative pain after day-case surgery. *Br J Anaesth* 1985;57:412–419.
7. Ouellette RD. Double-blind, multiple-dose comparison of buprenorphine and meperidine for postoperative pain following major abdominal surgery. *Curr Ther Res* 1989;46:352–365.
8. Ouellette RD, Mok MS, Gilbert MS, et al. Comparison of buprenorphine and morphine: a multicenter, multidose study in patients with severe postoperative pain. *Cont Surg* 1986;28:55–64.
9. Wang RIH, Johnson RP, Robinson N, Waite E. The study of analgesics following single and repeated doses. *J Clin Pharmacol* 1981;21:121–125.
10. Ahlstrom U, Fahraeus J, Quiding H, Strom C. Multiple doses of paracetamol plus codeine taken immediately after oral surgery. *Eur J Clin Pharmacol* 1985;693–696.
11. Mehlisch RD, Joy ED, Moore TE, et al. Clinical comparison of zomepirac with APC/codeine combination in the treatment of pain following oral surgery. *J Clin Pharmacol* 1980;20:271–278.
12. McQuay HJ, Carroll D, Watts PG, Juniper RP, Moore RA. Codeine 20 mg increases pain relief from ibuprofen 400 mg after third molar surgery. A repeat-dosing comparison of ibuprofen and an ibuprofen-codeine combination. *Pain* 1989;37:7–13.
13. Nystrom E, Gustafsson I, Quiding H. The pain intensity at analgesic intake, and the efficacy of diflunisal in single doses and effervescent acetaminophen in single and repeated doses. *Pharmacotherapy* 1988;8:201–209.
14. Quiding H, Oksala E, Happonen R-P, Lehtimaki K, Ojala T. The visual analog scale in multiple-dose evaluations of analgesics. *J Clin Pharmacol* 1981;21:424–429.

15. Quiding H, Oikarinen V, Sane J, Sjoblad A. Analgesic efficacy after single and repeated doses of codeine and acetaminophen. *J Clin Pharmacol* 1984;24:27–34.
16. Quiding H, Persson G, Ahlstrom U, et al. Paracetamol plus supplementary doses of codeine. An analgesic study of repeated doses. *Eur J Clin Pharmacol* 1982;23:315–319.
17. Stambaugh JE, Drew J. The combination of ibuprofen and oxycodone/acetaminophen in the management of chronic cancer pain. *Clin Pharmacol Ther* 1988;44:665–669.
18. Stambaugh JE, McAdams J. Comparison of intramuscular dezocine with butorphanol and placebo in chronic cancer pain: a method to evaluate analgesia after both single and repeated doses. *Clin Pharmacol Ther* 1987;42:210–219.
19. Stambaugh JE, Tejada F, Trudnowski RJ. Double-blind comparisons of zomepirac and oxycodone with APC in cancer pain. *J Clin Pharmacol* 1980;20:261–270.
20. Diamond S. Zomepirac in the symptomatic treatment of muscle contraction headache. *J Clin Pharmacol* 1980;20:298–302.
21. Mayer TG, Ruoff GE. Clinical evaluation of zomepirac in the treatment of acute orthopedic pain. *J Clin Pharmacol* 1980;20:285–291.
22. Honig S. Clinical trials in acute musculoskeletal injury states. *Am J Med* 1988;84(Suppl 5A): 42–44.
23. Laird NM, Ware SH. Random-effects models for longitudinal data. *Biometrics* 1982;38:963–974.
24. Zeger SL, Liang K-Y. Longitudinal data analysis for discrete and continuous outcomes. *Biometrics* 1986;42(1):121–130.
25. Wu MC, ed. *Proceedings of the workshop on methods for longitudinal data analysis in epidemiological and clinical studies,* September 1986;1–176.
26. Zeger SL, Liang K-Y, Albert PS. Models for longitudinal data: a generalized estimating equation approach (published erratum appears in *Biometrics* 1989;45:347). *Biometrics* 1988;44:1049–1060.
27. Jennrich RI, Schluchter MD. Unbalanced repeated-measures models with structured co-variance matrices. *Biometrics* 1986;42:805–820.

Advances in Pain Research and Therapy, Vol. 18,
edited by M. Max, R. Portenoy, and E. Laska,
Raven Press, Ltd., New York © 1991.

6

Multidose Analgesic Studies in Chronic Pain Models

John E. Stambaugh

*Department of Pharmacology, Thomas Jefferson University Medical College,
Philadelphia, Pennsylvania 19107; and Oncology and Hematology Associates, P.A.,
Haddon Heights, New Jersey 08035*

Although repeat-dose studies can employ many of the parameters used with single-dose studies such as verbal and visual pain descriptors, global evaluations, peak responses, and recording of side effects, past attempts to derive significant statistical data from such studies have been difficult. As a result, most repeat-dose study trials in the past have been reduced to safety studies, using in many cases an open-label design and rarely including enough statistical analysis to merit a major journal publication.

Single-dose data is not always applicable to clinical practice since most analgesics are used as repeat doses and responses can vary as the intensity of the pain and the patient's clinical status changes over time. In addition, repeated doses of an analgesic can lead to responses different from those observed in single-dose studies owing to cumulative toxicity or a delay in onset of action such as reported for codeine, d-propoxyphene, nonsteroidal antiinflammatory drugs (NSAIDs), and even morphine (1–4).

Our group's research has focused on the development of new methodology to compare analgesics in chronic pain conditions, specifically cancer pain and chronic musculoskeletal pain (5). The studies have combined the concepts used in single-dose studies with repeated-dose trials of 7 days or longer (6–8). From such studies, comparisons of single-dose versus repeat-dose efficacy and side effects can be made. In addition, these combined studies have further defined these chronic pain models and suggested alternative study designs.

STUDY DESIGN OF CHRONIC PAIN STUDIES

A complete discussion of the study designs that can be employed in chronic pain is not possible in this chapter since the published research is still limited in scope. A description of our cancer pain model is included in the commentary after Chapter 10 (p. 289) and depicts patients selected for these studies.

COMBINATION STUDY DESIGN OF SINGLE AND REPEAT DOSES IN CHRONIC PAIN

From single-dose and repeat-dose studies in chronic pain, it became apparent that matching results were not always obtained. Efficacy evaluations either improved or deteriorated for each of the drugs tested and side effect data appeared to explain the decreasing efficacy evaluations as the study was extended. Table 1 describes a randomized, double-blind study design yielding single-dose data in which each subject receives either a placebo, the reference compound(s), or the test drug(s). The study is a parallel design, and subjects who report adequate analgesia after the first dose then enter a 7-day repeat dosing evaluation period, receiving the same test agent. The repeat-dose portion of the study uses standard single-dose descriptors to define pain, and collects daily global ratings and side effect data throughout.

This study design allows comparison of initial analgesic efficacy to ongoing daily efficacy as determined by overall global ratings. In addition, a comparison of each agent's response in the single-dose phase can be accomplished using the statistics as described for single-dose studies. This particular study design could be further expanded to include last treatment single-dose hourly evaluations in which efficacy after the first dose and the last dose of the study could be compared to see if there is a difference in drug acceptance and analgesic scores. The design also allows the inclusion of pharmacokinetic data after single dose, after repeat doses during the 7-day evaluations, and after a last-dose evaluation. This study

TABLE 1. *Single-dose parallel study design followed by 7-day repeat-dosing evaluation—summary of events*

	Hours									Days						
	0	$\frac{1}{2}$	1	2	3	4	5	6	12	2	3	4	5	6	7	8
Physical exam	X															X
History	X															X
Laboratory	X															X
Vital signs	X			X					X	X	X	X	X	X	X	
Initial pain evaluation	X															
Analgesic ratings		X	X	X	X	X	X	X								
Visual +/− analogue scales																
Recording of adverse effects		X	X	X	X	X	X	X		X	X	X	X	X	X	X
Patient's global evaluation									X	X	X	X	X	X	X	X
Observer's global evaluation									X							X

From ref. 8, with permission.

has been conducted on both inpatients and outpatients, but an outpatient study requires careful patient selection to enhance compliance and a very prodigious observer to make daily calls for efficacy, toxicity, and overall global determinations.

RESULTS OF A SINGLE PLUS MULTIPLE DOSE
CLINICAL TRIAL IN CHRONIC PAIN

The results that can be obtained from this study design are exemplified in a recent publication describing a randomized, parallel double-blind trial comparing single doses and multiple doses of dezocine and butorphanol to placebo (8). The study required 60 subjects to separate the active agents from placebo and entry required a 24-month period. Comparisons of demographic data were done using a one-way analysis of variance.

STUDY CRITERIA

Chemotherapy regimens were permitted if the complete blood counts were stable with treatment. Analgesics, psychotropic drugs, and steroids that potentially could confound efficacy determinations were withheld for at least 4 hrs before initial administration of the study drugs. Patients with prior opioid exposure were not enrolled if their analgesic histories indicated potential opioid tolerance.

DOSING AND EVALUATION DESIGN SIMILAR
TO SINGLE-DOSE PARALLEL STUDIES

On a day that a patient reported moderate or greater pain, an initial dose of either placebo, butorphanol 2 mg or dezocine 10 mg was administered in a double-blind fashion by the nurse observer. At $\frac{1}{4}$, $\frac{1}{2}$, 1, 2, 3, 4, 5, and 6 hrs after administration of the first dose, observations of efficacy and safety and vital signs were recorded. For efficacy evaluation, the variables used were a verbal four-point pain intensity scale ranging from none (0) to severe (3), a verbal five-point pain relief scale ranging from worse (01) to complete relief (4), and a linear 100 mm visual analogue pain intensity scale ranging from "no pain" to "worse pain I've ever felt," on which the patients marked the line segment that best described the pain at that time.

If pain relief was insufficient after 2 hrs, the patient could be remedicated with either a standard analgesic or an additional dose of the same study medication at his or her request or the nurse observer's discretion, depending on the degree of relief experienced. These patients were assigned scores corresponding to baseline pain intensity or to no relief for the duration of the 6-hr observation period. If at the end of the initial drug administration period a patient's analgesic response was rated as satisfactory by the investigator and fair or better by the patient, he or she entered the multidose portion of the study (Table 1). If a patient reported a lesser response or significant side effects, he or she was withdrawn from the study.

THE REPEAT-DOSE PHASE OF THE STUDY DESIGN

In the repeat-dose portion of the study, the unit nurses administered the same medication that the patient had received initially for the next 7 days on an as-needed basis. Sedation and safety data and vital signs were recorded twice daily by the nurse observer. The patient recorded dosage times, daily global evaluations of efficacy, and the presence of side effects daily on a diary card throughout the study. Global efficacy evaluations were based on a four-point scale from poor (1) to excellent (4).

Patients were withdrawn if drug administration was associated with either inadequate (less than moderate) pain relief or clinically unacceptable toxicity. Otherwise, the study was terminated at the completion of the full 7-day period; the patients made a final global evaluation, and the investigator gave a global rating of satisfactory or unsatisfactory.

Statistical Evaluations

Weighted pain intensity differences and pain analogue intensity differences scores (i.e., each score multiplied by the fraction of 1 hr since the last reading) were added to determine cumulative efficacy measures. Individual total pain relief was calculated by adding weighted mean pain relief scores. Data for the groups were analyzed at each observation time by the generalized Cochran-Mantel-Haenszel procedure. Because of such factors as the lack of independence among observations after the first dose, statistical analyses of efficacy were restricted to the first dose given and to the global evaluations. The physician and patient global evaluations were also analyzed by the generalized Cochran-Mantel-Haenszel procedure as a measure of repeated-dose efficacy. Vital signs and laboratory data were compared using a paired t-test and the relative frequency of adverse effects among groups was compared by the X2 test supplemented by Fisher's exact test for pairwise comparison.

Results of Single Versus Repeat Doses

The mean pain relief scores for the three treatment groups are shown in Fig. 1. Results in this study for the three efficacy scales used showed higher scores for the dezocine and butorphanol compared to placebo. The mean scores for dezocine were higher than placebo on all scales up to 6 hrs, whereas butorphanol

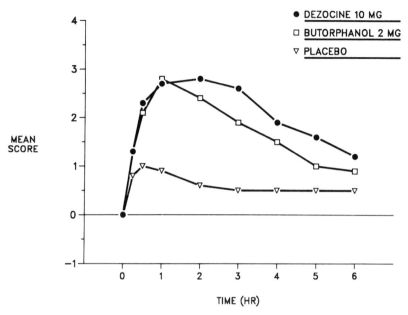

FIG. 1. Mean pain relief scores for the three treatment groups for 6 hrs after a single intramuscular dose. Higher scores indicate greater pain relief. (From ref. 8, with permission.)

showed significance to only 4 hrs. Dezocine showed an onset of action after 30 min while butorphanol showed analgesia after 15 min.

Evaluation of cumulative treatment failures (patients remedicated before the end of the initial 6-hr observation period) are shown in Fig. 2. This figure also suggests a longer duration of action for dezocine than for butorphanol. The daily mean scores for patients, the overall global evaluations, and the physician overall evaluations are shown in Table 2. The more favorable response was observed with dezocine relative to butorphanol. Both physician and patient evaluations indicated a significant ($p < 0.05$) advantage for dezocine over butorphanol and placebo. Mean doses of both treatment groups increased on day 2 but showed no trend to increasing doses or the development of tolerance.

A Placebo Effect May Not Persist in Repeat-Dose Evaluations

In the placebo group 90% withdrew on the first day of study as compared to 45% of the butorphanol-treated group (25% because of unsatisfactory pain relief) and 15% of the dezocine-treated group, all because of unsatisfactory relief (Table 3).

Fourteen subjects who received dezocine completed all 7 days, compared with only one who received placebo and four who received butorphanol. The percent of patients who withdrew from the entire study, regardless of reason, was sig-

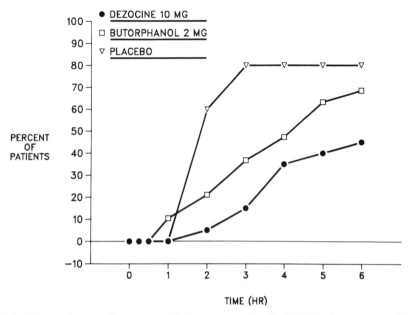

FIG. 2. Display of cumulative treatment failures versus time for initial treatment period. (From ref. 8, with permission.)

TABLE 2. *Mean scores for patient evaluations and physician evaluations*

Treatment	Patient evaluations[a]							Overall global	Physician overall global[b]
	Day 1	Day 2	Day 3	Day 4	Day 5	Day 6	Day 7		
Dezocine	3.2[c]	3.4[c]	3.3[d]	3.2	3.2	3.2[c]	3.3	3.0[c,d]	80[c,d]
n[e]	20	17	17	17	17	16	14		
Dose (mg)									
Mean	22.5	31.9	27.5	30.7	25.6	26.0	30.0		
Range	10–40	10–60	10–60	10–60	10–50	10–60	20–50		
Butorphanol	2.6[b]	2.8	2.4	3.0	2.8	3.0	3.0	1.9[c]	37
n[e]	20	11	10	8	6	4	4		
Dose (mg)									
Mean	3.7	5.0	6.7	6.0	4.5	5.5	7.3		
Range	2–8	2–10	2–10	2–8	2–8	2–10	6–12		
Placebo	1.2	2.0	NA	2.0	NA	1.0	2.0	1.3	11

NA, not available.
[a] Based on a scale of poor (1), fair (2), good (3), and excellent (4).
[b] Percentage of patients with a satisfactory evaluation.
[c] Significantly ($p < 0.05$) better than placebo.
[d] Significantly ($p < 0.05$) better than butorphanol.
[e] Number of patients at the beginning of the day.
From ref. 8, with permission.

TABLE 3. *Patients who withdrew from study*

Reason for patient withdrawal	Study day						Any study day
	1	2	3	4	5	6	
Dezocine (n = 20)							
Unsatisfactory pain relief	3 (15%)[a]	0	0	0	1 (5%)	0	4 (20%)[a]
Adverse experience	0	0	0	0	0	0	0[b]
Administrative	0	0	0	0	0	2 (10%)	2 (10%)[a,b]
Any reason	3 (15%)[a]	0	0	0	1 (5%)	2 (10%)	6 (30%)[a,b]
Butorphanol (n = 20)							
Adverse experience plus unsatisfactory relief	0	0	1 (5%)	0	1 (5%)	0	2 (10%)
Unsatisfactory pain relief	5 (25%)[a]	0	0	0	0	0	5 (25%)[a]
Adverse experience	4 (20%)	1 (5%)	1 (5%)	1 (5%)	0	0	7 (35%)
Administrative	0	0	0	0	1 (5%)	0	1 (5%)
Patient died (disease related)	0	0	0	1 (5%)	0	0	1 (5%)
Any reason	9 (45%)[a]	1 (5%)	2 (10%)	2 (10%)	2 (10%)	0	16 (80%)
Placebo (n = 20)							
Unsatisfactory pain relief	17 (85%)	0	0	0	0	0	17 (85%)
Adverse experience	0	0	0	0	0	0	0[b]
No further analgesia required	0	0	0	0	0	1 (5%)	1 (5%)
No further analgesia required/patient request	1 (5%)	0	0	0	0	0	1 (5%)
Any reason	18 (90%)	0	0	0	0	1 (5%)	19 (95%)

Note: Percentages are based on the number of patients enrolled in each therapy group.
[a] Significantly (p = 0.01) lower percentage than in the placebo group.
[b] Significantly (p = 0.01) lower percentage than in the butorphanol group.
From ref. 8, with permission.

nificantly higher in the placebo (95%) and the butorphanol groups (80%) than in the dezocine group (30%), and the difference between the dezocine and the other two groups was significant ($p < 0.01$). The percent of patients who discontinued the overall study because of an unsatisfactory response was significantly higher in the placebo group (85%) than in either the butorphanol (25%) or dezocine (20%) groups; pairwise comparisons showed a significant ($p < 0.05$) difference between placebo and both active therapy groups. In the entire study, 35% of the butorphanol-treated patients were withdrawn from treatment because of adverse experiences alone and two additional patients were withdrawn because of lack of efficacy and adverse effects. No patients in either the dezocine or placebo group discontinued as the result of adverse side effects.

Adverse Experiences Accounted for Dropouts

In the butorphanol group, the predominant adverse experiences included sedation, dizziness, confusion, anxiety, hallucinations, and dysphoria; several subjects had more than one side effect. Comparison of single- and multiple-dose safety data indicated that the butorphanol group had increasing toxicity to the point of eventual discontinuation of therapy. In contrast, multiple doses of dezocine did not lead to increased toxicity throughout the 7-day period, accounting for the significantly greater number of patients who completed the study. Psychotomimetic reactions to the butorphanol also increased in severity and frequency with multiple doses and accounted for patient discontinuance from the study. All four of the butorphanol-treated patients who reported psychoses discontinued treatment. Dezocine produced neither psychotomimetic reactions nor gastrointestinal upset, in contrast to the 15% of the patients who had nausea and vomiting with butorphanol. Overall, dezocine had fewer side effects than butorphanol with no limiting adverse effects from multiple doses.

The initial dose data also indicated that dezocine may have a longer duration of action (4 vs. 6 hrs) than the reference drug, with less toxicity. The repeat-dose phase of the study in the same subjects led to conclusions not easily reached by the single-dose study or from repeat-dose uncontrolled trials. The observed increase in sedation and psychotomimetic reactions after repeat doses of butorphanol primarily accounted for patient withdrawal during the 2- to 7-day period. The combined results of the initial and repeated doses indicate that in the management of cancer pain, dezocine should provide adequate analgesia for up to 7 days without the development of tolerance or limiting side effects. In addition, it would appear that 20 to 30 mg/day of dezocine in two to three divided doses is adequate to control moderate to severe cancer pain.

In Chronic Pain, the Placebo Group is a "No Treatment" Group

The results of this study suggest that in multiple-dose trials in chronic pain syndromes such as cancer in which there is reasonably effective standard therapy, a placebo group may be inappropriate. Even the rare placebo responder in this study obtained less analgesia than did subjects who received active drug. Comparisons of efficacy and toxicity data of an active drug with placebo in cancer pain was not possible after repeat doses because of withdrawal of the placebo group after the first day of administration.

THE "DOSE-REDUCTION" STUDY DESIGN

The dose-reduction study design is a placebo-controlled method for evaluating the analgesia resulting from the addition of a second analgesic to a standard. Single-dose studies have shown that aspirin-like drugs augment opiate analgesia (9). Such additive analgesia has recently been demonstrated in repeat-dose studies using the method of reducing the dose of a standard analgesic by the addition of a second analgesic to a controlled analgesic regimen (10).

The schema for a dose-reduction study design is shown in Table 4. In this design, the patient is stabilized on the control analgesic, for example a narcotic, and after an adequate stabilization period the test analgesic or a placebo is added. The ability of the second drug to reduce the dosage of the narcotic over a period

TABLE 4. *Dose reduction study design comparing placebo to test analgesic summary of events*

	Prestudy days							Poststudy days						
	1	2	3	4	5	6	7	8	9	10	11	12	13	14
Consent	X													
Physical	X													X
Evaluation of														
oxy/APAP use	X	X	X	X	X	X	X	X	X	X	X	X	X	X
Pain relief intensity	X	X	X	X	X	X	X	X	X	X	X	X	X	X
Hospitalized[a]						X	X	X	X	X	X	X	X	X
Final globals														X
Side effect data								X	X	X	X	X	X	X
Administration placebo														
vs test drug								X	X	X	X	X	X	X

[a] Optional, pending model and drug studied.
From ref. 10, with permission.

of observation is a demonstration of additive analgesia. Such an effect in chronic pain can be observed immediately with an agent with rapid onset of action or after prolonged administration of a slower-acting agent such as an NSAID.

RESULTS OF A DOSE-REDUCTION STUDY: IBUPROFEN OR PLACEBO ADDED TO OXYCODONE/ACETAMINOPHEN THERAPY

Subjects selected for the study were patients with moderate to severe pain caused by cancer metastatic to bone. Eligible patients experienced pain that was controlled by an oxycodone/acetaminophen (oxy/APAP) combination, requiring a minimum of four oxycodone/acetaminophen doses per day, and were anticipated to be hospitalized for treatment of their cancer. The 30 subjects who finally entered the hospital and completed the study were among 64 initially evaluated as outpatients for at least 5 days regarding daily as-needed oxycodone/acetaminophen requirement. All patients were screened for their ability to fill out the evaluation forms and accurately record their doses and responses.

Study Design—Ibuprofen Versus Placebo

During the prestudy days, a diary was used by the subjects to record daily oxy/APAP usage, pain intensity, and pain-relief scores. Study subjects who met all requirements of the study were hospitalized on or before day 6 of the study, and the use of oxy/APAP on days 6 and 7 of the observation period were recorded. Subjects were then randomized to receive, on day 8 of the study, either *ibuprofen,* 600 mg orally four times a day, or *placebo,* in combination with the as-needed oxy/APAP regimen for an additional 7 days. Daily oxy/APAP requirements were recorded and pain intensity and pain-relief evaluations were performed by the nurse observer each afternoon for days 6 through 14. Subject and investigator global evaluations were determined on day 14 of the study. Subjects were permitted an occasional rescue dose of an alternate parenteral analgesic throughout the study but were discontinued if more than one dose per 24 hrs was required. Changes in nonanalgesic medications and medical regimens during the study were limited as much as possible to create a stable baseline for evaluating both the efficacy and toxicity of the study medication and the oxycodone/acetaminophen usage.

Statistical Evaluation

A comparison was made between the daily oxy/APAP requirement during the first week and that during the second week using analysis of variance (ANOVA) and t-test analysis. Mean daily pain intensity and pain relief difference scores for the ibuprofen versus the placebo group were obtained by comparison of the daily efficacy evaluations performed before (days 6 and 7) and after (days 8 to 14) the addition of the study drug. Statistical analysis of the difference scores for the two groups was performed using ANOVA and student t-test analysis. Finally, the subjects' and investigator's global evaluations for the ibuprofen versus placebo groups were also compared by ANOVA and t-test analyses.

Results Observed—Ibuprofen Reduced the Requirements for Narcotic Analgesia

During the first 24 hrs of ibuprofen treatment, there was a reduction in the oxy/APAP usage from 8.9 to 7.4 pills (Fig. 3), significantly greater than the minimal change with placebo. A progressive reduction in opiate requirement was observed on each subsequent observation day, peaking after 5 days (day 12). This amounted to a 33% reduction in oxy/APAP usage during ibuprofen treatment. In the placebo group, the amount of oxy/APAP required to achieve pain relief actually increased and on day 12, the increase amounted to a 10% difference.

Figure 4 shows daily mean pain intensity differences and mean pain relief scores, respectively, for the ibuprofen versus placebo groups. Analysis of the subjects' pain intensity and pain relief indicated that the subjects receiving oxy/APAP and ibuprofen noted more analgesia than the group receiving oxy/APAP and placebo. Patient and nurse observer evaluations obtained at completion of the study also demonstrated enhanced analgesic efficacy in the ibuprofen group. Global ratings ranged from 1 (excellent) to 5 (poor). Mean patient global scores were 4.47 for placebo and 3.067 for ibuprofen ($p < 0.05$). Mean observer global scores were 4.467 and 3.133 for the placebo and ibuprofen groups, respectively ($p < 0.01$). Comparison of toxicity data of the two groups indicated that there were no differences in these 30 subjects as to observed side effects.

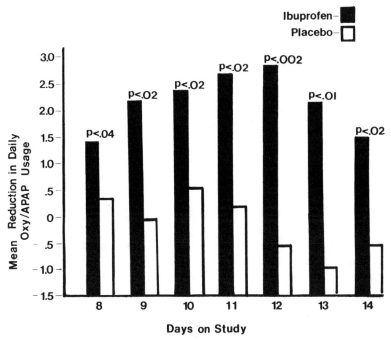

FIG. 3. Alterations of oxy/APAP use after the addition of 600 mg ibuprofen or placebo to regimen on day 8. Mean reduction scores were determined by comparing oxy/APAP pretreatment means of days 6 and 7 with treatment means for days 8 through 14. The *p* values indicate ANOVA of means of placebo versus ibuprofen for each study day. (From ref. 10, with permission.)

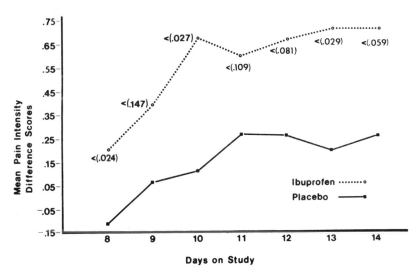

FIG. 4. Comparison of mean pain intensity differences of ibuprofen versus placebo in combination with oxy/APAP. Values in parentheses represent *p* values of ibuprofen versus placebo. (From ref. 10, with permission.)

This study demonstrates that ibuprofen reduces the opioid requirements of cancer patients with bone pain and that the time to initial onset of the analgesic effect of ibuprofen is less than 24 hrs, as verbal reports of analgesic efficacy were better and oxy/APAP dosage was reduced significantly in the subjects after 24 hrs. These findings confirm previous single-dose data that ibuprofen enhances analgesia and reduces opioid requirements in patients with cancer (11). However, this study further suggests that since the maximum analgesia occurs only by 5 days, repeated dosing might be necessary for full inhibition of prostaglandin mechanisms. Because of this delayed effect, it would appear that repeat-dose studies of NSAIDs are necessary to yield the most complete analgesic efficacy information.

OTHER STUDY DESIGNS CURRENTLY BEING EVALUATED

Alternative study designs used in our chronic pain model include a forced dose-reduction schema similar to the design shown in Table 3 in which the analgesic used to control the pain is slowly decreased by increments as a second agent versus placebo is added. Such a design allows titration of the analgesic downward after the second agent is added. Twice daily calls are necessary for evaluation of adequate analgesia and adjustment of the titrated component. Such a study design allows close approximation of the contribution of each component to the analgesic response.

Repeat-dose study designs employing chronic pain models also have been conducted comparing immediate (4 hrs) to sustained (8 to 12 hrs) release formulations. In such studies, the formulations are blinded after an open-label period during which the analgesic dose is determined using a titration technique. During the double-blind portion of the study, a placebo is used for the dummy doses required between the active sustained release formulas. Efficacy, toxicity, and pharmacokinetics data can be obtained from the study and crossover between immediate release to sustained release is possible.

SUMMARY

It is apparent that the above repeat-dose study designs used in the chronic pain model have greater potential to define clinical properties of an analgesic than any of the currently used single-dose models, since results observed will more accurately reflect the role that a particular analgesic (as well as the reference compound) could play in the management of chronic pain. It should be noted that many of the reference compounds have never been subjected to intensive long-term controlled studies and misusage in clinical practice may have resulted.

The study designs presented in this chapter are in the early stages of development and provide a nucleus from which further clinical trial designs might be elaborated. It is predicted that the single-dose studies eventually will play a lesser role in the evaluation of new analgesics and single-dose data will be used largely for determining the regimens to be used in repeat-dose studies.

The success of any clinical trial is based upon the personnel involved and a meticulous observer is needed to insure that day-to-day and week-to-week data is collected from as large a percent of the study's population as possible. The compliance in these studies is directly proportional to the control of the patients' treatment. If feasible, the physician-observer should be the attending physician for the subjects.

REFERENCES

1. Quiding H, Oikarinen V, Sane J, Sjoblad A-M. Analgesic efficacy after single and repeated doses of codeine and acetaminophen. *J Clin Pharmacol* 1984;24:27–34.
2. Caldwell JR, Germain BF, Lourie SH, et al. Ketoprofen versus indomethacin in patients with rheumatoid arthritis: a multicenter double blind comparative study. *J Rheumatol* 1988;15:1476–1479.
3. Hanks GW, Aherne GW, Hoskin PJ, Turner P, Poulain P. Explanation for potency of repeated oral doses of morphine. *Lancet* 1987;723–724.
4. Inturrisi CE, Colburn WA, Verebey K, Dayton HE, Woody GE, O'Brien CP. Propoxyphene and norpropoxyphene kinetics after single and repeated doses of propoxyphene. *Clin Pharmacol Ther* 1982;31(2):157–166.
5. Stambaugh JE. The evaluation of analgesics in chronic pain: repeat dose methodology. In: Mahon GM, ed. *Principles and techniques of human research and therapeutics—selected topics,* vol 2, Analgesics and NSAID. New York: Futura, 1985; Chapter 2.
6. Stambaugh JE, Sarajian C. Analgesic efficacy of zomepirac sodium in patient with pain due to cancer. *J Clin Pharmacol* 1981;21:501–507.
7. Stambaugh JE, Tejada F, Trudnowski RJ. Double-blind comparisons of zomepirac and oxycodone with APC in cancer pain. *J Clin Pharmacol* 1980;20:261–270.
8. Stambaugh JE, McAdams J. Comparison of intramuscular dezocine with butorphanol and placebo in chronic cancer pain: a method to evaluate analgesia after both single and repeated doses. *Clin Pharmacol Ther* 1987;42:210–219.
9. Houde RW, Wallenstein SL, Beaver WT. Clinical measurement of pain. In: de Stevens G, ed. *Analgesics.* New York: Academic Press, 1965;75–122.
10. Stambaugh JE, Drew J. The combination of ibuprofen and oxycodone/acetaminophen in the management of chronic cancer pain. *Clin Pharmacol Ther* 1988;44:665–669.
11. Ferrer-Brechner T, Ganz P. Combination therapy with ibuprofen and methadone for chronic cancer pain. *Am J Med* 1984;77:78–83.

Advances in Pain Research and Therapy, Vol. 18,
edited by M. Max, R. Portenoy, and E. Laska,
Raven Press, Ltd., New York © 1991.

Commentary

Repeated-Dose Clinical Analgesic Assays

Raymond W. Houde

*Pain Service, Department of Neurology, Memorial Sloan-Kettering
Cancer Center, New York, New York 10021*

As has been pointed out, there is no general agreement on how best to carry out
controlled repeated-dose clinical analgesic assays. The published literature on
studies of this type, particularly on short-term repeated-dose assays, is limited.
Few of the reports employ the same experimental designs or use the same language
as other reports. Dictionaries generally define the word "dose" as the quantity
of a drug, or other remedy, given or prescribed to be taken at one time. However,
in articles on repeated-dose analgesic assays, the terms "repeated-dose," "repeat-
dose," "multiple-dose," and "multidose" are often used simply to denote the
repeated administration of the study drugs, whether they are of the same or
different dosages. In addition, the terms are frequently used without clearly stating
whether they are in reference only to the administration of the drugs or to their
assessment as well.

DEFINITION OF TERMS

For the purposes of this discussion, the word "dose" will be used to refer solely
to the giving or taking of the drug, and "dosage" or "dose level" will be employed
to denote the amounts of drug in the doses. The doses will, of course, also include
both those that are actively monitored for their analgesic effects and those that
are not. To distinguish between the two circumstances, the term "administered
doses" will be used (for lack of a better term) to refer only to the doses given or
taken but not monitored, and the term "challenge doses" will be used to identify
the doses that are monitored. The terms "test drug" and "standard" will be
employed in the conventional ways, and "placebo" will be specified when a
dummy medication is a reference standard instead of, or in addition to, a known
active analgesic. Lastly, "study medication" will be used as a nonspecific term
to refer to any medication given as part of the study, whether merely as an
administered dose or as a challenge dose of either the test drug or standard (the
study drugs).

Monitored Dose Substitution

Rarely are all doses in a repeated-dose study actually monitored. Commonly, the monitored doses are single-dose challenges given as the last dose—sometimes along with the first dose and/or interspersed doses—of a series of administered doses. In fact, many so-called single-dose assays are also studies in which a solitary challenge dose of the study drug is substituted for an analgesic that the patient has already been receiving. Most single-dose assays carried out in patients with postoperative or chronic pain are, in reality, drug/dose substitution studies differing from repeated-dose studies only in that antecedent analgesics are not identified or are not the same drugs as the monitored study medications. Nevertheless, in these situations, as in repeated-dose and crossover designed studies, pharmacological as well as psychological carryover effects are inevitable—a fact that is often not fully appreciated. At the very least, the repeated-dose design insures control of the identity and dosage of the drug preceding the monitored study medication and that, in itself, is good reason for including short-term repeated-dose experimental designs in early Phase II analgesic drug assessments.

RATIONALE AND LIMITATIONS OF REPEATED-DOSE ASSAYS

The use of repeated-dose studies for the assessment of analgesic efficacy has been advocated for several reasons. The most frequently stated argument is that, in clinical practice, analgesic drugs are almost always administered or taken in series rather than as isolated single doses. Accordingly, it is felt that analgesic assays should be carried out under conditions that reflect clinical usage. Moreover, pharmacologists generally assert that a true comparison of the effects of two or more drugs cannot be made unless steady-state conditions prevail, and those conditions can only be approached or achieved by repeated or continuous dose administration. Lastly, it is obvious that cumulative effects, whether desirable or undesirable, can only become manifest after chronic or repeated administration of the drugs of interest.

There are, however, some caveats to be considered.

Drug Assessment and Clinical Usage

At the outset, we should not delude ourselves that the ways in which we carry out our controlled repeated-dose analgesic assays are likely to mirror the ways in which these drugs will be used clinically. Beyond our control, and yet capable of influencing our results, are a number of factors inherent in the nature of pain, the requirements for approval to undertake a clinical drug trial, and the ways in which medicine is customarily practiced. Patients solicited for studies of investigational drugs must be informed that they cannot be promised benefit to themselves by their participation, and they are expected to give their written consents on forms containing a mandatory statement of the institution's and investigator's responsibilities—a statement which, in a hospital consent form, could well read as follows:

> If you are injured as a result of your participation in this research study, emergency care, hospitalization, and outpatient care will be made available by the hospital and billed to you as part of your medical expenses. No money will be provided by the hospital as compensation for a research-related injury.

There are understandable reasons for such regulations, but even without discussing the potential impact on how representative the participants will be of the population of patients from which they are drawn, it should be obvious that these are not conditions that one associates with customary clinical usage of analgesics. Moreover, especially in short-term repeated-dose analgesic studies in an inpatient setting, the participants are likely to have some of their usual medications withheld, and to have to submit to repetitive interrogations and/or examinations by a research staff or nurses who are not primarily involved with the management of their disease or postoperative care. Even in the longer-term outpatient studies in which the principal investigators are more likely to be the patients' primary care providers, the demands of filling out repeated questionnaires and of adhering to protocols are not what the majority of patients ordinarily associate with their own or prescribed use of analgesics. In controlled analgesic assays, the focus is on assessing the analgesic merits and shortcomings of the test drug itself, to the exclusion of other factors capable of influencing the results. In clinical practice, physicians and other caregivers are not so constrained from employing other measures (e.g., suggestion, reassurance, rest, exercise) and they, and even the patients themselves, are not restricted from resorting to additional medications for treating pain and its associated symptoms.

Steady-State Requirements

Despite the desirability of conducting analgesic assays under steady-state conditions, even approximate steady states (plateau peak and/or trough plasma drug levels) are not readily attainable with repeated doses of analgesics in the clinical setting. To obtain relatively constant plasma concentrations of the study drugs and their active metabolites, the drugs must be given by-the-clock/around-the-clock (commonly referred to as ATC), without interruption or rescue medications, for at least five terminal elimination half-lives ($t_{\frac{1}{2}}$s) of the slowest cleared parent drug or active metabolite. Thus, apart from the necessary foreknowledge of the properties of the metabolites and of the pharmacokinetic attributes of the test drug and standard, and of their active metabolites, these studies are only feasible in patients with relatively constant pain and in whom the needs for medication for pain relief are predictable. There are few painful conditions to which these criteria would apply. In addition, to minimize the risk of intrusion of confounding factors, a repeated-dose study of this type would likely have to be a short-term assay of rapidly cleared test drugs and standards with no active metabolites.

Repeated-Dose Analgesic Assay Objectives

The decision of whether to employ a short-term as opposed to a long-term repeated-dose analgesic assay should be influenced by the objectives of the assay and, if a new drug, the investigational new drug (IND) stage of clinical investigation. Short-term repeated-dose assays are best used in early phase assessments of analgesic efficacy and relative potency, and they can be employed in virtually any population of pain patients in whom repeated doses of an analgesic may be required. On the other hand, long-term repeated-dose studies are more limited in their suitability for assaying analgesic potency, for which the demands for close control of outside influences are difficult to meet. Long-term repeated-dose studies, of necessity, require access to patients with chronic pain who, for the most part, are outpatients whose pain can be controlled with oral medications. In these circumstances, control of the use of concomitant medications, of variations in eating habits and other activities, and even of compliance with the study protocol is at best tenuous, and monitoring is commonly remote and on relatively insensitive global scales. Parenteral medications, especially opioids, are seldom suitable for controlled analgesic assays of this type, primarily because patients requiring these drugs for pain relief usually need closer monitoring than can be provided in an outpatient setting, and because long-term stays in hospitals, and access to patients in hospices and other chronic care facilities, tend to be limited. Consequently, long-term repeated-dose studies of analgesics are better suited for surveys of side effects, delayed cumulative effects and tolerance, drug interactions and idiosyncrasies, and other factors that contribute to judgments of the safety and patient acceptance of a drug, rather than for the assessment of analgesic power.

SHORT-TERM REPEATED-DOSE ASSAYS

Short-term repeated-dose assays are intended primarily for a truer assessment of analgesic efficacy of some drugs than can be provided by single-dose assays. They are, however, not expected to replace single-dose studies; there are some clinical situations where it is possible to compare analgesics in a fairly homogeneous population of patients who have not received prior analgesics, and where it is possible to carry out early Phase II assessments more expeditiously with single-dose studies than with short-term repeated-dose assays. The dental third molar extraction model, for example, has been used extensively, and with evident success, in assaying orally administered analgesics [primarily nonsteroidal antiinflammatory drugs (NSAIDs), acetaminophen, codeine, and their combinations] for their analgesic properties. In a few short-term repeated-dose assays in other postoperative pain models, estimates of the relative analgesic efficacy of fixed doses of opioids based on comparisons of the effects of the later or last in the administered series with those of the initial doses were generally in good agreement (1–3); however, this was not true in later, larger studies of the same and other drugs (4–6). In fact, one should expect that, since a meaningful assessment of the analgesic effectiveness of a drug can be judged only in terms of its effects relative to those of an established active standard drug, the relative analgesic potencies of test drugs and standards that have different durations of action will depend on when, in the course of repeated dosing, the comparisons are made.

How Long Should Repeated Doses Be Given?

In short-term repeated-dose studies, there will be less risk of interfering events and variations of pain, if the study medications are given for just as long as but no longer than necessary. An understanding of the pharmacokinetics of the test drug and standard can be a useful guide, not only for how long to give repeated doses of the study drugs, but also for how to design a most efficient study. For example, by basing the period of repeated dosing on five times the $t_{\frac{1}{2}}$ of the test drug or standard with the longest half-life, one can complete steady-state, cross-over, single-challenge dose comparisons of some drugs within a few days of repeated doses. Parenterally administered opioids, such as morphine and some of its congeners whose elimination half-lives are no more than 3 to 4 hr, have been successfully compared in this manner (Houde et al., *unpublished data*). On the other hand, some analgesics—such as methadone, propoxyphene, diflunisal, and piroxicam—have such long half-lives that it would require as much as a week or more to reach steady state by repeated dosing. In planning short-term repeated-dose analgesic assays of those drugs, it would probably be advisable to consider a parallel group (noncrossover) experimental design. This decision-making strategy, based on pharmacokinetic principles, should provide a more rational guideline for the design of studies of particular drugs than the setting of an arbitrary single period of x number of days for all drugs.

The variety of ways in which the administered doses and monitored challenge doses can be given in short-term repeated-dose analgesic assays is illustrated in Table 1. In discussing possible design options, it is helpful to consider separately the doses that are monitored for their analgesic effects (the challenge doses) and those that are not. Continuous monitoring of the administered doses at intervals comparable to those of the single-dose assays has rarely been practical, although some repeated-dose analgesic assays of this variety have been carried out for periods of up to 9 to 10 hrs (6–9). In the inpatient setting, the practical limits of assessments of that type are primarily determined by the patients' needs for uninterrupted sleep, and by the working schedules of the observers. In short-term repeated-dose studies in outpatients, continuous monitoring may extend

TABLE 1. *Alternative ways of employing administered and challenge doses of the study drugs in short-term, repeated-dose analgesic assays of either crossover or parallel-group designs*

Administered doses (repeated doses, not assessed for analgesic effect)
  Single dose-levels of the test drug *and* standard
    Double-blind *or* open-label
    By-the-clock (ATC) with/without rescues *or* on-demand (prn)
  Graded dosages of the test drug *and/or* standard
    Double-blind *or* open-label
    By-the-clock (ATC) with/without rescues *or* on-demand (prn)
  Titrated dosages of the test drug *and/or* standard
    Double-blind *or* open-label
    By-the-clock (ATC) with/without rescues *or* on-demand (prn)
Challenge doses (monitored for analgesic effect)
  Single doses of the test drug *and* standard
    Double-blind only
    Single *or* graded dose-levels
    Last doses in repeated-dose series are monitored, *or* last doses *and* interval *and/or* initial doses monitored
    On-demand (prn) only, for moderate or severe pain
  Repeated doses of the test drug *and* standard
    Double-blind only
    Single *or* graded dose-levels
    All repeated-doses are monitored
    By-the-clock (ATC) *or* on-demand (prn) administration

for longer periods, but the assessments are commonly less frequent, retrospective, and global. In most repeated-dose analgesic assays, monitoring is not continuous and the unmonitored administered doses are essentially staging or conditioning doses for the ensuing monitored challenge doses which are thus, in effect, substituted doses for ongoing therapy.

Double-Blind versus Open-Label Dose Administration

The most frequently used and most convenient method of administering the doses in these short-term assays is in the form of separate single dosages of the test drug and standard, given on demand (prn) for moderate or severe pain. The monitored challenge doses, on the other hand, may be of the same as the administered doses, or they may be graded dosages of either or both the test drug and standard, taken only for moderate or severe pain. Commonly, both the administered doses and the challenge doses are given double-blind. However, with appropriate designs, it is possible to achieve essentially the same result with open-label administered doses of the study drugs, followed by balanced, randomly assigned, double-blind challenge doses of the test drug and standard. These experimental designs are more complex and may be less efficient in terms of the numbers of patients required for a conclusive assay but, in some clinical settings and times (e.g., evening and overnight) when the study drugs must be administered by others than the research team nurses, it may be the more practical approach.

Dosage versus Dosing Titration

Adjustment of the administered doses to the differences in the needs of individual patients may be accomplished either by frequent titration of the dosages of the study medications given on an ATC schedule to each patient, or by employing single dosages of the test drug and standard and allowing each patient to receive the study medication prn. Alternatively, one may prescribe fixed single dosages given ATC with supplementary prn rescue doses for uncontrolled pain. In general, the ATC approach tends to be a less precise method of titration-to-need than the prn approach in that, especially when rescue medications are interposed, the ATC doses may be administered to patients with little or no pain (10). For that reason, if the assessment of analgesic effect is based on repeated ATC doses, estimates of equianalgesic doses of the test drug and standard can be at considerable variance from those obtained in other studies in which the challenge doses are given or taken only prn for moderate or severe pain (11). Most repeated-dose analgesic assays adhere to the latter approach with the dosages of the challenge doses of the test drug and standard fixed by protocol prior to the study and then given as single substituted doses either following or interspersed within the series of administered doses.

Standards and Controls

Every clinical analgesic assay must be designed to include an "internal control" (12) to provide assurances that, in that particular population and setting, the study will be capable of demonstrating the presence or absence of analgesic efficacy. Assay sensitivity of a study can be demonstrated by including challenge doses of both a placebo and a reference standard analgesic, and showing that they can be distinguished. Alternatively, one can employ graded-dosage challenges of the known effective standard for measuring assay sensitivity by showing that they can be distinguished by their corresponding graded effects. Since the challenge doses are commonly single substituted doses, the use of placebos can be justified, so long as appropriate rescue medication is available when needed. On the other hand, the use of placebos as repeated administered or challenge doses can rarely be condoned. In any case, the demonstration of graded dose-effects with challenges of graded dosages of the standard will usually dispense with the need for placebos, and when graded dosages of the test drug are also included, one has the additional advantage of being able to compare the side effects of the test drug and standard at equianalgesic dosages of the two drugs.

Design Options

Short-term repeated-dose analgesic assays can be conducted as either parallel group (noncrossover) or crossover studies. However, to take best advantage of this type of repeated-dose assay, the crossover design should probably be reserved for inpatient studies of parenterally administered drugs with short $t_{\frac{1}{2}}$s, in patient populations that are relatively nonhomogeneous (e.g., general surgery model, cancer patients, patients with chronic pain). Actually, with rare exceptions (13), virtually all of the short-term repeated-dose assays reported to date have been of the parallel-group design, without consideration of the drug kinetics or type of patient population. Although single dosages of the test drugs and standards are more convenient for administering the doses that are not closely monitored for their analgesic effects, graded-dosage challenges of either, or preferably both, of the test drugs and standards are possible and are more than worth the effort in terms of the information provided.

SUMMARY AND CONCLUSIONS

There is no single set of guidelines that would fit all possible ways of conducting repeated-dose analgesic drug assays. Short-term repeated-dose assays are particularly useful for determining the analgesic potency of drugs in virtually any population of patients in whom repeated doses of an analgesic may be required, whereas long-term repeated-dose studies are generally more suited for assays of the efficacy of orally administered analgesics in patients with chronic pain, and long-term repeated-dose studies are essential for evaluating cumulative effects and drug safety. However, the basic method of assessing analgesic potency used in the short-term assays can also be applied to the longer-term studies; single or repeated challenge doses that are closely monitored for their analgesic effects can be substituted at appropriate intervals in a series of any number of repeated doses that cannot be as closely monitored (and may thus be considered merely as staging or conditioning doses). The conceptual separation of the administered and the challenge doses can be helpful in planning repeated-dose studies.

The repeated doses that are not closely monitored for their analgesic effects may consist of either fixed single or graded doses, administered either prn or ATC with prn rescues, and given either as open-label medications or double-blind in a crossover or parallel-group design. The challenge doses of the study drugs, which are generally monitored in the same manner as in single-dose analgesic assays, must be given double-blind and in a randomized order appropriate to the crossover or noncrossover design of the study. Pharmacokinetic principles should be used as guidelines for determining the duration of repeated dosing and can be helpful in the consideration of the feasibility of a crossover versus a noncrossover design. In some major postoperative pain models, crossover designs may offer some advantages in dealing with problems of relative nonhomogeneity, but this design is likely to be practical only when assaying parenterally administered analgesics whose terminal elimination half-lives ($t_{\frac{1}{2}}$s) are less than 3 to 4 hrs.

The outstanding attribute of the short-term repeated-dose analgesic assay is that it guarantees that the medication preceding the challenge medication will be identified, controlled, and measurable in the same units as the drugs under investigation. Whenever possible, this type of assessment should be carried out as an integral part of early Phase II evaluations of new analgesics.

REFERENCES

1. Mok MS, Lippmann M, Steen SN. Multidose/observational, comparative clinical analgetic evaluation of buprenorphine. *J Clin Pharmacol* 1981;21:323–329.
2. Ouellette RD. Buprenorphine and morphine efficacy in postoperative pain: a double-blind multiple-dose study. *J Clin Pharmacol* 1982;22:165–172.
3. Wang RIH, Johnson RP, Robinson N, Waite E. The study of analgesics following single and repeated doses. *J Clin Pharmacol* 1981;21:121–125.
4. Ouellette RD. Double blind, multiple-dose comparison of buprenorphine and meperidine for postoperative pain following major abdominal surgery. *Curr Ther Res* 1989;46:352–365.
5. Ouellette RD, Mok MS, Gilbert MS, Wang RIH, Zeedick JF, Filtzer HS. Comparison of buprenorphine and morphine: a multicenter, multidose study in patients with severe postoperative pain. *Contemp Surg* 1986;28:55–64.
6. Quiding H, Persson G, Ahlstrom U, Bangens S, Hellem S, Johansson G, Jonsson E, Nordh PG. Paracetamol plus supplementary doses of codeine. An analgesic study of repeated doses. *Eur J Clin Pharmacol* 1982;23:315–319.
7. Quiding H, Oksala E, Happonen R-P, Lehtimaki K, Ojala T. The visual analog scale in multiple-dose evaluations of analgesics. *J Clin Pharmacol* 1981;21:424–429.
8. Nystrom E, Gustafsson I, Quiding H. The pain intensity at analgesic intake, and the efficacy of diflunisal in single doses and effervescent acetaminophen in single and repeated doses. *Pharmacotherapy* 1988;8:201–209.
9. Quiding H, Oikarinen V, Sane J, Sjoblad A-M. Analgesic efficacy after single and repeated doses of codeine and acetaminophen. *J Clin Pharmacol* 1984;24:27–34.
10. Twycross RG, Lack SA. *Symptom control in far advanced cancer: pain relief. Part 2, Pain control: analgesics. Part 3, Pharmacology.* London: Pitman, 1983;100–269.
11. Houde RW. Misinformation: side effects and drug interactions. In: Hill CS Jr, Fields WS, eds. *Drug treatment of cancer pain in a drug-oriented society. Advances in pain research and therapy,* vol 11. New York: Raven Press, 1989;145–161.
12. Modell W, Houde RW. Factors influencing clinical evaluation of drugs. *JAMA* 1958;167:2190–2198.
13. McQuay HJ, Carroll D, Watts PG, Juniper RP, Moore RA. Codeine 20 mg increases pain relief from ibuprofen 400 mg after third molar surgery. A repeat-dosing comparison of ibuprofen and an ibuprofen-codeine combination. *Pain* 1989;37:7–13.

Advances in Pain Research and Therapy, Vol. 18,
edited by M. Max, R. Portenoy, and E. Laska,
Raven Press, Ltd., New York © 1991.

Commentary

Multiple-Dose Analgesic Studies

Richard I. H. Wang

*Department of Pharmacology, The Medical College of Wisconsin,
Milwaukee, Wisconsin 53193*

It is well accepted that information regarding patient acceptability, long-term efficacy, carryover effects, tolerance, and dependence liability of an analgesic medication can only be ascertained after repeated doses. As pointed out by Stewart (see Chapter 5), the design of these multidose studies has not yet fully developed. Over the past 25 years our group has conducted seven multiple-dose analgesic studies. We would like to briefly comment on several specific points regarding multidose studies.

MULTIPLE DOSES ILLUSTRATING SIDE EFFECTS

Multiple-dose studies can detect side effects not detectable in single-dose studies. An example of this finding can be found in a double-blind, crossover study comparing the efficacy and safety of an investigational drug, Exp. 675, with meperidine and placebo in cancer patients with chronic pain (1). If the response of the patient to the first dose of the testing analgesic was satisfactory, the patient was given a second dose of the same medication for that day. After that dose, the patient was placed back on his regular analgesic medication. The study was discontinued after evaluating the ninth and tenth patients. Two patients dropped out owing to the development of hallucinations. One of them experienced 7 min of visual hallucinations 2 hrs after two doses of Exp. 675. The other patient developed more than 5 hrs of visual and auditory hallucinations starting 1 hr after the second dose of Exp. 675. Accompanying the hallucinations were hypertension, tachycardia, tachypnea, apprehension, dilated pupils, and tremors. The hallucinogenic effect of Exp. 675 had not been shown in previous single-dose studies.

DOSING REGIMEN AT FIXED INTERVALS

The first reported study in the literature using multiple doses was carried out comparing the analgesic efficacy of noracymethadol to morphine in cancer patients with chronic pain (1). In that study, using a double-blind, crossover design, morphine or noracymethadol was given in four repeated doses at 2 PM, 8 PM, 2 AM, and 8 AM. The patient was then crossed over to the other medication for four doses. The results of this multiple-dose study demonstrated not only the analgesic efficacy of the studied medications but also their acceptability and comparable side effects.

One interesting finding from this fixed-interval dosing regimen was that there were a number of patients having no pain at the zero hour (8 AM) on the fourth dose of either analgesic medication. A zero pain score at the initial time of interview can only produce either no change in score or even a negative score when the patient complains of pain in subsequent hours. If a clinically beneficial carryover analgesic effect of earlier doses of a medication can result in a zero or negative score for the next dose, this is a potential drawback of a fixed-interval regimen.

DOSING REGIMEN AT VARIABLE INTERVALS

Learning the possible shortcomings of fixed intervals, several other studies were carried out in an attempt to improve the study designs. The following design was found to be the best (2). The study used a double-blind, repeated dose, parallel design. Adult patients experiencing postorthopedic surgical pain of moderate to severe intensity were randomly divided into two groups, receiving initially either 0.3 mg of buprenorphine hydrochloride or 10 mg of morphine sulfate intramuscularly (IM). Like the usual treatment of patients with acute pain, each patient could receive up to six injections in each 24-hr period (a total of 1.8 mg buprenorphine or 60 mg morphine), spaced 2 to 8 hrs apart for up to 3 days on an as-needed basis for the relief of pain. No study analgesic medication was given unless moderate to severe pain had recurred, thus making negative relief scores less likely.

The method of evaluating and recording pain intensity, pain relief, sedation, vital signs, tissue reaction at the sites of injection, laboratory data, and concomitant medication was essentially the same as described elsewhere (3). Only the first daytime dose of each study day was evaluated and the results recorded. The initial dose on the first day (either 0.3 mg of buprenorphine or 10 mg of morphine IM) provided single-dose information whereas the second and the third day of evaluations provided data on repeated doses of the same analgesic medication. For comparative purposes, the early morning dose of each day is the most practical to evaluate on account of the variable intervals between subsequent repeated doses.

The results of the study showed that the mean total pain relief (TOTPAR) scores and the mean pain intensity difference scores (SPID) through 6 hrs and through 8 hrs were consistently higher on all treatment days (1, 2, and 3) for 0.3 mg of buprenorphine compared to morphine (Table 1). Also, the mean scores

TABLE 1. *Mean total pain relief (TOTPAR) and pain intensity difference (SPID) scores following the day's first dose at 0.3 mg buprenorphine or 10 mg morphine*

	Number of patients	TOTPAR		SPID	
		T6H	T8H	T6H	T8H
Day 1					
Buprenorphine	25	10.56	11.36	5.76	6.16
Morphine	25	10.20	10.72	5.40	5.68
Day 2					
Buprenorphine	11	12.82	14.46	7.00	7.91
Morphine	15	11.07	12.73	7.00	7.93
Day 3					
Buprenorphine	5	15.80	15.80	9.80	9.80
Morphine	4	13.50	15.50	5.75	6.75

for both buprenorphine and morphine were higher on days 2 and 3 than on day 1. The apparent increasing efficacy of the analgesics with repeated doses may have been owing to accumulation of drug from previous doses, decrease in perioperative inflammation, or psychological factors. It was also found that the test medications were well tolerated by most patients on the study. Only two of the 25 subjects receiving 0.3 mg buprenorphine requested discontinuation because of undesirable effects such as moderate sedation and nausea.

This study design incorporates flexibility in the amount of medication administered on an as-needed basis. This seems most appropriate because it is representative of the actual clinical situation in which patients take analgesic medications in repeated doses, with physicians determining the dosages appropriate for each patient. By giving the medication only on demand when pain has reached moderate to severe intensity, a baseline for comparative evaluation of analgesic medication is established.

All 50 patients participated on the first day of study (day 1) and 26 on day 2. Only nine participated on day 3 mainly because the other patients' pain had either subsided or dropped to a level unacceptable for analgesic evaluation. This population, therefore, is appropriate for no more than a 2-day study. If a longer period of study is needed, this type of multiple-dose design can be applied in a chronic pain population.

REFERENCES

1. Wang RIH, Sako K. Problems in analgesic studies using multiple doses. *Committee on Problems of Drug Dependence* 1967;4975–4984.
2. Wang RIH, Johnson RP, Robinson N, Waite E. The study of analgesics following single and repeated doses. *J Clin Pharmacol* 1981;21:121–125.
3. Houde RW, Wallenstein SL, Rogers A. Clinical pharmacology of analgesics 1. A method of assaying analgesic effect. *Clin Pharmacol Ther* 1960;1:163–174.

DISCUSSION (Chapters 5 and 6)

Dr. Thomas Kantor: When we have done multiple-dose studies, we have encountered the difficulty that unless one has a team of nurses working three shifts a day or the total cooperation of a hospital, it is very difficult to have the test doses given at night. Usually the attending physician would take over the pain management at night, which often confounded the study. In addition, multidose analgesic studies are notoriously difficult to interpret.

I don't agree with Patricia Stewart that you must do these multiple-dose studies under double-blind conditions. Why not just use the first dose as a double-blind comparison, and give the subsequent doses as an open study, to find out what the side effects are and whether the analgesic effect increases or decreases over time? That is what the clinician would really like to know.

Dr. John Stambaugh: I disagree with that because I think that reduces multiple-dose studies to safety studies. I think there is a need to make these studies double-blind efficacy trials. We must know whether there is efficacy after 7 days or 30 days. You can measure it.

Dr. Patricia Stewart: I would be interested in what the regulatory experts think about this. As sponsors, we would be loathe to rely on a pivotal study that wasn't double-blind.

Dr. John Harter: It would make me nervous, too. Open-label studies risk the introduction of the bias of the investigator, who has already seen a few patients, and of the patients themselves. The history of clinical trial methodology has shown us that when the blind inadvertently gets broken, it often influences the results for efficacy and side effects.

Dr. Mitchell Max: In chronic pain models, Dr. Stambaugh has shown that multiple-dose studies can effectively distinguish treatments according to efficacy and patient acceptability. In acute pain models, where pain declines within a day or two, it remains unclear whether repeated doses can add anything to the single-dose comparison in terms of distinguishing efficacy. What is the FDA looking for in asking for repeated dose efficacy studies in such acute pain models?

Dr. John Harter: The FDA has become quite interested in seeing data about multiple doses of analgesics in acute pain situations such as postoperative pain. Previously, we would get many studies of single doses in acute pain, and multiple doses in chronic pain states. In practice, though, people treated for acute pain get multiple doses, and we wanted to be able to advise physicians, through the package insert, about what happens on the second day. There are hints, for instance, that beyond the first dose, the difference you see between certain drugs disappears. On the other hand, I recently reviewed data for the NSAID meclomen that showed a better ability to discriminate between drug and placebo on the second dose than on the first. We would encourage people to try to get better at this methodology, and see what we can learn about efficacy with repeated doses.

Advances in Pain Research and Therapy, Vol. 18,
edited by M. Max, R. Portenoy, and E. Laska,
Raven Press, Ltd., New York © 1991.

7

N of 1 Trials

Henry J. McQuay

*Oxford Regional Pain Relief Unit, Abingdon Hospital, OX14 1AG Abingdon, Oxon,
United Kingdom*

Analgesic studies are necessary to demonstrate that a putative analgesic does indeed show the necessary biological activity and to compare the activity with that produced by existing analgesics. Initial tests of a novel analgesic may be performed as open-label studies. The reasons why these may be unsatisfactory are that improvements and deteriorations may be part of the natural history of the illness, symptoms, and signs. Also, results of investigations tend to revert to the mean, placebo effects may bias results, open assessment of subjective responses is far from ideal, and, importantly, patients may respond as they do because they are grateful (or simply polite). The methods for subsequent comparison with existing analgesics have been well studied, at least in single dose, but implicit in these designs is the assumption that the pain condition under study will be amenable to each of the classes of study analgesics, or that subgroups with different responses to those analgesics have been identified previously and the necessary stratification has been built into the design. A controlled alternative to open studies in initial trials would be an advance; so too would a design that allowed heterogeneous conditions to be tested without the prior knowledge required for stratification. The N of 1 design has the potential to fulfill these roles.

We were concerned about the lack of randomized controlled trial (RCT) data for treatment of neuropathic pain syndromes. This lack of data is well known (1), and the reasons why these syndromes are so difficult to study are discussed in this chapter. The study problems inherent in these pain syndromes are compounded by the difficulties introduced by the particular classes of drug that appear to be effective.

A high proportion of the chronic pain patients we see (>30%) are prescribed antidepressant or anticonvulsants to treat their pain, and we desperately need a way of rationalizing our prescribing in order to improve it. The N of 1 or single-patient design (2,3) seemed to us to be one way in which we could justify our clinical practice, both to ourselves and to the patients. This chapter describes why we made this decision and some of the practical difficulties that we encountered.

In chronic pain syndromes spontaneous improvements in pain can occur, and this improvement can be falsely ascribed to treatment unless care is taken in the trial design. The best known example is trigeminal neuralgia, where the symptoms may wax and wane. Neuropathic pain may also improve if the disease process destroys the nerve completely. This can happen in diabetic neuropathy and in pain owing to tumor compression of nerve.

In acute postoperative pain we have a workable analgesic trial methodology. It is not perfect, but it is capable of producing sensitive and reproducible results. A fundamental premise of single-dose studies in acute pain is that the analgesic sensitivity of the patients' pain is the same, in the sense that adequate doses of a standard "conventional" (aspirin through to morphine) analgesic, will reduce the pain intensity.

In chronic pain this premise may not be valid. Whereas the majority of chronic pain syndromes do show dose response to conventional analgesics, there are those syndromes that do not. These syndromes, where there is reduced or absent sensitivity to conventional analgesics, present a major problem for clinical trial design. Study designs that make no attempt to determine sensitivity to conventional analgesics and assume, extrapolating from classic single-dose acute pain designs, that all patients have the same sensitivity, and use conventional analgesics as the standard in the design, may well produce bizarre results.

We had experience of this some years ago in cancer pain. An injectable formulation of a nonsteroidal antiinflammatory drug (NSAID) was compared with placebo in a single-dose crossover. The NSAID was known to be an effective analgesic from single-dose studies of the oral formulation in postoperative pain. Some of the cancer pain patients were incapable, however, of detecting any analgesic effect difference between the active and the placebo, although the pain on injection from the active allowed them to distinguish the two injections. The study produced the result, when analyzed on a group basis, that the NSAID was ineffective compared with placebo in cancer pain. This was a nonsense result. The study included some patients who had marked benefit, and some who had none. The differential sensitivity of the patients to the NSAID is obviously clinically relevant, but is not amenable to between-group analysis. The caveat to this conclusion is that preliminary screening for a positive response to the drug class under test would allow classic designs to yield meaningful results, but again the interpretation would be on a group rather than an individual basis.

It is the variability of the response to conventional analgesics that makes neuropathic pain different and makes clinical trial design for these pain syndromes so difficult. This variability may be present in some nociceptive pain conditions, but in neuropathic pain the proportion of patients with such variable response is much higher (4–6). This variability may be a rightward shift in the dose-response curve to conventional analgesics, but with some pain conditions there may be an absolute rather than a relative change in the response. Even the rightward shift in the dose-response curve could wreck a parallel group design if the allocation of patients to the different groups in the study takes no account of the presence or possibility of such shift. In particular it is the choice of a conventional analgesic as reference or standard analgesic, with presumed equivalent sensitivity in all patients studied, that makes the design so difficult.

An example would be a crossover comparison of morphine (as the standard) and an alpha$_2$ adrenergic agonist (as the test analgesic) in a heterogeneous group of chronic pain patients, where heterogeneous means that the response to conventional analgesics such as morphine varies widely among the patients. If the alpha$_2$ agonist produces excellent pain relief in the patients who respond poorly to morphine but no pain relief in those who respond well, then the overall result will depend entirely on the relative numbers of each category entered into the study. A preponderance of morphine-sensitive patients will result in a false negative result for the alpha$_2$ agonist. If most patients entered into the study have reduced sensitivity to morphine, then a false positive result ensues, with the implication that the alpha$_2$ agonist is superior to morphine. We are all losers in this scenario because the appropriate role for potentially effective analgesics is not determined.

In neuropathic pain not only may response to conventional analgesics be altered but also analgesic response is found with drug classes not regarded conventionally as analgesics. The obvious examples of such unconventional analgesics are anticonvulsants (used, for instance, in trigeminal neuralgia), and the antidepressants. The advent of a whole variety of other drugs from different classes, such as clonidine, dipyridamole, etc., with claimed benefit in these pain conditions, emphasizes what may be the major objective, which is to develop clinical trials methodology in these problem pain conditions, and to develop methods that produce meaningful and clinically instructive results.

N OF 1 OR SINGLE-PATIENT DESIGNS

A potential solution to this study design problem is provided by the single patient or N of 1 design (7). N of 1 designs have been around for a long time (8,9); single-patient studies evolved because of the difficulty in assessing behavioral or other psychiatric interventions within the framework of traditional designs. The intention of the design is to test within a single patient whether or not a particular intervention improves matters clinically, and to make this judgment within a framework that affords some statistical analysis.

The use of the designs to study pharmacological interventions evolved as a method by which effective treatment for individual patients might be defined in circumstances where there were no relevant RCT results to guide treatment (10). The approach we have been exploring is to subvert this design, not only answering the individual patient question but also using it as a novel method to tackle the issue of design in the presence of heterogeneity.

A fairly basic question that has to be addressed early on is the distinction between traditional group crossover designs and the N of 1 crossover design.

Both designs are crossover. In the traditional design the hypothesis, that there is no difference between the treatments, is tested by the measured difference between the treatments for all the patients. The same hypothesis is tested in the N of 1 design, but an answer is sought for each patient. A statistically significant answer may be sought in the individual patient. The fundamental difference then is that in the N of 1 design the test being sought is within the *patient,* whereas in the traditional crossover it is a *group* response. The N of 1 design then has the potential to identify the subgroups required for a stratified traditional design.

The N of 1 design has potential in chronic pain studies both as an alternative to open-label initial testing, and as an alternative to the traditional crossover when the homogeneity of the patients' pain conditions is questionable. In that context a negative result for the group overall may obscure a therapeutic response in a subgroup. One way round this problem if group designs are really considered necessary would be to define the sensitivity of the patients to the drug class under test before embarking on the multiple-dose crossover. This contrasts with the possible definition of sensitivity *within* the N of 1 design.

BACKGROUND TO SINGLE-PATIENT DESIGNS

The classic illustration of the N of 1 design is the test of the claim that a woman could distinguish a cup of tea made with tea added to milk from one made with the milk added to the tea. How can this claim be tested? If eight cups of tea are made, four with milk added first, four with tea then milk, and the order of the presentation is randomized, the chance of identifying each cup correctly is 1/70 (8!/4!4!) [Fisher, quoted in (11)]. If the subject guessed correctly each time then a statistically significant result could be demonstrated within this single subject.

CLINICAL REQUIREMENTS FOR SINGLE-PATIENT STUDIES

The clinical equivalent of the cups of tea is to organize pairs of treatments, for instance of active drug and placebo (Fig. 1) (10). The necessary conditions (10) include random allocation to experimental or control treatment, double-

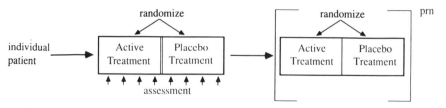

FIG. 1. "Replicated pairs" design for N of 1 study.

blind organization, measurement of the results of treatment, and formal statistical analysis to avoid false positive or negative results. Only then can the objections to open studies listed above be countered. To provide conventional medical significance at the $p < 0.05$ level, results from five paired crossovers would be the minimum requirement using the sign test, but using a paired t-test an α of less than 0.05 may be obtained from fewer than five pairs (10).

The basic ideal requirements are reversible action, rapid onset of effect, and rapid offset of effect. The conditions include random allocation, double-blind design, objective result measurement, and formal statistical analysis (10). Clinically relevant examples in the literature include studies of dyspnea (2), and metronidazole in ileostomy inflammation (3). The dyspnea study illustrates the approach to test the efficacy of a treatment in a single patient, but with insufficient treatment pairs to obtain statistical significance. The ileostomy case is perhaps the best-worked pharmacological case in the literature, with sufficient treatment pairs so that statistical significance was found supporting the use of metronidazole to control the inflammation.

For general clinical use of N of 1 designs the therapeutic target should be a valid measure of efficacy, sensible to both clinician and patient, and reversible. For analgesic studies, measures of pain intensity or relief meet the first and second objectives, but the reversibility clause imposes constraints on both treatments and pain conditions suitable for study by this method, as it would with conventional crossover designs. Treatments that produced infinite duration of relief would be unsuitable, as would conditions with unremitting increase or decrease in pain.

The speed of onset and offset of effect may also be very relevant to the trial design (7,10). Slow time of onset of effect is a relative rather than an absolute contraindication. If the time of onset is 3 days, the treatment periods for the crossover must clearly be well in excess of 3 days. This may be particularly pertinent for the use of unconventional analgesics such as antidepressants and anticonvulsants in chronic pain. Even with drugs whose onset of effect is anticipated to be rapid there may be a minimum necessary treatment period. False positive results and therapeutic responses from placebo may be obtained in the first week of the second treatment period of a crossover comparison where both treatments are ineffective (12), so that comparison of a novel agent with placebo may require as a minimum two 2-week treatment periods.

Prolonged duration of relief (or slow offset of effect) may also pose problems. While studying the effects of opioid antagonists in poststroke pain, we have found that occasionally patients obtained relief for 2 or more months after stopping the active treatment. Fixed treatment period duration of less than 2 months would lead to problems in this case, although this unexpected duration of efficacy might be considered as a nonreversible treatment and thus inadmissible to crossover study of either conventional or N of 1 design. Slow offset time raises the specter of carryover effects from one treatment to the next. There appears to be no absolute defense against this problem with either conventional or N of 1 crossover designs. A sufficient number (>3) of randomized crossovers may be the optimal strategy (11), and clearly this issue is more important as the duration of the effect that is carried over approaches the duration of the treatment period. If carryover is a particular concern, then designs that can estimate direct treatment effects even in the presence of substantial carryover effects should be considered (see pp. 87, 211–212).

WHEN IS THIS NOVEL DESIGN LIKELY TO BE USEFUL?

Single-patient designs can fulfill the clinical need to answer the question as to whether or not an individual patient does indeed benefit from a particular treatment. At its simplest the patient is provided with at least three (see ref. 10) paired treatments (active and placebo) and a method of judging analgesic efficacy. Not all designs, however, are restricted to a pattern of pairs. Given the caveats about treatment duration above, a clinically useful answer should emerge. Some of the practical difficulties encountered are discussed below. The approach may also help in identifying the efficacy of particular drugs or drug classes in pain syndromes that present particular trial design difficulty for conventional RCT studies, in preliminary studies as an alternative to the open-label design, and in determining stratification criteria for ensuing conventional designs.

PILOT STUDIES

We have been using the N of 1 approach in several chronic pain contexts. The most ambitious is to study antidepressant and anticonvulsant drug efficacy. A high proportion of the patients we see are prescribed antidepressants and/or anticonvulsants, and the limited RCT information provides little rational basis for individualizing treatment. We expected that the heterogeneity of pain syndromes for which these drugs are to be prescribed would not provide meaningful group analysis, so the primary design was on single-patient basis. We also prospectively designed a group analysis to see if the active drug had a general effect on a wide variety of pain syndromes. To provide better information on which to base our prescribing, we decided to use the single-patient design.

Antidepressant N of 1 Study

The sole criterion for admission to this ongoing study is that the patient is to be prescribed an antidepressant drug for pain management. The design is a paired comparison of a nonselective tricyclic antidepressant, dothiepin, at a single-dose level (75 mg) with placebo. Each randomized treatment pair takes 6 weeks, with 3 weeks on each treatment. Details of the pain conditions of the first 38 patients studied are given in Table 1. A variety of pain syndromes is included. In some cases tricyclic antidepressant treatment was prescribed because of the

TABLE 1. *Patient details in antidepressant study*

No.	Sex	Age (yr)	Height (cm)	Weight (kg)	Duration (months)	Diagnosis	Site of pain
1	M	34	175	92	15	Cervical pain	Cervical spine and arm
2	M	32	178	70	36	Groin pain	Groin, pubis, and penis
3	F	56	156	57	9	Back pain	Left buttock and leg
4	F	72	160	55	4	PHN	R axilla, scapula, and chest
5	F	69	163	76	18	PHN	R buttock, groin, knee to foot
6	F	73	165	83	120	Abdominal pain	Abdomen, back, chest, head
8	F	75	161	51	96	Perineal neuralgia	Perineum
9	M	56	184	95	60	Cervical pain	Neck, back of head, both arms
10	F	66	168	76	3	PHN	Thoracic region, L breast
11	F	35	156	51	60	Tension headaches	Neck and back of head
12	M	79	170	77	4	PHN	Dorsal area L foot
13	M	80	163	76	5	Postsurgical testicular pain	Testicles
14	M	48	180	99	60	Arachnoiditis	Back and R leg
15	F	19	170	70	56	Spinal stenosis	Lumbar sacral spine and legs
16	M	48	179	88	192	Back pain	Lumbar spine and R leg to foot
17	M	70	183	94	48	Postsurgical femoral neuralgia	Knee
19	F	41	163	71	163	Neck and arm pain	Neck and arms
20	F	71	158	54	5	PHN	L ribs and breast
21	F	60	151	41	11	Back pain	Back
22	M	48	188	91	72	Ependynoma	R leg
23	M	83	168	67	420	Old fracture cervical spine	R leg
24	F	62	171	70	48	Facial pain	L side face infraorbital
25	M	49	170	69	60	Perineal pain	Perineum, coccyx, rectum
26	M	38	173	73	12	Back pain	Lumbar spine, buttocks
27	F	73	158	79	24	Coccydinia	Back and legs
28	F	50	173	54	156	Abdominal pain	Abdomen and rib
29	M	44	183	101	5	Back pain	Back
30	M	86	170	72	14	PHN	T6 left side of chest
31	F	37	170	89	144	Back pain	L5S1 and leg
32	F	40	168	83	204	Back pain	Back, hips and leg
33	M	68	173	72	36	Testicular pain	Testicle
34	M	62	173	71	324	Back pain	Back and leg
35	F	65	168	65	6	Trigeminal neuralgia	Face, 3 divisions
36	F	51	168	83	36	Back pain	Back and leg
37	M	60	175	86	120	Arachnoiditis	Leg
38	F	59	178	108	60	Postsurgical scar pain	Face
39	F	55	154	65	36	Back pain	Back and leg
40	M	40	178	83	240	Facet joint degeneration	Back and legs
Mean (± SEM)		57 ± 3	170 ± 2	75 ± 3	80 ± 16		

deafferentation nature of the pain, in other cases because of the failure of conventional analgesics or treatments. Patients are permitted to take their regular analgesic drugs during the study. The study is run on an outpatient basis using daily diaries to record daily pain intensity (four-point categorical scale: none = 0, mild = 1, moderate = 2, severe = 3), daily pain relief (five-point categorical scale: none = 0, slight = 1, moderate = 2, good = 3, complete relief = 4), and daily side-effect incidence, with a weekly global rating (poor = 0, fair = 1, good = 2, very good = 3, excellent = 4). A global rating is obtained for each treatment period (poor = 0, fair = 1, good = 2, very good = 3, excellent = 4), and a patient preference after each pair of treatments. At the initial clinic visit current pain intensity and typical pain intensity over the previous week are recorded, with visual analogue scales for pain intensity and mood, an eight-word randomized word scale for pain intensity (13), and the McGill Pain Questionnaire. At subsequent clinic visits the same pain intensity measures are used, together with five-point categorical and 100 mm analogue ("no relief of pain" to "complete relief of pain") relief scales, global score for the first treatment, and mood and side-effect information. At the end of a pair of treatments patients are asked to make a preference judgment between the two treatments.

From the daily diary, pain intensity, and pain relief recordings, an area under the curve for pain intensity and for pain relief against time is calculated for each treatment week using the trapezoidal method. Incomplete recordings are omitted from analysis. To determine the sensitivity of the various outcome measures, the calculated data and the other analgesic raw data were compared for the two treatments using the Wilcoxon matched-pairs signed-ranks test. Preference significance was tested with the Chi-square test.

Although this study is still in progress and few patients have yet completed multiple crossovers, a preliminary analysis of the data revealed some serious logistical problems that may be inherent in an N of 1 study of pain treatments when long treatment periods are necessary. Only 21 patients completed the first paired comparison. The fate of the 38 patients recruited is shown in Fig. 2. Seven patients withdrew during the first treatment period, three on dothiepin and four on placebo. Ten then withdrew during the second treatment, again more on placebo (six) than on dothiepin (four), so that only 21 of the 38 patients completed both treatment periods. Of the 21 patients who completed, 11 expressed a preference, 8 for dothiepin and 3 for placebo. Of the 17 patients who did not complete, 10 expressed a preference, and all 10 were for dothiepin. Groups between treatment analysis demonstrated outcome measure sensitivity, with greater analgesic efficacy of dothiepin 75 mg compared with placebo being shown significantly on the McGill score ($p = 0.02$), global score for treatment ($p = 0.01$), global scores for the second and third weeks of treatment ($p = 0.01$ and $p = 0.03$) and area under the curve (AUC) pain intensity for week three ($p = 0.01$). There was a statistically insignificant increase in mood score with dothiepin. There was no significant difference in adverse events. When comparing the 21 patients who completed with the 17 who dropped out, to see for the future if there was any predictor, two statistically significant differences were seen in mood scores. The score before treatment was significantly lower (p = 0.006 t-test) in those who dropped out, 17.6 ± 6.2 (mean ± SEM), n = 11, compared with those who completed, 54.8 ± 11.1, n = 8. During placebo treatment mood score was also significantly (p < 0.001 t-test) lower in those who dropped out, 17.2 ± 4.9, n = 9 compared with those who completed, 51.6 ± 6.6, n = 8. There was no significant difference between the two categories for mood scores on dothiepin treatment or for the change in mood from before study for either treatment.

Although this preliminary analysis shows that the outcome measures provide adequate sensitivity, there are logistic and design problems. One logistic (and clinical) problem is the number of crossovers required to give a statistically significant answer within patient. If the treatment period duration necessary to establish efficacy is as long as 3 weeks, as appears from this and other published data to be the case for tricyclic antidepressants, then the minimum period (no allowance for washout) for a three-pair crossover would be 18 weeks. This is a long time to maintain this degree of compliance, as is evident from the attrition rate during the first pair of treatments, 21 completing of 38 admitted. A second problem is that patients obtaining clear clinical benefit after one crossover may be less than enthusiastic to continue with further paired comparisons with placebo. How are patients who prefer one of the treatments, and are unable to tolerate the other, to be managed through multiple-paired comparisons? It is apparent from Fig. 2 that patients withdrew from the study on both active drug and placebo. A clinically useful answer, however, either positive (greater efficacy on dothiepin, tolerable side effects, preference for dothiepin), or negative (no greater efficacy than placebo or intolerable side effects), might still be obtained despite failure to complete. The fact that 10 of the 17 patients who withdrew expressed a preference and all 10 preferred dothiepin emphasizes this point. One ethical solution might be to allow the patient to start the second of the two treatments early if the first is unsatisfactory. Defining early is not straightforward if onset of effect is slow. Defining early as 3 days, for instance, might mean that analgesic (or mood) effect of an antidepressant would not be perceptible. These problems are not insuperable, and we hope that the approach will both identify patients benefiting from the treatment and advance our knowledge. Support for this optimism comes from Guyatt and colleagues (10), who give an example of a patient tested for amitriptyline efficacy in fibrositis. After four pairs of treatments statistical significance was achieved with a paired t-test.

The design of the study presented here ducks the issue of dose response because we elected to compare one dose (75 mg) of dothiepin with placebo. Dothiepin 75 mg may not be the optimal dose for the patient, and might even be the no-effect dose for some patients. One possible way around this problem is open treatment before the study, to determine a dose at which effect, desired or not, is perceptible, and then to enter the double-blind crossovers using that dose and placebo. The second is to use the N of 1 approach to define the patients who may require a bigger dose. Those who detect neither benefit nor adverse effects

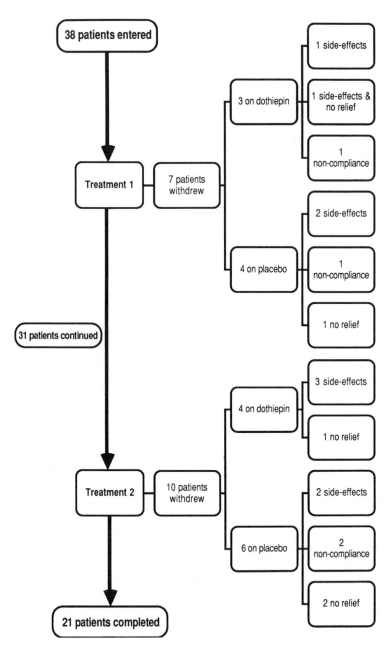

FIG. 2. Patient fate in dothiepin pilot study.

during the original study would enter a second study with an increased dose. These thoughts are summarized in Fig. 3. Adaptive randomization design variants such as the "play the winner" (14) or randomized urn (15) may have relevance in this context.

Naloxone in Poststroke Pain

It appears that efficacy of intravenous naloxone in poststroke pain (16) is predictive for efficacy of oral antagonists. The major difficulty is in obtaining

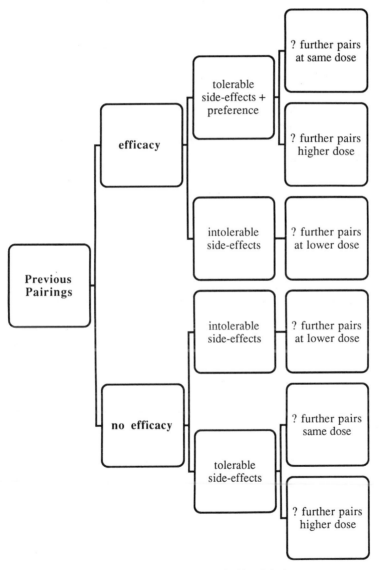

FIG. 3. "Replicated pairs" design, modified by clinical response.

unequivocal demonstration of efficacy, particularly in patients in whom communication difficulties and emotional lability are to be expected. We have been using the N of 1 approach to improve the specificity of our determination of the efficacy of intravenous naloxone. An example is a 60-year-old female with left-sided facial pain after a cerebrovascular incident in 1988. Intravenous 0.4 mg naloxone given open-label was thought to have improved her pain, but it was agreed that emotional lability left this conclusion in some doubt. Subsequent comparisons (three pairs; intravenous 0.4 mg naloxone and saline on successive days, using four-point categorical pain intensity and four-point categorical relief scores as outcome measures), showed no significant benefit from the naloxone compared with saline.

Our aim was to use the single-patient design both to aid treatment of the individual patient and as a research tool. The preliminary data presented here suggest that the outcome measures are both feasible and sensitive. The clinical answers have proved most helpful for management. One research issue as yet unresolved is the extent to which significant results determined within particular patients may be extrapolated to other patients. A second question is the legitimacy of using data from any completed treatment period obtained in an N of 1 study for subsequent group comparisons. Extended treatment periods and multiple treatment pairings will inevitably produce high attrition rates. Statistical methods for pooling data from all completed or partially completed treatments would be useful.

CONCLUSIONS

We do not yet have sufficient data to pass judgment on the utility of this approach. We believe that it is logistically feasible and offers considerable advantages over conventional designs, perhaps most obviously in the early stages of investigation of novel putative analgesics. We chose to work with this design in neuropathic pain, an area which is very difficult for conventional RCT design. We chose a difficult testbed, because of the lack of standard drugs of proven efficacy and because the drugs to be tested have slow onset of effect and present dose-response problems. Whether or not the design proves useful in neuropathic pain, there is no reason why single-patient designs should not be used for single-dose studies of conventional analgesics. One obvious context, where conventional crossover designs are logistically difficult, is in cancer pain patients. This may ultimately prove to be the most useful clinical role, using paired single-dose comparisons. Unfortunately few of our drug treatments are rapid in onset and rapid in offset, but for those which are, such as NSAIDs, the design could work well.

ACKNOWLEDGMENTS

Drs. Roy Bullingham, Andrew Moore, and Chris Nagle provided stimulus and advice; many of the ideas about the background of single-patient designs came from the work of Dr. D. Sackett. Sister Dawn Carroll actually ran the antidepressant study, and Dr. Cathy Stannard ran the opioid antagonist study. Dr. Chris Glynn allowed his patients to be studied. The studies were financed by Pain Relief Unit funds.

REFERENCES

1. McQuay HJ. Pharmacological treatment of neuralgic and neuropathic pain. *Cancer Surv* 1988;7: 141–159.
2. Guyatt G, Sackett D, Taylor WD, Chong J, Roberts R, Pugsley S. Determining optimal therapy—randomized trials in individual patients. *New Engl J Med* 1986;314:889–892.
3. McLeod RS, Taylor DW, Cohen Z, Cullen JB. Single-patient randomised clinical trial. *Lancet* 1986;1:726–728.
4. Tasker RR, Tsuda T, Hawrylyshyn P. Clinical neurophysiological investigation of deafferentation pain. In: Bonica JJ, Lindblom U, Iggo A, eds. *Advances in pain research and therapy,* vol. 5. New York: Raven Press, 1983;713–738.
5. Mazars GJ, Choppy JM. Reevaluation of the deafferentation pain syndrome. In: Bonica JJ, Lindblom U, Iggo A, eds. *Advances in pain research and therapy,* vol. 5. New York: Raven Press, 1983;769–773.
6. Arner S, Meyerson BA. Lack of analgesic effect of opioids on neuropathic and idiopathic forms of pain. *Pain* 1988;33:11–23.
7. Editorial. Single-patient trials. *Lancet* 1986;1:1254–1255.
8. Chassan JB. Stochastic models of the single case as the basis of clinical research design. *Behav Sci* 1961;6:42–50.
9. Chassan JB. Statistical inference and the single case in clinical design. *Psychiatry* 1960;23:173–184.
10. Guyatt G, Sackett D, Adachi J, Roberts R, Chong J, Rosenbloom D, Keller J. A clinician's guide for conducting randomized trials in individual patients. *Can Med Assoc J* 1988;139:497–503.
11. Edgington ES. Statistics and single case analysis. *Prog Behav Modif* 1984;16:83–119.
12. McQuay HJ, Carroll D, Moxon A, Glynn CJ, Moore RA. Benzydamine cream for the treatment of postherpetic neuralgia: minimum duration of treatment periods in a crossover trial. *Pain* 1990;40:131–135.
13. Tursky B. The development of a pain profile: a psychophysical approach. In: Weisenberg M, Tursky B, eds. *Pain: new perspectives in therapy and research.* New York: Plenum Press, 1975;171–194.
14. Zelen M. Play the winner rule and the controlled clinical trial. *Am Statist Assoc J* 1969;1:131–136.
15. Cornell RG, Landenberger BD, Bartlett RH. Randomized play-the-winner clinical trials. *Comm Statist A—Theory Methods* 1986;15:159–178.
16. Budd K. The use of the opiate antagonist naloxone in the treatment of intractable pain. *Neuropeptides* 1985;5:419–422.

DISCUSSION

Dr. Michael Cousins: I think that the N of 1 methodology, though cumbersome, may prove quite valuable in getting information in individual patients about the underlying mechanisms of pain. The results apply only in the particular patient studied, of course, but by getting this data in a sufficient number of patients, we may then be able to get a feeling for which disease processes and pain mechanisms are most responsive to certain classes of drugs. It might be misleading, however, to pool results from these diverse individuals in a group analysis if there is no basis for assuming that they are a group.

Dr. Mitchell Max: I see two important potential uses for the N of 1 methodology in clinical analgesic research. First, there are some patients who are clearly unique, in whom it is crucial to have therapeutic results of the highest certainty possible. For example, Cline and Ochoa have demonstrated that pain in several patients was caused by hyperactive C fibers by using microneurography, a procedure available in only a few laboratories. If one wished to study the effects of putative C fiber inactivators, one would never get 20, or even 5, similar patients. An N of 1 design might be the best way to make the most of the opportunity to demonstrate a therapeutic principle.

Second, for purposes of initial case reports of therapeutic results, the N of 1 design is a bit of an improvement over the usual standard practice of describing a single uncontrolled anecdote in a letter to a journal. At least repeated trials of drug and placebo in one or several individuals, accompanied by a graphic presentation of the resulting pain scores over time, will more readily rule out spontaneous improvement in pain.

Dr. John Harter: I agree that the N of 1 study is a great idea. Besides the use that has been suggested—to probe specific patient types—a group of patients studied in this manner might provide excellent data regarding the proportion of patients who respond to the drug.

Dr. Eugene Laska: Dr. McQuay and the discussants have pointed out that in N of 1 trials, the conclusions pertain to the individual subject tested. The "lady tasting tea," however, illustrates a principle more global than the conclusion about this particular lady. Having demonstrated that she could distinguish the order in which milk and tea were put into the cup, she proved the point that it is *possible* to have a lady who can distinguish the order in which these two elements are added to the cup. Mathematicians use this argument all the time, and call it "proof by example." So I propose that if a substance works in a single patient, this may be substantial evidence that the substance is an active compound, yielding conclusions beyond the individual in whom it was tested.

The replicated pair design that McQuay discussed is only one of the many possible N of 1 designs. Another that has received considerable attention in the statistical literature is known as the "two-arm bandit" problem. One stands at a slot machine and pulls the arm left or right in an effort to maximize the chances of winning the jackpot, by pulling the same arm after a payoff, and switching arms when there is no payoff.

In the clinical analogue, if a treatment worked for a patient, the treatment would be repeated in the next period, the alternative treatment given only if the first one failed. This may be a more satisfying solution to the ethical dilemma that McQuay describes, and may result in greater patient acceptance of the study.

There are many statistical complexities in interpreting N of 1 studies. If the FDA has taken a position questioning the value of two-period crossover studies, imagine the legion of potential objections to the carryover issues, covariate structures, and other problems of the multiple-period N of 1 study. If one wished to pool single-patient results into a group analysis, this would be even more problematic, and require careful statistical planning before beginning such a study. These issues are yet to be worked out, and I strongly encourage efforts to do this. But I think there is gain to be made in the single-patient study as well, without going through the pooled analysis.

Advances in Pain Research and Therapy, Vol. 18,
edited by M. Max, R. Portenoy, and E. Laska,
Raven Press, Ltd., New York 1991.

8

Neuropathic Pain Syndromes

Mitchell B. Max

*Neurobiology and Anesthesiology Branch, National Institute of Dental Research,
National Institutes of Health, Bethesda, Maryland 20892*

The design of analgesic studies in the various pain syndromes associated with disorders of the peripheral and central nervous system ("neuropathic pain") is an area particularly ripe for innovation. Patients with such conditions make up a large proportion of those whose pain remains intractable to standard therapies. Among the most common causes are the neuropathies associated with diabetes, cancer chemotherapy, and human immunodeficiency virus (HIV) infection; herpes zoster; cervical or lumbar nerve root compression owing to degenerative spine disease; malignant lesions of nerve, plexus, or root; nerve trauma, including amputation; and lesions of central pain pathways, including spinothalamic tract, thalamus, or thalamic radiations.

Given the large number of patients with these neuropathic pain syndromes, there is a stunning dearth of published data about their response to drugs and other specific treatment modalities (1). An exception is classic trigeminal neuralgia, where a widely accepted clinical definition has facilitated decades of therapeutic trials. Aside from trigeminal neuralgia, however, there are only one or two controlled trials supporting the use of each of several antidepressants, anticonvulsants, and miscellaneous agents in diabetic neuropathy and postherpetic neuralgia, a few trials pertaining to other neuropathic sydromes such as those following stroke (2) and spinal cord injury (3), and only a handful of reports describing extensive uncontrolled observations in neuropathic pain conditions (4,5). Table 1 lists drugs that are often recommended for the treatment of neuropathic pain conditions. Although neuropathic pain syndromes result from a wide variety of anatomical lesions and almost certainly encompass a mixed group of underlying neurophysiological abnormalities, little in the literature helps the clinician choose the right drug for the right patient, or even addresses the issue of patient heterogeneity. Reports rarely distinguish the response of different types of pain or pattern of neurological lesions. Whether the patient has burning, shooting, or aching pain, normal sensory exam or extreme hyperalgesia, acquired

TABLE 1. *Some drugs used to treat neuropathic pain*

Tricyclics	Amitriptyline
	Imipramine
	Desipramine
Anticonvulsants	Carbamazepine
	Phenytoin
	Clonazepam
Opiates	Oxycodene, morphine
NSAIDs	Ibuprofen, sulindac
Other drugs	Clonidine
	Lidocaine, mexilitene
	Fluphenazine
	Phentolamine, phenoxybenzamine
Topical agents	Local anesthetics
	Capsaicin

immunodeficiency syndrome (AIDS) or amputation, the clinician is likely to run through the same list of drugs in the same order.

Clinicians and neurophysiologists have long been fascinated by the rich phenomenology of pain arising from neural lesions. Neuropathic symptoms often include unusual sensations such as burning, electricity, feelings of bodily distortion, allodynia (pain evoked by innocuous stimulation to the skin), and hyperpathia (an exaggerated pain response persisting long after stimuli cease). Mechanisms remained a matter of speculation, however, until the past several years, when several research groups developed methods for selective stimulation and blockade of nerve fiber populations in humans (6–8) allowing pain mechanisms to be characterized in particular patients as, for example, altered central processing of $A\beta$ fiber input (7,8), hypersensitivity of C nociceptors (9), C-mediated hyperpathia (10), or sympathetically maintained pain (11,11a).

Until recently the pharmaceutical industry has played little role in research on neuropathic pain treatment. Most current treatments were developed for unrelated neuropsychiatric or medical disorders and serendipitously showed efficacy for neuropathic pain. An increasing role for industry is likely to be stimulated by the recent development of animal models of neuropathic pain that closely resemble human pain states (12,13). Multiple possible neural substrates of neuropathic pain have been identified in these animal models (14), including ectopic discharge from injured $A\beta$ and $A\delta$ fibers, alterations in a variety of peptides in primary afferent fibers and dorsal horn neurons, and degeneration of spinal neurons that may normally serve to inhibit pain. These advances may facilitate the development of novel compounds that could correct specific neural abnormalities. If matched to the correct subsets of patients, such drugs could find a vast potential market—millions of patients with these conditions may require treatment for months or years.

This chapter discusses the design of chronic drug trials in neuropathic pain syndromes. Single-dose studies have also been carried out in these syndromes

(15–17); these designs were thoroughly discussed in Chapter 4. Two major issues will be explored that are relevant to many of the other papers in Part III of this volume. The first is the general issue of effective methods for chronic studies of analgesics. As Stewart and Stambaugh pointed out in Chapters 5 and 6, these approaches have received relatively little attention relative to single-dose comparisons. The second issue relates to the development of diagnostic classifications for heterogeneous groups such as the patients with neuropathic pains. Current diagnostic categories, such as "distal symmetrical diabetic polyneuropathy" based on patterns of structural lesions, almost certainly lump together patients with a variety of underlying physiological mechanisms of pain that may have distinctly different patterns of response to various drugs. For example, studies that consider "distal symmetrical diabetic neuropathy" would have patients with burning, cold, lancinating, aching, numbing, steady, and brief pains, with or without allodynia, paresthesia, or hyperpathia, that might correspond to some or all of the mechanisms mentioned above.

This heterogeneity makes it critical to balance treatment groups, to avoid spurious treatment results that might arise if groups differed greatly in their mechanistic substrate for pain. Investigators must strive to define subgroups that may be good or poor responders, to make recommendations for more individualized treatment or speculate about mechanisms in a way to raise questions for basic research. Because we know so little about clinical pain mechanisms now, our explanations may well be wrong, but our empirical description of the patients and their symptomatic responses must be clear enough to allow future researchers to reinterpret the results. As we will discuss, the potentially great variability among patients also puts a premium upon getting the most information from each patient, encouraging the use of crossover designs, stratification, and post hoc "data dredging" to suggest hypotheses for further testing.

PURPOSE OF THE TRIAL: INFLUENCE ON DESIGN CHOICES

Clinical trials may serve a variety of purposes and audiences. Different types of evidence are required to convince the clinician who treats the patient, the basic neuroscientist choosing which neurotransmitter system to study, the regulatory official ruling on approval of a new drug application, or the third-party payer considering reimbursement for a treatment.

For this reason, anticipation of potential outcomes and criticisms from the intended audience is a crucial step in design, and for this reason any "rules" about study design must bend to consideration of study purpose. Schwartz and Lellouch (18) and Schwartz et al. (19) have distinguished two quite different purposes of clinical trials, which would, in pure form, give rise to what they term "explanatory" or "pragmatic" approaches. The main purpose in the explanatory approach is to elucidate a biological principle about the treatment and disease, whereas the pragmatic approach seeks to guide the clinician's empirical choice of treatment for similar patients. It may be useful to examine how these alternative orientations might affect design choices in a hypothetical painful neuropathy syndrome (Table 2.)

Main Question

In the explanatory approach, the investigator might ask, "What is the relative role of norepinephrine and serotonin in mediating pain relief seen with antidepressants?" In the pragmatic approach the clinician asks, "In everyday clinical practice, which treatment will provide a satisfactory result for the most patients?"

Patient Choice

Selection criteria will differ greatly under the two assumptions. In the explanatory model, patient choice is quite selective, perhaps limited to patients with touch-evoked pain that disappears after brief nerve compression that selectively eliminates normally innocuous $A\beta$ fiber input, implying that central nervous system (CNS) processing of "light touch input" had been abnormal (7,8). In contrast, patient choice in the pragmatic model is inclusive, with the intention of matching the wide range of patients seen by the clinician.

Treatments

In the explanatory approach, treatments are chosen to best support the biological principle under inquiry. Drugs with relatively specific mechanisms are favored. In the example, fluoxetine and desipramine, specific blockers of serotonin and norepinephrine reuptake, might be compared to each other because these two neurotransmitters are strongly implicated in pain-inhibiting processes. A

TABLE 2. *"Explanatory" versus "pragmatic" orientations of clinical trials: effect on design choices in hypothetical painful neuropathy trial*

Design issue	Orientation of clinical trial	
	Explanatory	Pragmatic
Main question	What neurotransmitter mediates analgesia?	What is the best treatment in clinical practice?
Patient choice	Selective A-beta mediated Definite neuropathy	Inclusive Probable neuropathy
Treatments	Pharm. specific Desipramine Fluoxetine	Clinical favorites, including combinations
Controls	Placebo	Other active medications
Dose	High; often fixed	Titrate as in clinic
Treatment conditions	Optimal	Corresponding to clinical practice
Analysis	Completers	Intent-to-treat

placebo group is desirable, because the detection of a drug-placebo difference will suggest an effect of the drug on the pathophysiology of pain, and establish assay sensitivity (see pp. 72–75). In the pragmatic approach, one compares the most effective available treatments to each other, or to a new treatment. Differences between treatments and placebo are of less interest, although a placebo may still be useful to document assay sensitivity. Drugs with less specific actions, or combinations of drugs, are more likely to be used in a pragmatic than an explanatory approach—in this case, perhaps an amitriptyline/fluphenazine combination might be compared to carbamazepine.

Treatment Conditions

In an explanatory approach, care is taken to maximize the chance of demonstrating efficacy, even at the risk of some toxicity—a "sledgehammer approach." A fixed, high dose of drug might be used, with meticulous instruction and telephone calls to maximize compliance. In the pragmatic study, actual clinical conditions are preferable—flexible dosage adjusted for side effects, and normal amounts of treatment supervision, which may decrease the frequency of adherence to the regimen.

Response

Patient response is carefully followed over time in the explanatory approach, as even a transient period of effectiveness may reveal an important biological phenomenon. In the pragmatic approach, a single response assessment at the end of a month of treatment may be quite adequate; if relief doesn't persist for a month, the treatment may not be worth prescribing.

Data Analysis

Choices regarding analysis may differ as well. In an explanatory approach, patients who do not take the full intended treatment are excluded from the main analysis, as their responses do not test whether a response is biologically possible. [Care must still be taken to minimize the number of dropouts, however, because an unequal dropout rate between treatments can bias the conclusions (20).] The pragmatic approach will include all patients for whom there was intent-to-treat; failure or inability to comply is relevant to the everyday usefulness of the treatment.

Controlled Trials Often Have Several Purposes

The dichotomous explanatory/pragmatic schema is an oversimplification, of course, intended to offer a perspective to discuss more complex cases. Usually, the investigator wishes to address both practical *and* theoretical concerns. For example, the controlled trials of Watson et al. (21) and Watson and Evans (22) in postherpetic neuralgia have a strong "pragmatic" flavor—they are shaped by experience in a large clinical practice (4), and use diagnostic groupings, drug titration, and assessment methods similar to those used by careful practitioners. At the same time, however, the investigators have chosen drugs with relatively selective actions on monoamine systems (22), allowing them to make the "explanatory" suggestion that serotonin reuptake blockade alone is not sufficient to relieve pain. In summary, despite the complexities of any clinical trial, the simple explanatory/pragmatic distinction may sometimes be helpful in considering individual aspects of design, because the schema tends to prompt reflection on the overall purpose of the study.

WHAT NEEDS TO BE KNOWN ABOUT A NEW DRUG TREATMENT FOR NEUROPATHIC PAIN?

In defining the clinical role for a drug, a number of questions must be answered in a sequence that facilitates a more efficient research program:

1. *What is the maximum safe and tolerated dose for chronic studies?* For drugs already marketed for other conditions (e.g., epilepsy, mood disorder, cardiovascular disease) this will usually be known from clinical practice. For investigational drugs, Phase I data is used to guide dosing (Chapter 2).

2. *Does the drug have efficacy in some patients with the particular neuropathic pain syndrome?* A placebo-controlled trial in a broad group of patients with the syndrome, titrating to maximal tolerated doses, may be helpful early in the course of the research program to see if the agent has potential value. If only a subset of patients respond, not an unlikely outcome in heterogeneous disorders like neuropathic pain syndromes, the overall treatment comparison may not show a significant difference, so care must be taken not to dismiss a treatment prematurely. Alternative approaches to demonstrating efficacy in a subgroup include conducting a preliminary open-label trial and then enrolling only the responders in a subsequent controlled trial, or carrying out preliminary N of 1 trials (see Chapter 7).

3. *What is the time-course of response?* At least one study early in the research program should follow patients on extended treatment, under either open-label or blinded conditions, to estimate the time course of response. Treatment periods should be long enough so that patients will approach maximal response, unless a significant incidence of dropouts or spontaneous change in the disease over that length of time mandates a compromise on study duration. This will help to maximize the power of subsequent studies to detect treatment differences. Figure 1, for example, from a study of amitriptyline, lorazepam, and placebo in postherpetic neuralgia (23), shows that pain continued to decrease through the 6th week of amitriptyline treatment. Any shorter treatment period would have resulted in a negative result.

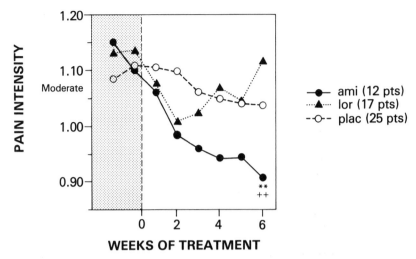

FIG. 1. Effects of lactose placebo, lorazepam, and amitriptyline on postherpetic neuralgia. Patients with postherpetic neuralgia received inert placebo (*open circles*), lorazepam (*triangles*), or amitriptyline (*filled circles*). Drugs were titrated up to limiting side effects, most commonly sedation, during first 3 weeks. Inert placebo did not affect pain, whereas amitriptyline was superior to placebo in week 6 (Newman-Keuls, $p < .01$). Lorazepam proved ineffective in last 2 weeks of treatment, when side effects had disappeared in most patients, but during dose escalation relief was similar to amitriptyline. This was probably an "active placebo" effect, although a transient "specific analgesic effect" of lorazepam cannot be ruled out. (From ref. 23, with permission.)

4. *Which patients tend to respond?* Careful pretreatment characterization of patients and poststudy "exploratory data analysis" or "data dredging" in initial open-label treatment or controlled trials will greatly enhance the value of subsequent trials. For the investigator, this information may be useful in balancing treatment groups for prognostic factors in subsequent trials, statistically adjusting treatment responses for appropriate variables, and in formulating subgroup hypotheses for further testing.

5. *What are the undesirable or toxic effects of the treatment?* This information is accrued over the entire research program, from Phase I toxicity testing to the periods of large controlled trials and initial clinical use. The modest-sized controlled efficacy trials that this chapter discusses may be used to quantitatively characterize the more common adverse reactions, but will miss many uncommon effects (24).

6. *What is the agent's dose-response curve for pain relief and toxicity?* Despite the substantial toxicity of some of the drugs used to treat neuropathic pain (25) there have been few published trials that prospectively examine dose response (26). In conditions that have a suitable physiological marker—e.g., acid secretion in ulcer disease—the dose-response curve can be estimated before undertaking chronic treatment trials. For agents that produce pain relief over days or weeks, however, only chronic clinical efficacy studies will provide useful information,

and the design of such studies will probably benefit from answers to questions 1 to 5 above.

CHOICE OF PATIENTS

As discussed above, the ideal population for an "explanatory" study would be relatively homogeneous regarding pain mechanism. At present, we can speculate about specific pathophysiologies in only a small portion of patients with neuropathic pain, but a growing number of clinical and laboratory criteria have been suggested to distinguish subsets of patients with similar pain mechanisms. These include quality and time-course of pain (e.g., trigeminal neuralgia), abnormal response to noxious and nonnoxious stimuli, response to regional sympathetic blockade or systemic α-adrenergic blockade (7,11,11a), response to sequential ischemic block of myelinated and unmyelinated nerve fibers (7,8,10,27), and microneurographic findings (9). The investigator interested in pain mechanisms should consider using variables like these as criteria for study entry, stratification, or post hoc exploratory analyses.

In many patients with neuropathic pain, however, there are no known procedures that evoke or relieve pain. Sometimes it is even difficult to say whether pain is related to a neuropathy. Aching pain in the feet of a patient with pedal neuropathy, in the absence of a definite orthopedic lesion, for example, may be related to some nonspecific rheumatic disorder. The presence of burning pain or allodynia makes the association with neuropathy more certain. The choice of whether to exclude or include these diagnostically uncertain cases will be influenced by the purpose of the study.

Many groups of researchers have chosen patient groups with a particular etiology for neuropathy, e.g., diabetes (28–32). Although this gives the reader of the study a familiar diagnostic handle, it should be kept in mind that pain mechanisms are not necessarily specified by the disease causing the neuropathy. Disease-based grouping may in some cases reduce variation among patients, who may have similarities in their patterns of neuropathy, other organ dysfunction, metabolism of drugs, and disease experience. If one chooses, on the other hand, to study patients with neuropathic pain caused by diverse diseases (17,33), even more care must be taken to stratify patient assignment to balance treatment groups for important variables (20,34) and to sift the data for associations. Where patient variables can be identified that correlate with outcome, their inclusion in the data analysis may increase the power of the study (35).

The investigator should also keep in mind that more restrictive entry criteria may make it harder to accrue the needed number of patients. This can be partially overcome by imaginative recruitment efforts. Letters to community physicians produce a modest but steady response, if supported by good follow-up and assurance that the research center is not "taking the patient away." Newspaper ads aimed at patients often yield a better response, while disease-oriented patient organizations such as the American Diabetes Association or the Reflex Sympathetic Dystrophy Association may be remarkably productive sources of volunteers. The source of patients may well affect response; for example, relatively untreated patients self-referred by local newspaper ads may have a higher response rate to a given drug than patients referred by neurologists or pain clinics. Most of the latter group have already failed to respond to the standard list of medications. The use of multicenter studies can overcome a shortage of patients in individual sites, but require extensive logistical work and rather rigid rules and procedures (34). Additional experience with more flexible single-center studies is needed before multicenter studies are widely used in these conditions.

OUTCOME MEASURES: PAIN AND PAIN RELIEF

A large number of scales and questionnaires have been used to measure pain in chronic studies. Cleeland (36) suggests that analyses of even the most complex of these measures with techniques such as factor analysis rarely distinguish more than three factors, which he denotes as (a) sensory intensity of the pain, (b) associated negative or positive mood, and (c) pain-related interference with activities.

Category scales, visual analogue scales (VAS), or the McGill Pain Questionnaire are the most commonly used measures of pain intensity in chronic pain treatment studies. Bradley and Lindblom's recent review (37) concludes that based on a very small literature, there is no evidence that any of these is superior to the others in a specific chronic pain population.

Category and VAS measures for pain and relief were extensively discussed on pages 57–64 and in the Commentaries following Chapter 4. In acute pain studies, relief category scales appear more sensitive than pain category scales in detecting drug treatment effects (38,39); the same advantage has been suggested for VAS relief scales over VAS pain scales (40, and pp. 97–100). Relief scales may lose this advantage in chronic studies, however, because any relief assessment requires a comparison with the memory of baseline pain, a more difficult task the longer the treatment period.

If one chooses pain rather than relief scales for chronic studies, the standard four-point pain category scale (e.g., none, slight, moderate, severe) is quite insensitive, largely because of the paucity of categories. The VAS may be more sensitive than the category scale (38), but this more abstract task may be confusing to some elderly patients and those with a poor grasp of English. In a study (41) where only written instructions were given, 11% of chronic pain patients failed to complete the VAS, although all used the category scale correctly. Most of these failures can be prevented by personal instruction (42).

The McGill Pain Questionnaire (43–45) has been extensively validated in acute and chronic pain conditions. Because it includes a large set of adjectives describing pain qualities (Fig. 2), the instrument may have particular value for distinguishing subgroups of patients with neuropathic pain (46,47). Its disad-

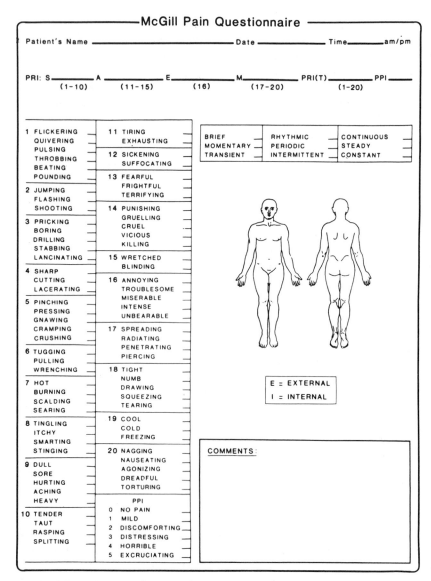

FIG. 2. McGill Pain Questionnaire. The descriptors fall into four major groups: sensory, 1 to 10; affective, 11 to 15; evaluative, 16; and miscellaneous, 17 to 20. The rank value for each descriptor is based on its position in the word set. The sum of the rank values is the pain rating index (PRI). The present pain intensity (PPI) is based on a scale of 0 to 5. (From ref. 45, with permission.)

vantages are that it takes about five minutes to complete, compared to seconds for VAS and category scales, requires a rich vocabulary, and confuses some patients (48,49).

An important issue is the frequency of pain assessment. Most studies of neuropathic pain have used single ratings before and after treatments, or at most weekly ratings. Like many other classes of chronic pain, neuropathic pain often fluctuates over hours or days (Fig. 3). Because single retrospective ratings covering a long period may be strongly affected by the pain level over the past day or two, treatment effects determined using the mean of daily ratings over a long period may be more robust; there will still be random fluctuations, but they will tend to average out over the study period.

For the primary pain outcome in chronic studies, our group has used weekly means of daily pain ratings, chosen from a 13-word list of pain intensity descriptors developed by Gracely et al. (50; Fig. 4). Each word has a numerical equivalent, established by cross-modality matching methods. The staff calls patients one to three times weekly to monitor drug dosage and check the diary ratings, and with such encouragement patients rarely wait until the end of the week to fill in the entire diary. Figure 5 shows the weekly means of the diary descriptors' numerical equivalents plotted against time in a comparison of amitriptyline to placebo in painful diabetic neuropathy (32). In that study, patients were also asked to rate their pain once weekly using the Gracely pain intensity

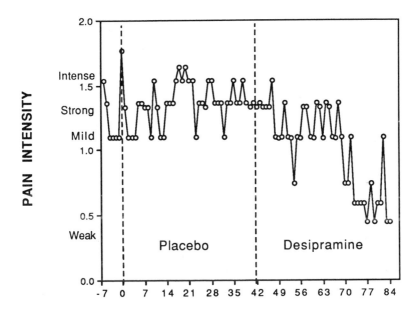

TIME, days

FIG. 3. Day-to-day fluctuation of pain in a patient with painful diabetic neuropathy. Daily pain intensity, rated with Gracely's 13-word ratio scale for pain intensity (several actual descriptors and numerical equivalents are shown) is plotted against time. *Horizontal dotted lines* separate initial drug-free baseline week from two 6-week treatments with active placebo and desipramine. Mean pain ratings calculated from diary scores tend to average out these random fluctuations in daily pain. Such measures may be more powerful in detecting treatment differences than single summary measures at the end of treatment; summary measures may be strongly affected by that day's level of pain.

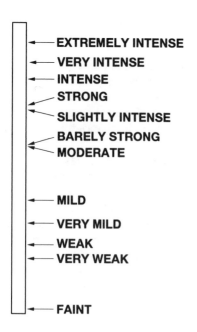

EXTREMELY INTENSE

VERY INTENSE

INTENSE

STRONG

SLIGHTLY INTENSE

BARELY STRONG

MODERATE

MILD

VERY MILD

WEAK

VERY WEAK

FAINT

NO PAIN SENSATION

FIG. 4. Gracely's verbal descriptor scale for pain intensity. Distances between descriptors reflect numerical values determined by cross-modality matching (50). In pain diaries using this scale, descriptors are simply listed, without a spatial display.

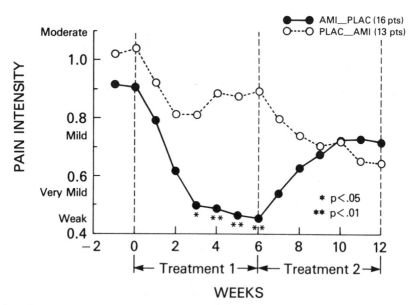

FIG. 5. Time course of analgesia, assessed using diary scores, in a crossover comparison of amitriptyline (AMI) to active placebo (PLAC) in painful diabetic neuropathy. Weekly means of numerical equivalents of pain intensity descriptors are plotted against time. Amitriptyline was effective compared with placebo in weeks 2 through 6 using within-patient comparison for all 29 patients ($p < .001$, paired t-test, weeks 3–6) but a between-group comparison showed a significant difference only in the first treatment period. Note initial response to benztropine/diazepam "active placebo," chosen to mimic amitriptyline dry mouth and sedation (*open circles,* first treatment). (From ref. 32, with permission.)

words and the McGill Pain Questionnaire; both scales showed a significant treatment effect, but with considerably less power (*unpublished data*). In four chronic studies (23,32,51,52), a five-point relief category scale (none, slight, moderate, a lot, complete) has been administered at the end of each treatment. Although these verbal ratings convey the range of patient outcomes in everyday language, in contrast to the weekly means of diary descriptor scores, which are abstract numerical values, in each case the global ratings have been less sensitive in detecting treatment effects than the mean of the final week's diary descriptor ratings.

Whatever the choice of pain intensity measures, the investigator might consider designating one scale as the primary outcome measure before the study begins; other pain measures would be labeled secondary. This may help avoid the "multiple comparison" dilemma that occurs if only some of the measures used show a significant result (20,53). For a primary measure, one might choose a scale likely to be sensitive to treatment differences and accepted as valid by other investigators, such as the scales discussed above. Secondary measures might include measures expressed in everyday language, such as the global relief category scale discussed above, patient satisfaction ratings, and various scales under investigation. Even with a sensitive scale, one may be hard-pressed to demonstrate an effect of an analgesic in patients who start the study with relatively low levels of pain. For this reason, one might specify a minimum level of pain for study entry. For example, one investigator (51) required patients to have either relatively constant mild pain, or at least 2 hrs a day of moderate pain. When there was some question about this, patients were asked if they had enough pain to notice a 50% reduction in severity.

Published neuropathic pain trials have said little about which types of pain get better, among the varied kinds of pain within any syndrome. Methods to assess the effect of the treatment on different qualities of pain are needed, both to individualize treatment and to distinguish the mechanisms of various types of pain. Despite anecdotal clinical lore that brief tic-like pains should be treated with anticonvulsants (5), and steady burning pain with tricyclics, in several trials (32,51) both kinds of pains were followed with separate relief category scales, and tricyclics were found to relieve brief pain as well as continuous pain. It would be of interest to individually follow other qualities, such as burning, cold, and sharp pains; the descriptor categories of the McGill Pain Questionnaire, for example, might be adapted for this use. In a study of postherpetic neuralgia (51) that used standard neurological examination methods before and after treatments, desipramine was observed to reduce allodynia, evoked by light touch, as well as patients' spontaneous pain.

Laboratory measures of pain sensation may provide insight into what treatment agents are doing in the nervous system. In a study of amitriptyline in diabetic neuropathy (32), for example, patients' perception of 3-sec noxious heat stimuli applied to neurologically normal forearm skin were assessed after amitriptyline and placebo treatment (Fig. 6). Although amitriptyline produced marked re-

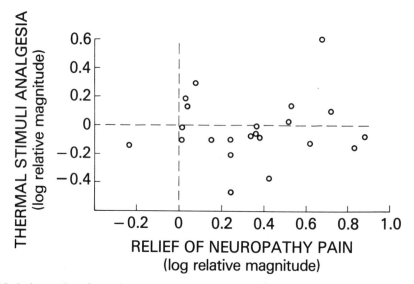

FIG. 6. Integration of experimental pain measures into a clinical trial. Within-patient differences in pain intensity after amitriptyline compared to placebo (32) are plotted for experimental heat stimuli and clinical diabetic neuropathy pain; each point is one patient. Numerical values indicate (placebo-amitriptyline) differences in final week's mean diary ratings using Gracely intensity descriptors. Positive values indicate relief with amitriptyline, relative to placebo; dotted lines demarcate zero change. Note that points cluster around *horizontal dotted line,* indicating that amitriptyline does not affect experimental heat sensation, even in patients on the *right side* of graph who reported marked relief of clinical pain.

duction in patients' neuropathic pain—most commonly burning of the feet—there was no change in their sensation of heat applied to normal skin, suggesting, for example, that amitriptyline does not exert a general inhibitory effect on neurons generating a subjective sensation of heat.

OUTCOME MEASURES: MOOD AND PAIN

Pain and mood are closely linked, but one can tease these out as separate phenomena in several ways. A number of investigators separately measured sensory intensity and affective aspects of pain (43,54,55). These two components have been reported to respond differentially to acute drug challenges with intravenous fentanyl and diazepam (55). As a measure of the affective dimension, our group initially used Gracely's ratio scale of 13 "pain unpleasantness" descriptors in addition to the sensory intensity list. Use of the affective list in chronic studies was subsequently discontinued because, apart from the affective descriptors' slightly greater association with daily mood ratings, the results with the two scales were virtually identical in two studies (23,32).

When treatments are known to affect mood, standard psychological measures (56) should be evaluated before and after treatments. Figure 7 shows the results

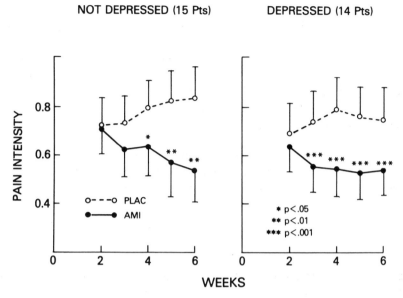

FIG. 7. Distinguishing drug effects on pain and mood. To examine question of whether amitriptyline relieves pain independently of its antidepressant effects, patients were assessed as "not depressed" or "depressed" by baseline psychiatric interview. Reduction in pain with amitriptyline, relative to placebo, was at least as great in the "not depressed" as in the "depressed" subgroup. Pain intensity values are from Gracely intensity descriptor scale, and combine ratings from both treatment periods to make a within-patient comparison. Week 1 is omitted because there was no washout period, and elimination of amitriptyline requires about 1 week. (From ref. 32, with permission.)

of the previously mentioned amitriptyline/diabetic neuropathy study (32) when patients were stratified according to a baseline psychiatric interview for depression. Patients assessed as not depressed had at least as much pain relief as those who were initially depressed, and pain relief scores were not significantly correlated with improvement in depression scores. These and similar data (21,23,56) have shown that amitriptyline can relieve neuropathic pain by mechanisms distinct from improvement in mood.

OUTCOME MEASURES: INTERFERENCE WITH ACTIVITIES

Published studies of neuropathic pain treatment have not included data on patient function. Bradley (57) recommends using disability measures that have been well validated in chronic pain patients; examples include the Sickness Impact Profile, Functional Status Index, Health Assessment Questionnaire, or Index of Functional Impairment (58–60). Because impaired function in some patients with neuropathic pain may be quite selective—for example, patients with neuropathic burning feet may reduce but not eliminate their walking—pilot studies should assess whether the measures selected are sensitive enough to pick up these functional limitations, or whether the investigator needs to design measures for functional outcomes of interest.

Measurements of overt motor behaviors have been shown to correlate well with subjective report in chronic low back pain, rheumatoid arthritis, and head and neck cancer (37,61). Because these measurements require rigorous training of observers, they have been used predominantly in pain syndromes in which verbal measures are not thought to be sensitive and reliable indicators of treatment efficacy. Subjective pain measures have been quite reliable in studies of diabetic neuropathy pain and postherpetic neuralgia, but behavioral measures may prove particularly valuable in populations that tend to rate pain consistently at the top of the scale (36), such as patients with causalgia or chronic radiculopathies.

OUTCOME MEASURES: ADVERSE EFFECTS

Some of the issues in the assessment of adverse effects are discussed in Chapter 4, pages 66–67. As in single-dose analgesic trials, there has been little quantitative scrutiny of adverse drug effects in chronic analgesic studies, particularly neuropathic pain trials, where some of the agents used have considerable toxicity.

In trials of new agents, the usual survey of volunteered side effects is often adequate. Many of the therapeutic questions in neuropathic pain, however, involve toxicity; e.g., can antidepressants with a narrower spectrum of actions than amitriptyline give equivalent pain relief but with less sedation, anticholinergic effects, and postural hypotension? In such studies prospective assessment of common side effects might be more sensitive to treatment differences than spontaneously volunteered reports, but these methodological issues need more research (20).

TREATMENTS, CONTROLS, AND PLACEBOS

A placebo is usually used to determine whether a drug has "efficacy," a derived concept defined as change with drug minus change with placebo. One can also establish a drug's efficacy without a placebo, by showing it to be superior to a standard drug known to relieve pain in the same population (see pp. 72–75). This is not yet practical in most neuropathic pain conditions because few agents are known to have any efficacy in specific populations. In conditions where there is a proven agent—e.g., amitriptyline in postherpetic neuralgia—this type of test may be too rigorous because it would take either a remarkable therapeutic advance or a very large sample size to significantly surpass the standard. More likely, an efficacious new drug will be statistically indistinguishable from the control. Skeptics would then deny any efficacy, suggesting that both new drug and control might be showing only placebo effects in this population (p. 75, Fig.

6G), a difficult claim to refute because marked placebo responses are not uncommon in chronic pain studies (62). A practical difficulty with including a standard control in a placebo-controlled study is that it is likely that most of the patients referred for the study have already tried the standard therapy without great success, and would be unwilling to take it again.

Hospital research committees sometimes question the ethics of giving placebos to patients in chronic pain studies. Most analgesic investigators consider this practice ethical as long as the patient has been fully informed of other proven treatments, and the patient chooses to accept the possibility of placebo treatment. A period of several weeks or even months of placebo treatment is not very different from standard care for many patients; Watson et al. (4) have reported that a majority of pain clinic patients with postherpetic neuralgia eventually stopped all treatments, finding them unsatisfactory. Some investigators include the possibility of short-acting rescue medications (e.g., a weak opiate or aspirin-like drug) for distressing levels of pain, although some patients with neuropathic pain syndromes do not get relief from standard analgesics (4,15,16).

Care must be taken to match all of the properties of the treatment drugs, e.g., pill size, shape, color, and taste (34). Most drugs that have been used to treat neuropathic pain have very obvious side effects, which would allow patients and investigators to easily distinguish drugs from inert placebos. Detection of side effects may increase patients' and staff's expectation that pain may be relieved, which in itself may result in reduction in pain report (16,63).

To avoid this bias, the investigator might consider an "active" placebo that mimics some of the side effects of the study drug of interest. In Fig. 5, the open circles represent diabetic neuropathy patients in a trial of amitriptyline (32) who were initially treated with an active placebo designed to mimic amitriptyline side effects: a mild anticholinergic drug (benztropine, 1 mg) and a sedative (diazepam, 5 mg). In weeks 1 and 2, the placebo-treated patients reported analgesia not dissimilar to those receiving amitriptyline, but pain returned toward the baseline in weeks 4 to 6. Figure 1 illustrates a study in which patients were titrated to maximum tolerated daily doses of amitriptyline 25 to 150 mg, lorazepam 0.5 to 6 mg, or inert lactose placebo (23). Although lorazepam was under study as a potentially therapeutic drug, pain relief was no better than inert placebo at 6 weeks, so it might be viewed in retrospect as an active placebo. For the first 3 weeks of the study, while all patients on active drugs were being titrated to limiting side effects (generally sedation), the lorazepam group reported less pain than the inert placebo group.

Although the use of an "active placebo" may reduce the risk of spuriously attributing efficacy to a new drug, one takes the chance that the masking agent itself might improve or worsen pain, potentially confounding the study results. For this reason, the investigator might choose the lowest dose of the agent that would produce detectable effects in most patients. Whether or not an active or inert placebo is used, the adequacy of the blinding can be checked by giving patients and/or staff a simple questionnaire (before the expected onset of pain relief), asking them to guess the identity of the medication and the reasons for this guess (64).

In studies comparing two or more active agents to placebo, the basic issues in design and interpretation are similar to those discussed above. If no placebo is used, the intent may be either to show the new drug to be superior to a standard— a difficult task as noted above—or to demonstrate that it is comparable in efficacy to the standard drug. Temple (65) has expressed concern that when the research objective is to show that there is no statistically significant difference between the two treatments, one may not have the same incentive for meticulous technique as in a placebo comparison where one aims to show a difference exists. In the former case, the investigator may be biased toward choosing patients, administering treatment, or recording outcomes in a way that increases variability and decreases the likelihood of a powerful response. To guard against this criticism, investigators should strive to maximize treatment effects and must quantitate the sensitivity of the methods by which they showed no difference, e.g., demonstrating narrow confidence intervals for estimates of the difference between treatments (66–68).

PARALLEL VERSUS CROSSOVER DESIGNS

Crossover Designs

Because the patients with neuropathic pain may be quite heterogeneous with regard to mechanism, a crucial principle of study design is to maximize the information gained from each patient. Crossover studies, in which a treatment comparison is made in each patient, are one way of meeting this need. Standard assumptions in crossover studies are that the disease is stable over the time of study, the effects of the proposed medications cease soon after discontinuing them, and there is no reason to believe that the treatments interact with each other. The controversies regarding the appropriateness of crossover designs are more extensively discussed in the commentary on pp. 84–87, here we will make a few remarks regarding their use in chronic studies of neuropathic pain.

Because the within-patient design reduces the variance relative to a between-patient comparison, and because the crossover design uses each patient several times, sample sizes can be smaller than would be required for parallel-group studies of the same power (69). This is an important practical advantage when carrying out the study in a single center.

The simplest and most commonly used crossover design is the 2×2 design (Table 3, left). It fulfills the goal, discussed above, of enabling the two treatments, or treatment and placebo, to be compared in each patient in a potentially heterogeneous group. Despite its popularity among clinicians, most statisticians would agree with Jones and Kenward (70) that "if we limit ourselves . . . to the

TABLE 3. *Alternative designs for two-treatment crossover study*

Standard 2 × 2	Alternative #1	Alternative #2
A-B	A-B	A-B-B
B-A	B-A	B-A-A
	A-A	
	B-B	

purely statistical properties of the 2 × 2 trial, then we would have to conclude that it is a design to be avoided." If the differences between treatments differ in the first and second periods, one cannot distinguish with any certainty whether this is owing to a carryover effect (persistence of a pharmacological or psychological effect of the first treatment into the second period), a treatment × period interaction (the passage of time affects the relative efficacy of the treatments, e.g., by the second period, patients who initially received placebo might be too discouraged to respond to any subsequent treatment), or a difference between the groups of patients assigned the two different orders of treatment.

Figure 5 illustrates several of these effects that occurred in an amitriptyline/placebo comparison in diabetic neuropathy (32). In the group receiving amitriptyline first (filled circles) analgesia persisted into the placebo period, particularly in weeks 7 and 8. The investigators had anticipated such a carryover effect, and specified the final week of each treatment as the primary outcome comparison, expecting that the first 5 weeks of the treatment would serve as a "washout period." An unexpected finding, however, was the difference between the effects of amitriptyline in the two periods. The group receiving the drug in the first period (filled circles, left) had a much greater decrease in pain than the group treated in the second period (open circles). This may have been caused by a difference between the patient groups—the group treated in the first period was able to tolerate almost twice the doses of amitriptyline—but such a post hoc explanation could only be tentative.

In the example in Fig. 5, the difference in treatment effect between periods did not call into question the conclusion that amitriptyline was superior to placebo. Cases where the treatment effect is greater in the second period than the first may be more problematic. Figure 8 illustrates a hypothetical case where administration of a drug affects pain little, but withdrawal of the drug increases pain. Drug and placebo will appear similar in the first period (or in a parallel study). In the second period, however, patients receiving the drug (following placebo) may have less pain than the patients receiving placebo, whose pain is worsened by withdrawal. The inclusion of data from the second period would risk spurious attribution of analgesic efficacy to the drug. Moreover, although statistical tests to detect carryover effects in the 2 × 2 crossover design are routinely used (53,71), they are not very sensitive because they rely on between-patient comparisons (69,72). For these reasons, regulatory agencies have been particularly reluctant to rely upon data from such designs.

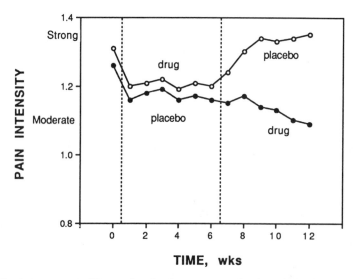

FIG. 8. Spurious treatment difference in a 2 × 2 crossover study: a hypothetical example. Although some carryover effects are "conservative," reducing the apparent drug-placebo difference (e.g., Fig. 5), a false attribution of efficacy could result if withdrawal of an ineffective drug causes the pain syndrome to worsen during the placebo period (*open circles*).

Fortunately, these statistical difficulties are largely limited to the 2 × 2 case. As discussed in Chapter 4, if the investigator adds several other treatment sequences (Table 3, center), or a third treatment period (Table 3, right), unbiased estimates of treatment effects are possible even in the presence of various types of carryover effects (73). For studies involving three or more treatments, there are a variety of designs that allow these effects to be distinguished (70). These designs also enable the estimation of the carryover effect, which may be interesting in its own right. Despite their superiority from the statistical perspective, however, the two alternative designs in Table 3 may have potential disadvantages compared to the standard 2 × 2, if the overriding goal is to examine treatment outcomes in individual patients. In Alternative #1, only half of the patients receive both of the treatments, so one cannot compare the treatments in every individual. In Alternative #2, one does compare the treatments in every patient, but if long treatment periods are required, addition of the third period risks a greater dropout rate. In most cases, the advantage of being able to estimate treatment, carryover, and period effects with greater certainty will favor the use of designs other than the 2 × 2 crossover.

Parallel Designs

Parallel study designs are preferable when there are strong concerns about carryover effects, when the natural history of the pain syndrome would make spontaneous improvement or worsening frequent over the longer time that a crossover design requires, or in other situations where within-patient variability is expected to be large compared to between-patient variability. Attention to several aspects of study design may mitigate the problems posed by the variability between patients with neuropathic pain (35).

A good baseline, consisting of at least several observations, is essential because it allows the investigator to subtract out baseline pain scores to yield pain intensity difference scores as the outcome variable. This usually increases the power of treatment comparisons, eliminating a large part of the variance (35,74). The baseline is generally determined under "no treatment conditions." Although this has been little used in chronic pain studies, in many studies of psychiatric, antihypertensive, and other drugs, all patients receive several weeks of a single-blind placebo "run-in" period. A significant proportion of patients improve considerably with placebo and are eliminated from the trial before randomization to active treatments. In studies of chronic pain, however, it might be inadvisable to screen out patients who responded to placebo unless they had such a marked placebo response that there was no longer enough pain to assess a further drug effect; many patients with chronic pain have modest responses to placebo (Figs. 1 and 5), and excluding all of these would make the study unrepresentative of a clinical population.

The investigator should also make an effort to balance the treatment groups for variables that predict response, whenever these predictors are known or suspected. If one wishes to examine response in specific subgroups, assignments must also be balanced appropriately. Groups can be balanced using stratification or various techniques of adaptive randomization (20,34; and pp. 70–71). In studies with sample sizes typical of neuropathic pain trials, 20 to 40 patients per group, these methods can significantly increase the power of a study (34) if the prognostic variables are well chosen and the statistical methods take the balancing method into account (35).

DETERMINING OPTIMUM DOSAGE

Only recently have any neuropathic pain trials prospectively examined the dose-response curve for relief of neuropathic pain (26). The relative neglect of dose-response studies is not surprising, since for most syndromes the prior question of whether an agent relieves pain at any dose has not been answered.

There is growing interest in the research issues involved in determining optimal dosing (see also Chapters 2 and 24). Pharmacologists first realized that this was a problem in the late 1970s, when it became clear that recommended doses derived from clinical trials of several hypertensive agents were as much as ten times the dose subsequently shown to yield near-maximal effect (65,75). Antihypertensive doses had initially been determined by a method used in many neuropathic pain trials (21,23,32): the physician gradually titrated the dose upward until an effect was seen or side effects prevented further escalation. This method is biased toward overestimating the recommended dose; if onset of relief is delayed, or if patients have spontaneous resolution, therapeutic success will be mistakenly attributed to the higher dose.

To correct for this bias, parallel dose-ranging designs have become the most common method used in the development of many classes of drugs. Separate groups of patients are randomized to one of several doses, a dose-response curve is prepared from the mean group responses, and the initial recommended dose is chosen from this curve. In a recent critique of dose-ranging methods, Sheiner et al. (76) argue that dosing recommendations are liable to be inaccurate unless they are based on knowledge of individual patients' dose-response curves, which require at least several doses to be tested in each patient. Individual dose-response curves are particularly important in defining guidelines for dose increments in patients with a suboptimal initial response. Sheiner's caveats are relevant to conditions such as neuropathic pain syndromes in which patients vary greatly in their responses to a given drug.

Current doses of drugs used to treat neuropathic pain are either based on anecdote or on studies that report only responses to a single-dose level; in many, the use of titration added the possible bias toward dose overestimation mentioned above. Several studies of antidepressant effects on postherpetic neuralgia (21,23) or diabetic neuropathy (32,77) retrospectively examined the relationship between drug dose, blood levels, and pain relief. A typical result is illustrated in Fig. 9. In a study of amitriptyline treatment of postherpetic neuralgia, there was a modest but statistically significant tendency for pain relief to be greater in patients who were titrated up to higher amitriptyline doses and higher tricyclic blood levels. This result suggests that nonresponders at lower doses may have benefited from dose escalation, although it remains possible that lower doses in some patients might have produced equal or superior pain relief (78). Another explanation for the positive association might be that patients with intractable pain were less able to tolerate side effects of high drug doses.

If a drug is superior to placebo, but retrospective dose-range analyses yield no significant association between dose or blood levels and therapeutic result, one can say little about choice of dosage. This lack of association certainly doesn't mean that "low doses are just as good as high doses." Perhaps, for example, many patients get pain relief linearly related to dose, including some who get relief at lower doses and stop escalating, while other patients are nonresponders who escalate to high doses without relief. The combination of these two populations might produce an apparently random assortment of doses and responses. Additional explanations for lack of an association might include variability in compliance, absorption, or metabolism, or for drug level-response data, variations in sample collection, storage and assays, or an unrecognized active metabolite.

To avoid the bias introduced by variable dose titration, one needs a prospectively planned dose-response study. [Alternatively and with somewhat more effort, one can prospectively titrate patients to several different *blood levels* of drug

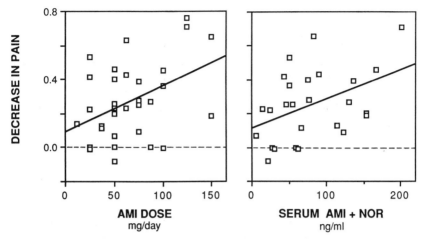

FIG. 9. Retrospective dose-response analyses yield limited information. In a study of amitriptyline in postherpetic neuralgia, decreases in pain intensity diary score (compared to week preceding amitriptyline treatment) are plotted against maintenance daily amitriptyline dose (*left*) and serum levels of amitriptyline and nortriptyline (*right*). *Horizontal dotted line* demarcates "no change in pain." Regression lines with positive slope (dose, $r = 0.43$; serum levels, $r = 0.44$, $p < .05$ for each) suggest that amitriptyline analgesia may increase with dose and serum tricyclic levels, over the ranges used in this study. These data are of limited use, however, in determining dose-increment strategy, for which single-patient dose-response curves are needed. In addition, the dose titration method used may bias toward recommending too high a starting dose. (From ref. 23, with permission.)

(26,79). Crossover designs, in which each patient takes a number of different doses in random order, allow an estimation of individual patients' dose-response curves while producing far less bias in dosing guidelines than parallel studies (76). A drawback of either crossover or parallel designs, compared to ascending titration, is that some patients will be assigned to doses that are too high for them, risking toxicity. Although the crossover mitigates the problem of between-patient differences, patients are still vulnerable to overdose.

Sheiner et al. (76) propose a return to ascending titration designs, with safeguards against overly rapid increases in dose and the use of better analytical methods to calculate optimal starting dose and dose increments. Because pain ratings are so susceptible to patients' expectations, however, such a method might still overrate the effects of higher doses; patients would be expecting more pain relief as the dose went up, which might bias them toward reporting more relief (see Chapter 3). An alternative method to obtain individual dose-response curves, yet avoid the risk of overdose posed by standard crossover designs, might be to titrate each patient to maximal response, a targeted drug blood level, or limiting side effects, and then enter responders into several randomly assigned treatment periods using various proportions of the maximum dose. Using such an approach, Sindrup et al. (26) studied individual responses to imipramine in patients with painful diabetic neuropathy, and showed the optimal plasma concentrations of imipramine and desipramine to be above 400 to 500 nM/L.

CONCLUSION

Therapeutic trials in neuropathic pain syndromes illustrate many of the challenges and opportunities in advancing the treatment of chronic pain. Newly developed animal models of neuropathic pain, receptor-specific drugs, and hypotheses regarding pain mechanisms herald the possibility of tailoring treatment to individual patients. Most clinical researchers collect data in a manner that illuminates the heterogeneity of neuropathic pain mechanisms, as well as develop effective methods for assessing responses to chronic analgesic treatment.

ACKNOWLEDGMENT

I would like to thank Drs. Gary Bennett, Ronald Dubner, Howard Fields, and Srinivasa Raja for their thoughtful comments on the manuscript.

REFERENCES

1. Maciewicz R, Bouckoms A, Martin JB. Drug therapy of neuropathic pain. *Clin J Pain* 1985;1: 39–49.
2. Leijon G, Boivie J. Central post-stroke pain—a controlled trial of amitriptyline and carbamazepine. *Pain* 1989;36:27–36.
3. Davidoff G, Guarracini M, Roth E, Sliwa J, Yarkony G. Trazodone hydrochloride in the treatment of dysesthetic pain in traumatic myelopathy: a randomized, double-blind, placebo-controlled study. *Pain* 1987;29:151–161.
4. Watson CPN, Evans RJ, Watt VR, Birkett N. Post-herpetic neuralgia: 208 cases. *Pain* 1988;35: 289–298.
5. Swerdlow M, Cundill JG. Anticonvulsant drugs used in the treatment of lancinating pain: a comparison. *Anaesthesia* 1981;36:1129–1132.
6. Lindblom U, Ochoa J. Somatosensory function and dysfunction. In: Asbury AK, McKhann GM, McDonald WI, eds. *Diseases of the nervous system: clinical neurobiology.* Philadelphia: W.B. Saunders, 1986;283–298.
7. Campbell JN, Raja SN, Meyer RA, MacKinnon SE. Myelinated afferents signal the hyperalgesia associated with nerve injury. *Pain* 1988;32:89–94.
8. Price DD, Bennett GJ, Rafii A. Psychophysical observations on patients with neuropathic pain relieved by a sympathetic block. *Pain* 1989;36:273–288.
9. Cline MA, Ochoa J, Torebjork HE. Chronic hyperalgesia and skin warming caused by sensitized C nociceptors. *Brain* 1989;112:621–647.
10. Ochs G, Schenk M, Struppler A. Painful dysaesthesias following peripheral nerve injury: a clinical and electrophysiological study. *Brain Res* 1989;496:228–240.
11. Raja SN, Treede RD, Tewes PA, Davis KD, Lin C, Campbell JN. A new diagnostic test for sympathetically maintained pain: systemic phentolamine administration (abstract). *Anesthesiology* 1989;71:A732.
11a.Campbell JN, Raja SN, Meyer RA. Painful sequelae of nerve injury. In: Dubner R, Gebhart GF, Bond MR, eds. *Proceedings of the Vth world congress on pain.* Amsterdam: Elsevier, 1988;135–143.
12. Bennett GJ, Xie Y-K. A peripheral mononeuropathy in rat that produces disorders of pain sensation like those seen in man. *Pain* 1988;33:87–107.
13. Wuarin-Bierman L, Azhnd GR, Kaufmann F, Burcklen L, Adler J. Hyperalgesia in spontaneous and experimental models of diabetic neuropathy. *Diabetologia* 1987;30:653–658.

14. Bennett GJ, Kajander KC, Sahara Y, Iadarola MJ, Sugimoto T. Neurochemical and anatomical changes in the dorsal horn of rats with an experimental painful peripheral neuropathy. In: Cervero F, Bennett GJ, Headley PM, eds. *Processing of sensory information in the superficial dorsal horn of the spinal cord.* Amsterdam: Plenum Press, 1989;463–471.
15. Arner S, Meyerson BA. Lack of analgesic effect of opioids on neuropathic and idiopathic forms of pain. *Pain* 1988;33:11–24.
16. Max MB, Schafer SC, Culnane M, Dubner R, Gracely RH. Association of pain relief with drug side effects in postherpetic neuralgia: a single-dose study of clonidine, codeine, ibuprofen, and placebo. *Clin Pharmacol Ther* 1988;43:363–371.
17. Kishore-Kumar R, Schafer SC, Lawlor BA, Murphy DL, Max MB. Single doses of the serotonin agonists buspirone and m-chlorophenylpiperazine do not relieve neuropathic pain. *Pain* 1989;37:223–227.
18. Schwartz D, Lellouch J. Explanatory and pragmatic attitudes in therapeutic trials. *J Chron Dis* 1967;20:637–648.
19. Schwartz D, Flamant R, Lellouch J. *Clinical trials* (Healy MJR, transl.). London: Academic Press, 1980.
20. Friedman LM, Furberg CD, DeMets DL. *Fundamentals of clinical trials,* 2nd ed. Littleton, Massachusetts: PSG Publishing Company, 1985.
21. Watson CP, Evans RJ, Reed K, Goldsmith L, Warsh J. Amitriptyline versus placebo in postherpetic neuralgia. *Neurology* 1982;32:671–673.
22. Watson CPN, Evans RJ. A comparative trial of amitriptyline and zimelidine in postherpetic neuralgia. *Pain* 1985;23:387–394.
23. Max MB, Schafer SC, Culnane M, et al. Amitriptyline, but not lorazepam, relieves postherpetic neuralgia. *Neurology* 1988;38:1427–1432.
24. Belville JW, Forrest WH, Elashoff J, Laska E. Evaluating side effects of analgesics in a cooperative clinical study. *Clin Pharmacol Ther* 1968;9:303–313.
25. Ray WA, Griffin MR, Schaffner W, Baugh DK, Melton LJ. Psychotropic drug use and the risk of hip fracture. *N Engl J Med* 1987;316:363–368.
26. Sindrup SH, Gram LF, Skjold T, Froland A, Beck-Nielsen H. Concentration-response relationship in imipramine treatment of diabetic neuropathy symptoms. *Clin Pharmacol Ther* 1990;47:509–515.
27. Ochoa J. The newly recognized painful ABC syndrome: thermographic aspects. *Thermology* 1986;2:65–66,101–107.
28. Cohen KL, Harris S. Efficacy and safety of nonsteroidal anti-inflammatory drugs in the therapy of diabetic neuropathy. *Arch Intern Med* 1987;147:1442–1444.
29. Dejgard A, Petersen P, Kastrup J. Mexiletine for treatment of chronic painful diabetic neuropathy. *Lancet* 1988;1:9–11.
30. Gomez-Perez FJ, Rull JA, Dies H, Rodriguez-Rivera JG, Gonzalez-Barranco J, Lozano-Casteneda O. Nortriptyline and fluphenazine in the symptomatic treatment of diabetic neuropathy. A double-blind study. *Pain* 1985;23:395–400.
31. Kvinesdal B, Molin J, Froland A, Gram LF. Imipramine treatment of painful diabetic neuropathy. *JAMA* 1984;251:1727–1730.
32. Max MB, Culnane M, Schafer SC, et al. Amitriptyline relieves diabetic neuropathy pain in patients with normal or depressed mood. *Neurology* 1987;37:589–596.
33. Langohr HD, Stohr M, Petruch F. An open and double-blind cross-over study on the efficacy of clomipramine (Anafranil) in patients with painful mono- and polyneuropathies. *Eur Neurol* 1982;21:309–317.
34. Meinert CL. *Clinical trials: design, conduct, and analysis.* New York: Oxford University Press, 1986.
35. Lavori PW, Louis TA, Bailar JC, Polansky M. Designs for experiments—parallel comparisons of treatment. *N Engl J Med* 1983;309:1291–1298.
36. Cleeland CS. Measurement of pain by subjective report. In: Chapman CR, Loeser JD, eds. *Issues in pain measurement.* New York: Raven Press, 1989;391–404.
37. Bradley LA, Lindblom U. Do different types of chronic pain require different measurement technologies? In: Chapman CR, Loeser JD, eds. *Issues in pain measurement.* New York: Raven Press, 1989;445–454.

38. Littman GS, Walker BR, Schneider BE. Reassessment of verbal and visual analog ratings in analgesic studies. *Clin Pharmacol Ther* 1985;38:16–23.
39. Sriwatanakul K, Kelvie W, Lasagna L, Calimlim JF, Weis OF, Mehta G. Studies with different types of visual analog scales for measurement of pain. *Clin Pharmacol Ther* 1983;34:234–239.
40. Wallenstein SL, Heidrich G, Kaiko R, Houde RW. Clinical evaluation of mild analgesics: the measurement of clinical pain. *Br J Clin Pharmacol* 1980;10:319S–327S.
41. Kremer E, Atkinson JH, Ignelzi RJ. Measurement of pain: patient preference does not confound pain measurement. *Pain* 1981;10:241–248.
42. Scott J, Huskisson EC. Graphic representation of pain. *Pain* 1976;2:175–184.
43. Melzack R. The McGill Pain Questionnaire: major properties and scoring methods. *Pain* 1975;1:277–299.
44. Melzack R, Katz J, Jeans ME. The role of compensation in chronic pain: analysis using a new method of scoring the McGill Pain Questionnaire. *Pain* 1985;23:101–112.
45. Melzack R, ed. *Pain measurement and assessment.* New York: Raven Press, 1983.
46. Melzack R, Terrence C, Fromm G, Amsel R. Trigeminal neuralgia and atypical facial pain: use of the McGill Pain Questionnaire for discrimination and diagnosis. *Pain* 1986;27:297–302.
47. Masson EA, Hunt L, Gem JM, Boulton AJM. A novel approach to the diagnosis and assessment of symptomatic diabetic neuropathy. *Pain* 1989;38:25–28.
48. Chapman CR, Casey KL, Dubner R, Foley KM, Gracely RH, Reading AE. Pain measurement: an overview. *Pain* 1985;22:1–32.
49. Daut RL, Cleeland CS, Flannery RC. Development of the Wisconsin Brief Pain Questionnaire to assess pain in cancer and other diseases. *Pain* 1983;17:197–210.
50. Gracely RH, McGrath P, Dubner R. Ratio scales of sensory and affective verbal pain descriptors. *Pain* 1978;5:5–18.
51. Kishore-Kumar R, Max MB, Schafer SC, et al. Desipramine relieves postherpetic neuralgia. *Clin Pharmacol Ther* 1990;47:305–312.
52. Max MB, Kishore-Kumar R, Schafer SC, et al. A randomized controlled trial of desipramine in painful diabetic neuropathy. *Pain* 1991, in press.
53. Pocock SJ. *Clinical trials, a practical approach.* Chichester, UK: John Wiley & Sons, 1983.
54. Price DD. *Psychological and neural mechanisms of pain.* New York: Raven Press, 1988.
55. Gracely RH, McGrath P, Dubner R. Narcotic analgesia: fentanyl reduces the intensity but not the unpleasantness of painful tooth pulp sensations. *Science* 1979;203:1261–1263.
56. Feinmann C. Pain relief by antidepressants: possible modes of action. *Pain* 1985;23:1–8.
57. Bradley LA. Assessing the psychological profile of the chronic pain patient. In: Dubner R, Gebhart GF, Bond MR, eds. *Proceedings of the Vth world congress on pain.* Amsterdam: Elsevier, 1988;251–262.
58. Bergner M, Bobbitt RA, Carter WB, Gibson BS. The Sickness Impact Profile: development and final revision of a health status measure. *Med Care* 1981;19:787–805.
59. Jette AM. Functional status instrument: reliability of a chronic disease evaluation instrument. *Arch Phys Med Rehabil* 1980;61:395–401.
60. Fries JF, Spitz P, Kraines RG, Holman HR. Measurement of patient outcome in arthritis. *Arthritis Rheum* 1982;25:1048–1053.
61. Keefe FJ. Behavioral measurement of pain. In: Chapman CR, Loeser JD, eds. *Issues in pain measurement.* New York: Raven Press, 1989;405–424.
62. Rull JA, Quibrera R, Gonzalez-Millan H, Castaneda OL. Symptomatic treatment of peripheral diabetic neuropathy with carbamazepine (tegretol): double blind crossover trial. *Diabetologia* 1969;5:215–218.
63. Gracely RH, Dubner R, Deeter WR, Wolskee PJ. Clinicians' expectations influence placebo analgesia (letter). *Lancet* 1985;1:43.
64. Moscucci M, Byrne L, Weintraub M, Cox C. Blinding, unblinding, and the placebo effect: an analysis of patients' guesses of treatment assignment in a double-blind clinical trial. *Clin Pharmacol Ther* 1987;41:259–265.
65. Temple R. Government viewpoint of clinical trials. *Drug Information J* 1982;16:10–17.
66. Detsky AS, Sackett DL. When was a "negative" clinical trial big enough? How many patients you needed depends on what you found. *Arch Intern Med* 1985;145:709–712.
67. Makuch RW, Johnson MF. Some issues in the design and interpretation of "negative" clinical studies. *Arch Intern Med* 1986;146:986–989.

68. Makuch R, Johnson M. Issues in planning and interpreting active control equivalence studies. *J Clin Epidemiol* 1989;42:503–511.
69. Louis TA, Lavori PW, Bailar JC, Polansky M. Crossover and self-controlled designs in clinical research. *N Engl J Med* 1984;310:24–31.
70. Jones B, Kenward MG. *Design and analysis of cross-over trials.* London: Chapman and Hall, 1989.
71. Fleiss JL. *The design of clinical experiments.* New York: John Wiley & Sons, 1985;263–290.
72. Brown BW. Statistical controversies in the design of clinical trials—some personal views. *Controlled Clin Trials* 1980;1:13–27.
73. Laska E, Meisner M, Kushner HB. Optimal crossover designs in the presence of carryover effects. *Biometrics* 1983;39:1087–1091.
74. Kaiser L. Adjusting for baseline: change or percentage change? *Stat Med* 1989;8:1183–1190.
75. Temple R. Dose-response and registration of new drugs. In: Lasagna L, Erill S, Naranjo CA, eds. *Dose-response relationships in clinical pharmacology.* Amsterdam: Elsevier, 1989;145–170.
76. Sheiner LB, Beal SL, Sambol NC. Study designs for dose-ranging. *Clin Pharmacol Ther* 1989;46:63–77.
77. Gram LF. Dose-response relationships in psychopharmacology. In: Lasagna L, Erill S, Naranjo CA, eds. *Dose-response relationships in clinical pharmacology.* Amsterdam: Elsevier, 1989;309–317.
78. Watson CPN. Therapeutic window for amitriptyline analgesia. *Can Med Assoc J* 1984;130:105–106.
79. Saudek CD, Werns S, Reidenberg MM. Phenytoin in the treatment of diabetic symmetrical polyneuropathy. *Clin Pharmacol Ther* 1977;22:196–199.

Advances in Pain Research and Therapy, Vol. 18,
edited by M. Max, R. Portenoy, and E. Laska,
Raven Press, Ltd., New York © 1991.

Commentary

Neuropathic Pain Syndromes

C. Peter N. Watson

*Irene Eleanor Smythe Pain Clinic, Toronto General Hospital, Toronto, Ontario,
Canada M5G 1L7; and Department of Medicine, University of Toronto,
Toronto, Ontario, Canada M5G 2C4*

As a clinical neurologist with an interest in chronic pain, I have carried out a number of different types of trials in a single center, chiefly in neuropathic pain. This experience I think has led to some improvement in design with each subsequent study. These studies have been done with very limited resources in funding and personnel. If the design is kept simple and effective we can usually incorporate it into the normal flow of clinical practice.

After formulation of the research question I think it is important to consult and work closely with a statistician to determine such matters as sample size, feasibility, exclusion criteria, and outcome measures. One possible danger with innovation is in making the study design excessively cumbersome and expensive, beyond the scope of a single center's resources in terms of manpower and economics. It seems to me that there are distinct advantages to keeping the design as simple as possible, confining a trial to a single center and minimizing the personnel involved there. Large multicenter studies may be required for adequate patient numbers, but have their own problems (1).

I shall assess Max's chapter with regard to those features that are important innovations, those aspects or types of trials that may still be useful because they are cost effective and less labor intensive, and raise the issue of whether some aspects of study design have been superseded and should, in fact, be discarded.

Max has nicely outlined the nature of the problem of neuropathic pain, both the large numbers of sufferers and our appalling ignorance of the natural history, mechanisms, and therapy of many of these disorders. But the phrase "critical to balance treatment groups" (p. 195) could be misinterpreted. This is fine if it refers to the process of stratified randomization; however, it could also be taken to refer to a deterministic balancing scheme not involving randomization. Balancing schemes not involving randomization are prone to bias and should be discouraged. It is also important to realize that small to moderate imbalances in treatment groups can be adjusted for in the subsequent statistical analyses, so perfect balance is not at all critical. The comments below on Max's paper are organized according to the section headings that he used.

PURPOSE OF THE TRIAL: INFLUENCE ON DESIGN CHOICES

With regard to the trial purpose and how this influences the choice of study design, I think it is important to emphasize the last point in this section, that the separation into explanatory and pragmatic is an oversimplification and may be somewhat artificial. This categorization should not discourage the clinician from considering explanatory aspects in the design and analysis of a clinical trial. It seems to me, in fact, that the direction for explanatory trials in some types of neuropathic pain may well evolve from this consideration in pragmatic studies. A crossover trial of all patients with a neuropathic pain for more than 3 months (pragmatic) with a selective noradrenergic agent versus a drug with mixed effect on noradrenaline and serotonin (explanatory) by gradual dose increments reveals relief with one agent in some, with the second drug in others, or relief with both or with neither. These observations may indicate different inhibitory mechanisms (explanatory). We may also for some time have no practical way to subgroup patients with neuropathic pain in explanatory trials and have to proceed in a "pragmatic" manner, taking all comers.

It is not unreasonable to assess completors in a pragmatic trial as a secondary analysis, as long as one is aware of the pitfalls. One of our open label trials (capsaicin in postherpetic neuralgia) had a high dropout rate owing to a side effect (burning) we later found to be fairly easily dealt with (2). The intent to treat analysis was not particularly impressive, whereas the efficacy analysis was closer to the result of a controlled trial that incorporated an approach to dealing with this untoward effect.

A placebo would still seem to be appropriate in a pragmatic trial when no clear standard of therapy or choice of treatment is apparent. I think it is possible to gain the impression that less frequent and careful follow-up may be adequate for a pragmatic trial. Frequent assessments are necessary also in this type of study, particularly with agents having untoward effects, to encourage compliance, deal with these side effects, and prevent dropouts.

With regard to study purpose and data analysis, Max comments that noncompliers are excluded in the analysis of an explanatory trial. As stated later in this commentary, the problem occurs with agents that have differential noncompliance rates. Excluding noncompliers who may be nonresponders may bias the results in favor of an ineffective agent. An effort to exclude noncompliers may be made prior to randomization, not after. Thus, one could use a 1-month trial of a placebo with a chemical tracer. Poor compliers would be excluded then, before the trial starts.

It is fairly well accepted now that the primary analysis in a clinical trial should include all patients on whom follow-up information is available, regardless of compliance status or whether there has been some deviation from protocol. This is because the "intent-to-treat" or "pragmatic" analysis is the only one that is protected by the original randomization. It is reasonable to conduct "explanatory" or "efficacy" analyses in which such patients are excluded, but these analyses should be regarded as strictly secondary. I do agree, however, that one could legitimately take either an explanatory or pragmatic approach to the design of the trial. This decision would affect the nature of the question posed, the characteristics of the patients enrolled, and the rigidity of the treatment protocol. But these are design, not analysis, issues.

WHAT NEEDS TO BE KNOWN ABOUT A NEW DRUG FOR NEUROPATHIC PAIN?

I think a couple of points are worth emphasizing with regard to what needs to be known about a new drug treatment for neuropathic pain. The first is the importance of measuring "effectiveness" in a pragmatic trial, that is, what is the regimen that works best in terms of compliance, side effects, lessening of disability, pain control, and patient satisfaction? A failure to adequately monitor and report some of these outcomes and determine who actually had a "good" response led me into some difficulty with a pharmaceutical company–sponsored trial. Based mainly on pain rating scale change, claims were made for marked clinical effectiveness in most patients. I did not believe this to be so. Because of this experience and articles I have had to review and have seen published, I think it is important that studies be designed and published so that both statisticians and clinicians can evaluate the results.

Pharmaceutical firms are important sources of study funding, particularly in Canada where other research funds are in increasingly short supply. An important issue is the development of guidelines for performing trials backed by the pharmaceutical industry. The industry has an obvious bias in desiring that its products be found effective and safe. It is important then to (a) participate in study design from the outset; (b) negotiate the level of funding at the outset regardless of outcome; (c) insist that the results be published regardless of outcome; and (d) insist on impartial, independent industry-funded analysis of the data (1).

With regard to following the time course of response, open-label, uncontrolled, extended observation may be limited because, although we can hope to choose a fairly stable population with chronic neuropathic pain by defining the duration of pain, for many of these conditions the extended natural history is unknown. For example, many patients with postherpetic neuralgia with a long duration of pain (>12 months) do continue to improve with time (50%); however, some in fact seem to get worse and fail to respond to initially successful treatment (20%)

(*unpublished data*). We need to know the natural history of other neuropathic pain problems and of specific subgroups, so that we can choose a relatively stable population for the duration of the trial.

CHOICE OF PATIENTS

With regard to choice of patients, I would agree that we should look toward subgrouping patients especially for explanatory trials if possible, but it is not practical or possible in some if not most neuropathic pains at present.

The concern about diagnostically uncertain neuropathic pain and broad disease-based groupings is worth reiterating. It would seem more profitable at least with the resources in our setting to choose a more stereotyped, restricted population with a clear-cut course and/or clinical findings implicating nerve injury. It is important to try to determine if adequate numbers of patients will be available over a reasonable time for a trial to be successfully completed. Two of our trials have foundered because of lack of availability and lack of aggressive recruitment. This information might be determined from published epidemiological data or from previous clinic data. It is important to underscore the recruitment ideas suggested in order to generate patients (pp. 200–201). We have found that colleagues and family physicians have short memories in this regard. Our best results have come from paid newspaper advertising, and from solicited columns by medical journalists in daily newspapers and weekly or monthly medical publications. This latter publicity has been gratis, but paid advertising may be incorporated into grant funding applications. If adequate numbers of a particular neuropathic pain problem are not available in one center then a trial involving two or more centers may need to be considered.

OUTCOME MEASURES—PAIN AND PAIN RELIEF

The use of a ratio scale such as the 13-category scale described, administered daily with three weekly phone call reminders and the calculation of a weekly mean, is a very meticulous way of monitoring pain intensity.

We have heard evidence that it is more powerful used daily than when used weekly or than the McGill questionnaire used weekly or a five-point pain relief category scale given at the end of treatment. It may, however, be too costly and labor intensive for some investigators. Even the McGill Pain Questionnaire given weekly is time consuming (5 min) and can be confusing to many chronic neuropathic pain patients, who are elderly, in discomfort, and may be of varied cultural backgrounds. As we have heard, convincing evidence is not available that it is superior to the visual analogue (VAS) or category scales for pain intensity. We do not have the resources to do means of daily ratings and this may be true of other small centers.

The VAS and category scales with personal instruction at weekly intervals remain a useful, simple, and economical, albeit perhaps less sensitive, means of achieving the same result in centers with more limited resources. These scales can easily be incorporated into the normal flow of office practice and can be supervised and scored at the same time and location reducing, the risk of loss of data. I would be interested to learn how the weekly 13-category scale compared with weekly VAS and categorical scales.

The repeated assessment of the sensory examination and sympathetic function is an important issue in both pragmatic and explanatory trials, since increased skin sensitivity (hyperesthesia, dysesthesia, allodynia) is an important aspect of the misery of neuropathic pain. A reduction in allodynia has been shown with desipramine in PHN (3), and VAS rating scale changes indicate a reduction with other antidepressants as well (unpublished data).

It is not inconceivable that areas of sensory impairment may also alter with treatment in either direction (capsaicin, for example, is neurotoxic and it is important to assess the possibility of increasing impairment of small primary afferent function). There is a need for the development of a standardized approach to the objective, quantified measurement of the extent of these areas of sensitized skin and sensory loss and the sensory thresholds to different modalities within the boundaries. The rapid and accurate measurement of signs of sympathetic over- and underactivity is also an important issue.

OUTCOME MEASURES: MOOD AND PAIN

Chronic pain and depression frequently coexist. Antidepressant drugs have been shown to relieve some types of neuropathic pain in some patients, apparently by an action independent of their antidepressant effect (4,5). Future studies will likely involve these or related agents and a reliable and facile measure of the absence or presence and severity of depression is therefore important. A variety of standard rating scales such as the Beck and Zung have been devised for use in a psychiatric population. Because of this, there are questions in these measures related to activity, sleep, fatigue, weight, and sexual activity. These are items that are likely to be affected by chronic pain as well as by depression. Thus a high score may occur leading to a factitious diagnosis of depression. Relief of pain may in a similar fashion lower the score because of these questions, although there may be no real change in mood. The Hamilton rating scale may be modified to 20 questions when those items related to somatic symptoms are removed, but it does take about 30 minutes to administer.

A psychiatric interview before and after treatment would help but it may be impractical for some investigators to coordinate schedules. A visual analogue scale for depression or a 0 to 10 scale are simple measures that can be used and are valid and reliable. The Hospital Anxiety and Depression Scale (6) is a reliable, easily used and scored self-report for the detection and severity of depressed mood that is free of these somatically oriented questions.

OUTCOME MEASURES: INTERFERENCE WITH ACTIVITIES

The comments are well taken regarding the validated disability measures. Guyatt et al. (7) have suggested that quality-of-life instruments that have been developed for the general population (The Sickness Impact Profile, etc.) may not detect clinically important changes in a specific disease. Different chronic pain states may affect different and quite specific aspects of life quality, such as the ability to tolerate clothing contact in postherpetic neuralgia, wear a brassiere with postmastectomy pain, tolerate a prosthesis with phantom or stump pain, or wear shoes with distal painful sensory neuropathies. Guyatt et al. (7) describe a strategy for developing questionnaires to measure disease-specific quality of life. This is based on previous work identifying principles for constructing instruments to measure within-subject change and assumes that such instruments must be based on what a subject feels is important. He provides two models: a "Rolls-Royce" model, requiring the two-stage development of a questionnaire with two patient samples to determine those relevant questions that indicate areas of difficulty that are frequent and important; and the "Volkswagen" model, using existing instruments with expert consultation to decide on the frequent and important items.

OUTCOME MEASURES: ADVERSE EFFECTS

Both the checklist (prespecified) and the record of events (volunteered) approaches are options for evaluating side effects. The former may lead to overreporting of events, but as indicated may be better for comparing two agents in this regard. Studies in neuropathic pain may be too small to pick up rare side effects and combining results in a meta-analysis may do this in the future.

TREATMENTS, CONTROLS, AND PLACEBOS

Although it is true that we do not have a standard of therapy for many neuropathic pains, a potential ethical concern does arise specifically with postherpetic neuralgia. Two controlled trials have shown amitriptyline superior to placebo (4,8), and it would be reasonable to consider this agent as such a standard treatment. The comments regarding problems comparing a new agent with a standard are well expressed. It has been suggested that it is not ethical to use a placebo control when a standard therapy exists [Friedman et al. (9) p. 62; Pocock (10), p. 92]. This seems particularly relevant to a severe pain problem. The skeptical view that both agents are placebo responses may be partially answered by referral to the previous two positive placebo-controlled trails of the standard treatment. If a new drug is not compared to placebo because of ethics, the question of how much of its effect is placebo cannot be answered because the trial will never be done.

Other benefits of an explanatory nature may result from comparing a new, perhaps more specific agent with a standard. For instance, maprotiline (noradrenergic) is effective in relieving postherpetic neuralgia in some patients who do not respond to amitriptyline (mixed noradrenergic and serotonergic) and vice versa, and some patients respond to both or neither. This may help us separate subgroups of these patients.

The use of an active placebo to mimic dry mouth and drowsiness is a clever way to blind for these side effects of antidepressant therapy, and the possible risks of this and the test for blinding have been discussed. The inert placebo is still acceptable in my view, although many patients will report side effects, particularly when elicited with a side effect checklist, so that it is often not clear that the patient is on an active agent. When resources are available an active placebo would seem to be an excellent innovation.

The double-placebo or double-dummy technique may be a useful method when two active drugs cannot be matched satisfactorily, in which case two different placebos can be produced, one for each drug. Patients are then randomized to receive drug A and placebo B or drug B and placebo A. Blinding can then be preserved though at the expense of involving more "pill taking," which might affect compliance. This method is also useful when two different routes of administration are being compared (example: a topical cream versus a tablet, such as topical capsaicin versus amitriptyline).

PARALLEL VERSUS CROSSOVER DESIGNS

The main criteria for considering a crossover have been stated. One may want to add that the agent not have extreme side effects that may result in a high dropout rate, since this has a larger effect in a crossover trial, and that the study be kept reasonably short to encourage compliance and avoid natural history effects for the same reason. The advantages and pitfalls of crossover trials are also well stated. As pointed out, this type of trial is vulnerable to the order effects mentioned. For many types of neuropathic pain, we do not know the natural history. Continued improvements and deterioration may occur at a rate higher than anticipated; for example, a longitudinal study of postherpetic neuralgia reveals that even with pain of long duration (>12 months), 50% of patients improve with time and 25% become more intractable (Watson et al., *unpublished data*).

It may be possible to reduce carryover order effects with a washout period, but the required length of time for "washing out" psychological effects in a placebo-controlled crossover trial is unknown. The problem may also be remedied in part by blinding the subjects not only to the drug but to the crossover point.

This is difficult if escalating doses are used and if the duration of the washout is disease-dependent. Two sorts of crossover rules are commonly used. A change in treatment may occur after a specified length of time ("time dependent") or when indicated by the clinical state of the patient, such as return of pain status to baseline ("disease-state dependent"). The most scientifically acceptable switch points depend on elapsed time. Initiating treatment in response to the appearance of symptoms (pain recurrence with disease dependent washout), makes it difficult to interpret observed treatment effects. Crossover designs will be impractical when a lengthy washout is necessary and where lingering effects from period 1 are present. This is a problem that Max has encountered and that we have found in some patients with a crossover trial of two antidepressants. I suppose one can only hope that enough patients remain in the trial without this problem to make the study useful.

It has been stated that "ultimately the crossover design remains vulnerable to psychologic carryover, and alternate designs should be considered when the measurement of treatment responses relies on subjective reports" (11). Because it is difficult and may be impossible to evaluate treatment differences when the ordering of treatments has an effect, an investigator obtaining a statistically significant sequence effect will not be able to say which treatment is effective. A method of statistical analysis has been prepared by Grizzle (12). This separates the analysis into two phases. The first evaluates the presence of a sequence effect. If this is significant, then analysis based on a crossover model will be biased. Standard practice says that when there is a carryover effect the results from the second period of the crossover must be ignored. Period 2 data are then discarded and analysis of period 1 data is made for treatment differences, using a parallel-groups comparison. This does not offer a complete solution because the sequence effect test is based on a between-subjects comparison that has low statistical power.

It may be difficult to rule out a sequence effect before conducting a trial. Performing a crossover study in the absence of confirmatory evidence on the grounds that it may be a more efficient way to proceed carries the risk of producing biased results. If one is unsure if data collected in a particular clinical context will support the assumption of a crossover analysis, then one should use a simple parallel-groups design.

PARALLEL-GROUPS DESIGN

When the assumptions of a crossover design are in doubt the simpler parallel-groups design is preferred. This requires more subjects but the problems of protocol violation and subject withdrawal are less. The incorporation of a series of baseline measures during a run-in period with placebo or no treatment is a useful measure to increase statistical efficiency, and probably without much time and effort. Doing the run-in on no treatment perhaps removes the concern about eliminating placebo responders. Is a placebo run of several weeks ethical if a comparison is made against a standard of therapy?

Although Max discusses stratification and adaptive randomization in the same paragraph (p. 213), I think it may be misleading to put stratification and adaptive randomization on the same footing as available methods of balancing treatment groups. Stratification is very simple to apply, whereas adaptive randomization is quite complicated operationally, since the probability of allocating a subject to the treatment group varies as the study progresses. Thus adaptive randomization is actually used far less frequently than stratification, mostly because of its cumbersome aspects.

CASE SERIES

The medical literature has a long tradition of reports of series of cases (longitudinal observational studies) that may be prospective as well as retrospective, and valuable information has been obtained in this matter. Having dredged a number of chronic pain conditions retrospectively I can attest to the labor and difficulty involved and the sparseness of useful data acquired. A more profitable approach would seem to prospectively collect the data in an organized fashion (13). This type of study is still useful, particularly in many chronic neuropathic pain problems, for which a search of the literature reveals little or no information about such basic data as demographics, subgroups, pain quality, physical findings, incidence, natural history, and treatment results.

HISTORICAL CONTROLS

Historical control studies are of course no substitute for a randomized control clinical trial. They do, however, in the author's view, continue to have a place in the investigation of new therapies for chronic neuropathic pain. They are quickly done and often a fairly inexpensive means of gaining an impression as to whether a new treatment seems to have an effect and whether the expense and labor of a randomized control trial is warranted. Since all new subjects will get the interventions, the time required to enter a given number of subjects will be approximately halved and the length compared to a crossover study will be similarly reduced. Since no patients receive placebo, there is no ethical question of treating pain with such an agent. Obvious bias enters into this type of trial on the part of subject and observer. It is important to treat a population with stable, chronic neuropathic pain of some duration to guard against the natural history of improvement that occurs, especially early on in such conditions as postherpetic neuralgia. It would be reasonable that a beneficial treatment effect be inferred if significant pain relief occurs in a population with chronic stable pain of more than 6-months duration over the short period of such a trial. Caution should be taken as well to not treat just patients who fail other treatments so that a factitiously negative result is obtained in a selected intractable group. As with a randomized control trial it is important to prepare a protocol beforehand carefully defining the disorder and population to be studied (age, pain duration, exclusion criteria), choosing reliable and valid outcome measures and limiting the study to one or two knowledgeable investigators in a single center with careful monitoring to discourage dropouts.

DETERMINING OPTIMUM DOSAGE

The difficulties with optimum dose determinations are well outlined. It is clear from our experience with antidepressants in neuropathic pain that dose overestimation for the best response is quite common, if one escalates even by small increments (10 to 25 mg) in a study every 3 to 5 days. This is not unexpected given the delay in onset of effect in many patients with this type of agent. This overestimation of dose and blood level associated with pain relief has been evident when after study completion we titrate the dose down in order to reduce side effects and determine the minimum effective analgesic dose and blood level. Less frequent dosage increments pose a problem particularly with crossover trials because they, of course, may make the trial excessively long and cause problems with compliance and dropouts. The range of doses (10 mg to 250 mg) seen in pragmatic trials with patients from the general population with neuropathic pain poses a major problem for planned dose-response studies crossing over different doses in random order, in terms of overdosage and lack of compliance because of side effects. Dose titration in order to achieve maximal analgesia and minimal untoward effects is a delicate business, particularly with antidepressants. One would at least have to stratify patients for age and give a lower range of doses to the older population.

The suggested alternative—ascending titration designs—is attractive, with free titration to maximum response or side effects and then assignment of responders to several treatments randomly of 25 to 100% of the maximum dose. We have been puzzled and disturbed by the frequent failure to recapture initial good responses on retreatment with the same dose. The reason for this is uncertain but it could be a result of the natural history (progression of disease), the placebo effect, tolerance, or some chronic change in receptors related to the drug.

It is also worthwhile considering here the issues of co-intervention and contamination. Co-intervention refers to treatments patients receive that are external to the drugs under study. Thus if a patient on a trial of amitriptyline versus placebo were given a prescription for opiates, this would be a co-intervention. The result is that this would bias treatment assessment. Contamination refers to patients in the control group inadvertently receiving the experimental treatment. Again treatment would be biased. Usually these problems occur because of physicians not related to the study being involved in the management of the patient.

REFERENCES

1. McKhann GM. The trials of clinical trials. *Arch Neurol* 1989;46:611–614.
2. Watson CPN, Evans RJ, Watt VR. Postherpetic neuralgia and topical capsaicin. *Pain* 1988;33: 333–340.
3. Kishore-Kumar R, Max M, Schafer SC, et al. Desipramine relieves postherpetic neuralgia. *Clin Pharmacol Ther* 1990;47:305–312.
4. Watson CPN, Evans RJ, Reed K, Merskey H, Goldsmith L, Warsh J. Amitriptyline versus placebo in postherpetic neuralgia. *Neurology* 1982;32:671–673.
5. Max MB, Culnane M, Schafer SC, et al. Amitriptyline relieves diabetic neuropathy pain in patients with normal or depressed mood. *Neurology* 1987;37:589–596.
6. Zigmond AS, Snaith RP. The hospital anxiety and depression scale. *Acta Psychiatr Scand* 1983;67: 361–370.
7. Guyatt GH, Bombardier C, Tugwell PX. Measuring disease—specific quality of life in clinical trials. *Can Med Assoc J* 1986;134:889–895.
8. Max MB, Schafer SC, Culnane M, et al. Amitriptyline, but not lorazepam, relieves postherpetic neuralgia. *Neurology* 1988;38:1427–1432.
9. Friedman LM, Furberg CD, DeMets DL. *Fundamentals of clinical trials,* 2nd ed. Littleton, Massachusetts: PSG Publishing Company, 1985.
10. Pocock SJ. *Clinical trials, a practical approach.* Chichester, UK: John Wiley & Sons, 1983.
11. Woods JR, Williams JG, Tavel M. The two period crossover design in medical research. *Ann Intern Med* 1989;110:560–566.
12. Grizzle JE. The two-period change-over design and its use in clinical trials. *Biometrics* 1965;21: 167–180.
13. Watson CPN, Evans RJ, Watt VR, Birkett N. Postherpetic neuralgia: 208 cases. *Pain* 1988;35: 289–297.

Advances in Pain Research and Therapy, Vol. 18,
edited by M. Max, R. Portenoy, and E. Laska,
Raven Press, Ltd., New York © 1991.

9

Cancer Pain

General Design Issues

Russell K. Portenoy

*Pain Service, Department of Neurology, Department of Anesthesiology and Critical
Care Medicine, Memorial Sloan-Kettering Cancer Center, New York, New York 10021;
and Department of Neurology, Cornell University Medical College,
New York, New York 10021*

THE DESIGN OF ANALGESIC STUDIES IN CANCER PAIN

Numerous surveys indicate that 30 to 50% of cancer patients undergoing active treatment and 70 to 90% of those with far-advanced disease have pain severe enough to warrant analgesic therapy (1,2). Unrelieved pain is experienced by 40 to 80% of patients treated in the home or routine hospital environment (1), despite the availability in most countries of the means necessary to successfully manage pain in more than three-quarters of these patients (3). Even in the hospice setting, in which symptom control is a major focus of care, over 10% of patients continue to experience unrelieved pain (4). There is, therefore, a compelling need to improve pain management in the cancer population.

Analgesic studies provide a foundation for progress in the treatment of cancer pain. Moreover, the diversity of pain and treatment approaches in the cancer population (2,5) offers a rich opportunity to evaluate virtually any analgesic intervention—from the simplest drug regimen to the most complex neuroablative procedure—in specific subgroups of patients. The diversity of pains and patients, however, is also the greatest obstacle to the realization of this potential. A detailed and sophisticated approach to methodology is prerequisite to successful research in cancer patients.

The Role of Analgesic Study Methodology in Cancer Pain

The application of analgesic study methodology to the cancer population can be evaluated from two distinct perspectives. First, cancer pain can be viewed as a reliable pain model similar to other models of clinical pain used in analgesic trials, such as postoperative pain or dental pain. Studies that use cancer pain in this way are typically focused on the analgesic potential of the treatment (usually a drug), rather than the merits of the approach for cancer pain management; they are usually carefully controlled clinical assays that are conducted over a relatively short time period and primarily assess pain and pain relief. Second, cancer pain can be approached as a unique clinical problem, for which studies are designed to address specific issues in pain management. These studies are often less well controlled, assess a longer timeframe, and may employ outcome measures (e.g., physical function) usually excluded in other analgesic trials.

These two perspectives highlight the potential limitations and advantages inherent in the use of cancer pain in analgesic trials. The methodological difficulties engendered by the heterogeneity of these patients are considerably greater than those encountered in other clinical pain settings. This suggests that studies focused on the analgesic potential of the treatment, rather than its role in cancer pain management specifically, are better undertaken in a different clinical setting unless there is some clear rationale for the use of cancer patients. This rationale may be a high likelihood that the treatment, if proven efficacious, will ultimately find use in the cancer pain population, or the desire to assess the intervention in patients of diverse characteristics who are evaluable in a single setting, thereby minimizing the influence of differences in hospitals or investigators that would otherwise occur if such factors were explored in multiple studies.

In contrast, the cancer pain population is clearly the appropriate model to resolve critical questions that relate to the utility of an intervention in the management of these patients. Most often, the overriding goal of the study conforms to one of three types: (a) evaluation of an intervention (usually a drug) proven efficacious in other pain models but now targeted to the cancer pain population; (b) evaluation of an intervention than is most often used in cancer pain patients, e.g., neurolytic procedures or chronic intraspinal opioid administration; or (c) evaluation of a treatment appropriate to pains that are relatively specific to cancer patients, e.g., bone pain. It should be evident that this perspective views analgesic study methodology in broad terms that extend considerably beyond the single-dose assays that have been the mainstay in the initial evaluation of analgesic drugs (see Chapter 4). An assessment of these methodological issues requires foreknowledge of the important unresolved issues in the clinical management of cancer pain.

Issues in the Pharmacotherapy of Cancer Pain

Three categories of analgesics are used routinely in the treatment of cancer pain: the nonsteroidal antiinflammatory drugs (NSAIDs), opioid analgesics, and adjuvant analgesics. The last category includes a diverse group of drugs, such as specific tricyclic antidepressants, anticonvulsants, corticosteroids, and many others, each of which has other specific indications but may be analgesic in selected circumstances (see Chapter 10).

In recent years, guidelines for the selection and administration of analgesic drugs for the treatment of cancer pain have been described repeatedly (6–10). Most of the elements in these guidelines derive from anecdotal experience, rather than controlled clinical investigation. Application of analgesic study methodology might yield substantial refinements in the pharmacologic understanding and clinical application of all categories of analgesic drugs. Indeed, each category raises a series of specific issues that potentially could be addressed through improved clinical studies.

Nonsteroidal Antiinflammatory Drugs

All NSAIDs (Table 1) are believed to be analgesic (11), although efficacy in cancer pain has been demonstrated for relatively few, among which are aspirin, acetaminophen, ibuprofen, ketoprofen, and flurbiprofen (12–17). Although others do not have established efficacy in these patients, they are commonly used in the treatment of mild to moderate pain (10). The following information, which is accessible through controlled analgesic trials, would be particularly useful in the clinical application of these drugs to the cancer population:

Confirmation that Other NSAIDs are Effective in Cancer Pain. Analgesic studies of specific NSAIDs that may have characteristics favorable in the cancer population would be useful. For example, choline magnesium trisalicylate, a nonacetylated salicylate, has been suggested to be as analgesic and antiinflammatory as aspirin in some conditions (18), but poses minimal risk of hemorrhagic or ulcerogenic complications (19,20). These properties, which would be beneficial

TABLE 1. *Nonsteroidal antiinflammatory drugs*

Chemical class	Generic name
p-aminophenol derivatives	Acetaminophen
Salicylates	Aspirin
	Diflunisal
	Choline Mg trisalicylate
	Salsalate
Proprionic acids	Ibuprofen
	Naproxen
	Naproxen sodium
	Fenoprofen
	Ketoprofen
	Flurbiprofen
Acetic acids	Indomethacin
	Tolmetin
	Sulindac
	Suprofen
	Diclofenac
	Ketorolac
Fenamates	Mefenamic acid
	Meclofenamic acid
Pyrazoles	Phenylbutazone

in medically ill patients who often have bleeding or ulcer diatheses induced by the disease or its treatment, must be confirmed in the cancer pain population.

Relative Efficacy in Cancer Pain Produced by Distinct Mechanisms. Confirmation is needed of the clinical observation that NSAIDs have especial benefit in patients with bone pain and little to no effect in those with neuropathic pain (21,22). The single study that specifically addressed the value of an NSAID, flurbiprofen, in patients with bone pain (13) was not designed to determine either the relative efficacy of this drug in pains of different mechanisms or the relative efficacy of this drug versus other NSAIDs in bone pain.

Relative Efficacy and Side Effect Potential of Different NSAIDs. Guidelines for the selection of NSAIDs in cancer patients are empiric. Comparative studies in the cancer population would provide a more valid basis for drug selection.

Evidence of Analgesia Additive to that Provided by Opioids. Evidence that the analgesia afforded by NSAIDs and opioids is additive has been obtained in some cases, including the combination of morphine with aspirin and methadone with ibuprofen (15,16). Replication with other NSAIDs would confirm that this phenomenon generalizes to other subclasses of these drugs, and determine the range of additive analgesia likely to accrue in different subtypes of cancer pain patients.

Efficacy and Side Effects from Long-Term Administration. Controlled repeated-dose studies of several weeks duration and careful open-label data collection for even longer periods will begin to evaluate the concern that toxicity attributable to NSAIDs may be cumulative in the medically complicated cancer pain patient.

Long-Term Effects of Combinations of NSAIDs and Opioids. The outcome of combined therapy over a long period should be assessed, both in terms of potential additive toxicity and opioid-sparing analgesic effect.

Adjuvant Analgesics

A large number of adjuvant analgesics have been used in the management of cancer pain (see Chapter 10). Relatively few have been evaluated in controlled clinical trials. Examples include studies of calcitonin for bone pain (23), methylphenidate for pain complicated by sedation (24), methylprednisolone (25) and imipramine (26) for pains associated with advanced cancer, and methotrimeprazine for unspecified cancer-related pain (27). These investigations have been very useful in developing guidelines for clinical practice (7,9,28). Many of the most accepted interventions, however, have never undergone rigorous study in the cancer pain population. Some of the specific issues that may be addressed through analgesic trials are as follows:

Evidence of Efficacy and Risk of Adverse Consequences. The risk/benefit ratio remains to be determined for most of the drugs commonly used as adjuvant analgesics.

Effects of Specific Adjuvants Combined with Opioids. The combination of specific adjuvants and opioid drugs needs to be assessed in terms of the potential for additive toxicity and opioid-sparing analgesic effect.

Efficacy of Adjuvants in the Treatment of Symptoms Other Than Pain. Other symptoms, such as lassitude, nausea, sedation, confusion, and constipation, are extremely prevalent in patients with cancer (29). Proven efficacy in one or more of these other symptoms, many of which occur as side effects of opioids or other drugs, would provide an additional indication for administration as an adjuvant in the cancer pain patient.

Opioid Analgesics

Opioid pharmacotherapy (Table 2) is the primary approach to the management of cancer-related pain (6–10). Information that would be particularly valuable to clinicians includes the following:

Relative Efficacy and Side Effect Profiles of Various Opioid Drugs. There have been no studies that systematically compare the various pure agonist drugs (Table 2) in terms of diverse opioid effects under conditions that approximate

TABLE 2. *Opioid analgesics*[a]

Opioids usually administered orally for moderate pain

    Codeine
    Oxycodone
    Hydrocodone
    Propoxyphene
    Meperidine
    Pentazocine

Opioids usually administered for severe pain

Morphine-like agonists

    Morphine
    Oxycodone
    Hydromorphone
    Levorphanol
    Methadone
    Oxymorphone
    Fentanyl
    Heroin

Agonist-antagonists

    Buprenorphine
    Butorphanol
    Nalbuphine
    Pentazocine

[a] See refs. 6, 7, 9, and 30 for discussion of pharmacology and guidelines for use in cancer pain management.

clinical usage. Although clinical experience suggests that the differences between drugs have less importance than intraindividual variability in the response to the various drugs, there have been no controlled trials to evaluate this proposition. Given the variability in the receptor selectivity and pharmacokinetics among these drugs (reviewed in ref. 30), it is entirely possible that drug-specific effects could be identified in controlled studies.

Influence of Patient Characteristics on Opioid Effects. Information of great clinical import could potentially be obtained from controlled studies that evaluated the influence on opioid pharmacokinetics and pharmacodynamics of specific patient characteristics, including demography (particularly age) and pathologic states (e.g., encephalopathy or renal insufficiency).

Influence of Pain Characteristics on Opioid Effects. It is likely that many specific characteristics of the pain, such as its temporal profile and mechanism, alter the likelihood of therapeutic response to the opioids. The most salient of these characteristics is probably pain mechanism. Considerable clinical experience and some rudimentary data from analgesic studies (31) suggest that pains owing to a neuropathic mechanism are relatively less responsive to opioids than other pains. This type of information has great practical relevance and can only be confirmed and quantitated in controlled clinical investigations.

Benefits and Risks of Alternative Routes of Opioid Administration. The clinical use of alternative routes of opioid administration (Table 3) has evolved remarkably in the last decade, propelled by pharmaceutical and technological advances, and by increasing recognition that most pain patients will be unable to tolerate oral dosing at some point during the course of disease (29). Additional modalities, such as transdermal administration, are expected to be available in the near future. Although some efforts have been made to establish efficacy through controlled investigations of several of these approaches, there have been few studies that address the clinical indications for each, the comparative efficacy and side

TABLE 3. *Routes of opioid administration*

Route	Comment
Oral	Preferred in the management of chronic cancer pain
Buccal	No commercial formulation
Sublingual	Buprenorphine available (not in U.S.) and proven efficacious
Intranasal	Intranasal butorphanol now in trials
Rectal	Morphine, hydromorphone and oxymorphone available; limited role in cancer pain
Transdermal	Commercial formulation (using fentanyl) expected soon
Intramuscular	
Subcutaneous	Can be administered as repetitive injection or continuous infusion, either with or without patient-controlled analgesia capability
Intravenous	Same as subcutaneous route
Epidural	Same as subcutaneous route; a variety of distinct methods of access are available
Intrathecal	Usually accomplished using an implanted pump
Intraventricular	

effects of one against another, or the most useful dosing regimen for those proven to be useful. Furthermore, there is a compelling need to obtain relative potency information for novel routes of opioid administration. For example, there are no data on which to base the size of the dose reduction needed during a switch from oral or parenteral dosing to epidural administration. It is apparent that analgesic studies might provide information that could greatly improve the selection and implementation of these alternative routes.

Other Issues Related to Relative Potency. There have been many carefully controlled single-dose studies designed to assess the relative potency of opioid drugs administered orally or intramuscularly (16,32–37; and Chapter 4). Additional relative potency studies are needed to address two important issues. First, the stability of relative potency estimates must be confirmed during repetitive dosing. The relative potency between oral and intramuscular morphine, for example, probably changes with repetitive dosing (38), and a similar phenomenon should be explored with other drugs and routes of administration. Second, there is a need to evaluate the possibility that relative potency among drugs or routes of administration may change systematically with specific patient-related factors (such as age, renal function, or body mass) or pain-related factors (such as mechanism).

Drug Efficacy at Maximally Tolerated Doses. Previous analgesic studies have not been designed to assess the maximal analgesic benefit that can be achieved from a therapy. This consideration is particularly relevant in studies of analgesic drugs. For example, the treatment of very severe pain or pain in a patient already tolerant to opioid effects would be limited with drugs that either possess a ceiling dose for analgesia or reliably demonstrate intolerable side effects with dose escalation. Although this assessment is problematic given the increased risk of toxicity associated with higher doses of analgesic drugs, the information that may be accrued from such studies is highly relevant to the clinical setting.

Comparison of Pharmacologic and Nonpharmacologic Approaches. Little attention has been focused on the methodology needed to evaluate nonpharmacologic methods of pain control in cancer patients. For example, the widely held conclusion that the safety and efficacy of celiac plexus blockade warrants early use in patients with malignant epigastric pain (39) has never been tested in a trial comparing this approach to the expert administration of oral pharmacotherapy or alternative pharmacologic approaches, such as epidural or intrathecal opioid administration. Systematic, long-term comparison of favorable and adverse effects would provide a scientific foundation for these and many other important clinical decisions that are presently resolved on empirical grounds alone.

Issues Related to Pain Mechanisms and Basic Pharmacology

In addition to the many therapeutic issues that may be addressed through the application of analgesic study methodology, these investigations offer opportunities for improved understanding of the basic mechanisms involved in clinical pain and the pharmacology of opioid drugs.

Pathogenesis of Pain

Analgesic studies in subgroups of cancer patients may provide a means to evaluate the underlying mechanisms of clinical pain. For example, there is suggestive evidence, derived from animal models, that specific pain mechanisms (e.g., visceral vs. somatic) may somehow involve the various opioid receptor subtypes in different ways (40). If confirmed, it may become possible to link the effects of various receptor-selective drugs to pain mechanisms in man. Similarly, studies may be able to confirm that the response to adjuvant analgesics with known modes of action may be an indication of specific mechanisms sustaining the pain. If enough evidence can be adduced from basic and clinical research to support the validity of these constructs, many such research applications can be envisioned.

Physiology of Endogenous Pain Modulating Systems

Analgesic studies may also be able to elucidate the physiology of endogenous pain modulating systems. For example, the constellation of effects mediated by specific opioid receptors may be illuminated by careful monitoring of analgesia and other effects in controlled clinical investigations of opioids with different receptor selectivities (41). Similarly, the function of specific opioid receptor systems at different levels of the neuraxis may be clarified by studies assessing the relative effects of receptor-selective opioids administered intraspinally (42). Changes in receptor function following exposure to opioid drugs, at least as it is reflected in the development of tolerance to various opioid effects, can likewise be investigated in studies employing repetitive dosing or sequential single-dose comparisons. The latter methodology has already been used to demonstrate that cross-tolerance between two opioid drugs is incomplete (16), and future studies may be able to further address the dynamics of tolerance, both as it relates to different drugs and various opioid effects. Finally, nonopioid, receptor-selective drugs can be used to determine the role of nonendorphinergic pathways in endogenous pain modulation; this process has already been undertaken with various serotonin (43) and adrenergic (44) receptor agonists.

APPROACH TO ANALGESIC STUDIES IN CANCER PAIN

Whether cancer pain is used as a pain model to scrutinize properties of a drug or is considered the clinical problem under investigation, the methodology employed must consider the specific needs and characteristics of the cancer patient.

Cancer pain is a multidimensional experience (45) that can be influenced by a large number of patient-related, pain-related, and disease-related factors (Table 4). The heterogeneity of these patients, particularly those with chronic cancer-related pain, distinguish them from others commonly recruited for analgesic studies. This heterogeneity must be addressed at every stage of the study, from selection of the study sample and design through the final analysis of the data.

Selecting the Study Sample

The study sample is first defined by inclusion and exclusion criteria that identify acceptable candidates for the study. For example, the investigator may decide to exclude patients of advanced age or those with abnormalities of hepatic or renal function. These selection criteria have important implications for the rapidity and quality of data collection. The potential benefits of numerous selection

TABLE 4. *Factors that contribute to the heterogeneity of the cancer pain population*

Pain-related factors	Pain characteristics
	Intensity and duration of chronic pain
	Pain intensity at study onset
	Quality
	Temporal pattern
	Precipitants
	Pain mechanisms
	Prior therapy
	Duration and extent of prior analgesic use
	Efficacy of previous analgesics
	Prior adverse effects from analgesics
Patient-related factors	Demographics
	Psychological factors
	Affective disorder
	Other psychiatric disorders
	Behavioral disturbances
	Cognitions, expectations, and fears
	Inteiiectual capacity
	Degree of placebo response
	Other historical factors
	History of chronic pain
	History of substance abuse
	History of psychiatric disorder
Disease-related factors	Related to neoplasm
	Type of tumor
	Extent of disease
	Previous antineoplastic therapy
	Ongoing antineoplastic therapy
	Other pathological processes
	Major organ dysfunction
	Number and severity of other symptoms
	Other treatments
	Concurrent use of centrally acting drugs
	Use of drugs that may be co-analgesic

criteria, such as improved reliability and a more homogeneous sample, must be balanced against the risk that patient accrual will be unduly slowed or that selection biases will be introduced that may invalidate the results or limit their generalizability. For example, exclusion of cancer patients with advanced age from a study of a new analgesic performed at a single community hospital may both markedly delay its completion and limit the clinical relevance of efficacy and safety data. The resolution of these issues depends largely on the intervention under study, and must be decided on a case by case basis.

Stratification on the basis of selected variables is advisable if it is likely that a factor will strongly influence the primary outcomes of the study, or if one of the primary study objectives is the assessment of the effect of the variable on treatment outcome. The need to stratify must be carefully balanced against the added complexity it may produce. In many cases, the use of post hoc adjustment using covariate analyses or other techniques can obviate the need for both stratification and stricter selection criteria (46). Post hoc analyses can assess the influence of independent variables on the outcome measures, and allow the investigator to evaluate the effect of combinations of these variables. These potential advantages cannot be realized, however, if the variables in question occur infrequently or distribute unevenly among study groups. Should the investigator perceive that it is critical for the success of the study to control for a factor, either because of a desire to understand it or the need to limit its impact, then such control should be implemented during data collection through the use of selection criteria or stratification procedures.

Careful records of the recruitment process must be maintained to ensure the appropriate application of selection criteria and provide the means to evaluate the possibility of selection bias through specific post hoc analyses. These records should include information about those patients who are screened and are found to be ineligible, those who are eligible but refuse to participate in the study, and those who are eligible and agree to participate. The first two groups, the "pretrial dropouts" (47), can comprise an extremely large proportion of the patients who are initially screened, and must be considered both in predicting the number of patients needed to achieve the appropriate sample size and in the interpretation of the data following the study (48). The information for all these groups should include, at the least, demographics, tumor-related data, and the findings on all the specific selection criteria elaborated for the study (e.g., renal function). The simplest method of record keeping involves the development of a worksheet in which appropriate information is requested and the screening procedures are outlined as a series of "yes-no" questions.

Important Factors in Patient Selection

Numerous factors that contribute to the heterogeneity of cancer pain patients may influence the outcome of analgesic studies (Table 4). These factors must be considered for selection criteria or stratification prior to the study, or for post hoc covariate analyses after data collection.

Factors Related to the Pain

Clinical experience strongly suggests that specific characteristics of cancer pain may influence the outcome of therapy. These features must be considered to be potentially important covariates in analgesic studies. Among the most important are pain mechanisms, temporal characteristics, baseline pain intensity, and prior opioid intake.

Stratification by pain mechanism, or covariate analyses using this factor, may help discern analgesic effects of specific interventions or determine the utility of various treatments in selected types of pain. The vast majority of cancer pains have some identifiable organic correlate, either nociceptive (related to ongoing activation of pain-sensitive primary afferent neurons) or neuropathic (related to an injury of neural tissue). Nociceptive pain, in turn, can be somatic or visceral. The operational definitions for these pain mechanisms are empirical, and should be stated clearly at the start of any analgesic trial that intends to assess this characteristic. For the purposes of these studies, definitions can be proposed as follows: *Somatic* pain is aching or throbbing, usually well localized, and attributable to a lesion in a somatic structure; if this structure is bone, the patient conforms to the category of bone pain. *Visceral* pain, which is a dull aching or cramping associated with a lesion in the viscera, can be further divided into the relatively better localized and usually aching pain associated with involvement of organ capsules and the poorly localized, usually intermittent cramping pain associated with obstruction of hollow viscera; these two subtypes should be distinguished in analgesic studies. *Neuropathic* pain is an unfamiliar, usually burning or stabbing pain associated with evidence of an appropriate injury to the peripheral or central nervous system.

The most salient temporal characteristic in analgesic studies is the existence of intermittent transient pains, such as those that may occur with movement. The analgesic efficacy of any therapeutic modality may be difficult to assess when these pains are frequent and severe. Single-dose drug trials typically minimize this problem by maintaining the patient in one comfortable position for the duration of the study. This does not eliminate the problem posed by studies with prolonged observation times or patients with spontaneous transient pains, such as those that may accompany nerve lesions. If transient pains are anticipated to be prevalent in the study population, their presence should at least be recorded. In some studies, it may be reasonable for the investigator to exclude patients in whom they are particularly prominent. Occasionally, it may be useful to consider quantitating the frequency and intensity of these pains as an additional outcome measure; for example, movement-related pain is such a common feature of bone pain that studies of new drugs for this syndrome should attempt to specifically evaluate treatment effects on these intermittent pains.

Baseline pain intensity must be recorded, since the ability of the study to distinguish the effects of different treatments may depend on the range of pain severities included in the study sample. For example, it is evident that a study performed in patients with relatively mild pain may be incapable of distinguishing among two or more interventions if all yield virtually complete analgesia during the study (see Chapter 4).

It is also essential to record the consumption of analgesic drugs prior to the study, including type and dose of drug, duration of treatment, and time of last dose. Preliminary data suggest that patients who have already achieved a high dose of opioid may be less likely to obtain analgesia from subsequent clinical interventions (49). The need for high doses of opioids may therefore indicate that the patient is less likely to discriminate analgesic effects from the intervention under study. Further research is needed to determine the validity of this proposition, but for the present, prior opioid exposure should be evaluated as a potentially important covariate in all analgesic trials, even those that do not evaluate drugs.

Prior opioid exposure is a particular concern in studies of opioid drugs. For example, both time since the last dose of the regularly scheduled opioid and the extent of prior opioid exposure have been demonstrated to have significant effects on the analgesia produced by single doses of opioids (50). It is likely that the results of repeated-dose studies would also be greatly influenced by previous opioid use. These effects may operate, at least in part, through the influence of tolerance (33). Although this is not a problem in studies that ignore pharmacodynamics (e.g., pharmacokinetic studies) or those that employ dosing to effect, variation in the degree of tolerance can greatly reduce the sensitivity of studies that assess opioid effects by increasing the variability in the observed response to the test doses of the drug. In some studies, this problem is best managed through the use of appropriate selection criteria. Specifically, the degree of tolerance in the study sample can be limited by selecting only those patients with a history of less than some agreed-upon level of opioid consumption (e.g., that equivalent to 30 mg intramuscular morphine per day for less than 1 week). Alternatively, a higher ceiling of prior opioid exposure can be chosen, and patients can be stratified by previous drug intake. In all these calculations, standard relative potency tables are used to estimate morphine equivalent milligrams (51).

Selection of patients with variable degrees of tolerance for clinical trials of opioid drugs can also be managed by flexibility in the test doses used during the study. Assuming that the relative potency of the test drug is known (compared to the opioid that the patients was taking prior to the study), doses of the study drug can be determined as a proportion of the patient's prior opioid exposure, rather than as a fixed milligram amount. For example, the test dose can be set as that equivalent to one-sixth the mean total daily opioid consumption in morphine equivalent milligrams during the 1 week prior to the study. The validity of this approach remains to be determined empirically. At the present time, the problem of prior opioid consumption should be managed on a study by study basis through the use of selection criteria, stratification, post hoc analyses, or flexible dosing.

The time since last opioid dose is a major consideration in single-dose studies of analgesic drugs, and may influence both patient selection and outcomes. Although a prolonged period following the last dose of the regularly scheduled analgesic, such as 6 to 8 hrs, would be valuable to avoid carryover effects and increase the likelihood that a large proportion of patients will be experiencing severe pain when the test drug is administered (thereby increasing the sensitivity of the assay; see Chapter 4), the investigator has the ethical obligation to prevent unnecessary suffering on the part of the patient. Moreover, it is likely that this approach will increase the proportion of pretrial dropouts, thereby prolonging the study and potentially reducing its generalizability. The investigator must develop criteria for the timing of drug administration that balances these concerns. It is usually best to incorporate both a time-since-last-dose criterion (e.g., at least 1 hr) and a pain criterion (e.g., at least moderate pain) in this process.

Factors Related to the Patient

A large number of patient characteristics (Table 4) must also be considered in the selection of appropriate candidates for study (16,33,34). Some are obvious, such as the exclusion of patients with a psychiatric disorder severe enough to compromise data collection. Other considerations are more subtle, however, and require greater flexibility. For example, the decision to recruit patients with specific tumor types depends on the question under study and the particular population available; studies of bone pain, for instance, may be most expeditiously performed by limiting patient recruitment to those with prostate, breast, and lung cancer.

Factors Related to the Disease

The types and severity of concurrent pathologic conditions must also be considered in patient selection for analgesic studies. Major organ failure, including pulmonary or renal insufficiency, cardiac or liver disease, or encephalopathy, may increase the risks to the patient of participation in the study, potentially undermine data collection, or bias against the perception of treatment acceptability even if analgesic effects are not obscured. It is important to recognize that all these disturbances occur on a continuum, which on one end comprise subclinical abnormalities, and on the other, severe clinical problems that obviously contraindicate participation in an analgesic study. At some point along this continuum is a degree of clinical dysfunction that so increases the likelihood of adverse effects or uninterpretable data that exclusion of the patient is warranted. Although it is sometimes worthwhile to define these exclusionary criteria precisely (e.g., calcium above 12 mg/dl), it must be recognized that successful recruitment necessarily relies on the clinical judgment of the investigator who screens patients for study. This is an inevitable source of variability, and a possible source of bias, which is reduced, but not eliminated, by careful randomization procedures.

The presence of acute or chronic encephalopathy (delirium or dementia, respectively) is particularly important in patient selection, since it may compromise the patient's ability to discriminate effects and is highly prevalent, multidetermined, and often subtle in those with cancer (52). Patient recruitment staff must become skillful in both screening cognitive function and determining the degree of impairment incompatible with the assessment of subjective effects like pain.

Selecting and Assessing the Important Variables

Although the most salient data derived from any analgesic study relates to pain and side effects, multiple facets of these outcomes can be assessed and a variety of other variables can also be evaluated. Accordingly, it is essential that the investigator select the independent and dependent variables of interest prior to the study, and define clearly the parameters of each that will be recorded.

The selection of variables to assess in an analgesic trial must resolve two competing interests: (a) the desire to collect information about patient experience that is as comprehensive and as detailed as possible, and (b) the need to maintain a high degree of clinical and statistical reliability and validity through the use of a limited number of simple measures that are easily completed by the patient. The resolution of these interests is guided by the overall goals of the study, as detailed below:

Assessment of Analgesic Efficacy

Pain measurement has been an active area of research for decades, and various reviews have clarified the most important clinical, methodological, and statistical advances (53–59). Several considerations are particularly relevant for studies in the cancer population.

Self-report as the "Gold Standard"

Despite the availability of physiological and behavioral measures, self-report is the accepted method of pain assessment in cancer pain. Although it may be necessary to consider alternatives (e.g., behavioral measures) in specific settings, most notably the evaluation of pain in very young children (60), self-report measures are feasible for the great majority of investigations. Similar to analgesic studies in other clinical settings, the measurement of pain in cancer patients has typically employed verbal descriptor scales (e.g., "none," "mild," "moderate," and "severe"), numerical scales (e.g., 0 to 10), or a visual analogue scale for pain (see Max and Laska, Chapter 4). Although some studies indicate that the visual analogue scale is most sensitive (57,58), others indicate only minimal differences in sensitivity between this type of measure and verbal descriptor scales (61). Other studies suggest that the change in pain intensity described by adjacent words on a verbal scale is not constant from one end of the scale to the other (58,62). Given these uncertainties and the ease of administration of both verbal rating scales and visual analogue scales, it is reasonable to use both types of measures in studies of cancer pain.

Clinical pain is a multidimensional experience that comprises both a sensory component and an affective response. Studies have demonstrated that patients can distinguish the sensory experience and unpleasantness of pain through the use of different verbal descriptor or visual analogue scales (63,64), and many surveys indicate the potential utility of multidimensional pain scales, such as the McGill Pain Questionnaire, in the assessment of patients with different types of pain (65). It should therefore be recognized that self-report pain severity measures that provide a single value actually reflect more than the sensory experience of pain alone (66), and that the use of multidimensional scales may be able to capture additional useful information about the pain. There is very little experience in the use of multidimensional pain assessment in cancer pain studies, and indeed, it may not be feasible to employ such instruments in studies (such as single-dose drug trials) that require frequent measurements. Future investigations that have relatively long observation periods (e.g., repeated-dose drug trials) should consider the use of these instruments.

Pain Relief Scale

Some patients appear more able to discriminate pain relief than change in pain intensity following an analgesic intervention. Pain relief measures, which may be categorical ("no relief," "slight," "moderate," "a lot," "complete") or numeric (percent of pain relief), or may employ a visual analogue format, are widely accepted as an important element in analgesic trials (61; and Chapter 4). More importantly, perceived pain relief may reflect a different aspect of experience than pain intensity. In cancer patients, for example, a pain relief visual analogue scale correlated more highly with mood than a pain intensity scale (67). Thus, the information provided by pain intensity and pain relief scales is not redundant, and it is reasonable to suggest that all analgesic trials in cancer pain should employ both.

Although a report of pain relief is likely to provide information, it must be emphasized that the interpretation of the relief measure may be problematic in studies other than the single-dose trials in which it was originally applied. In the latter studies, patients were asked to judge the degree of relief experienced at a particular moment, using a test dose administered minutes or hours before as the reference point for this determination. This task is clear and provides data with high face validity. In contrast, pain relief measurement in other types of studies, such as repeated-dose drug trials or trials of alternative routes of opioid administration, may reflect a more global experience, the precise components of which remain to be determined. Future investigations that employ global pain relief measures should try to characterize the factors that may contribute to this response.

Analgesic Use

As noted previously, it is extremely important to record the extent and duration of analgesic drug intake prior to the study. Equally important is the use of analgesic drugs during the study. Single-dose drug trials, whether in the cancer population or other clinical settings, typically obviate this consideration by proscribing the use of other drugs during the study period; indeed, the time to needed remediation is an important dependent variable in these designs. This approach can be implemented as well in studies of other analgesic modalities that assess a relatively brief period following the intervention, such as a trial of different local anesthetics in peripheral neural blockade.

Analgesic manipulation during the study cannot be avoided, and may become a critical source of variability, in studies that assess a longer timeframe, including repeated dose studies of analgesic drugs, and studies of nonpharmacological interventions that require longer than a few hours for data collection. In these situations, it is ethically necessary to prevent prolonged unrelieved pain by providing access to analgesic drugs, and consequently, a means must be developed to do so within the experimental exigencies of the study.

The most reasonable approach to the management of analgesic dosing during these studies employs a so-called "rescue" dose, the need for which can be used as an ancillary measure of analgesic efficacy (68–70). In this technique, patients are provided an opioid on an "as needed" basis (usually every 2 or 3 hrs) during the study period, either alone or in combination with a regularly scheduled analgesic regimen. If the latter is used, the patient's previous drug can be employed, but variability will be diminished if all patients are switched to a standard drug. Similarly, all patients should be given the same drug for the "rescue dose," if possible.

The dose of the regularly scheduled regimen should be set low enough to ensure that the patient's response to the intervention can be measured. A guiding principle in these studies, which has yet to be fully validated, is that the analgesic efficacy of the test treatment can be determined as *either* a reduction of pain or the need for fewer "rescue doses." Interestingly, studies of this type do not indicate that patients use the "rescue dose" to achieve a pain-free state (68); pain can therefore still be used as a valid dependent measure.

Thus, the baseline dose of analgesic administered during the study should be selected so that the patient who receives the study intervention either has an average pain intensity of moderate or greater (by personal choice, since access to "rescue doses" is provided), or, more likely, has mild pain but requires at least several "rescue doses" per day. It is therefore necessary to begin this type of study with a period during which the baseline dose can be adjusted until some preselected criteria are met. For example, the initial baseline dose can be set as that equivalent to one-third or one-half the total daily dose on the preceding day (or average daily dose during the preceding several days, if known), which can then be increased on a daily basis (e.g., by 50% per day) until average daily pain is moderate or greater and the patient desires no further "rescue doses" or average daily pain is less than moderate and between two and six "rescue doses" are consumed per day. Patients who fail to achieve this criterion within some pre-determined period, e.g., 5 days, are dropped from the study. Patients who do reach this criterion are given a 1- to 2-day period prior to administration of the study intervention, during which baseline data is collected. This dosing regimen is then maintained throughout the study.

A major problem with this approach is the management of patients with vary-ing degrees of prior opioid intake, whose opioid tolerance presumably varies, and hence, would have unpredictable effects from a standard "rescue dose." A "rescue dose" could only be considered a valid dependent measure of analgesic efficacy if it produced approximately the same proportionate effect in all patients under study, or there was sufficient balance among study groups that the vari-ability in these effects would not influence the outcome. As discussed previously, this problem can be managed either by implementing selection criteria that restrict the prior opioid exposure to some range, in which case all patients can have identical "rescue doses," or by adjusting the size of the "rescue dose" to be some proportion of the baseline opioid dose (e.g., 10% of the total daily opioid intake during the previous 24 hrs).

The quantitation of opioid consumption as a dependent measure of analgesic efficacy can also be accomplished with patient-controlled analgesia devices. In these designs (see Chapter 22), parenteral self-administration of small boluses of an opioid at frequent intervals using a programmable pump can provide several types of dependent measures, including total opioid consumed during the study period, number of bolus doses administered, and number of times the device is activated (whether or not drug is delivered). Further research is needed to validate the use of patient-controlled analgesia or "rescue doses" in analgesic research, but both approaches appear promising.

Assessment of Pain Characteristics Other Than Intensity

Pain has many characteristics other than severity, some of which are amenable to systematic quantitation during analgesic studies. For example, pain location and extent can be determined with a pain drawing, which can be scored with a template and compared across study conditions (71,72). Pain quality (e.g., burning, stabbing, aching, etc.) can be tabulated. The frequency of specific types of pain, such as paroxysmal lancinating pains or pains with certain activities (e.g., eating or standing) can be similarly recorded. At the present time, these aspects of pain are not routinely assessed during analgesic trials, and the importance of the information they could provide in cancer pain studies remains to be determined.

Assessment of Adverse Events

The importance of adverse events in the evaluation of new drugs has long been recognized (73), and numerous checklists for these effects have been devised (74). The more extensive of these (75,76) assess a variety of characteristics for each adverse symptom or sign that occurs following administration of the study drug, including severity, relationship to the drug, temporal characteristics (timing after a dose, duration, and pattern during the day), contributing factors, course, and action taken to counteract the effect. Symptoms can be listed *a priori* to ensure uniform terminology or can be recorded as they are reported by the patient or observed by the investigator. Each characteristic can be quantitated with scales of varying complexity. For example, the likelihood of a relationship between the adverse event and the study drug in clinical drug trials has been recorded on a categorical scale ("none," "remote," "possible," "probable," "definite"), according to the presence or absence of specific features (73); these may include a reasonable temporal relationship, foreknowledge that such an event may occur with the specific drug, improvement following discontinuation of the drug, and reappearance of the effect following repeated exposure.

The detailed assessment of adverse events can add considerably to the time and effort required for the evaluation of the study intervention. The degree to which the various characteristics are pursued should be determined by the overall goals of the study. The evaluation of a new type of analgesic drug, for example, may warrant this effort, whereas such detail may be appropriately neglected in lieu of other assessments in studies of accepted opioids, for which the side effect spectrum is well appreciated. Previous studies of opioid drugs in cancer pain patients have merely tabulated reported side effects (spontaneous or elicited), with or without some effort to categorize severity as mild, moderate, or severe (16). Occasionally, visual analogue scales have been used to achieve a more precise determination of a particular side effect, such as sedation (77). The investigator must carefully consider the type of data desired about adverse events and the impact that this assessment would have on attrition rates and the ability to assess other effects. In the absence of brief, validated assessment tools for adverse drug effects in the cancer population, or any tools designed to assess adverse consequences of nonpharmacologic analgesic interventions (e.g., nerve blocks), the investigator will need to fashion checklists or other types of report forms for each study, with the specific queries determined by the needs of the investigation.

Assessment of Associated Symptoms

Cancer patients experience a large number of symptoms other than pain (29,78). Evaluation of some of these symptoms can be used to clarify the clinical status of the study population, and thereby define the degree of generalizability of the results or judge the effect of the study intervention. Unfortunately, assessment tools for even the common symptoms, such as fatigue and nausea, have not been validated in analgesic studies. Although categorical, numerical, or visual analogue scales for virtually any symptom can be fashioned by the investigator and have high face validity, the tentative nature of such data must be recognized.

Assessment of Function

In clinical practice, the efficacy of an analgesic regimen is judged in part by evidence of improved patient function. Defined broadly, function encompasses psychological integrity (e.g., improved coping and mood), sociability, and physical activity. All these elements relate to the overall perception of quality of life, and quantitation of selected outcomes in each of these areas could provide very valuable information directly relevant to patient care.

Efforts to evaluate psychological function as an outcome in cancer pain studies have been limited to several measures of mood or specific affective disturbances that have been administered in single-dose studies (79). In this context, these measures reflect acute, treatment-related mood changes, which may or may not indicate long-term effects. Such effects may be better indicated by the use of these scales as global measures during studies with longer observation periods. A simple mood visual analogue scale has been found to correlate highly with a variety of psychometric instruments (67) and can be easily administered repeatedly during such studies. A questionnaire consisting of 15 contrasting word or phrase pairs (80) has also been used to assess mood in single-dose studies (79), but the degree to which this type of measure adds substantive information to the more simple analogue scale remains unclear. Other studies have attempted to assess various aspects of mood, using visual analogue scales for anxiety and depression (81,82) or formal depression inventories. The Hamilton Depression Inventory, for example, was used in a repeated-dose study of an adjuvant analgesic, methylprednisolone (83). All of these instruments are more cumbersome than a mood visual analogue scale, but each can provide additional information if successfully administered. The selection of psychometric measures must balance the burden to the patient with the desire to obtain detailed information about psychological functioning.

In addition to measures that assess mood, numerous validated instruments are available for the assessment of other diverse aspects of psychological and social functioning in cancer patients (84). Administered during analgesic trials, these scales can yield interesting information about personality traits, coping ability, health-related perceptions, cognitive style, social interactions, perceived social resources, or other characteristics (84). Again, the investigator must continually balance the desire for more data with the capacity of cancer patients, who are medically ill and often psychologically distressed, to reliably complete the instruments selected. Furthermore, studies are needed to determine if such information predicts the effects of the intervention in clinical usage.

Simple indicators of physical activity are also available, but like other measures, have seldom been used in analgesic studies. Validated measures of performance status exist, such as the Karnofsky Performance Status scale (85), or a simple categorical or visual analogue scale of perceived general activity can be devised. Related data that can be recorded easily by the patient in a diary include number of hours in bed, in chair, or walking, or hours engaged in activities of daily living, recreation, or work.

Finally, studies with longer observation periods may be amenable to a formal evaluation of quality of life. Although the ideal measure has not yet been developed, abundant research during the past two decades has yielded a large number of validated instruments that provide a multidimensional assessment (86–88). These have been successfully employed in clinical trials of antineoplastic agents, but with rare exceptions have not been adapted to analgesic trials (89). Such a measure may be useful in predicting the clinical acceptability of an analgesic intervention.

Acceptability of Treatment

A global determination of treatment acceptability, performed at the end of an analgesic study, may also provide a useful indication of the potential clinical utility of an intervention. In crossover trials, this may be accomplished by a question comparing one intervention against another ("Did you prefer treatment A or treatment B?"). All studies can incorporate a query about the future use of a treatment ("Would you be willing to continue treatment with this intervention?").

Assessment of Plasma Drug Levels

An understanding of pharmacokinetics is critically important in the management of analgesic drugs. Rational decisions about drug selection, route of administration, and dosing depend on knowledge of bioavailability, elimination half-life, metabolic pathways, and other factors. These data are collected early in the evaluation of new analgesic drugs (see Inturrisi, Chapter 24).

Clinical application of pharmacokinetic data, however, must recognize that the values obtained in Phase I and Phase II studies reflect population averages that may or may not be apropos to the individual patient. Indeed, the populations that often provide these pharmacokinetic data, e.g., healthy young volunteers, may be markedly different than the older, medically ill cancer patient who is ultimately a candidate for the drug. For example, the pharmacokinetics of opioid analgesics change in the elderly (90), and the failure to consider age in clinical judgments derived from pharmacokinetic data (e.g., size of loading dose, dosing interval, etc.) may yield unanticipated toxicity.

The remarkable interindividual variability in the response to an analgesic drug commonly observed in the clinical setting is at least partly attributable to this variation in pharmacokinetics. This suggests that measurement of plasma drug levels during drug trials may provide a critical covariate in the assessment of analgesic effects. Covariate analyses incorporating plasma levels may enhance the reliability of the effect data and increase the likelihood that group differences will be discerned. In studies that employ a route of administration other than the intravenous route, measurement of plasma drug levels also provides an indication of the rate and completeness of systemic absorption. Finally, measurement of plasma drug levels during repeated-dose drug trials can both ensure compliance with the analgesic regimen and determine effects at specific steady-state levels.

This type of information can be acquired through repeated sampling of blood at defined intervals after the dose in single-dose studies or sampling of several "trough levels" (at the end of a dosing interval) in repeated-dose studies. More sophisticated analyses are also possible. For example, modeling of the relationships between pharmacokinetic factors and effects has been accomplished through concurrent monitoring of plasma concentration and both analgesia and sedation during a intravenous infusion of methadone (77).

Selecting a Design

The selection of a design for analgesic studies in the cancer pain population must balance the desire for rigorous experimental control, which increases confidence in the reliability, validity, and generalizability of the results, with the need to ensure the feasibility of the trial and protect the interests of the patients who participate. To a large extent, this process is mediated by the predetermined goals of the study. For example, it may be appropriate to choose an open trial as the initial clinical evaluation of a new intervention that has no proven benefit, whereas no less than a randomized, double-blinded investigation using multiple control groups may suffice to determine therapeutic equivalence between two widely accepted analgesic interventions. Given the limited resources available for research, it is no more correct to undertake a large and expensive clinical trial in the first case than it would be to plan an open survey in the second.

The selection of a study methodology also clearly depends upon the specific intervention under study and both the patients and environment available for the investigation. For example, many fundamental aspects of experimental control are impractical or impossible in studies of many modalities employed commonly in cancer pain management, including invasive modalities of drug administration (e.g., intraspinal opioids), neurostimulation techniques (e.g., transcutaneous electrical nerve stimulation), neuroablative procedures (e.g., cordotomy or neurolytic nerve blocks), and psychological approaches (e.g., relaxation training).

Given these considerations, the investigator must be aware of the advantages and disadvantages of the many methodological options in studies of cancer pain. Some of the relevant properties of these designs can be summarized as follows:

Surveys of Current Practice

Although surveys of patients who have received or will be administered an available analgesic intervention cannot yield a rigorous determination of analgesic efficacy, they can provide insights into the variety and nature of the effects produced, and can be particularly useful in clarifying the range and prevalence of adverse responses to the intervention. Surveys also facilitate the development of hypotheses and help determine the methodology for future studies. This may be especially useful in the heterogeneous cancer population, wherein surveys can highlight the major sources of variability in the response to an intervention. If an approach has already achieved clinical acceptance, a survey can also help evolve clinically relevant guidelines for improving its implementation.

Although retrospective surveys are far more easily and rapidly performed than prospective surveys, they are more subject to bias, particularly when evaluating a subjective experience like pain. The use of supporting ancillary data, such as analgesic use, is helpful in these cases, but does not alter the much greater credibility of prospective data collection.

In all surveys, every effort should be made to limit bias. The survey should include all evaluable patients who undergo the intervention during a defined time period. This cannot eliminate bias inherent in the practices of the particular institution, or the variability that results from differences in clinical management across practitioners, but will limit systematic bias that could be introduced by restriction of the study sample to patients treated by selected services or physicians. Although aggressive case finding may increase the time required to complete a retrospective survey (as medical records are located), or necessitate the use of a telephone interview and mail contact during a prospective survey, the potential reduction of bias justifies these efforts. In prospective surveys, one source of bias can be assessed by recording the number and characteristics of "pretrial dropouts," patients who refuse the intervention under study, and comparing these patients to those successfully evaluated. Finally, if more than one investigator collects data, all should have uniform training and interrater reliability should be assessed.

The analysis and interpretation of survey data are enhanced by comparison with information acquired from patients who can act as a partial control for those who are administered the intervention in question. In retrospective surveys, this reaches its highest level in the well-conducted case-control comparison, in which there is careful matching of patients in an effort to isolate specific effects. Although the latter approach has not been applied in studies of analgesic interventions, many retrospective surveys have used statistical techniques to make similar comparisons. For example, a survey of nonsteroidal antiinflammatory drugs identified a differential effect of these agents on pains of various mechanisms (22). Prospective surveys of current practice can also include patients who can provide comparative data.

Open Trials

More reliable data can be obtained from open trials, in which an investigator prospectively administers an analgesic intervention to a sample of patients and carefully surveys effects. The best appreciated approach is the open-label drug trial. In the cancer population, open trials have provided useful information about many diverse interventions, ranging from oral morphine therapy to neuroablative procedures (91,92). The potential for selection bias and observer bias in this type of study is apparent, and similar to other surveys, the data obtained are best used to draw tentative inferences about analgesic efficacy, determine the issues that require further evaluation and the methods that may be best to address them, and provide baseline information about the type and prevalence of adverse consequences.

The potential utility of an open trial depends on the extent, uniformity, and reliability of data collection and the success of efforts to limit bias. Detailed information about analgesic effects, changes in associated symptoms, and adverse consequences should be collected from every patient. Uniformity in data collection is enhanced through preparation of patient report forms prior to the start of the study. If possible, a single observer should assess all patients, and this observer should be someone apart from the individual who administers the treatment. If more than one observer is used, tests of interrater reliability should be performed on the key measures of subjective response.

In open-label drug trials, the addition of a simple manipulation, dose ranging, can provide supplementary information. Dose ranging is an essential component in new drug development (Phase I studies), wherein its primary goal is the determination of an upper limit of safe dosing (see Chapter 2). Since subjective effects are critical to monitor in dose-ranging studies of analgesic drugs (providing an indication of the therapeutic ratio), and all studies of subjective effects must recognize the potential confound posed by the placebo response, open-label trials are not adequate to yield definitive information about the dose-response relationships of analgesic drugs (93). Nonetheless, systematic open-label trials of different doses can suggest the nature of some of these relationships and clarify the prevalence and types of adverse effects at different dosing levels.

It may be very useful to obtain plasma drug levels during an open-label drug trial, assuming the availability of a valid bioassay for the drug. If possible, blood should be sampled multiple times during a single-dose trial, thereby providing some notion of absorption time, peak concentration, and clearance. In repeated-dose studies, the most useful data is provided by sampling several trough levels (immediately prior to a dose) after enough time has elapsed to ensure that the steady state has been approached. If this can be done repeatedly at several different dose levels in the same patient, very important information about the linearity of kinetics during chronic dosing can be inferred from these data (see Chapter 24). The cancer population represents a unique opportunity to perform repeated sampling of plasma opioid concentration during prolonged treatment. Although random blood sampling cannot replace carefully conducted pharmacokinetic studies, these data may be very useful in designing future investigations, providing an indication of pharmacokinetic and pharmacodynamic variability, and presenting a rudimentary notion of the relationship between plasma concentration and effects.

An investigator who undertakes a prospective open study can apply an identical assessment procedure to more than one treatment administered to the study population. In effect, this is an open, nonrandomized comparative trial. Although subject to the same limitations as other open trials, these data are often more informative than comparisons gleaned from surveys of clinical practice or the use of historical controls.

Randomized Trials

Randomization of patients to various treatments within a study diminishes bias by distributing factors not otherwise controlled by the investigator according to the laws of chance (94–97). Along with blinding procedures and the use of carefully contrived control groups, randomization is a fundamental component of the controlled clinical trial, an approach that has been extensively used in the cancer population to evaluate single doses of analgesic drugs (16,33,34). As discussed previously, the purview of analgesic study methodology in cancer pain includes many situations in which randomization of treatments may be the only feasible, or the most reliable, experimental control available to the investigator. For example, blinding is not possible in most comparisons of nonpharmacologic interventions, such as cordotomy and chemical neurolysis, and selection of a control group is problematic. Occasionally, the use of randomization of treatments without other controls is undertaken purposely, usually when the goal of the investigation is not a definitive evaluation of treatment effects, but rather an exploration of trends that may help improve clinical management. For example, randomization of patients to receive oral morphine or methadone during a long-term repeated-dose open trial provided useful data about the risks and acceptability of these treatments (98).

Issues in the Randomization of Cancer Pain Patients

The process of randomization may be complicated by several factors in the cancer pain population. Ethical considerations may become problematic, since it is unjustifiable to randomize patients to a treatment that may risk prolonged unrelieved pain or adverse effects from a treatment if another, safer approach can be applied. Although this may appear to be a rather straightforward matter, many situations become confused in the cancer pain population by the availability of numerous treatments accepted on the basis of anecdotal evidence and the potential for serious adverse effects from unproved therapies in patients with concurrent medical disease. For example, celiac plexus blockade has become widely accepted in the routine clinical management of pancreatic cancer pain, despite the lack of any randomized trial comparing the long-term risks and benefits of this approach to other available analgesic modalities, including oral opioid therapy. Nonetheless, implementation of a randomized trial, in which a therapy widely considered to be routine would be withheld from patients in lieu of another, clearly raises a difficult ethical issue for the investigator. As discussed previously, these issues may be resolved through the use of designs that incorporate escape contingencies, such as "rescue doses" of opioids or early dropout rules. In some situations, however, there can be no resolution and the definitive study cannot be conducted.

Randomization of treatments may also become difficult in studies of diverse modalities, for which the clinical indications or the attendant risk/benefit ratio may vary in different types of cancer patients. If selection of the study sample does not reflect these considerations, randomization would not prevent the introduction of bias through dissimilar dropout rates or influences on outcome measures. For example, a randomized trial comparing subcutaneous infusion and intraspinal opioids, which would yield very useful clinical data, would likely draw on patients who had advanced disease and numerous medical problems; should those patients admitted into the trial be relatively predisposed to adverse effects from one or another of these treatments, the outcome may not be a valid reflection of the relative utility of the treatment in a properly selected patient, notwithstanding careful attention to randomization. The investigator in the cancer pain population, therefore, must not place undue faith in randomization as a means of obviating the problem of bias. The use of well-conceived selection criteria may reduce these problems, but does not eliminate them, and moreover, may then lead to results that have very limited generalizability.

Blinding

Randomized trials comparing two or more treatments can be open or blinded. Blinding clearly increases the validity of all subjective data and should be incorporated into analgesic studies if possible; double blinding of both study patient and the investigator who administers treatments is the preferred approach. As noted, blinding is feasible in most drug trials in cancer patients, but is impossible in many other types of analgesic studies, such as those assessing invasive procedures. When blinding can be performed, the risk of unblinding exists, and if possible, should be evaluated. An approach to determine the extent of this potential bias involves the use of a standard question at the end of the trial, in which the patient is asked to guess the identity of the treatment he or she was administered (94).

Randomized Trial with Comparison Against Control

The benefits and risks of an analgesic intervention in the cancer pain population can be greatly illuminated by comparison against a control treatment, the effects of which are presumed to be known. This allows the determination of relative effects, which are often far more interpretable, and clinically relevant, than absolute outcome measures (16,33). Several issues must be considered in the use of control groups for analgesic studies in the cancer pain population, as follows:

The Use of Inactive Controls. The investigator must choose between an inactive control that has no biologic activity or an active control that mimics one or more of the effects of the study drug. One type of inactive control is a no-treatment group. Studies that employ this control group are inherently unblinded, and hence, provide potentially biased information about subjective effects. Numerous other inactive controls are possible, the most refined of which is the placebo treatment in double-blinded analgesic drug trials. Single blinding is often possible when inactive controls are included in studies of nonpharmacologic approaches, such as a trial of transcutaneous electrical nerve stimulation that includes a sham stimulation control.

In some types of studies, inactive controls are proscribed by the potential risks involved. For example, placement of an epidural catheter for placebo administration or the insertion of a needle to stimulate a nerve block cannot be justified in this population. Furthermore, the use of an inactive control cannot be justified if patients could possibly experience prolonged severe pain or some other adverse effect as a result. Thus, placebo cannot be administered to patients who could already be physically dependent on an opioid, lest opioid withdrawal be precipitated, nor can it be used in repeated-dose analgesic trials unless the methodology includes an appropriate escape contingency, such as the "rescue dose."

Single-dose analgesic assays performed in the cancer pain population during the past three decades have generally managed concerns about a placebo control through the incorporation of an early escape into the design (16). In this approach, patients are given the study drug, which may or may not be placebo, and are told that they will be remedicated with their usual analgesic whenever pain returns and they request treatment. Often, an effort is made to define an interval, usually 2 hrs, during which the patient will be strongly encouraged to wait before medication is given. This recognizes that there may be a delay in occurrence of analgesia following administration of the study drug.

The Use of Active Controls. The term "active control" herein encompasses two approaches: (a) An "active placebo" is an intervention that is presumed to have no analgesic effect but produces other actions that are likely to mimic common side effects of the test treatment. This approach, which reduces the risk of unblinding, has seldom been incorporated in cancer pain studies, and with the exception of some single-dose trials, would be difficult to justify in a population that experiences numerous symptoms as a baseline and is predisposed to adverse effects as a result of advanced age, major organ dysfunction, and the use of concurrent medication. (b) An "analgesic standard" is an intervention with a known and reliable analgesic effect, which is measured during the study and compared with the effects of the test intervention. This approach can provide a clinically meaningful indication of relative effects, and as well, obviate concern about the use of a nonanalgesic control in cancer pain patients.

The use of analgesic standards is straightforward in single-dose analgesic trials (see Chapter 4). The procedure combines randomization of treatments and double-blinded administration of single or graded doses of a commonly accepted analgesic. Classically, morphine has been used in studies of the opioids and aspirin or ibuprofen has been used in studies of the NSAIDs.

The methodological issues become more complex in repeated-dose studies (see Chapter 6). These designs must include a method for ensuring adequate relief of pain throughout the duration of the study. A variety of approaches are possible. In one randomized, double-blind, placebo-controlled study that compared dezocine with an analgesic standard (butorphanol) and placebo during 7 days of administration, the approach incorporated several features: (a) the chronic dosing phase was administered only to those who had pain relief during an initial single-dose evaluation, (b) doses were administered on an as-needed basis during the chronic dosing phase, and (c) patients were withdrawn if less than moderate pain relief was reported or unacceptable toxicity ensued (99). This allowed a controlled comparison of repeated dosing without subjecting patients to the risk of unrelieved pain.

The major disadvantage of the latter approach is that inadequate pain control is managed through patient attrition, potentially resulting in the loss of a substantial amount of data. Another method, discussed previously, incorporates the administration of "rescue doses" of a known analgesic. This technique can also accommodate the use of placebo and should reduce the attrition rate while providing another dependent measure of analgesic efficacy (the quantity of "rescue" drug).

The use of analgesic standards in studies of nonpharmacologic interventions and many of the newer pharmacologic approaches (e.g., intraspinal opioids or subcutaneous infusion) requires careful consideration. In most cases, the investigator can select one or more of several distinct control groups. The choice depends on the particular questions that the study intends to address. For example, a study of subcutaneous morphine infusion might employ a control of continuous intravenous infusion if the goal is to better understand the effects of the subcutaneous route on time-action relationships and dose requirements of the drug; in contrast, a control group comprising patients administered regularly scheduled doses of oral morphine may be more appropriate if the goal of the study is to determine the role of subcutaneous infusion in the long-term management of cancer pain.

The Role of Titration in Drug Trials. The information available from controlled trials of analgesic drugs is greatly enhanced by the use of multiple dosing levels of the test drug, and if appropriate, the control drug as well. The advantages are best appreciated in single-dose trials, in which the use of graded doses can provide an indication of assay sensitivity and yield information that may allow the determination of relative potency and relative efficacy of the doses selected (see Chapter 4). Similarly, repeated-dose studies in chronic cancer pain can incorporate multiple dosing levels and potentially provide the same type of information about the dose-response relationship of the test drug on repeated administration.

An alternative approach to the use of multiple dosing levels is blinded dose titration of the test and control drugs. The specific procedures employed depend on the type of drug, the analgesic approach under investigation, and the investigator's understanding of the pharmacokinetics, time-action relationships, and side effect profile of the drug. If oral administration is used, blinded dose titration may involve instructions to increase the number of tablets at predetermined intervals; with other techniques, appropriate blinding procedures must be developed, such as increments in the infusion rate in studies that use this modality. If necessary, manipulations can be added that provide the means to treat unrelieved severe pain during the period of dose titration, such as the use of a "rescue dose."

The extent of titration in these studies must be operationally defined prior to the start of the study. With analgesic interventions using opioid drugs, the protocol should include a guideline for the cessation of titration when either "acceptable" analgesic occurs or intolerable side effects develop. With other drug classes, some other arbitrary limit must be set based on clinical experience or prior dose-ranging studies. If titration ensues until either a ceiling effect for analgesia is identified or intolerable side effects occur in all study groups, the study will be able to assess the maximum efficacy of the study drug compared to control, a finding with considerable clinical relevance.

Skill in the Administration of Treatments. Repeated-dose analgesic drug trials, studies of alternative routes of drug administration, and studies of nonpharmacologic cancer pain treatments all highlight another important consideration in the design of randomized trials. In all these studies, an analgesic technique must be implemented by the investigator; they are therefore dependent on the expert implementation of both the test intervention and the control intervention. This should be recognized as a potential source of bias that may skew outcome or limit the generalizability of the results. There is no simple resolution to this problem, but the investigator should try to ensure that guidelines for implementation of the intervention are stated *a priori* in the study protocol, that communication is maintained with the clinicians performing the study, and that the published report describes the approaches clearly.

Crossover versus Parallel-Group Designs. The decision to employ either a crossover or parallel-group design in randomized clinical trials of analgesic interventions remains controversial (see Chapter 4). In crossover trials, each patient acts as his/her own control, thereby eliminating the problems of between-patient variability. This reduces the variances within each study group and facilitates group comparisons (increasing study power and/or allowing smaller sample sizes). Recent studies (100) and two meta-analyses of single-dose drug trials performed in the postoperative pain setting (101,102) indicate that crossover designs are more efficient.

Notwithstanding these advantages, concerns exist about the potential for carryover effects, time-dependent effects, and order effects in crossover studies. In studies with a relatively long observation period, crossover trials may be more problematic owing to a high risk of attrition or time-dependent effects, the latter resulting from the rapid clinical changes that often characterize the patient with cancer pain. Likewise, the risk of carryover effects may be unacceptably high if the treatments under study produce prolonged changes. In the extreme case, it is obvious that permanent nerve blocks, or any other neuroablative procedure, cannot be evaluated in a crossover paradigm. These potential problems must be considered on a case by case basis. Unless they can be adequately addressed, a parallel-group design is more appropriate. Given the added efficiency of the crossover paradigm, however, consideration of this approach is warranted in virtually any trial.

Randomized Trial with Multiple Control Groups

The use of multiple control groups provides an opportunity to acquire additional important information about the intervention under study. These comparisons can better determine the relative efficacy and side effects of the treatment. The information obtained can have substantial clinical relevance.

Multiple control groups can also provide a measure of the sensitivity of the study to discern differences among treatment groups. In single-dose analgesic drug trials, the use of measures of assay sensitivity, specifically the combination of placebo and a single dose of an analgesic standard or graded doses of the analgesic standard, has become the accepted approach (see Chapter 4). Other types of cancer pain studies may also benefit from this technique. For example, the use of placebo plus a standard has been incorporated into a repeated-dose trial of an opioid in patients with advanced cancer, as described previously (99). Theoretically, repeated-dose studies could also use dose titration to demonstrate sensitivity by comparing observed effects at different dosage levels of the control drug, and other types of treatment trials could introduce multiple analgesic standards that accomplish a similar outcome. Finally, study sensitivity can also be assessed through power analyses performed after completion of the trial (103,104). Although it is likely that the use of multiple controls yields valuable additional information that power analyses cannot, it remains to be determined that this potential advantage justifies the cost and effort required to implement multiple control groups if the primary goal is to establish the sensitivity of the methodology.

CONCLUSIONS

Consideration of the many factors involved in the methodology for analgesic studies in cancer pain patients may improve the investigator's ability to address the key hypotheses and limit the "noise" inevitably introduced into the data by the variability within this population. The choice of an overall design and outcome measures represents only the first step in this process. A successful study ultimately depends on the management of numerous details, including the selection criteria and recruitment procedures, mode of administration of the study intervention, and methods of data collection. Sophisticated multivariate statistical techniques are now available routinely, and though these may allow manipulation of the data in ways that were previously impossible, these necessary approaches cannot substitute for critical methodological decisions and constant attention to quality control. With due consideration of these factors, clinical trials in patients with cancer pain may be able to successfully resolve most of the many clinical issues that remain to be addressed in the management of patients with cancer pain.

REFERENCES

1. Bonica JJ. Treatment of cancer pain: current status and future needs. In:Fields HL, Dubner R, Cervero R, eds. *Advances in pain research and therapy,* vol 9. New York: Raven Press, 1985;589–616.
2. Portenoy RK. Cancer pain: epidemiology and syndromes. *Cancer* 1989;63:2298–2307.
3. Ventafridda V, Tamburini M, DeConno, F. Comprehensive treatment in cancer pain. In:Fields HL, Dubner R, Cervero R, eds. *Advances in pain research and therapy,* vol 9. New York: Raven Press, 1985;617–628.
4. Kane RL, Berstein L, Rothenberg R. Hospice effectiveness in controlling pain. *JAMA* 1985;253:2683–2686.
5. Elliott K, Foley KM. Neurologic pain syndromes in patients with cancer. In:Portenoy RK, ed. *Neurologic clinics (Pain: mechanisms and syndromes).* Philadelphia: W.B. Saunders, 1989;333–360.
6. Portenoy RK. Pharmacologic management of cancer pain. *J Psychosoc Oncol* 1990;8:75–107.
7. Foley KM. The treatment of cancer pain. *N Engl J Med* 1985;313:84–95.
8. Cleeland CS, Rotondi A, Brechner T, et al. A model for the treatment of cancer pain. *J Pain Symptom Manag* 1986;1:209–216.
9. Twycross RG, Lack SA. *Symptom control in far advanced cancer: pain relief.* London: Pitman, 1984.

10. World Health Organization. *Cancer pain relief.* Geneva: World Health Organization, 1986.
11. Sunshine A, Olson NZ. Non-narcotic analgesics. In:Wall PD, Melzack R, eds. *Textbook of pain,* 2nd ed. Edinburgh: Churchill Livingstone, 1989;670–685.
12. Sunshine A, Olson NZ: Analgesic efficacy of ketoprofen in postpartum, general surgery, and chronic cancer pain. *J Clin Pharmacol* 1988;28:S47–S54.
13. Lomen PL, Samal BA, Lamborn KR, Sattler LP, Crampton SL. Flurbiprofen for the treatment of bone pain in patients with metastatic breast cancer. *Am J Med* 1986;80(Suppl 3A):83–87.
14. Cooper SH. Comparative analgesic efficacies of aspirin and acetaminophen. *Arch Intern Med* 1981;141:282–285.
15. Ferrer-Brechner T, Ganz P. Combination therapy with ibuprofen and methadone for chronic cancer pain. *Am J Med* 1984;77:78–83.
16. Houde RW, Wallenstein SL, Beaver WT. Evaluation of analgesics in patients with cancer pain. In:Lasagna L, ed. *International encyclopedia of pharmacology and therapeutics, section 6, Clinical pharmacology,* vol 1. Oxford: Pergamon Press, 1966;59–98.
17. Moertel CG, Ohmann DL, Taylor WF, et al. Relief of pain by oral medications. *JAMA* 1974;229: 55–59.
18. Belchman WJ, Lechner BL. Clinical comparative evaluation of choline magnesium trisalicylate and acetyl salicylic acid in rheumatoid arthritis. *Rheum Rehab* 1979;18:119–124.
19. Danesh BJZ, Saniabadi AR, Russell RI, Lowe GDO. Therapeutic potential of choline magnesium trisalicylate as an alternative to aspirin for patients with bleeding tendencies. *Scott Med J* 1987;32: 167–168.
20. Cohen A, Garber HE. Comparison of choline magnesium trisalicylate and acetylsalicylic acid in relation to faecal blood loss. *Curr Ther Res* 1978;23:187–193.
21. Hanks GW. The pharmacological treatment of bone pain. *Cancer Surv* 1988;7:87–101.
22. Ventafridda V, Fochi C, De Conno F, Sganzerla E. Use of nonsteroidal anti-inflammatory drugs in the treatment of pain in cancer. *Br J Clin Pharmacol* 1980;10:343–346.
23. Hindley AC, Hill EB, Leyland MJ. A double-blind controlled trial of salmon calcitonin in pain due to malignancy. *Cancer Chemother Pharmacol* 1982;9:71–74.
24. Bruera E, Chadwick S, Brenneis C, et al. Methylphenidate associated with narcotics for the treatment of cancer pain. *Cancer Treat Rep* 1987;71:67–70.
25. Bruera E, Roca E, Cedaro L, Carraro S, Chacon R. Action of oral methylprednisolone in terminal cancer patients: a prospective randomized double-blind study. *Cancer Treat Rep* 1985;69:751–754.
26. Walsh TD. Controlled study of imipramine and morphine in chronic pain due to cancer. *Proc Am Soc Clin Oncol* 1986;5:237.
27. Beaver WT, Wallenstein SM, Houde RW, Rogers A. A comparison of the analgesic effects of methotrimeprazine and morphine in patients with cancer. *Clin Pharmacol Ther* 1966;7:436–446.
28. Foley KM. Adjuvant analgesic drugs in cancer pain management. In: Aronoff GM, ed. *Evaluation and treatment of chronic pain.* Baltimore: Urban & Schwarzenberg, 1985;425–434.
29. Coyle N, Adelhardt J, Foley KM, Portenoy RK. Character of terminal illness in the advanced cancer patient: pain and other symptoms in the last 4 weeks of life. *J Pain Symptom Manag* 1990;5:83–93.
30. Foley KM, Inturrisi CE, eds. *Opioid analgesics in the management of clinical pain.* New York: Raven Press, 1986.
31. Arner S, Meyerson BA. Lack of analgesic effect of opioids on neuropathic and idiopathic forms of pain. *Pain* 1988;33:11–23.
32. Beaver WT, Wallenstein SL, Rogers A, Houde RW. Analgesic studies of codeine and oxycodone in patients with cancer. I. Comparisons of oral with intramuscular codeine and of oral with intramuscular oxycodone. *J Pharmacol Exp Ther* 1978;207:92–100.
33. Houde RW, Wallenstein SL, Beaver WT. Clinical measurement of pain. In: deStevens G, ed. *Analgetics.* New York: Academic Press, 1965;75–122.
34. Wallenstein SL, Houde RW. The clinical evaluation of analgesic effectiveness. In:Ehrenpreis S, Neidle A, eds. *Methods in narcotics research.* New York: Marcel Dekker, 1975;127–145.
35. Beaver WT, Wallenstein SL, Houde RW, Rogers A. A clinical comparison of the analgesic effects of methadone and morphine administered intravenously, and of orally and parenterally administered methadone in patients with cancer. *Clin Pharmacol Ther* 1967;8:415–426.
36. Kaiko RF, Wallenstein SL, Rogers AG, Grabinski PY, Houde RW. Analgesic and mood effects

of heroin and morphine in cancer patients with postoperative pain. *N Engl J Med* 1981;304: 1501–1505.
37. Wallenstein SL, Kaiko RF, Rogers AG, Houde RW. Crossover trials in clinical analgesic assays: studies of buprenorphine and morphine. *Pharmacotherapy* 1986;6(5):228–235.
38. Kaiko RF. Commentary: equianalgesic dose ratio of intramuscular/oral morphine, 1:6 versus 1:3. In:Foley KM, Inturrisi CE, eds. *Advances in pain research and therapy, vol 8, Opioid analgesics in the management of clinical pain.* New York: Raven Press, 1986;87–93.
39. Brown DL, Moore DC. The use of neurolytic celiac plexus block for pancreatic cancer: anatomy and technique. *J Pain Symptom Manag* 1988;3:206–209.
40. Schmauss C, Yaksh TL. *In vivo* studies on spinal opiate receptor systems mediating antinociception: II. Pharmacological profiles suggesting a differential association of mu, delta, and kappa receptors with visceral, chemical, and cutaneous stimuli in the rat. *J Pharmacol Exp Ther* 1983;228:1–12.
41. Kaiko RF, Wallenstein SL, Rogers AG, Canel A, Jacobs B, Houde RW. Intramuscular meptazinol and morphine in postoperative pain. *Clin Pharmacol Ther* 1985;37:589–596.
42. Moulin DE, Max MB, Kaiko RF, et al. The analgesic efficacy of intrathecal (IT) D-Ala-D-Leu-Enkephalin (DADL) in cancer patients with chronic pain. *Pain* 1985;23:213–221.
43. Kishore-Kumar R, Shafer SC, Lawlor BA, Murphy DL, Max MB. Single doses of the serotonin agonists buspirone and m-chlorophenylpiperazine do not relieve neuropathic pain. *Pain* 1989;37: 223–227.
44. Max MB, Schafer SC, Culnance M, Dubner R, Gracely RH. Association of pain relief with drug side effects in postherpetic neuralgia: single-dose study of clonidine, codeine, ibuprofen, and placebo. *Clin Pharmacol Ther* 1988;43:363–371.
45. Ahles TA, Blanchard EB, Ruckdeschel JC. The multidimensional nature of cancer-related pain. *Pain* 1983;17:277–288.
46. Meinart CL. *Clinical trials: design, conduct, and analysis.* New York: Oxford University Press, 1986;193–195.
47. Kaldor A, Gachalyi B, Vas A. Pre-trial drop-outs. *Eur J Clin Pharmacol* 1988;35:686.
48. Schwartz D, Lellouch J. Explanatory and pragmatic attitudes in therapeutical trials. *J Chron Dis* 1967;20:637–648.
49. Bruera E, MacMillan K, Hanson J, MacDonald RN. The Edmonton staging system for cancer pain: preliminary report. *Pain* 1989;37:203–210.
50. Wallenstein SL, Houde RW, Portenoy RK, et al. Clinical analgesic assay of repeated and single doses of heroin and hydromorphone. *Pain* 1990;41:5–14.
51. Houde RW: Misinformation: side effects and drug interactions. In:Hill CS, Fields WS, eds. *Advances in pain research and therapy, vol 11, Drug treatment of cancer pain in a drug-oriented society.* New York: Raven Press, 1989;145–161.
52. Silberfarb PM, Oxman TE. The effects of cancer therapies on the central nervous system. In: Goldberg RJ, ed. *Psychiatric aspects of cancer.* Basel: Karger, 1988;13–25.
53. Melzack R, ed. *Pain measurement and assessment.* New York: Raven Press, 1983.
54. Chapman CR, Loeser JD, eds. *Advances in pain research and therapy, vol 12, Issues in pain management.* New York: Raven Press, 1989.
55. Reading AE. Testing pain mechanisms in persons in pain. In:Wall PD, Melzack R, eds. *Textbook of pain,* 2nd Ed. Edinburgh: Churchill Livingstone, 1989;269–280.
56. Price DD. *Psychological and neural mechanisms of pain.* New York: Raven Press, 1988;33–34.
57. Huskisson EC. Measurement of pain. *Lancet* 1974;2:1127–1131.
58. Wallenstein SL, Heidrich G, Kaiko R, Houde RW. Clinical evaluation of mild analgesics: the measurement of pain. *Br J Clin Pharmacol* 1980;10:319S–327S.
59. Wallenstein SL. Measurement of pain and analgesia in cancer patients. *Cancer* 1984;53(Suppl): 2260–2266.
60. McGrath PA. Evaluating a child's pain. *J Pain Symptom Manag* 1989;4:198–214.
61. Littman GS, Walker BR, Schneider BE. Reassessment of verbal and visual analog ratings in analgesic studies. *Clin Pharmacol Ther* 1985;38:16–23.
62. Sriwatankul K, Kelvie W, Lasagna L. The quantification of pain: an analysis of words used to describe pain and analgesia in clinical trials. *Clin Pharmacol Ther* 1982;32:143–148.
63. Price DD, Harkins SW, Rafii A, Price C. A simultaneous comparison of fentanyl's analgesic effects on experimental and clinical pain. *Pain* 1986;24:197–203.

64. Price DD, Harkins SW, Baker C. Sensory-affective relationships among different types of clinical and experimental pain. *Pain* 1986;28:297–307.
65. Reading AE. A comparison of the McGill Pain Questionnaire in chronic and acute pain. *Pain* 1982;13:185–192.
66. Littlejohns DW, Vere DW. The clinical assessment of analgesic drugs. *Br J Clin Pharmacol* 1981;11:319–332.
67. Fishman B, Pasternak S, Wallenstein SL, et al. The Memorial Pain Assessment Card: a valid instrument for the evaluation of cancer pain. *Cancer* 1987;60:1151–1158.
68. Portenoy RK, Maldonado M, Fitzmartin R, Kaiko R, Kanner R: Controlled-release morphine sulfate: analgesic efficacy and side effects of a 100 mg tablet in cancer pain patients. *Cancer* 1989;63:2284–2288.
69. Cundiff D, McCarthy K, Savarese JJ, et al. Evaluation of a cancer pain model for the testing of long-acting analgesics. *Cancer* 1989;63:2355–2359.
70. Savarese JJ, Thomas GB, Homesley H, Hill CS. Rescue factor: a design for evaluating long-acting analgesics. *Clin Pharmacol Ther* 1988;43:376–380.
71. Margoles RB. The pain chart: special properties of pain. In:Melzack R, ed. *Pain measurement and assessment*. New York: Raven Press, 1983;215–225.
72. Margoles RB, Tait RC, Krause SJ. A rating system for use with patient pain drawings. *Pain* 1986;24:57–65.
73. Karch FE, Lasagna L. Adverse drug reactions. *JAMA* 1975;234:1236–1241.
74. Koeppen D, Mohr R, Streichenwein S. Assessment of adverse drug events during the clinical investigation of a new drug. *Pharmacopsychiatry* 1989;22:93–98.
75. Guy W, ed. *ECDEU assessment manual for psychopharmacology, (DOTES: Dosage Record and Treatment Emergent Symptom Scale).* Rockville, Maryland: National Institute of Mental Health, 1976;223–244.
76. Levine J, Schooler N, eds. *Systematic assessment for treatment emergent events (SAFTEE-GI).* Rockville, Maryland: National Institute of Mental Health, 1983.
77. Inturrisi CS, Portenoy RK, Max M, Colburn WA, Foley KM. Pharmacokinetic-pharmacodynamic (PK-PD) relationships of methadone infusions in patients with cancer pain. *Clin Pharmacol Ther* (in press).
78. Brescia FJ, Adler D, Gray G, et al. Hospitalized advanced cancer patients: a profile. *J Pain Symptom Manag* 1990;5:221–227.
79. Kaiko RF, Wallenstein SL, Rogers AG, Grabinski PY, Houde RW. Analgesic and mood effects of heroin and morphine in cancer patients with postoperative pain. *N Engl J Med* 1981;304:1501–1505.
80. Lasagna L, von Feisinger JM, Beecher HK. Drug-induced mood changes in man. I. Observation on healthy subjects, chronically ill patients, and "postaddicts." *JAMA* 1955;157:1006–1020.
81. Ventafridda V, Bonezzi C, Caraceni A, et al. Antidepressants for cancer pain and other painful syndromes with deafferentation component: comparison of amitriptyline and trazadone. *Ital J Neurol Sci* 1987;8:579–587.
82. Ahles T, Ruckdeschel JC, Blanchard EB. Cancer-related pain. II. Assessment with visual analogue scales. *J Psychosom Res* 1984;28:121–124.
83. Bruera E, Roca E, Cedaro L, Carraro S, Chacon R. Action of oral methylprednisolone in terminal cancer patients: a prospective randomized double-blind study. *Cancer Treat Rep* 1985;69:751–754.
84. Cella DF, Jacobsen PB, Lesko LM. Research methods in psychooncology. In: Holland JC, Rowland JH, eds. *Handbook of psychooncology: psychological care of the patient with cancer.* New York: Oxford University Press, 1989;737–749.
85. Schag CC, Heinrich RL, Ganz PA. Karnofsky Performance Status revisited: reliability, validity and guidelines. *J Clin Oncol* 1984;2:187–193.
86. Donovan K, Sanson-Fisher RW, Redman S. Measuring quality of life in cancer patients. *J Clin Oncol* 1989;7:959–968.
87. Van Knippenberg FCE, De Haes JCJM. Measuring the quality of life of cancer patients: psychometric properties of instruments. *J Clin Epidemiol* 1988;41:1043–1053.
88. Moinpour CM, Feigl P, Metch B, et al. Quality of life end points in cancer clinical trials: review and recommendations. *J Natl Cancer Inst* 1989;81:485–495.
89. Ferrell BR, Wisdon C, Wenzl C. Quality of life as an outcome variable in the management of cancer pain. *Cancer* 1989;63:2321–2327.

90. Owen JA, Sitar DS, Berger L, et al. Age-related morphine kinetics. *Clin Pharmacol Ther* 1983;34: 364–368.
91. Ventafridda V, Oliveri E, Caraceni A, et al. A retrospective study on the use of oral morphine in cancer pain. *J Pain Symptom Manag* 1987;2:77–82.
92. Brown DL, Bulley K, Quiel EL. Neurolytic celiac plexus block for pancreatic cancer pain. *Anesth Analg* 1987;66:869–873.
93. Schmidt R. Dose-finding studies in clinical drug development. *Eur J Clin Pharmacol* 1988;34: 15–19.
94. Kramer MS, Shapiro SH. Scientific challenges in the application of randomized trials. *JAMA* 1984;252:2739–2745.
95. Feinstein AR. An additional basic science for clinical medicine: II. The limitations of randomized trials. *Ann Intern Med* 1983;99:544–550.
96. Byar DP, Simon RM, Friedewald WT, et al. Randomized clinical trials: perspective on some recent ideas. *N Engl J Med* 1976;295:74–80.
97. Friedman LM, Furberg CD, DeMets DL. *Fundamentals of clinical trials,* 2nd ed. Littleton, Massachusetts: PSG Publishing Co., 1985;51–69.
98. Ventafridda V, Ripamonti C, Bianchi M, Sbanotto A, De Conno F. A randomized study on oral administration of morphine and methadone in the treatment of cancer pain. *J Pain Symptom Manag* 1986;1:203–208.
99. Stambaugh JE, McAdams J. Comparison of intramuscular dezocine with butorphanol and placebo in chronic cancer pain: a method to evaluate analgesia after both single and repeated doses. *Clin Pharmacol Ther* 1987;42:210–219.
100. Wallenstein SL, Kaiko RF, Rogers AG, Houde RW. Crossover trials in clinical analgesic assays: studies of buprenorphine and morphine. *Pharmacotherapy* 1986;6(5):228–235.
101. Forrest WH, James KE, Ho TY. Residual analgesic effects of morphine in 55 four-period crossover analgesic studies. *Clin Pharmacol Ther* 1988;44:383–388.
102. James KE, Forrest WH, Rose RL. Crossover and noncrossover designs in four-point parallel line analgesic assays. *Clin Pharmacol Ther* 1985;37:242–252.
103. Stolley PD, Strom BL. Sample size calculations for clinical pharmacology studies. *Clin Pharmacol Ther* 1986;89:489–490.
104. Peace KE, Schriver RC. P-value and power computations in multiple look trials. *J Chron Dis* 1987;40:23–30.

Advances in Pain Research and Therapy, Vol. 18,
edited by M. Max, R. Portenoy, and E. Laska,
Raven Press, Ltd., New York © 1991.

10

Cancer Pain: Chronic Studies of Adjuvants to Opiate Analgesics

Eduardo Bruera

*Palliative Care Unit, Edmonton General Hospital, Edmonton, Alberta, Canada T5K
0L4; and Department of Medicine, University of Alberta, Edmonton,
Alberta, Canada, T5K 0L4*

Opiate analgesics are the most important drugs for the treatment of chronic pain
(1,2). Although these drugs can control severe pain in most cases, they can cause
symptoms, or aggravate preexisting symptoms, such as nausea or somnolence
(1–3). This problem is particularly severe in the case of patients with advanced
cancer. The combination of severe pain, anorexia, chronic nausea, asthenia, and
somnolence in the same patient is a frequent finding in the daily treatment of
advanced cancer (3).

An adjuvant drug should be able to (a) increase the analgesic effect of narcotics
(adjuvant analgesia); (b) decrease the toxicity of narcotics; or (c) improve the
associated symptoms of terminal cancer. In some cases, when epidemiological
data suggest that patients are at high risk of developing toxicity after starting a
narcotic treatment (e.g., constipation after chronic narcotic therapy), the adjuvant
treatment should be started before there is any clinical evidence of toxicity.

Many drugs have been suggested to have adjuvant analgesic effects (Table 1).
Unfortunately, most of the evidence for the effects of these drugs is anecdotal.
Controlled clinical trials are needed to define the indications and risk/benefit
ratios of these agents, some of which have significant toxicity and could potentially
aggravate the toxicity of narcotics. Research is complicated by the multiple endpoints that need to be measured during such a trial. Although some of these
endpoints are likely to remain constant (e.g., constipation or pain), others are
likely to change as a function of time (sedation, nausea). The duration of the
clinical trial and the design will also be affected by the characteristics of the
adjuvant drugs being tested.

This chapter summarizes the current use of adjuvant drugs and the approaches
to clinical trial design. Emphasis will be placed on those drugs that should be
the focus of future research.

TABLE 1. *Drugs suggested to have adjuvant effects*

Nonsteroidal antiinflammatories	Antibiotics
Laxatives	Baclofen
Antiemetics	Amphetamines
Phenothiazines	Corticosteroids
Benzodiazepines	Diphosphonates
Tricyclic antidepressants	Calcitonin
Phenytoin	Clonidine
Carbamazepine	

CURRENT USE OF ADJUVANT DRUGS

Most patients with cancer pain receive adjuvant drugs (1,4–6). Our group studied the pattern of prescription of narcotics and adjuvant drugs in 100 consecutive patients admitted to a cancer center during 1980, 1984, and 1987. All patients in each year were consecutive admissions under the Department of Medicine and none of the patients had been seen by a pain specialist or a palliative care physician (4,5). Table 2 summarizes the patterns of use of adjuvant drugs during 1980 as compared to 1984 and 1987. The results show that more than two-thirds of patients received laxatives and nonnarcotic analgesics, almost half received hypnotics and antiemetics, and approximately one-third received psychoactive drugs. In a separate survey, we observed that the types of adjuvant drugs prescribed also differ between countries. Patients admitted to a South American cancer center received significantly fewer prescriptions for laxatives, hypnotics, and nonpharmacological treatments, and significantly more for tricyclic antidepressants and nonnarcotic analgesics, as compared to patients admitted to a North American cancer center (7).

Thus, most cancer patients receive more than one or two adjuvant drugs, in addition to narcotics. Unfortunately, very few of these drugs have been subjected to controlled clinical trials.

Nonnarcotic Analgesics

The main agents in this category are acetaminophen and the nonsteroidal antiinflammatory agents (NSAIDs). These drugs have different mechanisms of action and toxicity than narcotics, and therefore can be combined with narcotics unless otherwise indicated. These drugs are frequently administered to cancer patients in commercial preparations containing codeine or oxycodone. However, when patients need to be changed to stronger narcotics, such as morphine, hydromorphone, or levorphanol, nonnarcotics usually are not prescribed in addition to the narcotic and patients lose their potential advantageous effect (4,5). Because most cancer patients are elderly, and because hematologic and renal disorders are frequently present, peripheral prostaglandin inhibitors may be more difficult to use than acetaminophen.

Controlled trials have shown that nonnarcotics can provide analgesia additive to that of narcotics in cancer pain patients (8). There are also reports suggesting

TABLE 2. *Use of adjuvant drugs in 100 consecutive patients admitted to a North American cancer center during 1980, 1984, and 1987 respectively[a]*

	Number of patients receiving drugs		
Drugs	1980	1984	1987
Laxatives	65	69	66
Corticosteroids	8	11	14
Antiemetics	49	54	53
Psychoactive drugs	22	36	39
Hypnotics	47	49	48
Nonnarcotic analgesics	50	77	71

[a] See refs. 4, 5.

a particularly useful role for these agents in the treatment of patients with bone pain (9) and those in whom an inflammatory component contributes to their pain. There are no conclusive studies showing which nonnarcotic is more effective in cancer pain, and neither the proper dose nor route of administration has been established in prospective trials.

Tricyclic Antidepressants

These drugs are frequently used in hospice care (10) and in South American cancer centers (7), but very infrequently in North American cancer centers (4–11). Although they have a demonstrated effect in the treatment of postherpetic neuralgia (12), there is very limited evidence for a significant analgesic effect in other types of cancer pain. One placebo-controlled study in terminal patients suggested a decreased requirement of morphine for equal pain control in patients receiving imipramine (13). The tricyclic antidepressant's mechanism of action has been suggested to involve potentiation of descending inhibitory pathways (14), but one study also suggested that they may increase plasma morphine levels by enhancing its bioavailability (15). At least in patients with postherpetic neuralgia, their effect appears to be unrelated to mood changes (12).

The optimal drug and dosing regimen are unknown. However, most authors agree that the doses needed for analgesia are lower than those needed for antidepressant effects (1–6). The toxic effect of these drugs, mainly autonomic (dry mouth, postural hypotension) and central (somnolence, confusion), may contribute to the symptoms already present in debilitated patients. Because of their demonstrated success in postherpetic neuralgia, these drugs are usually tried in neuropathic pain syndromes, with uncertain success.

Corticosteroids

Uncontrolled studies suggested that corticosteroids could improve pain, appetite, and activity in patients with advanced cancer (16). In 1974, Moertel (17) randomized 116 patients with advanced gastrointestinal cancer to receive dexamethasone 0.75 and 1.5 mg four times daily or placebo in a double-blind trial. Although no significant tumor regression was observed, significant symptomatic improvement (mainly appetite and strength) was found after 2 weeks of treatment in patients receiving dexamethasone. Such improvement disappeared after 4 weeks of treatment. Toxicity was low, with one case of gastrointestinal hemorrhage.

We randomized 31 patients to methylprednisolone 16 mg bid versus placebo for 1 week (18). After that period a crossover took place and patients received the alternative treatment for another week. At the end of this double-blind trial, there was a significant improvement in pain, appetite, and activity. Patients blindly chose methylprednisolone as a more effective drug in 75% of cases. Subsequently, methylprednisolone was continued in an open-label trial. Unfortunately, after 3 weeks of treatment, all parameters except pain intensity were not significantly different from the baseline assessment. These results suggest that the effects of corticosteroids are significant but short-lasting (18). These studies could not establish if this is owing to a loss of the effect of corticosteroids with time or to the natural evolution of the disease.

The mechanism of action of corticosteroids in patients with terminal cancer is not clear, but may involve their euphoriant effects or the inhibition of prostaglandin metabolism. The optimal drug and dosing regimen have not been established. Corticosteroids may produce limiting side effects in cancer patients, particularly immunosuppression (candidiasis will occur in most patients), and psychiatric symptoms (restlessness, insomnia, agitation, psychosis), and with prolonged use of a fluorinated agent, myopathy may develop.

Phenothiazines and Benzodiazepines

Although these drugs have been frequently used in association with narcotics, there is very little evidence that drugs in either class have major adjuvant analgesic effects. Benzodiazepines do not appear to produce clinically useful analgesia, aside from their benefits as muscle relaxants in patients with muscle spasms (19). However, benzodiazepines are useful for short-term administration in situations characterized by anxiety and sleep problems, such as surgery (20), labor, or myocardial infarction (21). With the exception of methotrimeprazine, phenothiazines have not shown consistent analgesic effect, or potentiation of narcotics (21). Both groups of drugs can aggravate narcotic-induced sedation, thereby limiting the dose of narcotics that a patient is able to tolerate. Unless indications other than pain are present, these drugs should not be considered useful adjuvant analgesics at the present time.

Amphetamines

Somnolence is a frequent symptom in cancer patients, in some cases owing to a treatable metabolic disorder, in the majority owing to medications, most commonly narcotic analgesics. In the titration of narcotic dose, we usually try to find the "therapeutic window" between the upper dose level capable of causing sedation and the lower level in which there is recurrent pain. Unfortunately, in many patients such a window does not exist, and the dose needed for adequate analgesia is above that associated with intolerable somnolence.

Early research reported that amphetamine derivatives increase analgesia and decrease sedation in animals (22) and human volunteers (23), and increased arousal and decreased fatigue in normal adults (24). In 1977, Forrest et al. (25) conducted a double-blind study of dextroamphetamine in patients recovering from anesthesia. They found that a single dose of 5 or 10 mg of dextroamphetamine significantly potentiated the analgesic effects of morphine while decreasing sleepiness and increasing intellectual performance. In 1982, an open study in 18 cancer patients suggested that dextroamphetamine could improve pain, activity, and appetite in cancer patients, and thereby "enhance the comfort of terminally ill patients with cancer" (26). Our group decided to compare mazindol (a mild amphetamine derivative) 1 mg at breakfast, lunch, and at 4 PM versus placebo in a double-blind, crossover trial in a group of 26 patients with advanced cancer (27). Although a significant decrease in pain intensity and analgesic consumption was observed, there was also a significant decrease in appetite and food intake, an increase in anxiety, and serious toxicity in two cases (delirium). Because of the finding of some analgesic improvement in patients receiving mazindol, we studied patients receiving a higher dose of narcotics. The design was again double-blind, crossover, with a 3-day treatment period (28). In this study, we chose methylphenidate as the amphetamine derivative because of its shorter half-life and good tolerance in patients with geriatric conditions (29). Methylphenidate significantly decreased pain and sedation and increased activity in our patients. Toxicity was not significantly different from placebo and patients chose methylphenidate blindly as more effective in 20 cases (70%).

These data suggest that amphetamines should not be used indiscriminately for enhancing the comfort of terminal cancer patients. However, in a subset of patients they are able to decrease sedation and increase activity by antagonizing the side effects of narcotics. We have since used methylphenidate on 50 patients with narcotic-induced sedation and observed good results in an open trial (30). Toxic effects were very uncommon, but the induction of delirium and paranoid reactions in severe patients confirmed that they should be used only in selected patients. We routinely check cognitive function and review the past history for paranoid behavior prior to use.

Antiemetics

Chemotherapy-induced emesis has been very well studied in cancer patients, and effective treatments have been developed for acute emesis, delayed emesis, and anticipatory nausea. However, patients with advanced cancer frequently suffer severe chronic nausea and very limited research has taken place in this field. Chronic nausea correlates with cardiovascular (31) and gastrointestinal

(32) autonomic disturbances. Narcotic analgesics can aggravate nausea by central and peripheral effects (33). Antidopaminergic agents, such as metoclopramide or haloperidol, have been employed to treat chronic nausea, either orally or as continuous subcutaneous infusions (34,35). Unfortunately, because of the absence of studies that specifically address the problem of chronic nausea, most treatment is adapted from trials for chemotherapy-induced emesis, and this may compromise optimal therapy. For example, phenothiazines and antihistamines are commonly used for acute nausea, but can potentiate the sedating effects of narcotics and may not be appropriate for these patients. Newer and powerful antiemetics such as the modified benzamides (36) or antiserotonergic (37) have not been investigated for the treatment of chronic nausea or narcotic-induced emesis. At the present time, the best type and dose of antiemetic for the treatment of these symptoms is unknown.

Laxatives

Although there is a general consensus that laxatives are needed in patients receiving narcotic therapy, the best type and dose is unknown (38,39). Tolerance may not develop to the constipating effect of narcotics, unlike the sedation or nausea produced by these drugs, and most authors suggest that the use of laxatives should be continued for as long as patients continue to receive narcotics.

Other Drugs

Some other drugs have been suggested to have an analgesic effect in specific pain syndromes. For example, anticonvulsants, oral local anesthetics, and clonidine are used in neuropathic pain (40) and antibiotics are administered for the sudden aggravation of pain in ulcerated tumors (41). Studies are currently being conducted on drugs such as clonidine, calcium channel blockers, calcitonin, and baclofen. Most of the evidence available for the effects of these drugs results from anecdotal reports or open trials.

Future Research

Numerous studies of adjuvant drugs are needed. Some of the most important are as follows:

Nonnarcotic Analgesics

A better definition of the effects of these agents in different types of pain is needed (e.g., visceral, neuropathic, incidental, etc). Because of their different side effects and mechanism of action, a comparison between acetaminophen and

NSAIDs in cancer pain would be useful. Among NSAIDs, the best type and dose has not been defined as yet.

Tricyclics

Research on these drugs is complicated by their long latency to maximal effects and their high incidence of side effects. Although several controlled trials were started on these drugs as adjuvants for cancer pain, only one was published, in abstract form (12). A potential study on those drugs will be even more complicated in view of their recently suggested effect on the bioavailability of morphine (15). However, because they are frequently used as adjuvants by some groups and rarely used by others, these drugs should be studied in a controlled trial. Such a study could very likely require a multicenter effort.

Corticosteroids

The nature and duration of the effects of these drugs need better characterization. The best drug and dose of corticosteroid should also be established. The potential for additive toxicity suggests that they should not be combined with NSAIDs; a comparison of both drugs as narcotic adjuvants would be desirable.

Amphetamines

The indication of their use, as well as the proper type and dose, should be better defined.

Antiemetics

Comparative trials to assess effectiveness and toxicity should be performed among metoclopramide, haloperidol, prochlorperazine, and corticosteroids. The newer antiemetics, such as modified benzamides (36) or antiserotonergic drugs (37) should be tried as narcotic adjuvants. This is an area in which prospective studies are almost nonexistent.

Laxatives

Prospective comparative trials should be designed in narcotic-induced constipation to assess effectiveness, toxicity, and patient satisfaction and compliance. The last two endpoints are very important, given the need for long-term use of laxatives in patients receiving narcotics. These patients frequently experience anorexia and chronic nausea, both of which make the treatment more difficult.

Other Drugs

The rest of the drugs included in Table 1 have been suggested to have adjuvant analgesic effects. Osteoclast-inhibiting agents, such as diphosphonates (52) or calcitonin (53), are potentially useful drugs for bone pain. Antibiotic trials should be performed in patients with sudden aggravation of pain owing to ulcerated tumors (41). Because information on the potential adjuvant effects of these drugs is extremely limited, uncontrolled trials of different dosages of these agents should be tried before long-term, expensive controlled trials. These uncontrolled trials would help to define the type, duration, and endpoints of the controlled trial.

GUIDELINES FOR CLINICAL TRIALS IN ADJUVANT DRUGS

Clinical research on adjuvant drugs presents the investigator with a series of unique obstacles related to the characteristics of the drug under investigation, the patient population, and the nature of the effects that will be measured. The major considerations can be summarized as follows:

The Drug

As discussed previously, an adjuvant drug may be useful because it potentiates the analgesic effects of the narcotic (e.g., NSAIDs), or decreases narcotic-induced toxicity (e.g., laxatives), or does both (e.g., amphetamines). Thus, one constant characteristic of these trials is that patients are already receiving narcotic drugs. The interaction between the adjuvant drug and the narcotic is therefore a critical aspect of these studies. For example, the adjuvant drug may have effects on the bioavailability of the narcotic as suggested in a recent report demonstrating that orally administered imipramine can increase the bioavailability of morphine, possibly by reducing its rate of elimination (14). A study of an antiemetic that can increase gastric emptying also showed a change in the rate of absorption of orally administered narcotics (42).

In these two cases, the interaction between the narcotic and the adjuvant drug may significantly affect the final results. In the second case (antiemetics that increase gastric emptying) the potential bias can be easily eliminated by studying the antiemetic effects in patients receiving parenteral narcotics. In the first case (drugs that could increase the bioavailability of narcotics), one way of evaluating the potential for bias would be to measure plasma narcotic levels in patients followed until steady state is approached before and after the addition of the adjuvant. Another way would be to use a patient-controlled analgesic system to allow patients to adjust their dose to a stable degree of analgesia before and after addition of the adjuvant. If a lower dose of the narcotic yields a similar level of pain control in the absence of any change in blood level of the drugs, it can be assumed that the adjuvant narcotic works only by increasing the bioavailability of the narcotic. On the other hand, if less drug is needed to provide similar symptom control in the presence of a lower steady-state blood level of the narcotic, it can be assumed that there is a genuine analgesic potentiating effect.

One of the most sensitive areas of interaction between a narcotic and an adjuvant drug is that of increased sedation or confusion by the addition of the adjuvant. Comparisons between oral morphine solutions and the Brompton's cocktail (43) showed that the addition of other drugs in the cocktail did not result in analgesic potentiation, but did result in an increased incidence of central side effects. An increased level of obtundation or confusion in patients may result in decreased demand for analgesic drug, regardless of residual pain. Therefore, the simple measurement of "narcotic-sparing effect" (e.g., the degree of narcotic dose reduction following the adjuvant) is not an adequate measure of analgesic efficacy, particularly when the symptom assessment and the administration of the drugs are done by a third person. If the adjuvant drug has as possible side effects sedation or confusion (e.g., benzodiazepines, phenothiazines, antihistaminics), it is important to assess prospectively the cognitive status and the level of sedation of the patient during administration of the study drug and control. If the "narcotic-sparing effect" or the "blinded" choice by the patient and investigator are accompanied by a significant cognitive deterioration or increased sedation, it cannot be ruled out that the effects are just a consequence of increased central toxicity by the adjuvant drug.

If the adjuvant drug is likely to potentiate narcotic-induced sedation, patients should be asked at the end of the trial if they believe that they had received the adjuvant drug or placebo, and why, in order to assess the effectiveness of the blinding. One double-blind placebo-controlled crossover study of cyproheptadine by our group was canceled after 13 consecutive patients easily recognized the drug phase because of somnolence. This failure might have been avoided by doing a pilot study in a small number of patients. Some studies mask the sedating effect by controlling the results not only with a placebo, but also with other drugs with sedative effects (44,45). This is likely to improve blinding, but is also likely to make the trial longer and more complicated.

Long-Acting Drugs

For drugs with a long latency to maximal effect, such as tricyclic antidepressants, patients will need to receive the drug or placebo for several days before an assessment can take place. If a crossover design is tried under these conditions, the status of the patients' symptoms may change significantly before the completion of the trial. This change may relate to the development of tolerance to opiate-induced effects, including analgesia, sedation, or nausea, or to the development of new complications of the disease, such as confusion or bowel obstruction. In trials performed in advanced cancer patients, the number of nonevaluable patients at the end of the study may be large enough to invalidate the results. For these reasons, some investigators [e.g., Walsh (13)] choose a parallel-group design for the comparison of the effects of the adjuvant drug. There are problems associated with this choice: (a) the power of the trial decays very significantly; (b) a deterioration in the cognitive status or sedation in the patient population receiving the study drug may not be easily perceived; and (c) the final choice of the patient and investigator, as an overall assessment of satisfaction, is lost. Finally, it is important to consider that the long latency may not necessarily be true for all the effects of the drug. For example, although the antidepressant effect of tricyclics takes place approximately 2 or 3 weeks after starting the treatment, analgesic effects in postherpetic neuralgia takes place between 48 and 72 hrs after they are started (12). Similarly, although the maximal effect of an NSAID in the treatment of rheumatic conditions usually takes several weeks, its effect on cancer pain usually can be measured after just a couple of days (8).

Before embarking on a long and expensive controlled trial of a new adjuvant, it is extremely useful to perform a pilot uncontrolled trial in a small number of patients. This study can determine the onset of action and duration of the different effects of the new adjuvant. During this pilot trial, it is also possible to test different doses of the drug under study. Although the placebo effect is not systematically evaluated in these trials, they provide information about the characteristics of the drug and both the power and appropriateness of the trial that is being designed. Comparing the results of this trial with historical controls provides information very useful in planning the controlled trial.

Short-Acting Drugs

In the case of short-acting drugs, the design is much more simple. A double-blind, crossover trial is almost mandatory for proper assessment of these drugs. The power of this design is much higher than that of parallel design, and it allows for a blinded choice by patients and investigators. This blinded choice provides an overall estimation of the satisfaction with the new agent.

Some drugs should not be tested in a double-blind crossover trial, despite a short effect. Drugs with sedating effects may not be evaluated well this way, since the patient and investigator are much more likely to discriminate the effects and side effects of drugs in a crossover trial. Therefore, drugs with a significant number of side effects may need to be given in a very low dose or to be tested in a parallel-group design, in which the patient is not given the opportunity to compare the study drug with placebo. Other drugs that may not be used in a short-term crossover trial are those that have a rapid onset of action but a long-lasting effect. For example, a study of the effect of antibiotics on the pain of ulcerated tumors could not be designed as a crossover trial because of the significant effect that 3 or 4 days of antibiotic therapy would have on the natural history of local infection.

The Patient Population

Clinical trials should be performed in a population that resembles as much as possible the population that will clinically benefit from the use of the drug on a daily basis. Unfortunately, in an effort to better characterize the biological effects of certain agents and to simplify the clinical trial, investigators frequently study patients who are more stable than those who would ultimately benefit from the new treatment. One example of this problem is the development of long-acting morphine preparations. Most of the studies on these new agents were done in a population of very stable patients requiring an overall low dose of narcotics (46–48). The results from these trials cannot be applied to populations of patients with severe pain, who require much higher doses of narcotics and have significant impairment of the gastrointestinal motility. The bioavailability of the long-acting preparation may be significantly different in these patients than those in an earlier stage of the disease.

Sometimes, the characteristics of the drug preclude evaluation in the population that would most likely employ it. If this is the case, the investigators should report this fact in the "patients and methods" section and discuss the possible impact of the patient population on the final results of the study.

The patient population should be properly characterized using all known prognostic parameters. In the case of a crossover trial, this will help other investigators and clinicians to understand the population in which the trial was performed. In the case of a parallel-group trial, this information is even more important. These patients should be stratified according to the most important prognostic factors before randomization takes place. Factors that should be considered include pain mechanism (neuropathic versus nonneuropathic pain), temporal features of the pain (incidental versus continuous pain), high or rapidly increasing doses of narcotics, and severe psychological distress. A staging system has been proposed that considers all these prognostic factors (49). Patients with a history of severe alcoholism or drug addiction or with cognitive impairment should be detected before admission to the trial and considered ineligible. The statement "pain due to cancer," which is, unfortunately, considered an acceptable characterization of the pain syndrome by most medical journals (50) must be carefully explained in the reported results of these trials.

It is important to consider how many potentially eligible patients can be entered in the trial within a reasonable period of time. The assistance of a biostatistician is invaluable at this stage of the planning of a trial. By postulating what would be considered a clinically relevant difference between study drug and control, the number of cases needed to significantly reject a type II error (the possibility that a real adjuvant effect exists even if the study does not find it) can be estimated. The probability that the study will be able to reject this type II error is defined as the "power" of the study. As noted, study power is relatively less with a parallel-group design than a crossover design.

In some studies, large numbers of patients are required to answer some fundamental questions concerning the effects of different drugs. Even the largest individual centers may not be able to perform such trials. In cancer medicine, this problem has been overcome very successfully by the creation of cooperative groups. These groups are able to design a significant number of clinical trials, and all the member institutions cooperate by entering patients. Unfortunately, no such group exists for clinical research in pain.

If the problem under study occurs very rarely and patients remain stable for long periods of time, the "N of 1" design can be used. This has been discussed in depth by McQuay (see Chapter 7).

The Endpoints of the Study

An adjuvant drug given to a patient who is already receiving a narcotic analgesic can change the effects of the narcotic on the patient (e.g., analgesia, nausea, sedation, constipation, etc.) or have therapeutic and side effects of its own (in the case of a tricyclic antidepressant, for example, antidepressant effects occur with autonomic effects, dry mouth, hypotension, and arrhythmias). For these reasons, the effects of an adjuvant drug on a patient who is already receiving a narcotic can be extremely complex. Moreover, different effects can have a varying latency (in the case of a tricyclic, dry mouth and sedation can occur immediately, whereas analgesia requires 3 or 4 days, and mood effects can accrue for weeks), duration, and intensity.

From this, it is evident that no single study is able to fully characterize the adjuvant effects of a given drug. Short-term, intensive crossover trials will provide ample information on the acute effects of an adjuvant drug, but miss some of the important long-term effects. Less intensive, long-term studies will determine long-term effectiveness and side effects, but potentially miss early effects. Research on amphetamines provides a useful example of these problems. Forrest et al. (25) proved in an elegant double-blind study that a single dose of dextroamphetamine was able to potentiate morphine-induced analgesia and decrease sedation. However, it is not possible to conclude from this study that repeated doses of amphetamines are useful adjuvants for cancer pain. Our group found in two short-term crossover trials that amphetamines could decrease narcotic-induced sedation in cancer patients and potentiate analgesia (27,28), but significant toxicity and a rapid development of tolerance were detected. The results of our studies suggest that amphetamines can be useful adjuvants, at least for the short term, in some patients with pain owing to advanced cancer. However, from our studies it cannot be assumed that amphetamines will be useful during long-term administration.

The finding of a significant improvement in one or more isolated variables does not necessarily mean that an adjuvant drug will be clinically useful. For example, at the end of our double-blind, crossover trial of mazindol, patients had significantly better pain control and lower analgesic consumption on mazindol compared to placebo (27), but their overall preferences were equally distributed between "drug," "placebo," and "no choice." In the case of mazindol, the low level of patient satisfaction with the drug was probably owing to the significant anxiety and anorexia it caused (27). This fact could be determined because we were measuring several other variables in addition to pain. However, even the simultaneous measurement of several variables will not always provide an explanation for the observed global satisfaction or dissatisfaction. It is always possible that deterioration occurs in a variable that is not measured or that the patient's choice reflects improvement or deterioration of several variables combined, each of which does not independently reach statistical significance. A recent trial of clonidine in the treatment of anticipatory nausea in patients receiving chemotherapy is illustrative: Although clonidine was able to decrease anticipatory nausea, patients preferred not to receive it in subsequent courses of chemotherapy and the reasons for this remain unclear (51).

Although it is useful to combine objective variables (daily dose of narcotics, number of rescue doses, number of vomiting episodes, etc.) and subjective variables (pain intensity, nausea, somnolence, confusion, etc.) in these trials, it must be clear that the clinical usefulness of an adjuvant drug will depend on its ability to modify the subjective parameter. A "narcotic sparing effect" is only important for the patient's comfort if it is associated with decreased toxicity (e.g., decreased narcotic-induced toxicity without significant toxicity by the adjuvant), or improved pain control.

SUMMARY AND CONCLUSIONS

Patients with chronic cancer pain suffer from many distressing symptoms in addition to pain. Narcotic analgesics are very likely to improve pain, but will not improve and may actually worsen some of the other symptoms. Therefore, multidrug treatment will be unavoidable in this population. Unfortunately, the evidence for the efficacy of most of the adjuvant drugs is anecdotal. During recent years, efforts have been made to better characterize the effects of some of the adjuvant drugs. Although some improvement has occurred, prospective, well-designed clinical trials are badly needed in this area.

REFERENCES

1. Foley K. The treatment of cancer pain. *N Engl J Med* 1985;313:84–95.
2. *Cancer pain: a monograph on the management of cancer pain.* Health and Welfare Canada; Minister of Supply and Services, Ottawa, Ontario, Canada. H42-2/5-1984E.
3. Foley K, Portenoy R, MacDonald RN, Bruera E. Cancer pain. *Am Soc Clin Oncol Educational Booklet* 1988;79–82.
4. Bruera E, Fox R, Chadwick S, et al. Changing patterns in the treatment of pain and other symptoms in cancer patients. *J Pain Symptom Manag* 1987;2:139–51.
5. Bruera E, Brenneis C, Michaud M, et al. Influence of the Pain and Symptom Control Team on the patterns of treatment of pain and other symptoms in a cancer center. *J Pain Symptom Manag* 1989;4(2):112–116.
6. Twycross R, Lack S. *Symptom control for advanced cancer: pain relief.* London: Pitman, 1984.
7. Bruera E, Navigante A, Barugel M, et al. Treatment of pain and other symptoms in cancer patients. Patterns in a North American and a South American hospital. *J Pain Symptom Manag* 1990;5(2):78–82.

8. Ferrer-Brechner T, Ganz P. Combination therapy with ibuprofen and methadone for chronic cancer pain. *Am J Med* 1984;77:78–83.
9. Brodie G. Indomethacin and bone pain. *Lancet* 1988;2:1180.
10. Walsh T, Saunders C. Hospice care: the treatment of pain in advanced cancer. *Recent Results Cancer Res* 1984;89:201–211.
11. Derogatis L, Feidstein M, Morrow G, et al. A survey of psychotropic drug prescriptions in an oncology population. *Cancer* 1979;44:1919–1929.
12. Watson C, Evans R, Reed K, et al. Amitryptiline versus placebo in post-herpetic neuralgia. *Neurology* 1982;32:671–673.
13. Walsh TD. Controlled study of imipramine and morphine in chronic pain due to cancer. *Proc Am Soc Clin Oncol* 1986;5:237.
14. Feinman C. Pain relief by antidepressants: possible modes of action. *Pain* 1985;23:1–8.
15. Ventafridda V, Ripamonti C, De Conno F, et al. Antidepressants increase bioavailability of morphine in cancer patients. *Lancet* 1987;1:1204.
16. Shell H. Adrenal corticosteroid therapy in far-advanced cancer. *Geriatrics* 1972;27:131–141.
17. Moertel C, Shutte A, Reitemeir R, et al. Corticosteroid therapy in pre-terminal gastrointestinal cancer. *Cancer* 1974;33:1607–1609.
18. Bruera E, Roca E, Cedaro L, et al. Action of oral methylprednisolone in terminal cancer patients: a prospective randomized double-blind study. *Cancer Treat Rep* 1985;69:751–754.
19. Stimmel B. Barbiturates, nonbarbiturate hypnotics and minor tranquilizers. In: Stimmel B, ed. *Pain, analgesia and addiction.* Raven Press, New York, 1983;170–190.
20. Artru A. Midazolam potentiates the analgesic effect of morphine in patients with postoperative pain. *Clin J Pain* 1986;2:92–100.
21. Stimmel B. Tranquilizers. In: Stimmel B, ed. *Pain, analgesia and addiction.* Raven Press, New York, 1983;190–201.
22. Evans W, Beryner D. A comparison of the analgesic effect of morphine, pentazocine, and a mixture of metamphetamine and pentazocine in the rat. *J New Drugs* 1964;4:82–85.
23. Ivy A, Goetzl F, Burril D. Morphine-dextroamphetamine analgesia. *War Med* 1984;6:67–77.
24. Weiner N. Amphetamines. In: Gilman A, Goodman L, Gilman A, eds. *The pharmacological basis of therapeutics.* New York: Macmillan, 1980;159–162.
25. Forrest W, Brown B, Brown C, et al. Dextroamphetamine with morphine for the treatment of post-operative pain. *N Engl J Med* 1977;296:712–715.
26. Josh J, DeJongh C, Schnapper N, et al. Amphetamine therapy for enhancing the comfort of terminally ill patients with cancer. *Proc Am Soc Clin Oncol* 1982;C-210:55.
27. Bruera E, Carraro S, Roca E, et al. Double-blind evaluation of mazindol in enhancing the comfort of terminally ill cancer patients. *Cancer Treat Rep* 1986;70:295–298.
28. Bruera E, Chadwick S, Brenneis C, et al. Methylphenidate associated with narcotics for the treatment of cancer pain. *Cancer Treat Rep* 1987;71:67–70.
29. Katon W, Raskind M. Treatment of depression in the medically ill elderly with methlyphenidate. *Am J Psychiatry* 1980;137:963–965.
30. Bruera E, Brenneis C, Michaud M, et al. Use of methylphenidate as an adjuvant to narcotic analgesics in patients with advanced cancer. *J Pain Symptom Manag* 1989;4(1):3–6.
31. Bruera E, Chadwick S, Fox R, Hanson J. Study of autonomic insufficiency in advanced cancer patients. *Cancer Treat Rep* 1986;70:1383–1387.
32. Bruera E, Catz Z, Hooper R, et al. Chronic nausea and anorexia in advanced cancer patients: a possible role for autonomic dysfunction. *J Pain Symptom Manag* 1987;2:19–21.
33. Manara L, Bianchetti A. The central and peripheral influence of opioids on gastrointestinal propulsion. *Annu Rev Pharmacol Toxicol* 1985;75:249–273.
34. Bruera E, Brenneis C, Michaud M, et al. Continuous subcutaneous infusion of metoclopramide for the treatment of the narcotic bowel syndrome. *Cancer Treat Rep* 1987;71:1121–1122.
35. Billings A. Nausea and vomiting. In: Billings A, ed. *Outpatient management of advanced cancer.* Philadelphia: Lippincott, 1985;45–56.
36. Smaldone L, Fiarchild C, Rozencweig M, et al. Dose-range evaluation of BMY-25801, a non-dopaminergic antiemetic. *Proc Am Soc Clin Oncol* 1988;7:280.
37. Kris M, Gralla R, Tyson L, et al. Phase I study of the serotonin antagonist GR-C507 when used as an antiemetic. *Proc Am Soc Clin Oncol* 1988;7:283.
38. Manara L, Bianchetti A. The central and peripheral influences of opioids on gastrointestional propulsion. *Annu Rev Pharmacol Toxicol* 1985;25:249–273.

39. Billings A. Constipation, diarrhea and other gastrointestional problems. In: Billings A, ed. *Outpatient management of advanced cancer.* Philadelphia: Lippincott, 1985;69–72.
40. Maciewicz R, Boukons A, Martin J. Drug therapy of neuropathic pain. *Clin J Pain* 1985;1:39–49.
41. Bruera E, MacDonald RN. Intractable pain in patients with advanced head and neck tumors: a possible role for local infection. *Cancer Treat Rep* 1986;70:691–692.
42. Manara A, Shelly M, Quinn K, et al. The effect of metoclopramide on the absorption of oral controlled release morphine. *Br J Clin Pharmacol* 1988;25:518–521.
43. Twycross R. Effect of codeine in the Brompton cocktail. In: Bonica J, Ventafridda V, eds. *Advances in pain research,* vol 3. New York: Raven Press, 1979;627–632.
44. Woodcock A, Gross E, Gellery A. A comparison of diazepam and promethazine in the treatment of breathlessness in patients with chronic obstructive lung disease. *Br Med J* 1982;1:96–99.
45. Woodcock A, Gross E, Gellery A, et al. Effects of dihydrocodeine, alcohol and caffeine on breathlessness and exercise tolerance in patients with chronic obstructive lung disease. *N Engl J Med* 1981;305:1611–1618.
46. Hanks G, Twycross R, Bliss J. Controlled release morphine tablets: a double-blind trial in patients with advanced cancer. *Anaesthesia* 1987;42:840–844.
47. Walsh TD. Clinical evaluation of slow release morphine tablets. *Proc Am Soc Clin Oncol* 1985;4:266.
48. MacDonald RN, Bruera E, Brenneis C, et al. Long acting morphine in the treatment of cancer pain: a double-blind, crossover trial. *Proc Am Soc Clin Oncol* 1987;6:1054.
49. Bruera E, Macmillan K, MacDonald RN, Hanson J. The Edmonton staging system for cancer pain: preliminary report. *Pain* 1989;37:203–209.
50. MacDonald RN, Bruera E. Clinical trials in cancer pain. In: Foley K, Ventafridda V, eds. *Recent advances in pain research.* New York: Raven Press, 1989;16:443–449.
51. Fetting J, Stefanek M, Sheidlen J, et al. Noradrenergic activity in anticipatory nausea. *Proc Am Soc Clin Oncol* 1988;7:284.
52. Chung A, Chantrinia A, et al. Use of diphosphonate in metastatic bone disease. *N Engl J Med* 1983;308:1499–1501.
53. Vaughn C, Vaitkevicius K. The effects of calcitonin in hypendiemia in patients with malignancy. *Cancer* 1974;34:1268–1271.

Advances in Pain Research and Therapy, Vol. 18,
edited by M. Max, R. Portenoy, and E. Laska,
Raven Press, Ltd., New York © 1991.

Commentary

Chronic Studies of Adjuvants to Opiate Analgesics

T. Declan Walsh

*Palliative Care Service, Department of Hematology and Medical Oncology,
Cleveland Clinic Foundation, Cleveland, Ohio 44195-5236*

Polypharmacy is the rule rather than the exception in treating cancer patients, and it is interesting to compare the use of adjuvant drugs reported by Bruera from Edmonton, Canada, to those reported from St. Christopher's Hospice, London (Table 1), where all patients are seen by a palliative care physician (1). Although mandatory for optimal symptom control, polypharmacy may produce drug interactions and unwanted drug effects. Because of disturbed pathophysiology, pharmacokinetics may be altered in unexpected ways, and assessment of these interactions using pharmacokinetic or pharmacodynamic models is complex. Thus, studies that evaluate adjuvant drugs for analgesia in cancer should certainly be demonstrating efficacy, but just as importantly should define the side effect profile. Cancer pain research has suffered in the past from transferring inappropriate and misleading lessons about opioids from noncancer pain populations to the cancer population. The same applies to the adjuvant drugs, e.g., lessons learned from the use of corticosteroids in the rheumatoid arthritis population may or may not be relevant to the use of these drugs in cancer pain. Bruera mentions patient satisfaction and compliance in relation to the use of laxatives, but these are important criteria in the assessment of other agents, too. Such global assessments give a clinically powerful indicator of patient acceptability, and may also detect unanticipated side effects of medications not included in a standard checklist.

Cancer pain is not homogeneous, and though research into the use of adjuvant agents is needed, we must recognize that we are dealing with a complex phenomenon. A principal difficulty relates to the correct diagnosis of the cause of the cancer pain, particularly when the patient is suffering from more than one pain. Another difficulty lies in the frequency of incident pain, and how best to assess and evaluate its response to therapeutic intervention. We need a series of studies that is targeted for specific pain problems, e.g., brachial plexopathy, with appropriately delineated specific interventions and endpoints.

TABLE 1. *Adjuvant drugs used for symptom control in patients with advanced cancer*[a]

Drug	(%)
Phenothiazines	87
Corticosteroids	57
Night sedation	54
Antiemetics[b]	44
Daytime sedatives	35
Nonsteroidal antiinflammatory drugs	32
Antidepressants	19
Anticonvulsants	8

[a] n = 676.
[b] Excluding phenothiazines.

Although the therapeutic role of tricyclic antidepressants in cancer pain management is still unclear, it is noteworthy that we will have agents in the future with specific activities in relation to particular monoamine pathways. The bulk of the animal data supports the concept that compounds that potentiate monoamine activity in the central nervous system are likely to increase opioid analgesia, and may also have independent analgesic activity. It is unclear, however, if this effect is going to be therapeutically important. If, as demonstrated in one study (2), all that is achieved is a reduction in the total morphine dose that would have otherwise been required (for the same level of pain control), i.e., an opioid-sparing effect, it can be argued that this is a complicated means of achieving optimal pain control. It is noteworthy that the study that demonstrated opioid-sparing effects observed side effects in the tricyclic treatment group (imipramine/morphine) that were nearly identical to those in the placebo (placebo/morphine) group.

Side effects with corticosteroids are a problem, although I would disagree with Bruera and suggest that myopathy is a common and relatively early (if under-diagnosed) complication, rather than an outcome associated only with prolonged use. Although the corticosteroids have multiple actions, one important effect in advanced cancer may be inhibition of production of tumor necrosis factor (TNF). Many of the problems associated with advanced disease could be attributed to the activities of TNF. Inhibition of its production may be the reason for the multisystem and often dramatic improvements in well-being associated with the introduction of corticosteroids.

Insofar as the role of psychostimulants is concerned, although there are undoubtedly some patients in whom opioid-induced sedation occurs, I am unclear as to the frequency and severity of this problem. Nevertheless, the potential benefit from the introduction of methylphenidate is clearly shown in the elegant study by Bruera.

Some units caring for patients with advanced cancer routinely employ a prophylactic antiemetic prescribed at the same time that morphine is introduced. The incidence of opioid-induced nausea is unclear, but it is noteworthy that it appears more common in females. At St. Christopher's Hospice, a routine prescription of prochlorperazine 5 mg po q 4 hr was given along with each dose of morphine. Such doses of prochlorperazine are in the antipsychotic range, and the rationale for routine use of an antiemetic in this situation has never been clarified. At the Cleveland Clinic Foundation Palliative Care Service, it is our practice not to use antiemetics in this way unless nausea or vomiting ensue or there is a history of gastrointestinal intolerance to opioids. It should be noted that the incidence of morphine-induced nausea and vomiting may also be related to the vehicle or formulation for the morphine that varies considerably in different countries.

More common than opiate-induced nausea and/or vomiting, many cancer patients have symptoms of early satiety, suggestive of delayed gastric emptying, that may possibly be secondary to an autonomic neuropathy. This has been shown to be reversed by metoclopramide (3), although the clinical implications of this, and its potential effects on morphine pharmacokinetics are unclear.

Insofar as the design of clinical trials for adjuvant drugs are concerned, I wholeheartedly support Bruera's remarks, but wish to emphasize that these studies must be done in realistic clinical situations, and not in excessively artificial and constrained designs. If studies are to be meaningful and change clinical practice, they must reflect how drugs are given clinically, i.e., in combination and in repeated dosage. Furthermore, studies should be conducted in appropriate patient populations; for example, studies conducted in a hospice inpatient population may only be of relevance to that population and not to patients at much earlier stages of the disease. Visual analogue scales, although useful in patients with advanced cancer, are in my view fraught with difficulties that must be borne in mind in study design. Use of a psychotropic agent or opioid may in and of itself interfere with the patient's completion of the data required for the study of that drug. We have little information on psychometric assessment in this population. Assessment of performance status and measurement of quality of life is essential in studies of this population.

Difficulties exist with all study designs; obvious side effects, for example, may invalidate a crossover study. Some of these problems can be obviated by careful stratification of patients at the baseline and, if necessary, by weighting of specific criteria before entry to the study. It is very difficult to do "clean" studies in cancer patients. In my experience, study design, e.g., crossover or parallel-group design, are ultimately decided by pragmatic considerations, rather than statistical rigor. An important feature of the reporting of these studies is a description of the total number of patients who were evaluated for the study, with a breakdown of those patients who agreed to enter the study and those who actually fulfilled the predetermined study criteria. Studies should use appropriate drug administration, including flexibility of dosage for the agent under consideration, as well as predetermined criteria of efficacy and side effects. This will allow more realistic evaluation of the agent as it will be used in clinical practice.

Lastly, I would offer the comment that it is troubling to me that the major funding agencies for cancer research throughout the world have tended to neglect cancer pain research. Millions of dollars are spent annually in supporting investigation of potential chemotherapeutic agents that are unlikely ever to have any impact on cancer care. Little or no systematic research has been conducted in the symptomatic management of advanced disease, work that could have great benefits for the 500,000 people who die from cancer every year.

REFERENCES

1. Walsh TD, Cheater FM. Use of morphine for cancer pain. *Pharm J* 1983;231:525–527.
2. Walsh TD. Controlled study of imipramine (Im) and morphine (M) in chronic pain due to advanced cancer. *Proc Am Soc Clin Oncol* 1986;5:237.
3. Kris MG, Yeh SDJ, Gralla RJ, et al. Symptomatic gastroparesis in cancer patients—a possible cause of cancer-associated anorexia that can be improved with oral metoclopramide. *Proc Am Soc Clin Oncol* 1985;4:267.

Advances in Pain Research and Therapy, Vol. 18,
edited by M. Max, R. Portenoy, and E. Laska,
Raven Press, Ltd., New York © 1991.

Commentary

Issues for Chronic Pain Models with Specific Emphasis on the Chronic Cancer Pain Model

John E. Stambaugh

*Oncology and Hematology Associates, P.A., Haddon Heights, New Jersey 08035; and
Department of Pharmacology, Thomas Jefferson University Medical College,
Philadelphia, Pennsylvania 19107*

With the exception of arthritis, cancer pain represents the only chronic pain that has resulted in numerous reports of clinical analgesic trials. Whereas most chronic nonmalignant pain is not considered to be caused predominately by ongoing nociceptive activity, chronic cancer pain (Table 1) is primarily nociceptive pain since it is associated with increasing tissue damage from the cancer or the treatments (1–3). Indeed, cancer pain may be better described as long-standing acute pain.

Chronic cancer pain lends itself to repeat-dose studies. It should be apparent, however, that not all cancer pain is chronic and that all cancer pain is not alike. Recent studies have identified subgroups of patients with cancer pain who respond differently to analgesics. Even in the same patient, pain from one source may not respond in the same way as pain from another source. For example, comparison of osseous versus nonosseous pain, especially in studies evaluating nonsteroidal antiinflammatory drugs may be important.

Since cancer pain requires repeated and chronic doses of analgesics for control, studies of cancer pain can provide information about the frequency of dosing, drug tolerance, carryover effects, relative potency, pharmacokinetics, and cumulative side effects. In analgesic trials, cancer pain can be characterized with the same verbal, visual, and global descriptors used in single-dose acute pain studies. In addition, the very severe pain that may occur in cancer patients, which unfortunately too often represents a management dilemma in a clinical cancer practice, can be used to study potent analgesics, development of tolerance, and steady-state kinetics of continuous infusions of analgesics.

The use of the cancer pain model has certain unique restrictions not observed in other models. Accurate side effect data are difficult to obtain owing to the

TABLE 1. *Sources of cancer-related chronic pain—bone involvement is the major component*

Pain associated with the cancer
    Soft tissue infiltration
    Bone involvement
    Nerve compression
    Raised cerebral pressure, meningeal, brain or spinal cord metastasis
    Lymphedema
    Hollow viscus involvement; intestine, bladder, etc.
    Lung, liver, or other organ involvement
    Invasion into vascular structures—venous or arterial occlusion, thrombosis, rupture
    Muscle involvement with tumor
    Fractures, dislocations
    Eroding prosthesis, joints
    Edema; joint, ascites, pericardial, pleura
    Tumor surrounding edema
Pain owing to cancer therapy
    Postsurgical pain—acute vs chronic
    Paracentesis, thoracentesis, pleurodesis, instillation of sclerosing agents or chemotherapy
    Amputation
    Radiation-induced fibrosis, inflammation, edema
    Chemotherapy toxicity—neuropathy, stomatitis gastritis, colitis, ulceration at injection site
    Aseptic necrosis
    Infection
    Neuralgias; infectious, inflammatory
    Injection portal catheter, shunt, prosthesis complications
Pain in cancer patients unrelated to cancer or cancer treatment
    Degenerative bone disease, discogenic spine disease
    Noncancer surgery
    Chronic neuralgias
    Diabetic complications
    Gastritis, peptic ulcer disease
    Angina
    Headaches
    Others

alternative therapies, such as radiation and chemotherapy, that are simultaneously administered to these patients. Psychological disturbances, including severe denial, depression, and anxiety may occur and compromise pain assessment. Studies of opioid efficacy are more difficult in patients with a substantial previous exposure to opioids, although analgesia from increased doses or alternative analgesics can be determined.

Some inclusion/exclusion criteria for repeat dose chronic cancer pain studies are shown in Table 2. The exclusion criteria for cancer pain repeat-dose studies differ from the criteria that would be used for single-dose cancer pain studies. Patient selection factors that predict compliance with record keeping are extremely important in repeat-dose trials. Other criteria may be added according to the specific agent under study.

It is very important in cancer clinical trials to record demographics and clearly define underlying disorders, such as cardiac disease, liver disease, and kidney disease. These data are needed for inclusion/exclusion parameters and for posthoc or covariate analyses. To simply state the patient has no significant hepatic disease

TABLE 2. *Patient eligibility criteria for chronic cancer pain studies*

Inclusion criteria
  Male or female, age 18–75
  Moderate to severe chronic pain owing to cancer requiring analgesic medication
  Ability to comply with study requirements and to swallow and absorb oral medication (or take injectable analgesics)
  Able to understand the study purposes and to give informed consent
Exclusion criteria
  Analgesics received within 4 hrs of single-dose portion of the study medication administration
  History of narcotic abuse or tolerance, or receiving potent narcotics for pain relief that would interfere with study results
  Known sensitivity to narcotics or narcotic antagonists
  Concomitant, interfering, or potentially interacting medication within 4 hrs of the single-dose evaluations
  Concomitant chemotherapeutic medications (unless the blood count is stabilized on a maintenance dose)
  Clinically significant cardiac, hepatic, or renal disease or peptic ulcer—clinical parameters should be predefined using clinical and laboratory parameters
  Asthma or severe allergy disorders
  Neurological impairment or psychiatric disorder
  Childbearing potential
  Radiation therapy to the site of pain evaluation (radiation to alternate sites is permitted)

or liver disease is not adequate. Clinical and laboratory parameters should be established, both to better define the patient population in the study and exclude advanced disease states that would alter the results.

Attention to these sources of patient variability in the chronic cancer pain model will enhance the ability to identify treatment effects. The investigator must remember that cancer patients are not normal volunteers, and studies of cancer pain must include the mechanism for recording and analyzing details about the pain, medical condition, prior and current treatments, and psychological status that are not issues in a less ill population.

REFERENCES

1. Twycross RG, Fairfield S. Pain in far advanced cancer pain. *Prim Care Cancer* 1982;14:303–310.
2. Taddeini L, Rotschafer JC. Pain syndromes associated with cancer. *Postgrad Med* 1984;75:101–108.
3. Coyle N, Foley K. Pain in patients with cancer: profile of patients and common pain syndromes. *Semin Oncol Nursing* 1985;1:93–99.

DISCUSSION (Chapters 9 and 10)

Dr. Dwight Moulin: It is important to realize how highly selected are patients who agree to take part in cancer studies. For example, we were studying a novel narcotic analgesic and were able to recruit six patients from 450 potential candidates. It may be difficult to generalize from this patient population and assume that the results apply to the population as a whole.

Dr. Walsh: Some years ago, I was involved with a study that was going to be a potential multicenter study in patients with advanced disease. The Institutional Review Board wanted to take out everybody who had any abnormalities of either renal or hepatic function. When I suggested that those were the very people we wanted to include in the study, they were horrified. I think that these concerns about exclusion criteria are probably one of the major practical difficulties in getting these studies done expeditiously.

Dr. Raymond Houde: The numbers that we get consents on—and we try hard—ranges from about 1 in 7 to about 1 in 12 or 13 who are candidates for study.

Advances in Pain Research and Therapy, Vol. 18,
edited by M. Max, R. Portenoy, and E. Laska,
Raven Press, Ltd., New York © 1991.

11

Low Back Pain

Richard A. Deyo

*Back Pain Outcome Assessment Team, Northwest Health Services Research and
Development Field Program, Seattle VA Medical Center, Seattle, Washington 98108;
and the Departments of Medicine and Health Services, University of Washington,
Seattle, Washington 98195*

CLINICAL BACKGROUND

Low back pain is a pervasive symptom that will affect up to 80% of adults in the United States. Fortunately, the prognosis of acute low back pain is excellent. However, back pain is a symptom, not a diagnosis, and investigators must face the reality that a precise pathoanatomic diagnosis is in most cases unattainable (1). The differential diagnosis of the causes of back pain is lengthy, but serious etiologies such as osteomyelitis and metastatic cancer are unusual (2). Thus, the vast majority of patients have a "mechanical" cause of low back pain, implying that there is no primary infectious, neoplastic, or inflammatory process underlying the pain. Even imaging procedures are often unhelpful in distinguishing among the various mechanical causes of pain. This is true in part because many radiographic diagnoses, including some degenerative changes, spondylolysis, congenital anomalies (e.g., spina bifida occulta), and facet joint changes are found just as frequently in patients with no history of back problems as in those with low back pain (2). Sophisticated imaging procedures also pose difficulties in interpretation. For example, computed tomography, magnetic resonance imaging, and myelography all reveal herniated disks in 10 to 20% of normal persons with no history of low back pain (3–5).

There is even substantial controversy as to the existence of many commonly used diagnoses. For example, some observers argue against the existence of skeletal muscle "spasm" (6), and this is certainly not a reproducible finding even among specialists working in the same clinic (7). Nonetheless, "spasm" has often been used as an entry criterion in drug trials and ostensibly measured as an outcome. The existence of trigger-point syndromes is sufficiently controversial that separate chapters on this issue had to be written in an Institute of Medicine report on chronic pain syndromes (8). The existence of fibrositis as a distinct disease still generates controversy (9), as do the diagnoses of "disk disruption syndrome," "segmental instability," and "sacroiliac strain."

Thus, it may be appropriate for many studies of low back pain to select and describe subjects according to their medical histories and physical findings, rather than by unverifiable diagnoses. Several classifications have been designed for this purpose, typically incorporating as major features the chronicity of back pain, the presence or absence of neurologic deficits, and any history of prior back surgery. At the very least, it is valuable to distinguish between acute and chronic (greater than 3 months) pain syndromes, since nearly all observers would agree that the therapeutic approaches, both pharmacologic and nonpharmacologic, diverge substantially.

The prognosis of acute low back pain is excellent, with 60 to 80% of patients demonstrating substantial improvement within 2 weeks of onset (10–12). This rapid improvement can easily mislead the naive investigator, especially in the absence of appropriate control subjects. Only about 5% of patients will develop chronic pain syndromes persisting beyond 3 months (13). The prognosis for this group is much more guarded, however, and many develop pain "careers" that span many years. In this group, a variety of nonbiologic factors may complicate therapy, including psychological dysfunction, financial disincentives to improvement, hostile work environments, and dysfunctional family interactions.

Common Current Approaches to Drug Therapy

A variety of pharmacologic treatments are advocated for patients with low back pain, with selection often depending on clinical characteristics of the patient. The general categories would include pure analgesic medications, nonsteroidal antiinflammatory drugs (NSAIDs), "muscle relaxants," antidepressant medications, and a variety of injected drugs, including local anesthetics and corticosteroids.

For patients with acute low back pain or sciatica, the most commonly used medications are analgesics, NSAIDs, and muscle relaxants. For the patient with acute severe pain, narcotic analgesics are commonly used, but generally with a specific time limitation. There are few trials of these drugs specifically for patients with low back pain, but their general properties and a large body of clinical experience suggest that they are appropriate and efficacious in the face of acute severe pain, especially with sciatica. A variety of NSAIDs have been tested specifically for patients with low back pain, and these trials have generally demonstrated the superiority of these drugs over placebo treatments (14–16). Thus, convincing trials exist for diflunisal (14,15), naproxen sodium (14), and piroxicam (16), among others. It seems likely that most drugs in this category are efficacious, though many have not been specifically tested in this setting. The drawback of these trials has been that few provided an adequate description of the study subjects, so that it is difficult to know to whom the results are most likely to apply (17).

Muscle relaxant drugs are also widely used for acute pain, but there is greater controversy surrounding their use. In part, this is because of potential habituation to many of these medications, and uncertainty as to whether they have additive effects with analgesics or NSAIDs. Commonly used medications in this category include carisoprodol, diazepam, methocarbamol, and cyclobenzaprine. A newer drug, tizanidine, has recently been marketed for this purpose as well. Evidence for the efficacy for these medications is more scant and less consistent than that for NSAIDs, and has been subject to some unique methodologic pitfalls (17).

Antidepressant drugs are advocated primarily for chronic pain syndromes. Their use for chronic low back pain is in part based on their apparently successful application to other chronic pain syndromes, such as painful neuropathy and headaches. It remains unclear whether these drugs act through a primary analgesic affect, by treating subclinical depression, or by nonspecific methods, such as improving sleep. There is a relatively small literature addressing their use specifically for chronic low back pain, and the validity of this literature is often threatened by high dropout rates (18–20).

A bewildering variety of injected drugs have been used in the treatment of low back pain, administered in a bewildering variety of routes. These have included local anesthetics, corticosteroids, and narcotic analgesics, which may be administered intramuscularly, epidurally, or into putative trigger points. Most of these applications have never been tested in randomized clinical trials, and where such trials exist, they sometimes reach conflicting conclusions (21,22). These injection techniques have generally been used for patients with subacute (6 to 12 weeks) or chronic back pain syndromes.

Other Common Approaches

A variety of nonpharmacologic treatments are also widely employed for back pain and sciatica. Acupuncture and transcutaneous electrical nerve stimulation (TENS) are perhaps the most common of these treatments aimed exclusively at reducing pain. Other treatments purport to alter underlying pathoanatomic abnormalities (e.g., traction, spinal manipulation, and corsets), whereas others are mainly targeted at rehabilitation, such as exercise and physical therapy. Many of the same design issues that arise in drug trials are relevant to studies of these other modalities, and challenges such as blinding are even more problematical.

REVIEW AND CRITIQUE OF STANDARD APPROACHES TO STUDY DESIGN

Barriers Peculiar to Back Pain Research

There are some important peculiarities of research on low back pain that may jeopardize its validity and applicability. The problem of diagnostic ambiguity has been mentioned, and makes this problem different from many pain syndromes, such as those owing to cancer, arthritis, postoperative pain, or trauma. Although a definitive diagnosis may be impossible to identify in up to 85% of patients with low back pain (1), patients vary substantially in their clinical characteristics, and these must be carefully described for a reader to generalize study results.

Unlike the inpatient management of cancer pain or postoperative pain, a wide variety of cotreatments and over-the-counter remedies are available for most patients with low back problems. It is the rule rather than the exception for patients to obtain care for back pain from multiple sources, which may include chiropractors, over-the-counter drugs (e.g., aspirin, acetaminophen, ibuprofen), physical therapists, acupuncturists, primary care physicians, and specialists. Many patients use these sources of care simultaneously and unbeknownst to an investigator. Thus, there is a greater need than in most research areas to identify these cotreatments or attempt to limit them.

The favorable natural history of acute low back pain makes randomized controlled trials particularly important. It also requires frequent follow-up immediately after beginning a therapeutic intervention. Since most patients improve rapidly within weeks of onset of pain, two cohorts of patients may be virtually identical by the time of a 3- or 4-week follow-up. Nonetheless, there may be substantial differences between alternative treatments within the first few days of therapy, so that one group returns to usual activities several days faster than the other. This would be an important therapeutic benefit, but one that could be obscured if outcomes were only measured at a 3-week follow-up. Thus, either daily or multiple weekly measurements are often necessary after initiating therapy in trials for acute low back pain.

The favorable natural history of low back pain may also aggravate the problem of patient dropouts. If patients improve rapidly, they may lose interest in keeping return appointments or continuing study activities. Conversely, it often seems to be the case that patients being treated for chronic pain syndromes are impatient for improvement, and may drop out of a study if they perceive less than dramatic improvement. These patients have often undergone a variety of treatments from a variety of sources, and may be accustomed to making rapid judgments regarding the efficacy of new treatments. In any event, dropping out has been a major problem in many studies of therapy for low back pain, and strenuous efforts to retain subjects are generally necessary and appropriate.

Back pain is also somewhat unique in being an extremely common reason for seeking disability compensation. This appears to be a greater problem than for pain syndromes such as headache, which are unlikely to be recognized by the courts as occupation related. The historical, legal, and social reasons for this aspect of low back pain are complex, but they create problems that an investigator must acknowledge. There is a substantial body of literature suggesting that patients who are seeking disability compensation for low back pain problems respond less well to a variety of treatments, including rehabilitation, surgical intervention, and conservative treatments (23). Thus, investigators may want to identify patients with this social confounder and exclude them, stratify for this characteristic, or otherwise control for its presence in analyzing results. A more general problem is that social and demographic patient characteristics appear to have important prognostic significance in patients with low back pain, and these characteristics may also need to be measured and accounted for. Thus, factors such as educational status, income, and psychological characteristics measured on formal tests have a substantial influence on patient outcomes regardless of therapy (24,25).

The choice of outcome measures for studies of low back pain is problematical, as it is for many pain syndromes. Important outcomes may include not only pain relief, but changes in functional behavior and utilization (cost) of health care services. Quantifying these outcomes is not trivial, and substantial methodologic progress has been made in recent years (26).

A particular problem arises in the evaluation of drugs intended to treat muscle "spasm." As we have noted, the very existence of skeletal muscle spasm has been questioned, and the poor reproducibility of muscle spasm as a physical finding has been demonstrated repeatedly. To add to these problems, clinical trials have typically included patients with low back pain along with patients who have neck pain and even extremity pain syndromes in trials of "muscle relaxants." It may be hazardous to assume that overall results from such a study necessarily apply to the subgroup with low back pain, because the anatomic, physiological, social, and psychological considerations for low back pain differ substantially from other pain syndromes (17). One study that itemized results according to pain syndromes suggested that this concern is more than theoretical: the results for patients with low back pain were worse than for patients with other diagnoses (27).

Finally, low back pain may be a situation in which the use of crossover study designs is often inadvisable. The favorable natural history of acute low back pain, with very rapid improvement, may render crossover designs unfeasible. In the study of nonpharmacologic treatments, crossover designs may be especially hazardous because of difficulty in maintaining adequate blinding. For example, a patient who has experienced both true TENS and sham TENS will readily recognize the difference. Even among patients with chronic low back pain, there is a tendency toward gradual improvement in symptoms and function over time (28), creating potential hazards for a crossover trial. If these problems can be resolved, there remain several hazards of crossover designs that have been summarized elsewhere (29). The threat of patient attrition and the problem of psychological carryover effects may be the most problematical in this particular application.

Common Methodologic Flaws

We have previously reviewed a number of clinical trials for drug therapy and physical treatment of low back pain syndromes (17). We examined these studies for several methodologic criteria that are briefly summarized in Table 1, and include design features relevant both to internal validity (accuracy of results for the individuals within the study) and the applicability or generalizability of results. Table 2 presents the results of this methodologic review that examined clinical trials up until 1982 (17). The findings of this review would generally be true of published studies since that time, as well. The drug trials reviewed were often well designed, but with some common limitations related to the research barriers described above. There was rarely any attempt to assess or control co-interventions. Similarly, possible contamination of groups owing to availability of the same or similar medication from other sources was rarely considered. Compliance was measured in only about half the drug trials, and the adequacy of statistical power was never discussed in the small number of negative studies.

Perhaps the greatest limitation of the drug trials, however, was the failure to provide an adequate description of patients and outcomes. Because back pain

TABLE 1. *Criteria for assessing the validity and applicability of clinical research on conservative treatments for low back pain[a]*

Validity
  Random allocation: The best way to achieve equal distribution of prognostic factors between active treatment and control groups, and eliminate biases that lead to false results.
  Minimal patient attrition: Those who do very well or very poorly are most likely to drop out, biasing the remaining study sample. We required less than 15% attrition to meet this criterion.
  Blind outcome assessment: The best way to reduce investigator bias in measuring outcomes. Though patient blinding is also desirable, a blinded observer was the minimum to meet this criterion.
  Equal co-interventions: A wide variety of treatments for back pain are readily available and may be obtained by subjects in a clinical trial. Some effort to describe or insure equality of co-interventions was required.
  Compliance measured: Therapy cannot work if it is not received. Compliance with physical measures and lifestyle changes is often particularly poor. Inpatient studies were assumed to assure reasonable compliance.
  Minimal contamination: Unintended "crossovers" may occur if patients can obtain a study treatment elsewhere. A study was judged adequate if efforts were made to identify and quantify such "contamination" of study groups, and inpatient trials were assumed to have little contamination.
  Both statistical and clinical significance considered: A substantial clinical effect may fail to be statistically significant if the sample size is too small. For negative trials, some estimate of statistical power was required.
Applicability
  Good demographic description: At least age, sex, and referral source of patients.
  Good clinical description: Duration of pain, neurologic deficits, sciatica, prior surgery, and other entry criteria were considered. A study was required to have four of these five items to judge the clinical description as adequate.
  Treatment adequately described: Dose, duration, frequency, and a reproducible description of technique were required.
  Reporting all relevant outcomes: Four categories were considered: (a) symptoms and physiological changes, (b) functional status, (c) cost of care, and (d) patient perceptions or psychological measures. Reporting was judged adequate if at least one measure was included from three of the four categories.

[a] Adapted from ref. 17.

TABLE 2. *Prevalence of desirable study design features among articles on low back pain*

Study design feature[a]	No. of studies with feature/ total no. of studies (%)	
	Physical treatment trials	Drug therapy trials
Randomization	20/40 (50)	13/19 (68)
Minimal patient attrition	14/20 (70)	11/13 (85)
Blind outcome assessment	13/20 (65)	10/13 (77)
Assurance of equal co-interventions	2/20 (10)	1/13 (8)
Compliance measured[b]	5/20 (25)	6/13 (46)
Contamination reported[c]	5/20 (25)	5/13 (38)
Report of statistical power if no difference between treatments found	0/7 (0)	0/3 (0)
Adequate demographic description	9/20 (45)	7/13 (54)
Adequate clinical description	10/20 (50)	2/13 (15)
Adequate description of intervention	9/20 (45)	13/13 (100)
Most relevant outcomes reported	3/20 (15)	3/13 (23)

[a] With the exception of randomization, all study features were considered only for the 33 randomized trials.

[b] Compliance for inpatient trials was assumed to be good, and this criterion was said to be met.

[c] Contamination was assumed not to occur in inpatient trials, and the criterion was said to be met.

Reproduced with permission from ref. 17.

syndromes are quite heterogeneous in their duration, clinical findings, and prognosis, these details are important in generalizing reported results (28). Furthermore, since back pain may be cared for in a variety of settings and by wide variety of specialists, it is important to describe the source of patients in a clinical trial. Those seeking specialist care may often be a highly selected group which is substantially different from an unselected primary care population. Although most studies provided some demographic description of study subjects, the source of patient enrollment was often omitted. Furthermore, the clinical description of study subjects was generally inadequate, often lacking details such as the duration of pain, presence or absence of sciatica, neurologic deficits, or prior surgical intervention. Finally, the reporting of relevant outcomes was problematical. Though some may argue that only pain relief is a relevant outcome for therapeutic drug trials, others believe that the subjective experience of pain relief is most important if it results in changes in daily functioning, patient satisfaction, or cost of care. These latter outcomes were infrequently reported in most therapeutic trials.

In trials of nonpharmacologic therapy, design threats to the internal validity of results were generally more common than among drug trials. The clinical description of study subjects was often somewhat better, but other details necessary for generalizing study results were as poorly reported as they were for drug trials.

RECOMMENDED APPROACHES TO CLINICAL TRIAL DESIGN

Classification of Patients

Rather than insisting on exhaustive diagnostic efforts prior to study entry (which may often be clinically ill-advised), investigators should select and describe patients according to a standard clinical classification that describes patients in some detail. The Quebec Task Force on Spinal Disorders has proposed one such classification that incorporates the duration of symptoms, the presence of neurologic findings, the patient's work status, and, when available, results of various diagnostic tests (Table 3) (30). More widespread application of such a classification would greatly enhance our ability to generalize the results of analgesic trials for low back pain. Even simpler classifications, such as that of Mathew and his colleagues (31) would be valuable. These authors described patients as having (a) simple low back pain (no evidence of nerve root entrapment); (b) root pain, suggesting disk prolapse or spinal stenosis; (c) spinal pathology, including malignancy infection or inflammatory disease (a group typically excluded from therapeutic trials in low back pain); and (d) abnormal illness behavior, typically including chronic pain patients who may have substantial psychologic overlay in response to their back problems. In general, we would recommend against combining patients with neck pain or extremity pain with patients who have low back pain in studies of analgesics or other classes of medication.

Prognostic Stratification

There is a great need for better characterization and prediction of the prognosis of patients with low back pain. Existing studies emphasize the importance of

TABLE 3. *Quebec Task Force classification of spinal disorders*

Class	Symptoms	Duration	Work status
1	LBP, no radiation	<7 days	Working
2	LBP, radiation to thigh	7 days to 7 weeks	Not working
3	LBP, radiation to calf, foot	>7 weeks	
4	LBP, radiation to leg, + neurological deficit		
5	Presumed radicular compression on plain x-ray (spinal instability or fracture)		
6	Confirmed radicular compression (CT, myelogram, or MRI)		
7	Spinal stenosis		
8	Postsurgical status, <6 months		
9	Postsurgical status, >6 months Asymptomatic Symptomatic		
10	Chronic pain syndrome		
11	Other diagnoses		

LBP, Low back pain; CT, computerized tomography; MRI, magnetic resonance imaging.

several sociodemographic and psychological characteristics in patient recovery. Thus, aside from clinical classification, it may be valuable in designing a clinical trial to provide some prognostic stratification on other factors that are relevant to future outcomes. We have previously suggested, for example, that a simple four-point index combining data on prior episodes of back pain, educational status, and a self-rating of overall health may define subgroups of patients with substantially different prognoses (24). With or without detailed diagnostic information, these factors may help to define relatively homogeneous patient groups for analyzing treatment effects.

Use of Factorial Designs

Because multiple treatments are often prescribed for low back pain, the use of factorial designs may be particularly useful in understanding any additive or synergistic effects (32). Although such effects may sometimes raise complex analytical issues (33), the use of factorial designs may be the best way to identify interactions or additivity between two treatments. In a factorial study, subjects are simultaneously randomized to receive each of two (or more) independent treatments or their respective control groups. In a "two by two" factorial design, four treatment groups would result: placebo, drug A, drug B, and both A and B. Examples for which a factorial design might be useful would be studies of combination therapy with an NSAID plus a muscle relaxant, or an NSAID plus an antidepressant. Factorial designs may be helpful in identifying additive effects of such regimens, and where no interaction occurs, one may have in effect two clinical trials for the price of one, with nearly equivalent statistical power. Like crossover designs, factorial designs bring with them a variety of complexities that one avoids with simple parallel designs, but the benefits may in some cases be substantial. This may be the best way to evaluate the multimodal treatment regimens often advocated for the management of low back pain. For the reasons described above, we would generally recommend avoiding crossover research designs in the study of low back pain.

Outcome Measures

For trials aimed primarily at reducing the symptom of pain, it may seem unnecessary or inappropriate to measure other patient outcomes. However, we have previously documented that there are important dissociations between outcomes such as pain relief, physiologic measures, and functional measures (26). It is hazardous to assume that pain relief will be associated with other benefits such as improvement in daily functioning. Thus, although pain relief in itself is a worthy goal, clinicians managing patients with low back pain will generally want to know about other benefits, including possible changes in patient behavior and effects on the cost of care. A variety of functional status measures for patients with low back pain have been devised and tested, and these are reviewed elsewhere (26). Several, such as the Sickness Impact Profile (34), the Oswestry Disability Questionnaire (35), and the Roland and Morris adaptation of the Sickness Impact Profile (36), appear to be reliable, valid, and responsive to clinical changes.

Blinding

Careful efforts at blinding are justified, even for trials of nonpharmacologic therapy. This can be difficult to accomplish, but many notable examples of blinded trials of physical treatments are available. Examples include the use of sham TENS units with pulsating "on" lights, the use of hands-on therapy such as massage as a control for spinal manipulation, the use of "misplaced" needling as a control for acupuncture, and the use of subtherapeutic weight as a control for traction. In general, trials that employed vigorous efforts at blinding (with control treatments mimicking the active intervention) have found less difference between alternative treatments than trials that compared obviously different forms of therapy.

A related issue concerns the time and attention patients receive from therapists or research personnel. It seems likely that personal interaction alone has important therapeutic benefits, which we use to our advantage in the clinical setting. In a clinical trial, however, such attention may be a confounding factor if patients in one treatment group receive more time and attention from health care providers. Thus, trials that compare an innovative therapy with a waiting-list control seem destined to show major advantages for the treatment group. Similarly, a treatment involving multiple visits with hands-on interaction from a physical therapist may have an unfair advantage over a drug treatment that involves less frequent visits and no physical contact.

QUESTIONS FOR FUTURE RESEARCH

A wide variety of important questions remain to be addressed with regard to the pharmacologic treatment of low back pain. One important question concerns the role of combination treatments, such as a NSAID plus muscle relaxant, or a NSAID plus antidepressant therapy. Some recent trials suggest that there may be an advantage to combination therapy (37), but these trials have been reported with such scant detail and inadequate patient description that both their validity and generalizability remain uncertain. Combined therapy appears to be common in practice, but may result in more frequent patient side effects than single drug therapy. It therefore deserves to be more rigorously scrutinized.

Uncertainty and controversy persist with regard to the role of muscle relaxant drugs for acute low back pain. Many experts eschew their use, though some clinical trials suggest they are efficacious at least for some patients. The limitations of existing trials have already been described. There is a need for more rigorous trials with objective entry criteria and thorough patient descriptions. It remains unclear whether these drugs add anything to analgesic or nonsteroidal therapy alone. There is also a need to examine alternative prescribing patterns for potentially habit-forming drugs such as muscle relaxants. A small bit of evidence for outpatients with acute low back pain suggests that time-limited therapy produces better patient outcomes than pain-contingent therapy (38). Thus, prescriptions for a fixed duration that are not extended in the face of persistent patient symptoms may be advisable. Such considerations apply equally to the use of narcotic analgesics. Nonetheless, there is a need for better data comparing time-contingent versus pain-contingent outpatient treatment and examining the effects of strictly circumscribed prescriptions.

There is growing evidence for the efficacy of tricyclic antidepressants for chronic low back pain, but the existing trials are far from definitive. The validity of these studies has been jeopardized by high dropout rates, in part a consequence of the frequent side effects from these medications. Thus, further studies with rigorous design and efforts to prevent dropping out are necessary. Trials of nonsedating drugs such as desipramine may help in this regard, and trials comparing different antidepressant drugs are needed. Physiologic hypotheses for their mechanism of action have suggested that some may be superior to others (39), although a small number of head-to-head comparisons have failed to demonstrate advantages of one drug over another (40). It also remains to be determined if tricyclic drugs are effective only in persons with chronic pain and depression or in patients without measurable depression as well.

The proper role of corticosteroid drugs (oral, intramuscular, or epidural) and other injected drugs remains entirely unclear. Trials of these forms of therapy have been hampered by uncontrolled designs, small sample sizes, nonrandom allocation, and, predictably, conflicting results. Well-designed clinical trials of epidural steroid injections should have a particularly high priority because of their growing popularity and invasive nature. The numerous potential side effects of corticosteroid therapy demand better evaluation of its use by other routes as well. The widespread use of trigger-point injections clearly requires rigorous controlled evaluation.

Finally, there is a need for ongoing methodological research with regard to conduct of clinical trials for low back pain. A major issue in this regard is the development of more accurate indexes for classification and prognostic stratification of patients. This will be essential to help define homogeneous groups of patients in a situation for which diagnostic ambiguity is the rule (and is likely to remain so for the foreseeable future). Further innovation is also necessary in the arena of outcome assessment, with a particular need for innovations in measuring functional ability and health care utilization. Because of the rapidly evolving course of acute low back pain, refinements in the use of home diaries may be important for capturing early symptomatic and functional improvements.

The ambiguities and difficulties of studying low back pain have made it an "orphan condition" both with regard to clinical care and research. Because low back pain is so common, however, more and better research in this area is a high priority, and this is one area in which achieving adequate sample sizes should generally be quite feasible.

REFERENCES

1. White AA, Gordon SL. Synopsis: workshop on idiopathic low-back pain. *Spine* 1982;7:141–149.
2. Deyo RA. Early diagnostic evaluation of low back pain. *J Gen Intern Med* 1986;1:328–338.
3. Hitselberger WE, Witten RM. Abnormal myelograms in asymptomatic patients. *J Neurosurg* 1968;28:204–206.
4. Weisel SE, Tsourmas N, Feffer H, Citrin CM, Patronas N. A study of computer-assisted tomography in the incidence of positive CAT scans in an asymptomatic group of patients. *Spine* 1984;9:549–551.
5. Weinreb JC, Wolbarsht LB, Cohen JM, Brown CEL, Maravilla KR. Prevalence of lumbosacral intervertebral disk abnormalities on MR images in pregnant and asymptomatic nonpregnant women. *Radiology* 1989;170:125–128.
6. Johnson EW. The myth of skeletal muscle spasm. *Am J Phys Med Rehabil* 1989;68:1.
7. Waddell G, Main CJ, Morris EW, et al. Normality and reliability in the clinical assessment of backache. *Br Med J* 1982;284:1519–1523.
8. Osterweis M, Kleinman A, Mechanic D, eds. *Pain and disability: clinical behavioral and public policy perspectives.* Washington, DC: National Academy Press, 1987.
9. Hadler NM. Miscellaneous putative causes of shoulder region pain: thoracic outlet syndromes and fibrositis: clinical concepts that withstand the onslaught of logic poorly. In: Hadler NM ed. *Medical management of the regional musculoskeletal diseases.* Orlando: Grune and Stratton, 1984;123–126.
10. Roland M, Morris R. A study of the natural history of back pain, part II: development of guidelines for trials of treatment in primary care. *Spine* 1983;8:145–150.
11. Dillane JB, Fry J, Kalton G. Acute back syndrome—a study from general practice. *Br Med J* 1966;2:82–84.
12. Chavannes AW, Gubbels J, Post D, Rutten G, Thomas S. Acute low back pain: patients' perceptions of pain four weeks after initial diagnosis and treatment in general practice. *J R Coll Gen Pract* 1986;36:271–273.
13. Frymoyer JW. Back pain and sciatica. *N Engl J Med* 1988;318:291–300.
14. Berry H, Bloom B, Hamilton EBD, et al. Naproxen sodium, diflunisal, and placebo in the treatment of chronic back pain. *Ann Rheum Dis* 1982;41:129–132.
15. Hickey RFJ. Chronic low back pain: a comparison of diflunisal with paracetamol. *NZ Med J* 1982;95:312–314.
16. Amile E, Weber H, Holme I. Treatment of acute low-back pain with piroxicam: results of a double-blind placebo-controlled trial. *Spine* 1987;12:473–476.
17. Deyo RA. Conservative therapy for low back pain: distinguishing useful from useless therapy. *JAMA* 1983;250:1057–1062.
18. Pheasant H, Bursk A, Goldfarb J, Azen SP, Weiss JN, Borelli L. Amitriptyline and chronic low back pain: a randomized double-blind crossover study. *Spine* 1983;8:552–556.
19. Alcoff J, Jones E, Rust P, Newman R. Controlled trial of imipramine for chronic low back pain. *J Fam Pract* 1982;14:841–846.
20. Jenkins DG, Ebbutt EF, Evans CD. Tofranil in the treatment of low back pain. *J Int Med Res* 1976;4(suppl 12):28–40.
21. Cuckler JM, Bernini PA, Wiesel SW, Booth RE, Rothman RH, Pickeus GT. The use of epidural steroids in the treatment of lumbar radicular pain. *J Bone Joint Surg* 1985;67A:63–66.
22. Dilke TFW, Burry HC, Grahame R. Extradural corticosteroid injection in management of lumbar nerve root compression. *Br Med J* 1973;2:635–637.
23. Walsh NE, Dumitru D. Financial compensation and recovery from low back pain. *Spine State-of-the-Art Reviews* 1987;2(1):109–121.
24. Deyo RA, Diehl AK. Psychosocial predictors of disability in patients with low back pain. *J Rheumatol* 1988;15:1557–1564.

25. Barnes D, Smith D, Gatchel RJ, Mayer TG. Psychosocioeconomic predictors of treatment success/failure in chronic low-back pain patients. *Spine* 1989;14:427–430.
26. Deyo RA. Measuring the functional status of patients with low back pain. *Arch Phys Med Rehabil* 1988;69:1044–1053.
27. Cowan IC, Mapes RE. Carisoprodol in the management of musculoskeletal disorders: a controlled trial. *Ann Phys Med* 1963;7:140–143.
28. Deyo RA, Bass JE, Walsh NE, Schoenfeld LS, Ramamurthy S. Prognostic variability among chronic pain patients: implications for study design, interpretation, and reporting. *Arch Phys Med Rehabil* 1988;69:174–178.
29. Woods JR, Williams JG, Tavel M. The two-period crossover design in medical research. *Ann Intern Med* 1989;110:560–566.
30. Quebec Task Force on Spinal Disorders. Scientific approach to the assessment and management of activity-related spinal disorders: a monograph for clinicians. *Spine* 1987;12(suppl 7):S22–S30.
31. Mathew B, Norris D, Hendry D, Waddell G. Artificial intelligence in the diagnosis of low back pain and sciatica. *Spine* 1988;13:168–172.
32. Chalmers TC. A potpourri of RCT topics. *Controlled Clin Trials* 1982;3:285–298.
33. Brittain E, Wittes J. Factorial designs in clinical trials: the effects of non-compliance and subadditivity. *Stat Med* 1989;8:161–171.
34. Berger M, Bobbitt RA, Carter WB, Gilson BS. The Sickness Impact Profile: development and final revision of a health status measure. *Med Care* 1981;19:787–805.
35. Fairbank JCT, Davies JB, Mbaot JC, O'Brien JP. The Oswestry low back pain disability questionnaire. *Physiotherapy* 1980;66:271–273.
36. Roland M, Morris R. Study of the natural history of back pain, part I: development of a reliable and sensitive measure of disability in low-back pain. *Spine* 1983;8:141–144.
37. Basmajian JV. Acute back pain and spasm: a controlled multicenter trial of combined analgesic and antispasm agents. *Spine* 1989;14:438–439.
38. Fordyce WE, Brockway JA, Bergman JA, Spengler D. Acute back pain: a control-group comparison of behavioral vs. traditional management methods. *J Behav Med* 1986;9:127–140.
39. Ward NG, Bokan JA, Phillips M, Benedetti C, Butler S, Spengler D. Antidepressants in concomitant chronic back pain and depression: doxepin and desipramine compared. *J Clin Psychiatry* 1984;45(3, sec 2):54–59.
40. Ward NG. Tricyclic antidepressants for chronic low back pain: mechanism of action and predictors of response. *Spine* 1986;11:661–665.

Advances in Pain Research and Therapy, Vol. 18,
edited by M. Max, R. Portenoy, and E. Laska,
Raven Press, Ltd., New York © 1991.

12

Osteoarthritis

Thomas G. Kantor* and Daniel E. Furst**

*Rheumatic Diseases Study Group, New York University
Medical Center, New York, New York 10016;
**Department of Medicine/Rheumatology, University of Medicine and Dentistry of
New Jersey, New Brunswick, New Jersey 08903; and Ciba-Geigy Pharmaceuticals,
Summit, New Jersey 07901*

Pain is the single most important symptom that brings patients to see a rheumatologist and the most important initial function that physicians wish to perform is to relieve the pain (1). Only recently, however, has a major rheumatology text addressed pain in a separate chapter (2). As yet there has been relatively little effort to study chronic arthritic pain in analgesic trials. This chapter reviews what has been done in the past and considers what may be done in the future, focusing on pain in osteoarthritis.

HISTORICAL CONSIDERATIONS

Prior to 1965, the slow acceptance of gold therapy for rheumatoid arthritis spurred Bayles and Hall (3) to make classifications of rheumatoid disease using anatomic and functional criteria, but they almost completely ignored pain as a scoring parameter. Steinbrocker and Blazer (4) then devised a similar scoring system with a "therapeutic score card" that included pain and tenderness. However, pain was allowed a 5% proportion of the total score.

Meanwhile, a protocol for proving antiinflammation in arthritis was devised by Lansbury (5). He further attempted to compress the various components of his index into a single value by weighting them according to an arbitrary value system. One of the components, an articular index, incorporated tenderness and degree of pain on joint motion. This quantified a system Lansbury had suggested two years earlier and also another evaluation system described by Wallace and Ragan (6). Quantification was determined by assigning weighted scores to each joint according to its size. Lansbury's system was meant for rheumatoid arthritis and was not considered for osteoarthritis.

In 1965, it was generally believed that aspirin was a simple analgesic with respect to arthritis pain. However, in that year and the subsequent year, two studies (7,8) proved that aspirin actually reduced inflammation in rheumatoid arthritis. Dolor being one of the Galenian tenets of inflammation, it became generally accepted that the reduction of inflammation resulted in reduced pain. Pharmaceutical firms then began a search for compounds more potent than aspirin and it became obvious that protocols would have to be devised to test such compounds.

These conceptions were obvious for the inflammatory arthridities but left the problem of osteoarthritis in abeyance. Based on pathologic studies, Europeans called the disease "osteoarthrosis" whereas Americans persisted with the term "osteoarthritis," implying an inflammatory component. This controversy still continues. However, the studies of Ferreira (9) in Vane's laboratory showed that the pain-reducing qualities of aspirin and the nonsteroidal antiinflammatory drugs (NSAIDs), and to a great extent, the modulation of inflammation in joints, were owing to the same mechanism—the reduction of prostaglandin synthesis by inhibition of the enzyme cyclooxygenase. Thus, the "osis-itis" argument has been rendered moot.

As further therapeutic advances took place, the need for more precise and simple measurements of improvement became evident and Ritchie and her associates (10) devised an articular index using a semiquantitative measure of tenderness for each joint. This differed from the Lansbury index by simply adding up the number of tender joints with a partial attempt to quantify the degree of tenderness. Again, these various measurement devices were less suitable for osteoarthritis where only one or two joints might have been involved.

During the preceding decade, Beecher's conceptions of subjective response measurement had been introduced (11) and successfully utilized by Lasagna (12) to differentiate analgesic drugs from placebo under double-blind conditions and to separate doses of analgesics from each other. These methods were established in postoperative pain models that looked only at a single dose. Subjective response methodology had been further developed by Houde et al. (13) who assigned numerical scores to verbal categories chosen by the patient to describe his degree of pain and pain relief. Huskisson (14) introduced the Visual Analogue Scale (VAS) as another refinement of the measurement of pain. These subjective response quantifications of pain allowed therapeutic trials to be successfully performed in osteoarthritis and other inflammatory arthridities such as reactive arthritis and the spondyloarthropathies.

From the 1960s on, under the pressure of third-party evaluations of disability in arthritis and low back pain, various functional and behavioral methods of evaluation were suggested (15–25). Most of these used the newly documented subjective response measurements of pain quantity, usually the visual analogue scales.

THE ANATOMY OF PAIN IN ARTHRITIS

The study of the neural basis of arthritic pain became fully established in the 1970s when peroxidase staining methodology allowed correlation between peripheral nerve endings and the cell bodies of their neurons in other anatomical locations. The nerves that carry the pain signal are the lightly myelinated A delta fibers and thinner and unmyelinated C fibers (26–28). Their nerve endings are found in the capsules and tendon attachments around joints and their corresponding cell bodies are in the dorsal ganglia alongside the spinal cord. Recent findings have suggested pain nerves in the synovium as well (29).

Other small unmyelinated or partially myelinated nerves in the synovium and in the border region between the cartilage and synovium are part of the autonomic nervous system. Sympathetic fibers are more numerous than parasympathetic fibers (30). Although such nerves are not ordinarily considered to be nociceptive in that they are efferent in function, there is evidence that they may stimulate unmyelinated C fibers (31). Blockade of the sympathetic nervous system either by local anesthetics or systemic pharmacologic agents has been shown to diminish pain in rheumatoid arthritis (32). Because pain in rheumatoid arthritis depends largely on acute inflammatory processes and the activity of the primary disease, it is harder to dissect out the activity of analgesics from drugs that affect the disease. For this disease, it would be difficult to conclude whether or not a new class of NSAID would be helpful in other painful conditions. Therefore, we focus this chapter on osteoarthritis because it is less confounded by inflammatory events and because there are more studies to draw upon. The lessons learned from osteoarthritis may also be applied to the more difficult challenge of rheumatoid arthritis analgesic studies.

ARTHRITIS AS A PAIN MODEL

Choosing the Patient Group

Inflammation is an integral part of the pathogenesis of most rheumatic diseases, including rheumatoid arthritis, seronegative spondyloarthropathies, the numerous vasculitides, systemic sclerosis, crystal-induced disease, and arthritis associated with infections (33). The inflammatory process releases a number of substances that affect pain, such as bradykinin, histamine, and prostaglandins (33). Further, the destructive effects of inflammation and its concomitant oxygen radical release may cause tissue damage, which also results in pain. Thus pain and inflammation are inextricably intertwined.

Of the rheumatic diseases, osteoarthritis, back pain associated with osteoarthritis, and the seronegative spondyloarthropathies and various forms of "soft-tissue rheumatism" are probably those associated with the least inflammation (34–37). Pain associated with back pathology contains many noninflammatory or pauciinflammatory neuropathic elements. Measurement and trials of neuropathic pain and back pain are discussed in Chapters 8 and 11. Whereas "soft-tissue rheumatism" includes a number of very common symptom complexes (such as repetitive strain injury), this heterogeneous group of diseases is not well enough defined to be readily used as a model of rheumatic disease pain.

Even osteoarthritis involves elements of inflammation and may represent a group of diseases rather than a single entity (38). In one study of osteoarthritis of the hip or knee, 87% of patients were noted to have inflammation at joint replacement surgery (39). There are inflammatory and erosive forms of osteoarthritis (40). In fact, osteoarthritis probably represents the final common pathway of a number of pathogeneses, including congenital disease, metabolic disease, crystal-induced disease, and trauma (38). Although most clinical trials of osteoarthritic pain do not consider the pathogenesis of the illness, it is probable that some consideration of this factor should be included in future trials, in order to decrease variability of response. Thus, for example, it would be useful to exclude osteoarthritis associated with clinical calcium pyrophosphate deposition disease, and metabolic diseases such as hemochromatosis, ochronosis, hyperparathyroidism, diabetes mellitus, severe congenital hip disease, and erosive osteoarthritis.

Other diagnosis-related attempts to decrease heterogeneity and increase model sensitivity have included definition of disease severity and requirement for a certain degree or frequency of analgesic or antiinflammatory therapy as entrance criteria. The Cooperative Systematic Studies of Rheumatic Disease Group, a multicenter group of academic rheumatology centers, is presently studying naproxen versus acetaminophen in osteoarthritis of the knee (H. J. Williams, *personal communication*). Entrance criteria for this study included specific criteria of symptomatic disease (e.g., knee pain for at least 25 days plus x-ray evidence of osteoarthritis), and the need to have used a "therapeutic dose" of NSAID for at least 3 months prior to study entry (e.g., indomethacin 75 mg a day or more). Exclusion criteria included hemochromatosis, recent knee injury, or concomitant rheumatoid arthritis.

In addition to considering etiology, it is usual to consider the pattern and extent of joint involvement in trial design. Most commonly, osteoarthritis of the knee or of the hip is used in clinical trials of osteoarthritis (41–44). Although occasional clinical studies have used a mixed population of osteoarthritis patients involving back, hands, or other weight-bearing joints, these studies are not as sensitive for delineating analgesic effects of drugs. Although each of the above maneuvers will, potentially, decrease heterogeneity and increase model sensitivity, these restrictions may limit the generalizability of the results and impede patient recruitment. Thus, a balance needs to be struck between the "ideal" study and the most reasonable one to accomplish the stated objectives.

Measurements of Response

Measurements of response include those that more or less directly measure pain and those that measure pain indirectly. In addition, the investigator may choose from a series of functional measures that include consideration of psychological components of patient response.

Traditionally, visual analogue scales or categorical pain scales are done periodically to assess pain intensity or pain relief (see pages 57–64). In osteoarthritis, visual analogue scales are often used for estimations of patient pain, patient global response to the medication, and the physician global response to the medication (41–44). In addition, palpation of the joint for tenderness is frequently done, using a categorical scale of 0 (no tenderness) to 3 (severe tenderness) (41–44). The rationale for these particular measures rests on their relative simplicity, their derivation from studies of rheumatoid arthritis, and their ability to distinguish drug effects (41–44). Dolorimeters or algometers are semiobjective, potentially valuable devices for measuring joint tenderness (45–46). These devices utilize a spring-loaded plunger to apply reproducible amounts of measurable pressure to exactly specified anatomical locations on the joint surface. Although theoretically very attractive, these devices have not been adequately tested in osteoarthritis.

Another series of measurements used in some studies include measurement (in seconds) of time to walk 50 feet, measurements of range of motion of the affected joint, grip strength and swelling (either on a categorical or continuous scale), and duration of morning stiffness and time to onset of fatigue (49). These may be viewed as derivative measurements of pain, as they worsen if pain increases and improve if pain decreases. The validity of most of these measures is unknown in osteoarthritis, although their validity has been studied in rheumatoid arthritis (47,48). The coefficient of variation for joint tenderness in rheumatoid arthritis is approximately 27%, for morning stiffness it is 100%, and for time to onset of fatigue, 38% (48).

In 1983, a review of osteoarthritis trials by Altman and Hochberg (49) indicated that only 30% of trials assessed joint tenderness, 24% of trials measured joint swelling, and 22% of trials utilized 50-foot walking time. Walking time has not been reliable in some arthritis trials, although it occasionally is a sensitive measure (50). It is possible that 50-foot walking time has been a poor discriminator because it has been used in all patients in some trials, ranging from those with severe problems requiring walking aids and to those without any significant disability. These two subgroups would obviously increase the variance and decrease the sensitivity of the walking time.

Although joint swelling is a reasonable, if inexact, measure in diseases with large inflammatory components, osteoarthritis is not one of those and swelling is not likely to be a sensitive indicator of response in this disease. Likewise, morning stiffness is a lesser component of osteoarthritis, as compared to rheumatoid arthritis, and combined with its large coefficient of variation, makes morning stiffness an unlikely candidate for use in osteoarthritis pain trials. Grip strength has been tested by Lee et al. (51) and found to vary by 10 to 20 mm Hg when different physicians test the same patient. It is also very dependent upon the time at which the testing is done (52). Although grip strength may be a reasonable measure for pain in trials of hand osteoarthritis, it obviously will not be useful for those studies involving only the knee, hip, or other joints of the lower extremity.

Future research in measurement of osteoarthritic pain should involve validation and delineation of better pain scales and better quantitation of semiobjective measures such as walking time. Thus, different pain characteristics might be examined in osteoarthritis, using scales such as the McGill Pain Questionnaire (53). This questionnaire is excellent for examining different qualities of pain, although it is somewhat lengthy and complicated to administer. Daily "pain postcards" or pain visual analogue scale diaries could also be used. In the former case, the pain severity visual analogue scale, done at the same time each day, may be sent by the patient to the investigator on a daily basis; this would prevent patients from examining their previous day's result. A visual analogue pain diary would allow the patient to enter data daily and send results in periodically (e.g., weekly or biweekly). Other analogue scales and indices are being developed and validated, such as the index of severity for hip disease (54).

Although 50-foot walking time is a simple measure of lower extremity function, more exact and quantitative methods to measure walking have been developed. Electronic walkways that measure many aspects of the stride (e.g., length of stride, time on any given extremity, or speed and acceleration), have been developed and used in orthopedic models (56). They could easily be tested as indirect measures of analgesia, since decreased pain should lead to increased function and "better" stride.

Several minicomputer systems are now being developed for patient use (55); hand-held computers are programmed to record dosages, effects, and assessments. Such minicomputers could be uploaded into a PC at each clinic visit allowing daily, weekly, or even hourly outpatient data to be analyzed.

Design Issues

A primary characteristic of osteoarthritis is its chronicity. Within this chronicity, however, there may be a certain degree of waxing and waning of symptoms (57), particularly as activity levels change. Thus, a trial that lasts up to 3 months may be characterized by some shifting baseline, making crossover trials problematic (57). In general, then, parallel trials are recommended in studies of the treatment of pain in osteoarthritis even though the "N" per data point will be necessarily large. It is appropriate to allow a prestudy flare, to "normalize" the baseline characteristics of patients and to corroborate responsiveness to medication (41–47,49,58). This may be done by having the patient stop his therapy and return when his symptoms have worsened. In longer studies, consideration can be given to a poststudy flare. This latter flare of disease can be compared to the prestudy flare to corroborate lack of change in underlying disease activity. Should differences between pre- and poststudy flare exist, they can be used to attempt to compensate for the change in activity (50,58). Although these latter considerations have not been utilized in osteoarthritis, they might be considered in the improvement of future trial design.

As is true of most analgesic trials, double-blind methodology and randomization are appropriate. As is also true of other trials using pain models, it is appropriate to have both a positive control (active medication) and negative control (placebo) in trials when possible. Long-term trials using placebo may be difficult but occasionally can be accomplished using numbers of tablets of rescue medication such as acetaminophen as a measure of response (55). One strong justification for the use of placebo in osteoarthritis is the potentially large placebo response in trials of rheumatic diseases; depending on the degree of difference, placebo response can be surprisingly high. For example, 29% of placebo-treated patients experienced a 20% response in four trials of second-line agents in rheumatoid arthritis (59) and 19% of placebo-treated patients experienced more than 50% improvement in their swollen joint count in another study (60). This degree of placebo response makes it important and, frequently, possible to do placebo-controlled trials in patients with moderate osteoarthritis. Dose-response studies are possible in this model (58) and can make it possible to demonstrate assay sensitivity even when a placebo group is not used (see pp. 72–75, this volume).

In rheumatoid arthritis, a shifting baseline has been well documented (48,50,58). Although these fluctuations are not as well documented in osteoarthritis, it is advisable to do at least two baseline measurements whenever a new measurement scale (semiobjective, or even objective) is being tested in analgesic trials of osteoarthritis to validate the stability and the responsiveness of the new measures.

Some investigators have suggested that in osteoarthritis, pain relief increases with the second or third dose of an analgesic compared to the initial dose (FDA, *personal communication*). On the other hand, induction of drug metabolism could potentially decrease response after chronic dosing. For example, salicylate concentrations decreased 23% during one month of continuous therapy, secondary to induction of salicylate metabolism (61). In addition, multidose trials in other pain models have shown a certain amount of psychological carryover dependent on the perceived potency of the first dose (62,63). These interesting questions could be approached by using a single-dose methodology imposed upon a chronic dosing design (see Chapter 4). Thus, patients can be placed in a chronic dosing study but have selected pain measurements done for the first 4, 6, or 12 hrs after the first dose of double-blind medication; this could be done again after the second or third dose and/or as many times as seems appropriate thereafter. For example, in a parallel, 3-month, double-blind study of medications that will be given three times a day, one might wish to assess pain hourly for 6 hrs after the first dose of drug, one week later, and at the end of the trial.

Pitfalls to Avoid in Trial Design to Measure Pain in Osteoarthritis

It is important to monitor the use of other drugs that may affect pain. Amitriptyline and other antidepressants, for example, are active in pain syndromes such as fibromyalgia and may affect pain outcome secondary to their effects on perception of pain or anxiety (64). Their use should be avoided, or stratified, or included as a covariate in the analysis.

Although placebo treatment and allowance for "disease flare" may increase the sensitivity of the trial, they may not always be possible. In that situation, a dose-response study or one using only "positive" controls may need to be considered. To achieve sufficient power to detect a modest advantage over a standard analgesic often requires a large sample size.

In multiclinic protocols, there is great value in having the co-investigators meet before the trial. Discrepancies among investigators with respect to exact methodology must be addressed at that time and their resolution written into the protocol. For example, weight-bearing osteoarthritic joints tend to become more painful with use, thus worsening as the day goes on, so agreement must be reached that all clinics see their patients at approximately the same time of day (57).

It should go without saying that the appropriate dose range and regimen need to be considered when embarking on analgesic trials in osteoarthritis. It would, for example, be inappropriate to compare 800 mg/day of ibuprofen with 750 mg/day of naproxen, as these are not equipotent doses of medication.

As is true in all longer-term studies, the influence of dropouts upon results must be considered prior to starting the trial. The anticipated dropout rate may alter the objectives of the trial, the number of patients in each group that needs to be recruited into the trial, or the analysis of the investigation.

Other Issues

Although it is not the purpose of this review to examine specific drugs, some general aspects of drug design and purpose should be considered. For example, there is interest in the differential effect of drug enantiomers upon efficacy and toxicity (65). If one or several of the drugs being tested is a racemic mixture, consideration of the effect of one or the other enantiomer on the drug trial may be worthwhile.

Whereas purely analgesic drugs in osteoarthritis are not usually aimed at this disease's underlying pathogenesis, other drugs may be developed that affect the underlying pathology of this disease. Such drugs will, ultimately, decrease pain (66). Should one be interested in testing such a drug, it would be important to be sure that background medications are the same across study groups. In rheumatoid arthritis, for example, it is probably best to use the same nonsteroidal antiinflammatory drug for all study groups. This is because the efficacy of a given NSAID is different among different individuals and because the incidence and severity of side effects from NSAIDs are not necessarily the same (67).

SUMMARY

Osteoarthritis is a chronic pain model that has been shown to be useful in assessing analgesics. However, a number of aspects of study design and response measurement are still in need of improvement. This chapter has critically reviewed the reasons that osteoarthritis is being used as a chronic pain model, the common outcome measures in analgesic trials, and considerations in study design. Some of the major pitfalls in studying pain in osteoarthritis were briefly reviewed, and a number of suggestions were made for potential investigation and improvement in the future.

Important methodologic issues for research in this area include: (a) better understanding of the pathogenesis of osteoarthritis in order to more effectively distinguish patient subsets that might respond to a given therapy; (b) development of more sensitive, accurate, and objective tools to measure change in chronic pain (computerized techniques, gait measurement, objective serum correlates); and (c) a better understanding of the variation in chronic pain and influences on it (diurnal variation, effect of repeated dosing, degree of psychological input, external stressors that affect chronic pain).

REFERENCES

1. Bombardier C, Tugwell P, Sinclair A, et al. Preference for end point measures in clinical trials. Results of structured workshops. *J Rheumatol* 1982;9:798–801.
2. Moore ME. Pain and rheumatic disease. In: Katz WA, ed. *Diagnosis and management of rheumatic diseases,* 2nd ed. Philadelphia: JB Lippincott, 1988.
3. Bayles TB, Hall MG. Yardstick for rheumatoid arthritis applied to patients receiving gold salt therapy. *N Engl J Med* 1943;228:418–421.
4. Steinbrocker O, Blazer A. A therapeutic score card for rheumatoid arthritis. A standardized method for appraising results of treatment. *N Engl J Med* 1946;235:501–506.
5. Lansbury J. Report of a three year study on the systemic and articular indexes in rheumatoid arthritis. Theoretic and clinical considerations. *Arthritis Rheum* 1958;1:505–522.
6. Wallace SC, Ragan C. The problem of therapeutic evaluation in rheumatoid arthritis. *Arthritis Rheum* 1958;1:20–30.
7. Fremont-Smith K, Bayes TB. Salicylate therapy in rheumatoid arthritis. *JAMA* 1965;192:103–106.
8. Boardman PI, Hart FD. Clinical management of the anti-inflammatory effects of salicylate in rheumatoid arthritis. *Br Med J* 1967;240:200–213.
9. Ferreira SH. Prostaglandins, aspirin-like drugs and analgesia. *Nature* 1972;240:200–213.
10. Ritchie DM, Boyle JA, McInnes JM, et al. Clinical studies with an articular index for the assessment of joint tenderness in patients with rheumatoid arthritis. *Q J Med* 1968;147:393–406.
11. Beecher HK. Quantitative effects of drugs. In: *Measurement of subjective responses.* New York: Oxford University Press, 1959;189–200.
12. Lasagna L. Analgesic methodology. A brief history and commentary. *J Clin Pharmacol* 1980;20:373–376.
13. Houde RW, Wallenstein SL, Rogers A. Clinical pharmacology of analgesics: a method for studying analgesic effects. *Clin Pharmacol Ther* 1960;1:163–174.
14. Huskisson EC. Visual analog scales. In: Melzack R, ed. *Pain measurement and assessment.* New York: Raven Press, 1983;45–67.
15. Schmidt AJM, Gierlings REH, Peters ML. Environmental and interoceptive influences on chronic low back pain behavior. *Pain* 1989;38:137–143.
16. Turk DC, Meichenbaum D, Genest M. *Pain and behavioral medicine: a cognitive-behavioral perspective.* New York: Guilford, 1983.
17. Lee P, Jasani MK, Dick WC, et al. Evaluation of a functional index in rheumatoid arthritis. *Scand J Rheumatol* 1973;2:71–78.
18. Fordyce WE. *Behavioral methods for chronic pain and illness.* St. Louis: Mosby, 1976.
19. Yelin E, Meenan R, Nevitt M, et al. Work disability in rheumatoid arthritis: effects of disease, social and work factors. *Ann Intern Med* 1980;93:551–560.

20. Brown JH, Kazis LE, Spitz PW, et al. The dimensions of health outcomes. A cross-validated examination of health status measurement. *Am J Public Health* 1984;74:159–161.
21. Anderson KO, Keefe FJ, Bradley LA, et al. Prediction of pain behavior and functional status of rheumatoid arthritis patients using medical status and psychological variables. *Pain* 1988;33:25–32.
22. Anderson JJ, Firschein HE, Meenan RF. Sensitivity of a health status measure to short-term clinical changes in arthritis. *Arthritis Rheum* 1989;32:844–850.
23. Hagglund KJ, Haley WE, Reveille JD, et al. Predicting individual differences in pain and functional impairment among patients with rheumatoid arthritis. *Arthritis Rheum* 1989;32:851–858.
24. Melzack R. The McGill Pain Questionnaire. Major properties and scoring methods. *Pain* 1975;1:277–299.
25. Burckhardt CS. The use of the McGill Pain Questionnaire in assessing arthritis pain. *Pain* 1984;19:304–314.
26. Georgopoulos AP. Functional properties of primary afferent units probably related to pain mechanism in primate glabrous skin. *J Neurophysiol* 1974;39:71–83.
27. Torebjork HE. Afferent C units responding to mechanical thermal and chemical stimuli in human non-glabrous skin. *Acta Physiol Scand* 1974;92:215–390.
28. Harkness IAL, Higgs ER, Diepp PA. Osteoarthritis. In: Wall PO, Melzack R, eds. *Textbook of pain.* London: Churchill Livingstone, 1984;215–224.
29. Konttinen YT, Gronblad M, Hukkanen M, et al. Pain fibers in osteoarthritis: A review. *Semin Arthritis Rheum* 1989;18(suppl 2):35–40.
30. Bedalamente MA, Cherney SB. Periosteal and vascular innervation of the human patella in degenerative joint disease. *Semin Arthritis Rheum* 1989;18(suppl 2):61–66.
31. Fields HL. Painful dysfunction in the nervous system. In: Fields HL, ed. *Pain.* New York: McGraw-Hill, 1987;133–169.
32. Levine JD, Fye K, Heller P, et al. Clinical response to regional intravenous guanethidine in patients with rheumatoid arthritis. *J Rheumatol* 1986;13:1040–1043.
33. Ruddy S, Lewis RA, Kozin F, et al. The inflammatory response. In: Kelley WN, Harris ED Jr, Ruddy S, Sledge B, eds. *Textbook of rheumatology.* Philadelphia: WB Saunders, 1989;241–416.
34. Mankin HJ, Brandt KD. Pathogenesis of osteoarthritis. *ibid.,* 1469–1479.
35. Lipson SJ. Low back pain. *ibid.,* 508–525.
36. Bennett RM. Fibrositis. *ibid.,* 541–553.
37. Savarese JJ, Thomas GB, Homesley H, et al. Rescue factor: a design for evaluating long-acting analgesics. *Pain* 1988;43:376–380.
38. Howell DS, Woessner Jr JF, Jimenez S, et al. A view on the pathogenesis of osteoarthritis. *Bull Rheum Dis* 1979;29:996–1001.
39. Goldenberg DL, Egan MS, Cohen AS. Inflammatory synovitis in degenerative joint disease. *J Rheumatol* 1982;9:204–209.
40. Peter JB, Pearson CM, Marmor L. Erosive osteoarthritis of the hands. *Arthritis Rheum* 1966;9:365–388.
41. Gengos DC, Neu DC, Miola SR. Evaluation of sustained-release indomethacin in osteoarthritis. *Semin Arthritis Rheum* 1982;12:142–146.
42. Brooks PM, Cleland LG, Haski AL, et al. Evaluation of a single daily dose of naproxen in osteoarthritis. *Rheum Rehab* 1982;21:242–246.
43. Kaklamanis PH, Sfikakis P, Demetriades P, et al. Double-blind, 12-week comparison trial of diflunisal and acetylsalicylic acid in the control of pain of osteoarthritis of the hip and/or knee. *Clin Ther* 1978;1(suppl A):20–24.
44. Brown BL, Johnson J, Hearron MS. Double-blind comparison of flurbiprofen and sulindac for the treatment of osteoarthritis. *Am J Med* 1986;80(suppl 3A):112–117.
45. McCarty DJ Jr, Gatter RA, Phelps P. Dolorimeter for quantification of articular tenderness. *Arthritis Rheum* 1965;8:551–559.
46. Device may be obtained at: Pressure Threshold Meter, Pain Diagnostics and Thermography Inc., 223 East Short Road, Suite 108, Great Neck, NY 11023.
47. Anderson JJ, Felson DT, Meenan RF, et al. Which traditional measures should be used in rheumatoid arthritis clinical trials? *Arthritis Rheum* 1989;32:9:1093–1099.
48. Lansbury J, Baier HN, McCracken S. Statistical study of variation in systemic and articular indexes. *Arthritis Rheum* 1962;5:445–456.
49. Altman RD, Hochberg MC. Degenerative joint disease. *Clin Rheum Dis* 1983;9:681–693.
50. Day RO, Furst DE, Dromgoole SH, et al. Relationship of serum naproxen concentration to efficacy in rheumatoid arthritis. *Clin Pharmacol Ther* 1982;31(6):733–740.

51. Lee P, Baxter A, Dick WC, et al. An assessment of grip strength measurement in rheumatoid arthritis. *Scand J Rheumatol* 1974;3:17–23.
52. Wright V. Some observations on diurnal variation of grip. *Clin Sci* 1959;17–23.
53. Melzack R. The McGill Pain Questionnaire. In: Melzack R, ed. *Pain measures and assessment.* New York: Raven Press, 1983;41–47.
54. Lequesne MG, Mery C, Samson M, et al. Indexes of severity for osteoarthritis of the hip and knee. *Scand J Rheumatol* 1987;(suppl 65):85–89.
55. Turner RA, Jr, Brindley DA, Mitchell FN. Nabumetone: a single-center three-week comparison with placebo in the treatment of rheumatoid arthritis. *Am J Med* 1987;83(suppl 4B):36–39.
56. Gabel RH, Johnston RC, Crowninshield RD. A gait analyzer/trainer instrumentation system. *J Biol* 1979;12:543–549.
57. Mankin HJ. Clinical features of osteoarthritis. In: Kelley WN, Harris ED Jr, Ruddy S, Sledge CB, eds. *Textbook of rheumatology.* Philadelphia: WB Saunders, 1989;1491–1500.
58. Furst DE, Caldwell J, Klugman M, et al. Serum concentration and dose-response relationships for carprofen in rheumatoid arthritis. *Clin Pharmacol Ther* 1988;44:186–194.
59. Paulus HE, Egger MJ, Ward JR, et al. Analyzing improvement in individual rheumatoid arthritis patients during treatment with slow-acting drug based on the responses of placebo-treated patients. *Arthritis Rheum* 1990;33:477–484.
60. Furst DE, Koehnke R, Burmeister L, et al. Increasing methotrexate effect with increasing dose in the treatment of resistant rheumatoid arthritis. *J Rheumatol* 1989;16:313–320.
61. Day RO, Furst DE, Dromgoole SH, et al. Changes in salicylate concentration and metabolism during chronic dosing in normal volunteers. *Biopharm Drug Dispos* 1988;9:273–283.
62. Laska E, Sunshine A. Anticipation of analgesia—a placebo effect. *Headache* 1983;13:1–11.
63. Kantor TG, Sunshine A, Laska E, et al. Oral analgesic studies of pentazocine HCl, codeine, aspirin and placebo and their effect on subsequent administration of placebo. *J Clin Pharm Ther* 1966;7:447–454.
64. Scudds RA, McCain GA, Rollman GB, et al. Improvements in pain responsiveness in patients with fibrositis after successful treatment with amitriptyline. *J Rheumatol* 1989;19(Suppl):98–103.
65. Jamali F, Mehvar R, Pasutto FM. Stereospecific aspects of drug action and disposition: therapeutic pitfalls. *J Pharm Sci* 1989;78:695–715.
66. Moskowitz RW, Davis W, Sammarco J, et al. Experimentally induced degenerative joint lesions following partial meniscectomy in the rabbit. *Arthritis Rheum* 1973;16:397–405.
67. Paulus HE, Furst DE. Aspirin and other nonsteroidal anti-inflammatory drugs. In: McCarty DJ, ed. *Arthritis and allied conditions,* 11th ed. Philadelphia: Lea & Febiger, 1989;507–543.

Advances in Pain Research and Therapy, Vol. 18,
edited by M. Max, R. Portenoy, and E. Laska,
Raven Press, Ltd., New York © 1991.

13

Sickle Cell Disease

Lennette J. Benjamin

*Comprehensive Sickle Cell Center, Montefiore Hospital Medical Center and
Department of Medicine, Albert Einstein College of Medicine, Bronx, New York 10467*

The paucity of pain research in sickle cell disease reflects the neglect that pervades the management of this disease. There is no treatment for the underlying disease. The studies of agents that prevent or treat vaso-occlusive phenomena are few in number (1–3); only two such agents have shown modest efficacy, and none has progressed to general clinical usage (4–6). Given the absence of specific therapies for sickle cell disease, the treatment of pain takes on greater significance. Yet, it is only recently that publications about pain have even included sections on the management of sickle cell pain (7–9), or publications on sickle cell disease have devoted chapters to pain management (10,11).

Pain syndromes in sickle cell disease are diverse, and can be divided into those secondary to sickle cell disease itself, those associated with therapy, and those owing to causes independent of or indirectly related to the disease or therapy (Table 1). Acute painful episodes cause sickle cell patients to seek hospital-based care more than any other event. It is generally reported that approximately 20% of the patients account for 80% of the hospitalizations for acute painful episodes (10–13). More than 50% of patients experience significant acute or chronic pain. A small number of patients report that they are always in pain. The acute painful episode or so-called painful crisis is perhaps the most devastating manifestation of the disease. Chronic pain is usually the most debilitating.

To consider analgesic study design issues in sickle cell disease, it must be recognized that the patients, the disease, and the pain are very heterogeneous (14–16). Not only is there enormous interpatient heterogeneity, there is intercrisis and intracrisis variability within a given individual. The average duration of painful crises has been reported to be from 4 to 6 days with a range of a few hours to weeks depending upon the occurrence of co-morbidities and a multitude of extrinsic and intrinsic stimuli (12). Although very little is known about the specific predisposing pathophysiologic factors that initiate acute painful episodes, it is generally recognized that these events are attributable to ischemic tissue

TABLE 1. *Types of pain in patients with sickle cell disease (SCD)*

Acute pain associated with SCD
  Painful crisis
  Hand-foot syndrome
  Arthritis
  Acute chest syndrome
  Splenic sequestration
  Bowel infarction and necrosis
  Intrahepatic sickling
  Priapism
Chronic pain associated with SCD
  Arthropathies
  Aseptic necrosis
  Vertebral body collapse
  Leg ulcers
Pain associated with therapy
  Withdrawal
  Constipation—fecal impaction
  Gout
  Loose hip or shoulder prostheses
Pain not related or indirectly related to SCD or therapy
  Trauma
  Infection
  Arthritis
  Headaches
  Cholelithiasis
  Cholecystitis
  Peptic ulcer disease

injury or infarction resulting from the obstruction of blood flow by sickle erythrocytes. The myriad reactions that accompany the initial vaso-occlusion and tissue injury contribute to the pain syndrome, including vasospasm, inflammation at the site of injury, and local elaboration of histamine, bradykinin, serotonin, prostaglandins, substance P, and potassium ions (8,12). In addition, pain is strongly influenced by psychological factors (17,18). The psychological components of a chronic illness are compounded by devastating, unpredictable, recurrent acute pain. Repeated episodes can lead to both organ damage and chronic pain.

The treatment of pain in sickle cell disease has been based largely on anecdotal and empirical observations. The pharmacokinetic and relative potency guidelines that are used may not be appropriate because they have been derived from studies in other pain models, such as postoperative pain and cancer pain (19). Pharmacokinetics can be altered by organ dysfunction, common in sickle cell disease. For example, as a result of intrahepatic sickling, many sickle cell patients have impairment of liver function (12,13). Furthermore, the hyposthenuria (impaired ability to concentrate urine) that results from renal damage and often occurs very early in the course of the disease can be a factor in the clearance or excretion of certain drugs (12,20). In addition, acute-phase proteins are increased during acute pain (21,22). One of these, alpha-1 acid glycoprotein, has been shown to bind some analgesics (23) including meperidine in the treatment of acute sickle pain (24). Thus, the disposition, elimination, bioavailability, half-lives, and clearances of selective agents might be altered in some or all sickle cell patients.

Diurnal variations in sickle cell patients' clinical response to meperidine have been reported (25). Another study that compared serum concentrations following a 100 mg dose of meperidine in sickle cell patients experiencing acute pain (crises) to control patients receiving 100 mg meperidine prior to incision and drainage reported lower peak drug concentrations in the sickle pain group (26). The authors questioned whether this difference could explain, at least in part, the relatively poor pain control often noted in sickle cell patients. The safety profiles of drugs might also be altered.

A broad range of clinical studies of pain and related issues in sickle cell disease are needed including descriptive studies that determine the prevalence and incidence of pain and characterize its type, intensities, origins, and mechanisms, as well as efficacy studies directed to the various types of pain. Pharmacokinetic studies of commonly used drugs should be evaluated during crisis and steady state. Relative potency assays of single and repeated doses should be performed to elucidate whether the equianalgesic dosages determined from single-dose analgesic studies in other pain states are applicable to the sickle cell patient population. New drug preparations, routes, and methods of drug delivery should be evaluated for their potential in enhancing effective usage of analgesics during sickle cell painful crisis and for the chronic pain.

Finally, more attention should be given to the suffering or psychosocial components of pain and to therapeutic modalities such as relaxation, behavior modification, hypnosis, and other techniques that address stress issues. Of paramount importance are epidemiological studies to determine the true prevalence and incidence of drug dependency and "addiction" in sickle cell disease. In other disease states it has been shown that whereas tolerance and physical dependence are predictable pharmacologic effects of repeated administration of narcotics (27), medical use of these agents rarely lead to drug abuse or iatrogenic narcotic addiction (28). The few reports in sickle cell disease that have dealt with this subject do not make the distinction between these entities and are lacking in a clear definition of addiction (8,11,29). The tendency to define the entire patient population by its worst cases and to erroneously categorize patients as "addicts" largely owing to a lack of clarity in definition of terms severely compromises the management of pain in a large number of individuals.

PAIN ASSESSMENT

The design of analgesic trials in sickle cell pain depends upon pain assessment. Pain should be characterized in such a way that therapy can be tailored to the individual needs of the patient. Monitoring of treatment should specify the pain parameters that will be measured.

Types of Pain

The types of pain syndromes in sickle cell disease are depicted in Table 1. Each type of pain depicted here is directly or indirectly related to either vaso-occlusion or therapy. The acute painful vaso-occlusive event (painful crisis), the most devastating and commonly encountered pain syndrome seen in sickle cell disease patients of all ages, is characterized by the abrupt unpredictable onset of pain for which there is no other explanation. It is self-limiting but can be recurrent and is characterized by exacerbations, subsidences, and migrations from one site to another within a given episode. This pain is often severe and involves extremities, especially joints, the lower back, the abdomen, or the chest. The associated magnetic resonance imaging (MRI) finding of infarctive changes in bone and soft tissue in lower extremities of patients experiencing acute pain episodes (30) as well as biochemical changes that have been reported (3,21,30,31) support the explanation of pain based upon ischemia, infarction, and inflammation.

The hand-foot syndrome, or dactylitis, occurs more commonly during early childhood, (6 months to 4 years), and is often the first manifestation of the disease. It occurs as a result of symmetrical infarcts of metacarpal and metatarsal bones owing to obstruction of developing blood vessels to the distal limbs, and clinically appears as painful dorsal swelling of the hands and feet. Acute inflammation of joints can occur in the context of both preceding types of pain. In addition, as a result of repeated episodes of vaso-occlusion, acute flare-ups of arthritis can appear as isolated events.

The acute chest syndrome can occur alone or in association with acute painful crises. Its hallmark is pleuritic chest pain. Pulmonary infiltrates may be associated with infarction, infection, fever, tachypnea, and/or hypoxia. Splenic sequestration also occurs in young children with many forms of sickle cell disease as well as in older individuals with syndrome such as S-C or S-B+ thalassemia in which the spleen has not been repeatedly infarcted and remains large and functional. Splenic sequestration in children can be catastrophic, with a sudden decrease in hemoglobin concentration and possibly circulatory collapse. In older individuals its onset is, in general, more insidious. Obviously, an effort to maintain circulatory integrity, reduce spleen size, or if necessary, to remove the spleen, are therapies for this cause of pain that take precedence over any other symptom-related intervention. Intrahepatic sickling or hepatic sequestration occur more commonly in adults and must be differentiated from pain owing to cholelithiasis or other conditions in which there is obstructive jaundice. Abdominal pain can also be secondary to bowel infarction and necrosis, which is known to occur but is not often documented. Priapism is a painful continuous erection that occurs as a result of sickling in the sinusoids of the penis. It may last from hours to days or may be intractable. Therapy is directed toward relieving the obstruction.

Chronic pain is most commonly associated with bony changes (aseptic necrosis of humeral or femoral heads or vertebral collapse) or chronic recurrent leg ulcerations. Either of these can severely compromise mobility and represent major management problems. In addition to the significant psychological responses to these sequelae, chronic pain also results as a consequence of the suboptimal or inappropriate management of acute or chronic pain.

The design of a study of acute pain, which is characterized by marked fluctuations (Fig. 1), will differ greatly from a study of chronic pain, which is in general consistent and stable. Similarly, the design of a study of painful crisis, for which there is only symptomatic therapy with hydration and analgesics, will differ from acute pain owing to priapism or splenic sequestration, which in addition to symptomatic care, may require blood transfusion and/or surgical intervention.

Origin and Mechanisms of Pain

The classification of patients' pain may have important therapeutic implications. If possible, it is highly desirable to characterize pain in terms of its origin (32). There has been a dramatic increase in our knowledge of the sites and mechanisms of both pain and analgesia (33–35). The typically deep pain experienced during vaso-occlusive episodes as a result of nociceptive stimuli can either be somatic or visceral. Chemical messengers and mediators of inflammation

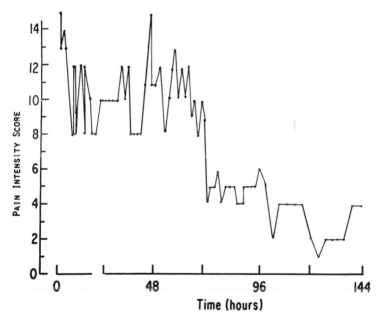

FIG. 1. Representative pain profile in a sickle cell patient experiencing painful crisis. The scale for assessment of intensity was 0 = pain-free; 0.5 = residual soreness; 1 = mild pain; 2 = moderate pain, and 3 = severe pain. The pain intensity score is the sum of the intensity scores for each site.

elaborated as a result of damage to tissue can amplify the pain by activating and sensitizing nociceptors. The nature of biochemical mediators differs depending on the target tissue (36). Although the technology for assessing these differences has not advanced to widespread use, it may become possible to utilize this knowledge to assess mechanisms regarding the somatic and visceral sites of injury (see Chapter 25). From this approach should emerge more specific information regarding the pain picture in sickle cell disease to which more site- and mechanism-directed therapies could be employed.

Somatic pain is probably the most frequent type of pain encountered in sickle cell disease. It involves primarily the deep structures such as muscles, tendons, ligaments, periosteum, bone marrow, joints, and arteries. This pain can be focal or referred. Stimuli in sickle cell disease that evoke visceral pain are the sudden abnormal distension seen in splenic and hepatic sequestration, vasospasm, and anoxemia or hypoxia of visceral musculature. Visceral pain is generally vague, poorly localized, diffuse, characterized by dull aching, and often associated with nausea, vomiting, and sweating. Vaso-occlusion frequently recurs in certain viscera, e.g., spleen, lungs, liver (12), and thus, there may be a greater ability to localize the injury in this disorder than in others characterized by visceral pain. Some patients have visceral pain of sharper quality that is more localizable and is felt closer to the site of the injured viscera. This subtype of visceral pain is rarely associated with nausea or vomiting and it is frequently associated with muscle spasms, tenderness, and hyperesthesia.

There is reason to believe that inflammation contributes to the intensification of the pain experienced during acute vaso-occlusive episodes. When ordinarily nonnoxious stimuli are inflicted upon inflamed tissues, pain of considerable intensity can be evoked. Thus, inflammation may significantly lower the threshold of either somatic or visceral pain. Biochemical alterations in the acute phase response, coagulation, and fibrinolytic systems are consistent with inflammatory changes and have been noted during the acute painful episodes (21,30). These substances as well as histamines, bradykinins, prostaglandins, and substance P, could contribute to pain, not only at the injured site but also in surrounding structures such as the periosteum, the pleura, or blood vessels (37). Thus, drugs that inhibit particular inflammatory mediators should be investigated as analgesics or co-analgesics in sickle cell disease–related pain.

Psychological factors may also contribute greatly to the pain (17,18,32). Following several painful crises, some sickle cell patients develop fear, fail to readjust, and become intensely fixed on the possibility of another painful crisis. In these instances organic pain may be psychogenically amplified, and emotional difficulties may be focused on this pain. The treatment of this psychogenic component is pivotal to the success of therapy (38,39). Drug-taking behavior may also contribute to psychogenic perpetuation of pain. This can occur in the context of the vicious cycle caused by undermedication during acute pain and overmedication during chronic pain. A psychological event, particularly stress, can also be the primary factor that precipitates an acute painful crisis (12,32). The importance of the psychological factors are such that pain assessment, whether clinical or investigational, should include psychological measurement.

Pain Measurement

In most clinical analgesic studies, pain is generally measured by categorical and visual analogue scales that have been validated and determined to be reliable and sensitive in studies of cancer pain and postoperative pain in adults (40; and see Chapter 4). Pain assessment should consist of both cognitive and affective components. The Memorial Pain Assessment Card (MPAC) is a simple instrument that uses several category and visual analogue scales (VAS) to evaluate pain intensity, pain relief, and mood or psychological distress (41,42). Patients are asked to rate the pain and relief at each site in addition to the overall rating. We are currently assessing this methodology, along with human figure drawings (43) on which painful sites are marked, in both clinical management and clinical trials of pain in sickle cell disease. The segmental distributions of the shadings should also delineate origins of pain (32). Although category and VAS measures of pain and relief have been formally validated in acute pain and chronic cancer pain, their sensitivity and reliability have not yet been examined in patients with pain owing to sickle cell disease.

The establishment of sensitive and reliable assessment tools in this disorder is important not only in the evaluation of analgesics but also in the evaluation of drugs that prevent or treat painful crises. In the absence of objective measures that correspond to clinical state, the therapeutic effects of antisickling agents have been measured by assessing effects on the intensity and duration of pain (3,44). Thus, improved analgesic study methods may further enhance the key role that pain measurement plays in assessing clinical response to agents that intervene in the pathophysiology of the disease. Another result of pain assessment and measurement may be to uncover pain that is neither somatic nor visceral. For example, neuropathic pain that results from actual injury to nerves is refractory to the traditional therapies of somatic or visceral pain.

CLINICAL TRIALS IN SICKLE CELL DISEASE: NEEDS AND POTENTIAL METHODOLOGIES

Parenteral Nonsteroidal Antiinflammatory Drugs (NSAIDs): A Potential Alternative to Narcotics

It is generally agreed that pain management in sickle cell disease is fraught with obstacles centered around issues of narcotic misuse. Misgivings of health care personnel about administering narcotic analgesics, misunderstandings as to the relevance of tolerance and dependency, and preoccupation with the question of addiction are major contributing factors to poor management of pain in sickle cell disease. Thus, the elimination or diminution of the need for narcotic analgesics could revolutionize the medical approach to controlling acute pain in the sickle cell patient. One pharmacologic alternative would be an effective non-narcotic analgesic. This drug should have a short onset and a long duration of action; it should be easily administered and have a parenteral formulation. Lysine acetylsalicylate (LAS), a water soluble derivative of aspirin, appears to be such an agent. Both LAS and another parenteral NSAID preparation, ketorolac, have been shown to have efficacy similar to that of morphine in relieving postoperative pain (45,46). In relative potency studies, 1.8 g of LAS has been estimated to be equivalent to 10 mg morphine or 75 mg of meperidine.

The evaluation of LAS can be used to illustrate an approach to the design of studies to evaluate new analgesic agents in sickle cell disease. In our studies of this drug the pain model selected for study was acute vaso-occlusive painful crisis of moderate to severe intensity. Patients were eligible if the pain had not been controlled by usual home measures, had persisted for a minimum of 4 hrs, and upon presentation at the hospital required potent parenteral dosing or its equivalent for pain control.

The objectives of the initial study were to determine if the drug could be given at safe and effective doses in pain crisis, to gain experience with the drug, and to determine a dosing range prior to embarking on a double-blind study. In addition to the usual considerations in patient selection, disease-specific and drug-specific criteria were essential for inclusion into the study, (e.g., a normal bleeding time and no untoward effects of aspirin challenge during an asymptomatic period). Patients who had been prescreened and had signed informed consent forms during the asymptomatic period were entered into the study as they presented in painful crisis.

An open-labeled crossover dose titration design was chosen (47). The patient was treated with the test medication (LAS) or the standard analgesic (meperidine). Patients were individually titrated to optimal analgesia with single or multiple doses of the first medication by bolus dosing alone or in combination with continuous infusion. Optimal analgesia was defined as mild to no pain and good to complete relief of pain (Fig. 2). After achieving this level of relief, patients were observed until moderate to severe pain returned. At that time, they were crossed over to the other medication and the process was repeated. The patients received

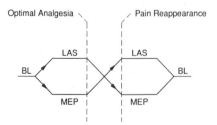

FIG. 2. Trial design: pilot open-label crossover dose titration study of lysine acetylsalicylate (LAS) and meperidine (MEP) in the treatment of acute sickle pain (crises). BL, baseline.

LAS or meperidine as needed to a maximum 24-hr dose of 9 g of LAS. Salicylate levels were assayed for the corresponding points of optimal analgesic.

The starting pain was comparable for both treatments (Table 2). Nine crisis events were studied. Two of the patients who received LAS first required no further medication. Five patients who were crossed over achieved optimal analgesia with both drugs, and in these patients, the duration of optimal analgesia was at least as long with LAS as with meperidine. The patients' global evaluations of the quality of the pain relief provided by the two medications were comparable. The salicylate levels at optimal analgesia were within the safety range of the drug (<300 μg/ml). The adverse reactions noted were minimal.

This was an open study and no placebo was used. It is recognized that such a design can give only preliminary evidence that LAS is effective. We learned that LAS as given is safe and has the potential for efficacy in sickle cell crisis. Moreover, global evaluation showed that the patients perceived LAS as being as satisfactory as meperidine in the relief of pain. The drug was easily administered and patients responded well whether receiving the medication by bolus dosing or by continuous infusion. There were dose-dependent effects. The concentrations of LAS in the blood at optimal analgesia were at levels considered to be safe and were high enough to provide both analgesic and antiinflammatory effects. Accordingly, dosing and scheduling for the double-blind study could be based upon an increasing potential for efficacy within the safety limits of the drug.

Based upon these considerations, follow-up studies have been started using two types of study designs. First, the possibility of a narcotic-sparing effect is being examined in a double-blind placebo-controlled parallel study (Table 3). In order to perform a placebo-controlled analgesic study, a backup rescue regimen is essential. The patient receives either LAS or placebo and is titrated to optimal analgesia with morphine or meperidine. Patient-controlled analgesics (PCA) can be used to deliver the rescue doses in such studies (see below).

Narcotic Analgesics

Data are needed to clarify the relative analgesic effectiveness of the two or three narcotic agents most commonly used in the management of sickle cell

TABLE 2. *Pilot dose titration studies of lysine acetylsalicylate (LAS) in acute sickle cell pain*

	LAS	Meperidine
Starting pain		
2 = moderate, 3 = severe	2.4 ± 0.6 (9)[a]	2.3 ± 0.6 (7)
Duration of optimal analgesia	5.4 ± 2.8 (5)	2.8 ± 1.3 (5)
Global score of analgesic		
0 = worst, 10 = best	8.5 ± 1.4 (5)	7.2 ± 1.3 (5)
Salicylate levels at optimal analgesia μg/ml	130 ± 41 (8)	

[a] Mean ± standard deviation (number of episodes).

TABLE 3. *Trial design: randomized double-blind placebo-controlled parallel study of the narcotic sparing effect of lysine acetylsalicylate (LAS) during acute painful events in sickle cell*

Treatment group	Number of episodes	Treatment 1 Time 0 Drug/Dose	Treatment 2 Hours 1–24 Drug/Dose	Treatment 3 Hours 24–48 Drug/Dose
1	25	LAS 1.8 gm bolus	LAS 1.8 gm bolus + LAS 0.45 gm/hr	LAS 0.9 gm bolus + LAS 0.225 gm/hr
2	25	Placebo bolus infusion	Placebo bolus + continue	Placebo bolus + continue infusion
1 and 2	50	—	(Hours 1–48) Meperidine 50–100 mg gl/hr prn	

pain, and to explore potential advantages of newer methods of delivery, such as patient-controlled analgesia, and preparations such as sustained-release morphine.

Relative Potency and Efficacy Studies

Most clinicians use meperidine rather than morphine as a first-line drug in painful vaso-occlusive crises. The reasons for this are unclear but seem to be based on traditional use of these drugs in clinical practice. Controlled studies to determine the relative potency and pharmacokinetics of these drugs have not been performed in individuals with sickle cell disease. Many physicians have been influenced directly or indirectly by early teachings that meperidine has low or no addicting properties, that it is as effective an analgesic as morphine, and that it causes fewer side effects such as respiratory depression and vomiting. Although these claims have not been proved, meperidine remains the most prescribed narcotic.

Many patients also communicate a preference for meperidine over morphine, perhaps because they have been given this drug in the past. They perceive morphine as having a greater risk of addiction. To them, meperidine seems to be associated with fewer side effects. Ironically, meperidine is more hazardous, in fact, and is associated with seizures caused by its toxic metabolite, normeperidine (48). There have been reports of seizures in sickle cell patients while being treated with meperidine (49). However, there are some patients who report that meperidine is the only short-acting narcotic that gives them pain relief without significant adverse effects. Based upon clinical experience and the lack of available data, it is premature to suggest that parenteral meperidine has no place in the management of sickle cell pain. Because it is known that myoclonus and seizures are associated with the dose and repetitive administration, efforts should be made to minimize the risks (49) until carefully controlled studies are performed. This author's opinion is that although parenteral meperidine may prove to have certain advantages for acute treatment, oral meperidine should not be used. Meperidine usage, when required, should be reserved for parenteral dosing in the hospital. The widespread use of oral meperidine contributes to the development of tolerance and higher normeperidine levels result when parenteral dosing becomes superimposed, placing the patient at higher risk for seizures. Combination therapy with promethazine (Phenergan) should also be avoided because the phenothiazines lower the seizure threshold for meperidine.

Comparisons of morphine and meperidine might provide insight into a major management problem: the tug of war between patients who insist that meperidine works best and physicians who insist that morphine is the best drug. Although there is a recent report of a double-blind study that showed that morphine and butorphanol were equally effective in controlling acute sickle cell pain (50), and there are uncontrolled studies reporting the efficacy and toxicity of oral morphine (51), and morphine or meperidine by bolus or continuous infusion (52), there are no blinded controlled studies that evaluate these two agents in this disorder.

In addition to parallel designs as reported above, crossover studies should be strongly considered as a means of reducing the effects of interpatient and intercrisis variability (53). As noted earlier, the average duration of crisis is about five days. In most individuals, pain of comparable intensity, upon allowing the pain to reappear, can be treated within a 48-hr study period (see Fig. 1). It is generally at around 72 hrs that the pain begins to subside. This design can be very efficient as fewer patients are needed, since the patients can serve as their own controls. Moreover, experiments can be performed in a much shorter time period, thereby lessening the likelihood of disease variation.

Patient-Controlled Analgesia Utilizing Parenteral Narcotics

When narcotic medication is given by the intramuscular route, there are peaks and troughs that may cause wide swings of analgesia, sedation, and pain (54). The desired effect is to maintain the patient in the range of analgesia without periodically raising the plasma drug concentration high enough to produce adverse effects, such as respiratory depression. With "as-needed" dosing, the patient makes a report of need to the nurse, who in turn must proceed through several steps before medicating the patient. The issue in pain management is always whether the patient receives what is needed. Pain studies often report what the patients received by design without being reflective of need (27). Table 4 shows meperidine dosing over the first 4 days of hospitalization in a patient during routine care and on two different protocols. Dose titration, whether in open or blinded studies, attempts to take into account patient variability. Patient-controlled analgesia can be utilized to overcome some of these problems as they present in management of acute vaso-occlusive pain.

As with the study of a new drug, it is also important to pilot a new method of drug delivery to gain experience regarding its capabilities and its limitations, as well as to discern whether the dosing range of a drug is altered. In collaboration with the anesthesiology pain service, we sought to explore the potential for the use of PCA in acute vaso-occlusive pain (55). The primary objectives were to

TABLE 4. *Total daily meperidine doses (mg) during the first four days of regular care or drug study protocols in an individual experiencing multiple acute painful episodes (crises)*

| Events | Crisis date | Study severity | Medication | Meperidine doses (mg) by day | | | | Duration |
				1	2	3	4	
Antisickling protocol								
1	1/82	Severe	Drug	1,425	1,140	850	570	4
2	8/82	Moderate	Placebo	1,000	1,300	1,075	250	4
3	12/82	Moderate-Severe	Placebo	1,500	1,600	1,375	1,523	6
Regular care								
4	12/83	Severe	—	1,700	1,500	1,050	675	6
5	12/86	Severe	—	1,800	1,550	1,325	1,050	10
Analgesic study								
6	3/87	Severe	?	650	650	1,450	1,650	7
7	6/87	Severe	?	900	1,250	2,300	2,300	9

determine a dosing regimen that provided timely administration of analgesics according to patients' needs. A dosing formula was derived from trial and error dose titrations based on prior analgesic history of patients who were at least 24 hrs into the painful episode. Specifically, the total amount of medication received in the previous 24 hrs (usually meperidine) was converted to the analgesic equivalent of the planned PCA drug (usually morphine) and increased by 50%. We found that PCA alone did not permit uniform control of pain and that better pain control was achieved if the PCA was delivered with a continuous infusion of the medication. Thus, one-third of the calculated 24-hr dose was administered by continuous infusion and two-thirds of the total dose was allocated for PCA. The PCA dose divided by eight gave the incremental dose and the lockout interval was set at 8 to 10 min.

This dosing regimen was tested on 25 patients. Although an effort was made to place all patients on morphine, six patients could not be switched from meperidine and two were treated with hydromorphone. The narcotic had to be increased in 9 (36%) of the patients. This group included all six patients who remained on meperidine. Five of these six responded favorably to the increased regimen. Of the 17 patients who were placed on morphine, all stayed within the dosing formulation except for three in whom the medication had to be increased. The medication was discontinued because of side effects or poor pain control in two patients in the morphine group and one patient on meperidine. Overall, PCA was safe and effective and it was the preferred mode of pain medication for 84% of the patients and 100% of the health care providers.

A preliminary study such as this provides a frame of reference and guidelines for dosing for additional studies of relative potency and efficacy and studies of pharmacokinetic variability. In addition to use as a primary analgesic method, PCA can be utilized to more effectively deliver "rescue" analgesia medication during the studies that compare other drugs. An example might be a study comparing oral slow release morphine preparations (56) with morphine administered by continuous infusion (57).

PCA might also permit the evaluation of agents such as fentanyl, sufentanil, or alfentanil, whose usage to date has been limited by a very short half-life (51). The evaluation of this group of compounds would be especially interesting in tolerant patients in whom all other narcotic analgesics with rapid onset and short duration of action have been exhausted in the treatment of acute pain. We have administered fentanyl by PCA to a few patients in whom all other short-acting narcotic analgesics alone or in combination with antiinflammatory agents and/ or tricyclics have failed to control pain. Because of positive results, a pilot study is underway to establish a dosing range for this family of drugs. Finally, subcutaneous and epidural PCA might be explored in patients with sickle cell disease whose venous access is limited or in whom localized pain accessible by these routes has been refractory to traditional measures. Various methodologies in PCA are presented in Chapters 22, 23, and the commentary on p. 525.

SUMMARY

There are many acute and chronic pain syndromes in sickle cell disease. The assessment of pain regarding its type, origin, mechanisms, and measurements are essential for the design and evaluation of appropriate and effective therapies for pain experienced by individuals with sickle cell disease. Pharmacokinetic, pharmacodynamic, and epidemiologic studies are needed of both traditional and new pharmacologic and nonpharmacologic therapies. In particular, parenteral NSAIDs have potential as alternatives to narcotics. Patient-controlled analgesia, which permits the timely administration of analgesics according to patient needs, shows promise as a valuable investigative and clinical management tool. Although neglected in the past, the clinical management of pain in sickle cell disease is receiving increasing attention in the medical literature. It is even conceivable that sickle cell disease may have a role as an acute pain model in which analgesics are studied. Such a role would probably attract more clinical scientists to this area of pain research. Nonetheless, the immediate need is for studies that will provide information with clinical utility in this disorder.

REFERENCES

1. Alouch JR. The treatment of sickle cell disease: a historical and chronological literature review of the therapies applied since 1910. *Trop Geogr Med* 1984;36:51–52.
2. Mentzer WC. A review of clinical trials in sickle cell anemia. In: Beuzard Y, Charache S, Galacteros F, eds. *Approaches to the therapy of sickle cell anemia (approaches to therapeutiques de la drepanocytose).* Paris: Les Editions INSERM, 1985;141:115–127.
3. Benjamin LJ. Conventional and experimental approaches to treatment of pain crisis. In: Mankad VN, Moore RB, eds. *Sickle cell disease: pathophysiology, diagnosis and treatment.* Prager Scientific, 1990; In press.
4. Begue P, Bertrand E, Bonhamme J. Action de la Dihydroergotoxine sur la Crises Drepanocyaire Resultates d'une Estude Multicentrique en Double-Aveugle Nealisse en Afrique Fransophone. *Noun Presse Med* 1978;7:2449–2452.

5. Benjamin LJ, Berkowitz LR, Orringer E, et al. A collaborative, double-blind randomized study of cetiedil citrate in sickle cell crisis. *Blood* 1986;67(5):1442–1447.
6. Cabannes R, Sangare A, Cho YW. Acute painful sickle cell crisis in children: a double-blind placebo-controlled evaluation of efficacy and safety of cetiedil. *Clin Trial J* 1983;20:207–218.
7. Hardy WR. Sickle cell anemia as a problem in pain management. In: Marc LC, ed. Pain control. *Practical aspects of patient care.* New York, Masson, 1981;1–11.
8. Benjamin LJ. Pain in sickle cell disease. In: Foley KM, Payne R, Decker BC, eds. *Current therapy of pain.* Ontario: 1989;90–104.
9. Shapiro BS. The management of pain in sickle cell disease. *Pediatr Clin North Am* 1989;36(4): 1029–1045.
10. Payne R. Pain management in sickle cell disease: rationale and techniques. In Whitten CF, Bertles JF, eds. Sickle Cell Disease. *Ann NY Acad Sci* 1989;565.
11. Charache S, Lubin B, Reid CD. Management and therapy of sickle cell disease. U.S. Department of Health and Human Services, 1985; NIH Publication, #85-2117.
12. Vichinsky EP, Lubin BH. Sickle cell anemia and related hemoglobinopathies. *Pediatr Clin North Am* 1980;27:429–447.
13. Davis JR, Vichinsky EP, Lubin BH. Current treatment of sickle cell disease. In: Bluck L, Conte TE, eds. *Current problems in pediatric.* 64.
14. Nagel RL, Fabry ME. The many pathophysiologies of sickle cell anemia. *Am J Hematol* 1985;20: 195–199.
15. Schechter AN, Noguchl CT, Rodgers GP. Sickle cell disease. In: Stamatoyannopoulos G, Nienhus GAW, Leder P, Mayerus PW, eds. *The molecular basis of blood diseases.* Philadelphia: WB Saunders, 1987;179–218.
16. Ingram V. Molecular and cellular pathogenesis, clinical, and epidemiological aspects. In: Bunn HF, Forget BG, eds. *Hemoglobin: molecular, genetic, and clinical aspects.* Philadelphia: WB Saunders, 1986;453–564.
17. Whitten CF, Fishhoff J. Psychosocial effects of sickle cell disease. *Arch Intern Med* 1974;133: 681–689.
18. Nadel C, Portadin G. Sickle cell crisis: psychological factors associated with onset. *NY State J Med* 1990;14:171–180.
19. Inturrisi CE. Effects of other drugs and pathologic states on opioid disposition and response. In: Benedetti C, Giron G, Chapman CR, eds. *Advances in pain research and therapy.* New York: Raven Press, In Press.
20. Keltel AG, Thompson D, Itano HA. Hyposthenuria in sickle cell anemia: a reversible renal defect. *J Clin Invest* 1958;35:998.
21. Benjamin LJ. Biochemical and cell alterations in sickle cell anemia: crisis markers and therapeutic monitors. In: Beuzard V, Charache S, Galacteros F, eds. *Approaches to the therapy of sickle cell anemia.* Paris: Les Editions INSERM, 1985;451.
22. Becton DL, Raymond L, Thompson C. Acute-phase reactants in sickle cell disease. *J Pediatr* 1989;115(1):99–102.
23. Abramson FO. Methadone plasma protein binding: alterations in cancer and displacement from alpha 1-acid glycoprotein. *Clin Pharmacol Ther* 1982;32:652–658.
24. Williams WD, Chung H. Protein binding diminishes the efficiency of meperidine. *Blood* 1985;66(Suppl):67A.
25. Ritschell WA, Bykadi G, For DJ, et al. A pilot study on disposition and pain relief after i.m. administration of meperidine during the day and night. *Int J Clin Pharmacol Ther Toxicol* 1983;21:218–223.
26. Abbuhl S, Jacobson S, Murphy JG, Gibson G. Serum concentration of meperidine in patients with sickle cell crises. *Ann Emerg Med* 1986;15:433–438.
27. Inturrisi CE. Management of cancer pain pharmacology and principals of management. *Cancer.* 1989;63:2308–2320.
28. Marks RM, Sachar EJ. Undertreatment of medical inpatients with narcotic analgesics. *Ann Intern Med* 1973;78:173–181.
29. Rayport M. Experience in the management of patients medically addicted to narcotics. *JAMA* 1954;156:684–691.
30. Mankad VN, Williams JP, Harpen M, et al. Magnetic resonance imaging of bone marrow in sickle cell disease: clinical, hematologic and pathologic correlations. *Blood* 1990;75(1):274–283.
31. Benjamin LJ, Jones RL, Peterson CM, Zellers R, Harpel P. Hemostatic alterations in sickle cell anemia: objective markers of vaso-occlusive crisis. *Blood* 1985;66(5)Suppl 1:318A.

32. Bonica JJ. Introduction. Pathophysiology of pain. *Current concepts in postoperative pain.* New York: H.P. Publishing Co., 1978;1–15.
33. Payne R. Anatomy, physiology, and neuropharmacology of cancer pain. In: Foley KM, Inturrisi CE, eds. *Medical clinics of North America: cancer pain.* Philadelphia: W.B. Saunders, 1987;153–168.
34. Martin WR. Clinical evidence for different narcotic receptors and relevance for the clinician. *Ann Emerg Med* 1986;15:1026–1029.
35. Malliani A, Pagani M, Lombardi F. Visceral vs somatic mechanisms. In: Melzack R, Wall PD, eds. *Textbook of pain.* London: Churchill Livingstone, 1989, pp. 128–140.
36. Wall PD. Introduction. In: Melzack R, Wall PD, eds. *Textbook of pain.* London: Churchill Livingstone, 1989;1–18.
37. Campbell JN, Raja SN, Cohen RH, Manning DC, Khan AA, Meyer RA. Peripheral neural mechanism of nociception. In: Melzack R, Wall PD, eds. *Textbook of pain.* London: Churchill Livingstone, 1989;22–45.
38. Vichinsky EP, Johnson R, Lubin BH. Multidisciplinary approach of pain management in sickle cell disease. *Am J Pediatr Hematol Oncol* 1982;4:328–333.
39. Gil KM. Coping with sickle cell disease pain. *Ann Behav Med* 1989;11:49–57.
40. Houde RW. Methods of measuring clinical pain in humans. *Acta Anaesthiol Scand* 1982;74:25–29.
41. Wallenstein SL, Houde RW. The clinical evaluation of analgesic effectiveness. In: Ehrenpreis S, Neidle A, ed. *Methods in narcotics research.* New York: Marcel Dekker, 1975;127.
42. Fishman B, Pasternak S, Wallenstein SL, Houde RW, Holland JC, Foley RM. The Memorial pain assessment card: a valid instrument for the evaluation of cancer pain. *Cancer* 1987;60:1151–1158.
43. Gil KM, Phillips G, Abrams MR, Williams DA. Pain drawing and sickle cell disease pain. *Clin J Pain* 1990; In Press.
44. Cooperative Urea Trials Group. Clinical trials of therapy for sickle cell vaso-occlusive crisis. *JAMA* 1974;228:1120–1124.
45. Kweekel-de-Vries WJ, Speirdijk J, Mattie H, Hermans JMH. A new soluble acetylsalicylic acid derivative in the treatment of post-operative pain. *Br J Anaesth* 1974;46:133–135.
46. Yee JP, Koshiver JE, Allbon C, Brown CR. Comparison of intramuscular ketorolac tromethamine and morphine sulfate for analgesia of pain after major surgery. *Pharmacotherapy* 1986;6(5):253–261.
47. Benjamin LJ. Intravenous lysine acetylsalicylate for the treatment of acute pain in sickle cell disorders: potential alternative to narcotics. *Clin Res* 1989;37(2):335A.
48. Kaiko RF, Foley KM, Grabinski PY, et al. Central nervous system irritability effects of meperidine in cancer patients. *Ann Neurol* 1983;13:180–185.
49. Tang RS, Shimomura SK, Rotblatt M. Meperidine-induced seizures in sickle cell patients. *Hosp Formul* 1980;15:764–772.
50. Gonzalez ER, Ornato JP, Ware D, Bull D, Evens RP. Comparison of intramuscular analgesic activity of butorphanol and morphine in patients with sickle cell disease. *Ann Emerg Med* 1988;17(8):788–791.
51. Friedman EW, Weber AB, Osborn HH, Schwartz S. Oral analgesia for treatment of painful crises in sickle cell anemia. *Ann Emerg Med* 1986;15:43–47.
52. Cole TB, Sprinkle RH, Smith SJ, Buchanan GR. Intravenous narcotic therapy for children and severe sickle cell pain crises. *Am J Dis Child* 1986;140:1255–1259.
53. James KE, Forrest WH, Rose RL. Crossover and noncrossover designs in four-point parallel line analgesic assays. *Clin Pharmacol Ther* 1985;47:242–252.
54. Bennett RL, Griffen WD. Patient controlled analgesia. *Contemp Surg* 1983;23:75–84.
55. Kepes E, Kaplan R, Claudio M, Benjamin LJ. Patient controlled analgesia (PCA) dosing in sickle cell crisis. *World Congress on Pain* 1990.
56. Khojasteh A, Evans W, Reynolds RD, Thomas G, Savarese JJ. Controlled-release oral morphine sulfate in the treatment of cancer pain with pharmacokinetic correlation. *J Clin Oncol* 1987;5:956–961.
57. Schecter NL, Berrien FB, Kat SM. The use of patient-controlled analgesia in adolescents with sickle cell pain crises: a preliminary report. *J Pain Symptom Manag* 1988;3:109–113.
58. Mather LE. Clinical pharmacokinetics of fentanyl and its newer derivatives. *Clin Pharmacokinet* 1983;8:422–426.

Advances in Pain Research and Therapy, Vol. 18,
edited by M. Max, R. Portenoy, and E. Laska,
Raven Press, Ltd., New York © 1991.

14

Sports Injuries

David S. Muckle

*Department of Orthopaedic Surgery, Middlesbrough General Hospital, Middlesbrough,
Cleveland TS5 5AZ England; and Honorary Consultant, Football Association, England*

Sports injuries are universally common and, in this respect, offer frequent and valid opportunities for study, especially in designing a clinical trial. However, major problems may be encountered when undertaking such a study and the most relevant of these will be briefly considered before proceeding to the main methodological issues.

At the outset, it must be acknowledged that it is difficult to assess the true injury rate in any sport, for any age group, to any area of the body, and in any country. The most obvious problem is one of overall quantification, for many minor injuries are self-treated and thus go unreported.

Then there is the difficulty of accurate assessment. Even in the most professional clubs and organizations, injuries are often poorly recorded in the case notes. For example, the bland statement "a sprained ankle" does little to denote which ligamentous complex is damaged and to what degree. Or as a further example, one of the most commonly injured areas in sport is the knee. A review of high school football injuries (1) reported a total injury rate of 22.9 per 100 participants, with almost 80% having knee injuries. Ligamentous problems were the most common. Although more frequent in numbers, the long-term disability of ligamentous injuries (5%) was much less than that owing to meniscal injuries (25%). Thus, the initial assessment of any knee problem may require detailed investigations (e.g., an arthrogram or arthroscopy) to accurately differentiate between these two conditions before a knee "injury" can be admitted to a study. However, with the clinical presentation of both ligamentous and meniscal injuries being very similar in the earliest stages, these investigations, although important, are costly, invasive, and could affect the outcome of drug therapy. Thus, trials based on a clinical diagnosis of knee trauma alone could flounder on the basis of accuracy.

A further problem may arise when the patient requires hospital treatment because the computer-filed data on sports injuries may be loosely coded under a variety of headings (e.g., orthopedic, general surgery, neurosurgery, etc.). Owing to inadequately detailed cross-referencing, less serious injuries may be missed and thus the data become limited in value for both prospective and retrospective studies.

In this respect, multiple injuries are often incompletely recorded and coded, with more major injuries overshadowing what appear to be minor problems (for example, a ligamentous injury in a joint adjacent to a fracture is commonly overlooked in the initial assessments and may only come to light when training is resumed months later).

It is an obvious fact (but worth noting) that sporting pursuits and the numbers participating vary greatly from country to country. For example, injuries owing to skiing are relatively uncommon in Great Britain, whereas hockey injuries are more frequent in India and football injuries in North America. Thus, each country's trials will have a different emphasis and bias. Each one may require a different strategic approach and direct comparisons may not always be easily made, or be relevant.

How great is the sports injury problem? This question is difficult to answer accurately. Each year in Great Britain some 5 million people suffer such an injury. On an individual basis this approximates to 12% of the population, but this figure is distorted because many patients have more than one injury annually. Several other countries give total figures of between 5 and 12%. However, these are the patients who seek medical advice, usually in the accident and emergency departments or in the local sports injury clinics.

Fortunately, serious injuries are rare, but demanding of resources. In the author's study, at least 10% of the admission to an orthopedic ward in 1987 were owing to soccer-induced fractures and dislocations.

Mild to moderate sports injuries are more common although the so-called mild injuries may be underestimated, for the reasons mentioned above. Moderate injuries are often those which are referred to the outpatient clinics of sports doctors and, because hospital admission and complex therapies are not usually required, become the basis of many clinical trials.

One of the earliest studies to assess the overall problem was by Weightman and Brown (2,3). They ascertained the frequency of injury per 10,000 hrs of match play. However, when looking carefully at their figures it is apparent that certain variations occurred in their study that could influence trial data. For example, although soccer was reported as having the highest injury rate (36.5 per 10,000 hrs) and swimming the lowest (0.3), the latter is deemed paradoxically the most dangerous sport owing to the associated mortality rate from drowning. Rugby football, although less serious in frequency terms (30.5) compared to soccer, was more serious with regard to the severity of injury, with a hospital admission rate of 52.8% for rugby injuries and 29.8% for soccer.

These perturbations between mild, moderate, severe, and lethal injuries require an exacting analysis of the problems peculiar to each sport. They indicate that rigid criteria for admission to a trial are needed before any critical statistical evaluation can be made.

Some sports are difficult to analyze for analgesic trials because of the relatively high incidence of severe multiple injuries that need complex treatments; for example, boxing, where injuries are the rule rather than the exception, motorcycle or car racing, and hang gliding. Although skiing is another sport bedeviled by serious injuries that would (in some respects) make it difficult to study, the numbers involved in skiing injuries are enormous—it has been reported that over 225,000 fractures occur in the United States annually—and this volume of clinical data readily gives adequate numbers for many statistical subgroups. Thus, skiing injuries have been commonly used in analgesic and antiinflammatory trials, especially ankle sprains (4).

Age is also a factor that must be taken into consideration, for sports injuries are more frequent in the young than often suspected. Eriksson (5) showed that 42% of skiing injuries were found in the under-fifteen age group. Thus, it is important to segregate juvenile and adolescent injuries from the mainstream analysis because their response to therapy may vary considerably compared to adults. Not only do most injuries heal more rapidly in the young (for example, a lower radial fracture can heal within 3 to 6 weeks compared to at least double that period in the adult), but also children may have different background conditions that can affect their participation in a clinical trial. For example, it has been reported that in a health study of 300 high schools in Washington State an allergic condition was recorded in almost 66% of questionnaire forms (6) and many of these pupils would have required intermittent or long-term therapy.

Very serious injuries are obviously barred from analgesic investigations. An obvious example is injury to the cervical cord with its associated neurological sequelae, as found in football injuries (7).

Another feature that is often forgotten and must be taken into consideration in the design of a clinical analgesic study is that an assessment of efficacy made in training or practice may differ from an assessment made in the match play situation.

Training/practice injuries are common. One study has shown that in a review of 11,349 rugby injuries in France, 12.5% occurred in training and 46% were found when the players resumed playing after the summer break (8). The author has seen a similar summer peak with preseason training at soccer, accounting for almost a fifth of the annual total. However, not all injuries are as frequent in training/practice as in the game situation. In a study of 1,877 high school football injuries, 65% were seen in practice matches; but when compared on a time unit basis, the games were usually more dangerous, both for the type of injury and to the playing position involved. Significantly more contusions occurred during the game, whereas more sprains occurred in practice. Also, quarterbacks and linebackers were injured more often in games, whereas wide receivers were injured more often in practice (9).

Thus, there can be a variation not only in number, type, and severity between practice/training and match play situations, but there can be a more positive (or even negative) reaction to recovery if a match is imminent, as distinct from the lack of motivation when only further training sessions are pending—in essence, the player may be keen to play but not to train and thus distort the subjective analyses.

Soft-tissue injury is a broad field and encompasses sports injuries. It is pertinent to inquire whether any injury is truly sports specific. There is no doubt that some injuries may occur more frequently in sport (e.g., hamstring tearing) but no injury is only sports-induced and similar injuries can occur both in the home or at work. The demand on a soft-tissue injury may be almost as great under these conditions, for many occupations and domestic duties impose repetitive and intense activities. Thus, advances in the therapy of sports injuries should have a beneficial effect on all soft-tissue trauma treatments, and any information gathered from clinical trials should have a positive extrapolation to the treatment of other conditions, such as postoperative, dental, and malignant pain.

These initial questions must be taken into consideration when planning the design of an analgesic or antiinflammatory trial. Methodological issues are discussed in depth below. First, however, it is useful to briefly consider the complex biochemical and pathophysiological processes involved in traumatic inflammation.

BIOCHEMISTRY

Complex cellular and biochemical events occur with traumatic inflammation and most attention has focused on the metabolites of arachidonic acid, otherwise known as prostaglandins (10). An understanding of these events is necessary to rationalize the use of antiinflammatory or analgesic agents in sports injuries.

Prostaglandins belong to a group of unsaturated 20-carbon carboxylic acids derived from arachidonic acid. Trauma, heat, bacteria, and a wide range of chemicals activate phospholipase A_2, thus releasing arachidonic acid from the cell wall, so it can now pass through two different pathways: (a) the cyclooxygenase pathway and (b) the lipoxygenase pathway.

The cyclooxygenase pathway gives rise to prostacyclin (PC = PGI_2), thromboxanes, and the prostaglandins (PGs); the latter cause a dilatation in most vascular tissues and their presence increases the pain caused by other chemicals such as kinins and histamine. Thromboxane (THX) induces aggregation of platelets and white cells to the blood vessel walls. Prostacyclin can disperse such aggregated cells. However, PGs are not potent chemotactic agents or vascular permeability promoters.

The second pathway—lipoxygenase—gives rise to leukotrienes (LTs). They are potent chemotactic agents for phagocytosis and also increase capillary permeability.

Thus, the by-products from arachidonic acid cause the chain or cascade reaction of inflammation—namely pain, vasodilatation, increased capillary permeability, and a chemotactic action on white cells.

However, there are pharmaceutical agents that will antagonize these pathways, the first historically being an extract from the common willow—salicylic acid, or its derivative, aspirin. The cyclooxygenase system was found to be blocked by aspirin (10) and later by many nonsteroidal antiinflammatory agents. But their action on the second pathway (LTs) is debatable although indomethacin, for example, may be an exception.

The action of the commonly used corticosteroids (either in a short-acting preparation or in a long-acting form) is more complex, and they probably act via the internal mechanism of the cell to inhibit phospholipase A_2. Thus, there is a time delay in the onset of the steroid antiinflammatory effect.

The part played by oxygen free radicals in the acute inflammatory process has been outline by Blake et al. (11). Prostaglandins are themselves formed by enzyme reactions catalyzed by oxygen free radicals, and both polymorphonuclear leukocytes and macrophages are also activated to produce large quantities (12). The drug treatment for these radicals is still in its infancy. The fibroblasts are also affected by PGs; both E1 and F1α increase collagen biosynthesis and may be responsible for excessive scar formation after injury.

EARLY TRIALS AND METHODOLOGICAL ISSUES

Thus, three important and seemingly unrelated factors occurred in the late 1960s, all of which highlighted the relevance of analgesic studies in patients with sports injuries—namely, the discovery of the action of the prostaglandins and other chemicals in soft-tissue trauma; an increased awareness in and a demand for a more effective drug therapy for the injured athlete; and a better surveillance of these injuries by doctors, physiotherapists, coaches, and others interested in sports injuries. It was fairly common knowledge that certain of the butazone derivatives (especially phenylbutazone) were efficacious in soft-tissue injuries sustained by horses during racing. Various trials of these compounds were carried out in athletic injuries (13) and although it was thought that soft-tissue injuries on the whole could be treated by drug therapy, data from human studies were inconclusive. Indeed, most investigations in the 1960s occurred in nonrandomized, relatively uncontrolled trials using a variety of enzyme preparations such as Ananase and chymoral (14–16) and indomethacin (17,18).

Many problems beset these early clinical trials and most are now considered only in a historical context. For example, in 1973 indomethacin was studied in only 15 professional footballers (19) and a comparison was made with another 15 having a placebo. No difference was found between the groups although the numbers concerned are obviously too few and the injuries too general for a valid statistical analysis. In a study on 30 professional athletes in which three subgroups were identified, Santilli et al. (20) claimed statistical superiority of piroxicam over placebo and ibuprofen. However, this trial suffered another problem, namely of using a relatively ineffective dose of a drug, i.e., ibuprofen (900 mg daily).

Clyman (21), in an overview assessment of the rationalized use of antiinflammatory agents in sports injuries, felt that statistically reliable, well-controlled, double-blind studies were difficult to accomplish in basically healthy young athletes where the natural course of the clinical problem was rapid and uncomplicated.

Thus, what are some of the basic problems in designing a clinical trial? The following discussion clarifies the general difficulties described in the introduction with reference to the author's experiences following the initial study, which began in 1970 (22).

The first and most important decision to be made concerns the type of injury or injuries that should be the basis of the study. There are several key questions to be answered. Will the injury respond to the medication, either by its nature or severity? For example, if the investigator chooses to study the broad topic of "sprains," there will be a multitude of patients from sports, industry, and the home. However, are all sprains to be included? A sprain of the medial ligament of the knee may behave very differently from one of the lumbosacral spine. Thus the group "sprains" becomes subdivided into "knee sprains." However, will such an injury respond to antiinflammatory agents, as in the author's study on ibuprofen (23)? If the answer is yes, the next decision may be to include only acute sprains, thereby excluding acute-on-chronic and chronic injuries that may not respond, or may behave in an entirely different manner. So the subgroup becomes "acute medial ligament sprains of the knee." However, the word "sprain" is too imprecise for any detailed study. It includes a minor tear of the collagen and elastin framework of the medial ligament (grade I), right through to an incomplete rupture (grade II). A complete rupture would not be considered as pertinent to the study. But the clinical diagnosis of a sprain is a difficult assessment, for objective signs, other than a localized area of tenderness, may be nonexistent. A partial tear would probably be associated with an effusion in the knee from a synovial reaction and would not have leakage of contrast dye when introduced in arthrogram, as observed in a complete rupture. Thus, the subgroup now becomes "acute medial ligament sprains of the knee with an effusion." The injury has now been more clearly defined, but other factors must be taken into consideration.

First and foremost, one must ask if this sprain is an isolated injury or part of a complex problem. It has been the author's experience that injuries to large complex joints rarely occur in isolation. In the case of medial collateral knee ligament injuries, there may be other ligamentous damage (for example, to the anterior cruciate in approximately 30% of cases and to the medial meniscus in approximately 40% of cases). These complex injuries may have to be excluded from the study or included as a further subgroup. In addition, the patient may have had a similar injury previously and thus the response to medication may be compromised. Also, there may be long-standing degenerative changes within that knee joint that would affect the outcome of the study.

Thus, for a clearly defined grouping the patients should have suffered "an acute grade II sprain of the medial collateral ligament of the knee, with effusion, in a joint free of previous trauma and showing no other injury problems or degenerative changes." Clearly such rigid criteria will severely limit the rate of entry of patients into the study unless the injury is relatively common.

The investigator must next turn his attention to the pool of patients from which the studied group is to be drawn and must precisely define the type of patient and particular injury required for investigation. Clearly, a time scale should be placed on the trial (for example, 9 months or 1 year), and the investigator must see a sufficient number of these sports injuries (for example, acute knee injuries) within this period. What is a sufficient number? There should generally be at least 50 patients, and preferably 60, if only one or two parameters are to be studied. Statistical advice should be sought if necessary. Sometimes 100 or 120 patients might be required—50 or 60 in each group. The patients should be healthy, so that concomitant drug medication interactions or blurring of the trial drug effectiveness will not be a problem. For example, patients entering an analgesic study should not be on long-term medication with analgesic compounds, for the admission of such patients will be of no value in an acute assessment, and cross-reactions may cause problems.

Luckily in sports medicine, the patients are usually healthy and generally not taking medications, although concurrent therapy can be a problem. In most sports injuries trials patients ranging from adolescence to the late 40s are used, although age does not bar one from the study. Usually there is no problem in mixing female and male data (unless a hormonal compound is used), but it is advisable to measure body weight and height, for there may be possible difficulties with side effects that are dose/weight related; for example, a 112-pound woman might require much less of the drug than a 280-pound man.

Once the type of injury and the type of patient has been selected, the trial protocol has to be established. One must first ascertain how quickly should the drug be administered after injury and for how long.

One of the attractive features of having a clinical trial with professional sports people is that most are seen shortly after injury, often immediately in the larger sport organizations and tournaments. Thus, treatment can begin at once. Also, assessments can be made regularly, for example, each day, and compliance is high. (It has often been stated that in military studies, compliance is a function of rank and usually total! A similar phenomenon is seen in large sporting organizations.) Drug therapy commonly lasts for a week but can be continued longer; however, compliance falls in studies beyond 7 to 14 days and the incidence of side effects may rise.

The response of the study can be assessed in two ways, subjective and objective. It goes without saying that the most enlightened studies are double-blind and, in general terms, the author only recommends this type. On the analysis only a relatively short number of parameters are recorded at regular and frequent intervals—in the case of the knee, the degree of pain, swelling, and restriction of movement. The patient must be given clear guidelines on the assessments to be made (for example, none, mild, moderate, or severe). These results will be ranked for statistical (nonparametric) analyses later. Summary pain scores can be assessed as a total group score daily and any change analyzed, or as an alternative method, the average improvement on an individual basis from the baseline score can be employed (24).

Complex assessments such as measuring swelling, goniometer recording for joint movements, etc., are usually too involved for the ordinary patient and are thus futile. A pocket-sized and simply illustrated booklet should be provided for the recordings by the patient—too small a booklet is regularly lost whereas large cumbersome files with complex and multiple carbon-copy pages tend to be discarded. The subjective assessment should be at regular intervals (4, 6, 12, or 24 hrs) taking into account the variations in diurnal rhythm, if necessary. There are problems with rigidly fixing recordings to certain times rather than certain time intervals, for a injury assessed at noon the following day could be at 27 hrs if the accident had occurred at 9 AM the previous day or at 13 hrs if it happened at 11 PM. This disparity could affect the results in short-term trials (for example, 3- to 5-day studies). Thus, if possible, it may be wisest to assess the injury at time intervals (for example 24 hrs later, if possible). Since football and rugby players are generally injured in the afternoon between 3 and 5 PM, the regularity of their assessment at a certain part of the day is another attractive feature of using such athletes in clinical studies.

Some aspects of the objective analyses can be fraught with problems. For many years, it was assumed that the size of a bruise, hematoma, or muscle group (for example, the quadriceps in the thigh) could be accurately measured, either directly or by comparison with the uninjured limb. However, basic clinical observations and recently computerized tomography scanning have revealed that a comparison of muscle girth at a given point in a limb could give inaccurate results; there are natural differences that are especially noticeable in the dominant limb of professional players in football, soccer, and rugby. A difference of several inches might be found in the upper thigh.

Also, the measurement of bruising and swelling can be imprecise. Bruising from a deep (or intramuscular) hematoma might never reach the surface, remaining encapsulated within a muscle group, or may escape as an intermuscular hematoma and pass along fascial planes to a site remote from the original injury; thus, a hematoma of the popliteal space can spread down the calf. In addition, the concurrent muscle atrophy after injury might disguise the underlying swelling; for example, as the vastus medialis muscle becomes smaller, the swelling beneath becomes greater, and the thigh measurements remain the same.

The author, in his initial study (22), adopted the simple approach of assessing a return of function. In a trial of ibuprofen versus aspirin the professional players were seen daily, and pain and swelling were ranked as none, mild, moderate, or severe, and the return to training and eventually match play were noted. The known parameters of recovery for each player (namely, running, jumping, and lifting capabilities) could also be determined by comparison with the preseason and preinjury data in the notes that had been recorded regularly as part of the club's routine fitness program.

The radiological assessment of soft-tissue injuries is difficult. Plain films give little of value unless used in a certain way, for example as a stress test on a ruptured ligament to differentiate between a partial and complete rupture. Xerox films outline muscle groups, but direct quantification is difficult. Technetium bone scan with Tc 99 isotope may show pooling in the bone around damaged joints and increased uptake when minor stress lesions are found, as may occur in the ankle and midtarsal bones in professional kicking sportsmen. An arthrogram may give details of capsular and ligamentous damage, including stretching (for example, in the shoulder after recurrent dislocation), but does not allow volumetric or any other quantifiable analysis. Ultrasonics can be used in the presence of a large cystic lesion and can delineate meniscal injury within the knee. Computerized tomography will show soft-tissue injury, such as meniscal tears (25) and swelling, as will magnetic resonance imaging (MRI). At present, the interpretation of MRI data may be difficult; Watanabe et al. (26) have outlined the common pitfalls in knee investigations when normal anatomical structures are a predictable source of false-positive diagnoses of internal derangement. However, the detailed biochemical interpretations from the newer generation of MRI scanners make this technique particularly attractive for research work in the future.

An arthroscopic examination of joints (especially the knee and shoulder) allows a direct ranking of intraarticular lesions, but this procedure is invasive, difficult to justify on a repeated basis, and dependent on costly support staff (e.g., anesthetists, nurses, etc.). Eventually, this invasive method will be replaced by special radiographic techniques, as exemplified by MRI.

Laboratory tests as parameters of fitness include: (a) VO_2 max. (the maximal oxygen uptake indicates endurance and the capacity of the body tissues to consume oxygen during the period of activity); (b) the vital capacity (the volume of gas that can be expired forcibly after deep—maximum—expiration, which roughly represents the usable capacity of the lungs; (c) the heart rate during and after exertion, plus the recovery interval for a return to preexercise levels; and (d) the 12-min Cooper training run, or other performance indicators such as agility run times, flexibility reach, vertical jump height, bench press maximum and other weight tests, and bicycle and treadmill ergometry studies (such as the 6-sec sprint), which can be linked to a microcomputer and give accurate and reproducible data. Thus, over a period of time, repeated studies can give a physiological profile and provide a means of assessing fitness, as well as determining recovery after either injury or illness. For example, an assessment of functional disability used in the United States in rheumatoid arthritis is based on the Stanford Health Questionnaire (27); such tests may be a useful guide in predicting outcome and therapeutic response.

SOME RELEVANT STUDIES

In 1970, a trial was commenced using the newly discovered propionic acid derivative ibuprofen (23). This drug had been shown to have antiinflammatory properties in animal studies using ultraviolet and arachidonic acid–induced erythema, carageenan foot edema, and adjuvant arthritis. Sixty professional soccer players entered a double-blind trial, 30 in each group (22). Immediately after a soft-tissue injury to the lower limb the player received the standard therapy of cold compress, elastic or crepe support, and limb rest and elevation. No plaster of paris immobilization was given. In addition, the injured player received a pack containing a 5-day supply of either ibuprofen or soluble aspirin. All major injuries (fractures and dislocations) were excluded, as were those needing joint aspiration, ultrasound, and shortwave diathermy. By concentrating on moderate injuries in players with known parameters of recovery it was established that ibuprofen had a significant antiinflammatory effect in reducing the severity and duration of pain while allowing both training and match playing earlier than in the group on aspirin.

Bourne and Bentley (28) conducted another double-blind study involving 60 undergraduates suffering from acute soft-tissue injuries sustained during various amateur sporting events. A significantly greater number receiving ibuprofen recovered within 5 days of the trial than those receiving acetaminophen (paracetamol). In a study of 178 patients with soft-tissue injuries that compared ibuprofen, placebo, and propoxyphene hydrochloride, the ibuprofen group was significantly superior in analgesic and antiinflammatory properties (29). Bouchier-Hayes and Jones (30) found that naproxen had a similar benefical action in the treatment of sports injuries, and another study demonstrated that naproxen (825 mg daily) was equipotent to indomethacin (75 mg daily) in 114 soft-tissue injuries (31). Nabumetone (1 g daily) was as effective in pain relief as naproxen (1 g daily) in sports injuries (32).

Diclofenac has also been shown to be efficacious in several studies in nonarticular rheumatism and soft-tissue injuries. Diclofenac 100 mg daily was as effective as ibuprofen 1,600 mg daily in 50 patients with shoulder pain from periarthritis (33). A placebo-controlled trial demonstrated that diclofenac 150 mg daily and oxyphenbutazone 600 mg daily were similarly efficacious in sports injuries to the knee (34).

The author has also carried out trials using flurbiprofen in professional soccer players (24). In 52 players given either flurbiprofen 50 mg three times daily or aspirin 1,200 mg three times daily for 6 days, there was enhanced recovery after flurbiprofen (24,35). The analysis of pain scores was done by comparing the total daily pain score for all individuals in each group; and because the pain scores for the two treatment groups were almost identical at the beginning of treatment, it was not necessary to look at the improvement in pain score but rather a pain score for any one day could be evaluated.

Flurbiprofen has been show to have a significant effect when given immediately after meniscectomy (36). In a study of 100 patients undergoing either partial or total meniscectomy, half received 400 mg daily of flurbiprofen and the other half received 4 g acetaminophen (paracetamol) daily for 7 days immediately after surgery. Once again the criteria for selection were strict. All patients with previous knee problems (such as chondromalacia of the patella or femoral condyles, loose bodies, osteoarthrosis, etc.) were excluded, as were patients having had a previous meniscectomy. The degree of pain and swelling was assessed by the investigator as none, mild, moderate, or severe. Knee flexion and knee power were also evaluated, as were the length of disability and the time to full recovery. In the patients who underwent a partial meniscectomy and who received flurbiprofen, recovery was rapid; by the third day, pain and swelling were significantly reduced compared to the acetaminophen-treated group. Full knee flexion and muscle power had returned by the 21st day after antiinflammatory therapy, significantly sooner than with acetaminophen. Similar findings were found after total meniscectomy, but the recovery was slightly slower, i.e., 5 days for pain and swelling abatement, and 1 month for full recovery. On average, patients were able to resume full activities 22 days earlier with flurbiprofen. A recent trial by the author in 60 patients undergoing knee surgery demonstrated that diclofenac 75 mg IM followed by 150 mg a day orally for 7 days had better analgesic effect in the postoperative setting than pethidine 50 mg IM plus acetaminophen (paracetamol) 3 g daily for 7 days. The antiinflammatory effects of diclofenac were also statistically significant compared to pethidine/acetaminophen (37).

Since many surgeons now use arthroscopic methods to treat sports injuries, a study was undertaken of 139 patients who had undergone a meniscectomy in this way (38). Those receiving a prostaglandin inhibitor (naproxen sodium, 67 patients in all) had significantly less pain, less synovitis, less effusion, and a more rapid return of movement and quadriceps function than patients in the placebo group, 72 in all. Patients taking naproxen had significantly less pain at rest up to 21 days. The median time for returning to sporting activities was 56 days in the placebo group compared to 22.5 days in the active treatment group.

Many reports have shown the safety of nonsteroidal and analgesic compounds (39,40). The Committee on the Safety of Drugs in 1988 noted a distinct relationship between the half-life of the drug and the incidence of side effects. Serious adverse reactions per million scripts in the first 5 years after introduction showed azapropazone (87.9) and piroxicam (68.1) to have the highest incidence (half-life of 20 and 35 hrs, respectively), compared to ketoprofen (38.6), flurbiprofen (35.8), and ibuprofen (13.2) (half-life of 6 hrs or less). However, most side effects are mild to moderate in nature and the difference between compounds in short-term sports injuries studies is not usually great. For example, one study showed a similar incidence of side effects in patients taking piroxicam compared to flurbiprofen (41) despite the above findings. In the author's experience with testing a range of analgesic and antiinflammatory compounds, the incidence of side effects is between 3 and 5%. Surprisingly, in hospitalized patients the incidence was less than 2%; this observation is perhaps related to regular drug administration, adequate fluid intake, and perhaps a reduction in alcohol intake.

In the future, there is no doubt that more selective agents will be designed to block the pathophysiological detrimental effects of the soft-tissue reaction, thereby further enhancing recovery. More investigations are needed to unravel the basic problems in chronic conditions (such as recurrent hamstring tears and tennis elbow). Also, improved quantification by biochemical and bioengineering field testing and radiological methods will further enhance clinical studies. In the latter respect, the exciting advances in magnetic resonance imaging are important. The advantages of such advances are not confined to the sporting fraternity, but are directly applicable to all soft-tissue injuries, including those in other specialities such as dental surgery, plastic and hand surgery, etc. However, the development of newer analgesic and antiinflammatory treatments will continue to demand a strict, carefully planned, and logical approach to clinical trials, probably more so than has often been the case in the past, in order to have any meaningful value.

REFERENCES

1. Pritchett JW. A statistical study of knee injuries due to football in high-school athletes. *J Bone Joint Surg* 1982;64A:240–242.
2. Weightman D, Brown RC. Injuries in rugby and association football. *Br J Sports Med* 1974;8: 183–186.
3. Weightman D, Brown RC. Injuries in eleven selected sports. *Br J Sports Med* 1975;9:136–139.
4. Crane J, Gibson T, Busson M. A comparative study of ibuprofen and indomethacin in ligamentous injuries of the ankle. *Br J Clin Pract Suppl* 1970;6:92–94.
5. Eriksson E. Symposium on ski trauma and skiing safety. *Orthop Clin North Am* 1976;7:1–2.
6. Smilkstein G. Health evaluation of high school athletes. *Physician Sports Med* 1981;9:73–80.
7. Mueller F, Blyth CS. Annual survey of catastrophic football injuries: 1977 to 1983. *Physician Sports Med* 1985;13:75–81.
8. Allemandou A. A statistical review of injuries. In: O'Connell TCJ, ed. *Injuries in rugby football and other team sports.* Dublin: Irish Rugby Football Union, 1976;81–91.
9. Culpepper MI, Niemann KMW. A comparison of game and practice injuries in high school football. *Physician Sports Med* 1983;11:117–122.
10. Vane JR. Inhibition of prostaglandin synthesis as a mechanism of action for aspirin-like drugs. *Nature New Biol* 1971;231:232–235.
11. Blake DR, Allen RE, Lunec J. Free radicals in biological systems: a review orientated to inflammatory processes. *Br Med Bull* 1987;43:371–385.
12. Babior BM. Oxygen-dependent microbial killing by phagocytes. *N Engl J Med* 1978;298:659–668.
13. Blazina ME. Oxyphenbutazone as an adjunct to the conventional treatment of athletic injuries. *Clin Med* 1969;76:19.
14. Blonstein JL. Oral enzyme tablets in the treatment of boxing injuries. *Practitioner* 1967;198: 547.
15. Boyne PS, Medhurst H. Oral anti-inflammatory enzyme therapy in injuries in professional footballers. *Practitioner* 1967;198:543.
16. Shaw PC. The use of trypsin-chymotrypsin formulation in fractures of the hand. *Br J Clin Pract* 1969;23:1.
17. Buelvas PR. Action of indomethacin in acute traumatic musculo-skeletal disorders. Abstr. IV Pan Am *Congr Rheum Excerpta Medica Found Int Cong Series* 1967;143:99.
18. Leclerc FP, Autissier D. The use of indomethacin in the treatment of limb injuries and their sequelae. *Gaz Hop Paris* 1969;1:31.

19. Huskisson EC, Berry H, Street FG, Medhurst HE. Indomethacin for soft-tissue injuries: a double-blind study in football players. *Rheumatol Rehab* 1973;12:159–160.
20. Santilli G, Tuccimei U, Cannistra FM. Comparative study with piroxicam and ibuprofen versus placebo in the supportive treatment of minor sports injuries. *J Int Med Res* 1980;8:265–269.
21. Clyman B. Role of non-steroidal anti-inflammatory drugs in sports medicine. *Sports Med* 1986;3: 242–246.
22. Muckle DS. Comparative study of ibuprofen and aspirin in soft-tissue injuries. *Rheumatol Rehab* 1974;13:141–147.
23. Adams SS, Cliffe EE, Lessel B, Nicholson JS. Some biological properties of 2-(4-isobutylphenyl)-propionic acid. *J Pharm Sci* 1967;56:1686.
24. Muckle DS. A double-blind trial of flurbiprofen and aspirin in soft-tissue trauma. *Rheumatol Rehab* 1977;16:58–61.
25. Manco LG, Kavanaugh JH, Lozman J, Colman ND, Bilfield BS, Fay JJ. Diagnosis of meniscal tears using high-resolution computed tomography. *J Bone Joint Surg* 1987;69A:498–502.
26. Watanabe AT, Carter BC, Teitelbaum GP, Bradley WG. Common pitfalls in magnetic resonance imaging of the knee. *J Bone Joint Surg* 1989;71A:857–862.
27. Wolfe F, Kleinheksel SM, Cathey MA, et al. The clinical value of the Stanford Health Assessment Questionnaire Functional Disability Index in patients with rheumatoid arthritis. *J Rheumatol* 1988;15:1480–1488.
28. Bourne M, Bentley S. Enhanced recovery from sports injuries: a comparison of ibuprofen and paracetamol. *Br J Clin Pract* suppl. IXth Europ Cong Rheumatology 1979;6:72–77.
29. Goswick CB Jr. Ibuprofen versus propoxyphene hydrochloride and placebo in acute musculo-skeletal trauma. *Curr Ther Res* 1983;34:685–692.
30. Bouchier-Hayes T, Jones CW. The treatment of sports injuries: a comparison between naproxen and indomethacin. A Royal Army Corps multicentre study. *Practitioner* 1979;223:706–710.
31. Backhouse CI, Engler C, English JR. Naproxen sodium and indomethacin in acute musculoskeletal disorders. *Rheumatol Rehab* 1980;19:113–119.
32. Muckle DS, Rotman H. A report on a study on the assessment of the effectiveness of nabumetone in the treatment of sports injuries by comparison with naproxen. *Roy Soc Med Int Cong Symp Series* 1985;69:187–191.
33. Famaey JP, Ginsberg F. Treatment of periarthritis of the shoulder: a comparison of ibuprofen and diclofenac. *J Int Med Res* 1984;12:238–243.
34. Van Heerden JJ. Diclophenac sodium, oxyphenbutazone and placebo in sports injuries of the knee. *South African Med J* 1977;52:396–399.
35. Muckle DS. Flurbiprofen for the treatment of soft tissue trauma. *Am J Med* 1986;80(suppl 3A): 76–80.
36. Muckle DS. Open meniscectomy: enhanced recovery after synovial prostaglandin inhibition. *J Bone Joint Surg* 1984;66B:193–195.
37. Muckle DS, Rotman H, Brookes J. The assessment of intramuscular diclofenac sodium in patients after partial meniscectomy. *J Orthop Rheum* 1989;2:211–217.
38. Ogilvie-Harris DJ, Bauer M, Corey P. Prostaglandin inhibition and the rate of recovery after arthroscopic meniscectomy. *J Bone Joint Surg* 1985;67B:567–571.
39. Hutson MA. A double-blind study comparing ibuprofen 1800 mg or 2400 mg daily and placebo in sports injuries. *J Int Med Res* 1986;14:142–147.
40. Walker JW, VandenBurg MJ, Currie WJC. Differential efficacy of two non-steroidal anti-inflammatory drugs in the treatment of sports injuries. *Cur Med Res Opin* 1984;9:119–123.
41. Rosenthal M. The efficacy of flurbiprofen versus piroxicam in the treatment of acute soft tissue. *Rheumatism* 1984;9:304–309.

Advances in Pain Research and Therapy, Vol. 18,
edited by M. Max, R. Portenoy, and E. Laska,
Raven Press, Ltd., New York © 1991.

15

Oral Surgery

James A. Forbes

*Department of Psychiatry, Johns Hopkins University School of Medicine,
Baltimore, Maryland 21205*

New analgesics are often evaluated in patients who have had oral surgery. There
are no special problems managing pain in these patients; this model allows one
to quickly and reliably estimate a drug's profile of efficacy and safety before
using it to treat other types of pathologic pain, e.g., pain following orthopedic
surgery.

My associates and I have conducted over 50 studies using oral surgery outpatients as subjects. Many were evaluations of investigational new drugs and
have served as pivotal studies in New Drug Application (NDA) submissions;
others were reevaluations of drugs already approved for marketing. The presentation that follows outlines the oral surgery analgesic model as I see it, describes
to some extent how to conduct a clinical trial with these patients, and discusses
what I consider some important issues related to this model. Although the paper
does cite representative work from the archival literature, by necessity it is heavily
dependent on the studies my associates and I conducted. In the first place, it is
impractical to access and analyze the raw data of other investigators. If the data
were available there would still be the question of how the data were collected.
That is important since, in my opinion, the outcome of an analgesic trial is a
function of the administration of the study, e.g., instructions to the patient. I
believe these studies are susceptible to investigator-induced bias, as is any evaluation of a subjective phenomenon. This paper is not a review of the literature
concerning the oral surgery outpatient analgesic model, nor do I consider it the
definitive description of this model. It is a collection of observations made by a
technician.

Journal citations would suggest that most researchers date the oral surgery
outpatient analgesic model with Cooper and Beaver's 1976 article in Clinical
Pharmacology and Therapeutics (1). However, the oral surgery outpatient model

preexisted Cooper's research; investigators such as Lokken et al. (2), Hepso et al. (3), Sveen and Gilhuus-Moe (4), Ahlstrom and Lantz (5), Ruedy and Bentley (6) and numerous others recognized the value of working with this group of patients. Indeed, essentially all of the elements of the model described by Cooper and Beaver (1) and Cooper (7) were present in the design employed earlier by Ruedy and Bentley (6).

Cooper's goal was ". . . to develop an outpatient model which approaches the sophistication of current inpatient models" (7). He thought investigators had far less control of outpatients than did their colleagues who used inpatients as subjects. Specially designed data collection forms and precise instructions were implemented to combat this problem. Patients who had impacted third molars surgically removed were selected as subjects, since he felt these patients were homogeneous with respect to the etiology of pain. In addition, they were young, healthy, intelligent, and available. Few of these patients had preexisting pain; however, the majority required analgesic medication following this oral surgery procedure. Cooper initially thought a well-designed data collection record would obviate the need for a research nurse; however, he subsequently utilized a nurse to instruct patients preoperatively and interview them at a postoperative follow-up. Cooper's early research established the oral surgery outpatient analgesic model as a systematic method for evaluating analgesic efficacy and adverse effect liability, employing a trained "nurse-observer," standardized instructions, and a standardized Patient Self-Rating Record (PSRR).

SURGICAL PROCEDURE

Although early clinical trials of analgesics in dental pain often included patients who were heterogeneous with respect to the type of surgical procedure, current studies tend to employ subjects who have had similar surgery. Usually, subjects are outpatients who have had at least one impacted third molar (wisdom tooth) removed by an oral surgeon. The procedures described herein have also been applied to patients who have had other dental surgery, e.g., periodontal surgery (8), and a variation of these procedures has been applied to inpatients who have had dental surgery (8,9). Initially, I will discuss outpatients who have had impacted third molars removed.

Typically, patients requiring third molar surgery are referred to an oral surgeon by a general dentist. Although 90% of these patients have a preoperative consultation and return for surgery at a later date, some patients have the consultation and surgery on the same day. A brief health history and radiologic examination to determine the number and type of impactions are completed as part of the consultation. Patients usually remain for a brief observation period after surgery to make sure there are no significant negative effects of surgery or anesthesia. Patients who have general anesthesia remain longer than those who have local anesthesia and must have a driver to take them home following their recovery.

There is a follow-up examination 5 to 7 days after surgery to remove sutures. Additional visits may be required if the patient has a postoperative complication, e.g., dry socket or bleeding. On the day of surgery patients are generally given a prescription for an analgesic; usually it is a narcotic-containing combination, e.g., hydrocodone 5 mg with acetaminophen 500 mg. Approximately 90% of the patients having third molars removed use an analgesic (10–12) and some patients medicate for 5 to 6 days postoperatively (13,14).

STUDY PROCEDURES

In our studies, potential subjects are interviewed preoperatively by a nurse-observer. A detailed description of the nurse's training and role in the study is presented in Chapter 26. Patients are excluded if they are pregnant or lactating; have any history of hypersensitivity or serious adverse reaction to any agent similar to the study medications; have any clinically significant condition that would affect the absorption, metabolism, or excretion of the study medications; or require concomitant medication that might confound quantitating analgesia. Long-term users of analgesics or tranquilizers are also excluded. Based on personal interviews, the nurse-observer selects patients who are able to communicate fluently and are willing to participate in the study. The purposes and procedures of the study are explained to potential subjects in detail on the day of surgical consult and day of surgery. Patients must give written informed consent. The participation of minors requires the written informed consent of a parent or legal guardian, in addition to that of the minor.

On the day of surgery, after a briefing on the study procedures, each patient receives a packet of materials: a Patient Self-Rating Record-1 (PSRR-1) to be used to evaluate the study medication; the study medication; a common kitchen timer; a supply of a standard analgesic, e.g., Phenaphen with codeine No. 3 (codeine phosphate 30 mg with acetaminophen 325 mg, A.H. Robins Company) to be used as a backup if additional pain relief is needed after taking the study medication; and a Patient Self-Rating Record-2 (PSRR-2) to be used as a diary for the backup analgesic or to evaluate doses subsequent to dose 1 in repeat-dose studies (PSRR-1 and PSRR-2 are presented in Figs. 1 and 2). Patients are instructed to take the study medication when they have steady pain that is moderate or severe and in their opinion requires treatment. The time and intensity of their baseline pain is recorded when they medicate. Then they are required to complete the following statements at periodic intervals, e.g., hourly, for the duration of the study period or until remediation is necessary: My pain at this time is: none (0), slight (1), moderate (2), severe (3); my relief from starting pain is: none (0), a little (1), some (2), a lot (3), complete (4); my starting pain is at least half gone: no (0), yes (1).

At the end of the evaluation period, e.g., hour 8 in an 8-hr study, or at the time the patient takes backup analgesic, the patient makes an overall evaluation

Study: 88-08 Patient's Number__________ Patient's Initials__________

If you have moderate or severe pain, and need to take medication for that pain, tear open the envelope attached and take all of the medication with a glass of water. Record the severity of your starting pain (moderate or severe) and the time you took the medication. At the end of 1/2 hour then at the end of each hour, record the time and answer the questions for the next 8 hours.

ANSWER WHEN YOU TAKE THE MEDICATION

My starting pain is: ☐ slight ☐ moderate ☐ severe

I took the medication at: TIME __________ ☐ AM ☐ PM

No pain |——————————| Worst pain

Set the timer for 30 minutes

ANSWER 1/2 HOUR AFTER TAKING THE MEDICATION TIME: __________ ☐ AM ☐ PM

My pain at this time is: ☐ none ☐ slight ☐ moderate ☐ severe

My relief from starting pain is: ☐ none ☐ a little ☐ some ☐ a lot ☐ complete

My starting pain is at least 1/2 gone: ☐ no ☐ yes

No pain |——————————| Worst pain

Set the timer for 30 minutes

ANSWER 1 HOUR AFTER TAKING THE MEDICATION TIME: __________ ☐ AM ☐ PM

My pain at this time is: ☐ none ☐ slight ☐ moderate ☐ severe

My relief from starting pain is: ☐ none ☐ a little ☐ some ☐ a lot ☐ complete

My starting pain is at least 1/2 gone: ☐ no ☐ yes

No pain |——————————| Worst pain

Set the timer for 1 hour

•
•
•

ANSWER 8 HOURS AFTER TAKING THE MEDICATION TIME: __________ ☐ AM ☐ PM

My pain at this time is: ☐ none ☐ slight ☐ moderate ☐ severe

My relief from starting pain is: ☐ none ☐ a little ☐ some ☐ a lot ☐ complete

My starting pain is at least 1/2 gone: ☐ no ☐ yes

No pain |——————————| Worst pain

HOW WOULD YOU RATE THE STUDY MEDICATION YOU RECEIVED FOR PAIN?

☐ EXCELLENT ☐ VERY GOOD ☐ GOOD ☐ FAIR ☐ POOR

DID YOU HAVE ANY OTHER EFFECTS FROM THE STUDY MEDICATION? ☐ NO ☐ YES

If you had other effects from the study medication, list the other effect(s) and the time you first noticed it.

__________ Patient's Initials Date __________ Nurse Observer Date __________ Investigator Date

FIG. 1. Patient Self-Rating Record 1 (PSRR-1)—front and back.

of the study medication as poor (0), fair (1), good (2), very good (3), or excellent (4), taking into consideration the onset, level and duration of relief, and any other effects experienced. Adverse effects are noted on the self-rating record. Patients are asked (a) to give the study medication at least 2 hrs to manifest an effect before taking the first dose of the backup medication, (b) not to remedicate

Pt. No. ________

Initials ________

# Taken	DOSE 2	DOSE 3	DOSE 4	DOSE 5	DOSE 6	DOSE 7	DOSE 8	DOSE 9	DOSE 10	DOSE 11	DOSE 12	DOSE 13	DOSE 14	DOSE 15
DATE:														
Month														
Day														
Year														
TIME:														
Hour														
Minutes														
	am	am	am	am	am	am	am	am	am	am	am	am	am	am
	pm	pm	pm	pm	pm	pm	pm	pm	pm	pm	pm	pm	pm	pm
PAIN NOW:														
None	0	0	0	0	0	0	0	0	0	0	0	0	0	0
Slight	1	1	1	1	1	1	1	1	1	1	1	1	1	1
Moderate	2	2	2	2	2	2	2	2	2	2	2	2	2	2
Severe	3	3	3	3	3	3	3	3	3	3	3	3	3	3
RELIEF THIS DOSE:														
None	0	0	0	0	0	0	0	0	0	0	0	0	0	0
A Little	1	1	1	1	1	1	1	1	1	1	1	1	1	1
Some	2	2	2	2	2	2	2	2	2	2	2	2	2	2
A Lot	3	3	3	3	3	3	3	3	3	3	3	3	3	3
Complete	4	4	4	4	4	4	4	4	4	4	4	4	4	4
OVERALL OPINION THIS DOSE:														
Poor	0	0	0	0	0	0	0	0	0	0	0	0	0	0
Fair	1	1	1	1	1	1	1	1	1	1	1	1	1	1
Good	2	2	2	2	2	2	2	2	2	2	2	2	2	2
Very Good	3	3	3	3	3	3	3	3	3	3	3	3	3	3
Excellent	4	4	4	4	4	4	4	4	4	4	4	4	4	4

Patient's Initials ________ Nurse Observer ________ Investigator ________

Date ________ Date ________ Date ________

FIG. 2. Patient Self-Rating Record 2 (PSRR-2)—front.

as long as they are having any relief, (c) not to remedicate if their pain is less than moderate, and (d) to complete the next evaluation of the study medication before remedicating.

PATIENT CHARACTERISTICS

Table 1 summarizes patient characteristics for 20 analgesic trials my associates and I have conducted. These studies represent approximately one-third of the analgesic trials we have conducted over the past 15 years.

The average age was approximately 22 years; over half of the patients were female; and over 95% of the patients were Caucasian. Race is not a factor in selecting patients for our studies; the low percentage of non-Caucasian patients may be due to socioeconomic factors, since the surgical procedure is usually elective and is relatively expensive for patients who do not have insurance coverage. The length of the surgical procedure varies from site to site due to differences in the technique of the surgeon, the type of anesthesia, the number and type of impactions, and whether other procedures, e.g., a concomitant simple extraction, were completed. The number of teeth removed is relatively homogeneous except for sites 5 and 6, two sites that are no longer utilized. There seemed to be a tendency at site 5 to withhold patients with fewer than four impactions from the study. At site 6 the oral surgeons frequently elected to remove half of the patient's impactions at one surgical session, then remove the others at a later date. This is no longer common practice since it is more costly for the patient and more importantly, exposes the patient to additional risk, if general anesthesia is employed.

The ratio of sutures to extractions differs markedly between the sites with site 5 using on average 0.59 sutures/extraction versus site 6 which used 3.22 sutures/extraction. This appears to be simply a function of the surgeon's technique. The time from the end of the surgical procedure until the patient medicated varied from 2 hrs 36 min to 3 hrs 2 min. This time is probably longer than the time from surgery until the onset of pain in the usual, nonstudy private practice, since these patients were asked to wait until their postoperative pain met certain criteria.

Over half (59%) of the patients medicated with moderate pain. It is unclear how we get patients with severe pain. That is, do these patients have moderate pain and delay medicating until the onset of severe pain? Do they go directly from slight or no pain to severe pain? Or do they fail to understand the meaning of the descriptor "moderate"? Based upon interviews with patients, we know that trauma at the operative site, e.g., from eating, can cause the patient to go from no pain to severe pain.

Table 2 summarizes the compliance of these study patients. Less than 1% of the patients have been lost to follow-up; most of them were individuals who did not return for suture removal, returned to college and could not be located, gave a false address, etc. Eighty-nine percent of the patients entered had steady mod-

TABLE 1. Summary of demographic data, parameters related to the surgical procedure, and baseline pain intensity[a]

	Site 1	Site 2	Site 3	Site 4	Site 5	Site 6	Total
Number valid	542	915	833	415	333	164	3,202
Age (yrs)	21.0	22.0	22.1	21.6	22.2	22.7	21.9
(range)	(15–44)	(15–54)	(15–54)	(15–46)	(15–41)	(15–45)	(15–54)
Sex							
Male	229 (42%)[b]	364 (40%)	357 (43%)	192 (46%)	141 (42%)	64 (39%)	1,347 (42%)
Female	313 (58%)	551 (60%)	476 (57%)	223 (54%)	192 (58%)	100 (61%)	1,855 (58%)
Height (cm)	169.7	170.4	170.7	172.4	170.5	170.3	170.6
Weight (kg)	65.2	65.6	65.3	63.8	65.7	65.9	65.2
Length of surgical procedure (min)	35.9	30.0	25.0	21.2	22.4	20.1	27.3
Number of impactions	2.9	2.6	2.9	2.7	3.5	1.9	2.8
Number of sutures	5.3	2.5	5.8	5.1	2.0	6.2	4.3
Time from procedure until taking study medication (hrs)	2.8	3.0	2.6	3.1	2.7	3.0	2.8
	2.4	2.4	2.5	2.3	2.3	2.5	2.4
Baseline pain intensity							
Moderate	309 (57%)[b]	543 (59%)	436 (52%)	282 (68%)	237 (71%)	79 (48%)	1,886 (59%)
Severe	233 (43%)	372 (41%)	397 (48%)	133 (32%)	96 (29%)	85 (52%)	1,316 (41%)

[a] Mean values are reported unless otherwise specified.
[b] Frequency and percentage.

TABLE 2. *Compliance with instructions for oral surgery studies (frequency and percent reported)*

	Site 1	Site 2	Site 3	Site 4	Site 5	Site 6	Total
Number entered	676	1,141	1,093	491	403	217	4,021
Lost to follow-up	3	7	4	3	0	3	20
	(<1%)	(<1%)	(<1%)	(<1%)	(0%)	(1%)	(<1%)
Did not medicate	90	86	150	39	51	26	442
	(13%)	(8%)	(14%)	(8%)	(13%)	(12%)	(11%)
Number medicated	583	1,048	939	449	352	188	3,559
	(86%)	(92%)	(86%)	(91%)	(87%)	(87%)	(89%)
Number invalid[a]	41	133	106	34	19	24	357
	(7%)	(13%)	(11%)	(8%)	(5%)	(13%)	(10%)
Number valid[a]	542	915	833	415	333	164	3,202
	(93%)	(87%)	(89%)	(92%)	(95%)	(87%)	(90%)

[a] The percentage of valid and invalid is based on the number of patients who medicated.

erate or severe pain and felt they needed medication to relieve their pain. Eighty percent of all patients entered provided valid efficacy data. These data indicate a high degree of compliance. Table 3 summarizes the reasons efficacy data were invalidated.

NURSE-OBSERVER

The typical analgesic study employs a trained research nurse, generally referred to as a "nurse-observer" or "analgesic study nurse," who selects patients, instructs them concerning the study procedures, issues study medication and materials,

TABLE 3. *Reasons for invalidating efficacy data[a]*

Reasons for invalidating	Number of patients invalidated n = 357
Remedicated before a specified time[b]	122 (34%)
Remedicated with "some" or more relief	48 (13%)
Remedicated with "slight" pain	37 (10%)
Did not complete evaluations	37 (10%)
Evaluations too far off schedule	36 (10%)
Did not follow instructions	29 (8%)
Took backup medication instead of study medication	11 (3%)
Took only part of study medication	9 (3%)
Data lacked internal consistency	8 (2%)
Medicated for reason other than postoperative pain	6 (2%)
Vomited study medication	4 (1%)
Given local anesthesia after taking study medication	3 (<1%)
Took study medication several days after surgery	3 (<1%)
Took another analgesic with the study medication	2 (<1%)
Ratings made by person other than patient	1 (<1%)
Rated one side of mouth only	1 (<1%)

[a] Frequency and percent reported (based on total number of invalid patients). A total of 4,021 patients entered studies at six sites; of these 20 were lost to follow-up, 442 did not medicate, and 3,559 took study medication. Of those who took study medication, 3,202 had valid efficacy data and 357 had invalid efficacy data.
[b] 2 hrs for all except one study, which had a 1-hr time limit.

debriefs patients at the postoperative follow-up visit, and follows the patient until any adverse effects or postoperative complications are resolved. The nurse-observer controls the day-to-day activity of the clinical trial (see Chapter 26). Each time the nurse-observer enters a study patient she is completing what Sidman would call an "exact replication" of the experiment completed on the previous patients (15); each patient receives the same instructions, study materials, etc. Therefore, differences in outcome, i.e., analgesic efficacy, are hopefully due to drug effect as opposed to other factors.

ROLE OF THE ORAL SURGEON

The oral surgeon's primary responsibility is to complete the required surgery and follow the patient's progress in order to assure complete recovery. If there is a nurse-observer, the role of the oral surgeon in the study is intentionally limited for scientific reasons. In order to standardize the study for all patients, all information concerning the study procedures is presented by the nurse-observer. Instructions from more than one source has a tendency to increase variation in response.

ANTICIPATORY SET

It is necessary for legal, ethical, and scientific reasons that the patient know what drugs are being evaluated in a study. The legal and ethical aspects of this issue are generally understood; however, the scientific rationale for full disclosure is not obvious to all. The patient must understand what drugs are being studied and the potential analgesic response to each in order to prevent having a biased anticipatory set favoring a particular response. For example, if one were evaluating 1,000 mg diflunisal, 650 mg aspirin, and placebo it would be quite easy to leave the patient with the impression that his dose of study medication would be diflunisal, if one discussed that treatment longer and more enthusiastically than the aspirin standard.

In the aforementioned case, the nurse-observer must emphasize, "You will get only *one* of the three treatments: diflunisal, aspirin, or placebo. I do not know and you will not know which medication you will get. You could have complete relief for 8 hrs, no relief at all, or a medium amount of relief for a few hours." Patient responses indicate they do not expect a specific result following these instructions; instead, they are open to any treatment outcome. They also understand their chance of receiving placebo is 1 out of 3.

PATIENT SELF-RATING RECORD

In a single-dose analgesic trial, ratings of the study medication are recorded on a Patient Self-Rating Record (PSRR-1, Fig. 1). The nurse-observer gives the patient detailed verbal instructions concerning the use of the PSRR; the brief instructions printed on the PSRR are only to remind the patient of the instructions from the nurse-observer. Patients are told to read the statements aloud at baseline and each interval evaluation and select the response that best describes their condition at that time. It is suggested that the patient think about the baseline or starting pain, rate relief from starting pain, and indicate whether the starting pain is at least half gone (50% relief). They are told not to think about the ratings at the previous evaluation; we are interested in their current status.

A single dose of the study medication is attached to the top right corner of PSRR-1. The starting, or baseline, pain and time of medicating are recorded in the first box on the PSRR; patients who check "slight" for baseline pain are considered invalid. The PSRR in Fig. 1 also requires the patient to rate pain intensity using a 100-mm visual analogue scale (VAS) with anchor points of "no pain" and "worst pain." Printed instructions indicate the time interval for evaluations and remind the patient to set the timer.

We have used booklets, with a separate page for each interval evaluation, instead of the single-page PSRR-1. Some think this format prevents the patient from referring to the ratings for the previous hour; however, our experience indicates that patients using booklets make more mistakes, e.g., skipping pages. My associates and I think the single-page PSRR-1 is the easiest presentation for the patient and it has worked very well in many studies.

Typically, evaluations are completed at hourly intervals over a 4- to 12-hr period. The length of the evaluation period is a function of the expected duration of action of the study medication as determined by previous clinical trials, animal data, etc. For example, evaluations of diflunisal at therapeutic dosage levels would call for 12 hrs of evaluation, whereas routine formulations of aspirin, acetaminophen, and codeine could be evaluated in a 6-hr study (16). Occasionally there is a need to complete an evaluation at an interval other than one hour. We have conducted studies of effervescent compounds in which evaluations were completed at 15-min intervals during the first hour (17). One potential problem that exists when using aperiodic evaluation intervals is that patients may become confused and complete subsequent evaluations off schedule. In studies with an evaluation at 30 min in addition to hourly ratings, we have found two to three times as many patients are off schedule, necessitating the invalidation of their efficacy data.

Special care must be taken when conducting studies requiring 12 hrs of evaluation. In addition to the problem of asking the patient to complete 12 interval evaluations, there is a potential problem related to the time of day the surgery is completed. For example, if a patient's surgery was completed at 3 PM he might be expected to take study medication at 6 PM, since the mean time from the end of surgery until taking medication is approximately 3 hrs (see Table 1). If the study medication was effective for 12 hrs, the hour-12 evaluation would be scheduled for 6 AM the morning following administration of the medication. In general, requiring evaluations during normal sleep times is a problem. In our units, patients in 12-hr studies must have completed surgery by 1 PM. This rule helps, but patients still fall asleep despite having a kitchen timer to use to standardize evaluation intervals and awaken themselves if asleep. In some 12-hr studies, 25% of the patients receiving effective medications were asleep for one or more observations.

There is also a practical issue related to the conduct of a 12-hr study. If entry is restricted to patients who have completed surgery by 1 PM, or earlier, the nurse-observer will usually lose a significant number of patients since most oral surgery practices schedule surgery in the afternoon as well as the morning. In our own units we must have two studies ongoing; morning patients are assigned to the 12-hr study and afternoon patients participate in a trial with fewer evaluations, e.g., 6 hrs. This increases the time required to conduct a given clinical trial and leads to consideration of multisite studies.

The study medication is attached to PSRR-1 in order to increase the probability that the patient will take the correct medication first and use the appropriate form. We prefer that the study medication be packaged in transparent blister packs, so it can be screened for damage and deterioration.

RATING SCALES

Most oral surgery outpatient analgesic studies employ more than one measure of efficacy; usually, there is at least some evaluation of the level of pain and its relief. The rating scales we employ were chosen because other experienced investigators had used them successfully (18,19). We have continued to use them since they have worked and there is no obvious reason to change our system. In addition, there is great reluctance to change scales, or the descriptors within a particular scale, after having amassed a data base of approximately 10,000 patients. Since the same scales and procedures have been employed routinely, we are able to compare data from different studies within an analgesic site, as well as compare different sites, making reasonably accurate predictions concerning the relative analgesic efficacy of drugs.

Figure 3 presents the percentage of patients having 50% relief plotted across time in hours. These curves represent combined data from a number of our studies. We have families of time-effect curves (TECs) for different drugs at different dosage levels. In my opinion, composite data such as these represent the best estimate of performance of a single dose of the drug at *our* analgesic research sites. We can quickly obtain an estimate of the analgesic effect of a new test drug by conducting a double-blind pilot study with a small number of patients and comparing the results to the family of curves in our data base. In this case, the test drug could be compared to placebo, aspirin 650 mg, ibuprofen 400 mg, and diflunisal 1,000 mg. This procedure has allowed us to accurately predict the relative performance of some analgesics prior to completing a full-scale study. If we changed our rating scales, e.g., added a category of "very severe pain," it would be difficult to compare new data to our old data base.

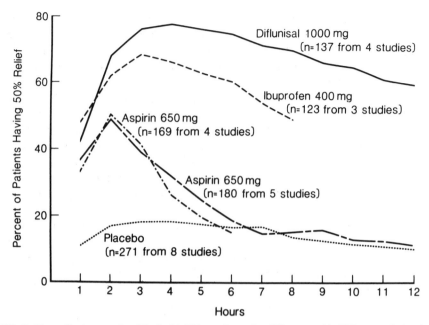

FIG. 3. Time-effect curves for diflunisal 1,000 mg, ibuprofen 400 mg, aspirin 650 mg, and placebo, with data combined across studies. The percentage of patients having 50% relief on the ordinate is plotted against time in hours on the abscissa.

The VAS is sometimes used along with, or in lieu of, the usual categorical ratings (see pp. 60–61). Wallenstein (20), in a classic study in cancer patients, demonstrated a linear relationship between categorical ratings of pain relief and concomitant estimates of relief using a VAS. We have confirmed this linear relationship between categorical and VAS ratings of pain intensity in oral surgery outpatients (Fig. 4). Comparisons between the two types of ratings were made at baseline and at hour 2 of the study; the distance between descriptors, in VAS units, was remarkably uniform.

These VAS ratings of pain intensity were compared to patient ratings of 50% relief; 209 patients made 1,306 ratings. Approximately 90% of the ratings were in agreement; that is, when baseline pain was rated as one-half gone VAS pain had decreased by 50% or more, and when baseline pain was rated as not one-half gone VAS pain had not decreased by 50%. Less than 10% of the time, starting pain was rated half gone and VAS pain had decreased less than 50%. Fewer than 1% of the patients indicated their pain was not half gone when VAS pain had decreased by 50% or more. This demonstrates consistency between the two types of scales, VAS versus categorical, and two different measures of analgesia, i.e., pain intensity and 50% relief.

Categorical or visual analogue scales can be used to evaluate effects other than analgesic efficacy, such as anxiety and relaxation (21). One must be careful se-

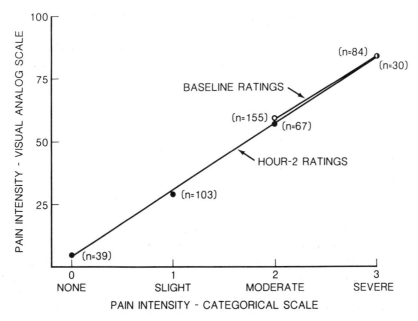

FIG. 4. Pain intensity at baseline and hour 2. Visual analogue scale ratings on the ordinate are plotted against categorical scale ratings and descriptors on the abscissa.

lecting the descriptor or adjective for such measures and the nurse-observer must brief the patients thoroughly, so that there is common understanding among patients concerning the effect being measured.

MEASURES OF EFFICACY

Measures of efficacy, typically estimates of total and peak analgesia, are derived from patients' subjective reports using some variation of the aforementioned rating scales. In our own studies, we are able to evaluate the hourly pain intensity difference score (PID), sum of the pain intensity difference score (SPID), peak PID score, hourly pain relief score, total pain relief score, peak pain relief score, total hours of 50% relief, the patient's overall evaluation of the study medication, and the number of hours until remediation with a backup or rescue analgesic. Hourly scores are added to obtain the SPID and total relief; these are simply estimates of the area under the time-effect curve. SPID and total relief may be weighted if aperiodic time intervals, e.g., 30- and 45-min evaluations, were employed in a study with routine hourly evaluations. The peak score for these measures is the highest interval score. Patients who do not remediate by the end of the study are assigned a time-until-remediation score equal to the last scheduled evaluation; this is a conservative procedure and would underestimate the mean time until remediation.

TABLE 4. *Correlation between measures of analgesic efficacy*

	Baseline pain	SPID[b]	Peak PID[b]	Total relief[b]	Peak relief[b]	Hours of 50% relief[b]	Patient's overall evaluation[b]
Baseline pain	—	—	—	—	—	—	—
SPID	0.28[b]	—	—	—	—	—	—
Peak PID	0.29[b]	0.87	—	—	—	—	—
Total relief	0.06	0.86	0.75	—	—	—	—
Peak relief	−0.04[c]	0.78	0.85	0.87	—	—	—
Hours of 50% relief	−0.07	0.80	0.69	0.92	0.80	—	—
Patient's overall evaluation	−0.05	0.72	0.71	0.81	0.78	0.80	—
Hours until remedication	−0.09[a]	0.70	0.57	0.80	0.66	0.77	0.66

[a] Statistically significant r: $p < 0.05$.
[b] Statistically significant r: $p < 0.01$.
[c] Minus signs indicate negative correlation.

Table 4 summarizes the correlation between measures of analgesic efficacy. Correlations were statistically significant for all measures and ranged from 0.69 to 0.92. Approximately 85% of the variation in total relief can be accounted for by knowing the number of hours the patient's baseline pain was half gone. We could pick one of these measures of effect, e.g., 50% relief, and conduct an assay-sensitive trial without great loss. Baseline pain was not significantly related to treatment outcome for these patients except for measures of SPID and peak PID, which are a function of starting pain, and the number of hours until re-medication.

SCORING SYSTEM

From the statistical point of view it would be ideal if patients evaluated the study medication for the entire study period regardless of their level of pain and its relief. By doing so, each patient would provide the investigator with a complete matrix of efficacy data, that is, a score for each scale for each time point. This is neither realistic nor humane, since patients who have inadequate pain relief, e.g., patients treated with placebo or an ineffective dose of active medication, cannot be expected to endure hours of discomfort for the sake of science. In addition, some institutional review boards (IRBs) do not want us to ask the patient to wait until relief has ended and/or pain has returned to the baseline level. So, we are often left with the problem of dealing with an incomplete data matrix owing to the patient remedicating before the end of the study or for some other reason, e.g., falling asleep. Before a study is initiated the investigator must decide how incomplete data will be handled, and provide the rationale for that decision.

Patients in most analgesic studies are probably given some instructions concerning remedication with the backup or rescue medication. Unfortunately, most analgesic studies reported in the archival literature do not specify these instructions. The instructions should be such that the patient gives the medication time to be absorbed, and does not take additional analgesic if he or she is having satisfactory relief. We routinely ask patients (a) not to remedicate before hour 2 of the study, (b) not to remedicate as long as they are having *any* relief, and (c) not to remedicate if their pain is less than moderate. An informal review of our own data suggests that the time of remedication, one measure of efficacy, is a function of these instructions. For example, the attrition rate owing to remedication will be higher if instructions indicate that remedication is permissible after completing 1 hr of the study than if patients were asked to wait 3 hrs. In the first instance, patients might remedicate before the medication has had an opportunity to show any effect. It is likely that the time-effect curves for sulindac, a drug with a slow onset of action, would look very different for patients who waited 3 hrs before remedicating than for patients who waited 1 hr. A drug with a rapid onset of action, e.g., 400 mg ibuprofen, would be affected to a lesser degree.

In addition, if the instructions concerning remedication only refer to the time element, e.g., "Wait at least 2 hours . . .," we would probably see more patients remedicating with relief than if patients were instructed, "Wait at least 2 hours, and do not take the backup medication as long as you are having *any* relief from the study medication." When the results of clinical trials differ markedly, it may be difficult to determine whether these differences were owing to the chemical effect of the drugs or mostly owing to investigator-induced effect (22,23). Likewise, differences between studies may be a function of the scoring system used even if instructions to the patients were identical.

The scoring system is basically a set of rules to determine, before the double-blind has been broken, which patients have valid efficacy data and how missing evaluations, regardless of cause, will be handled. This information should be specified in the study protocol. In our studies, patients must have completed the hour-2 evaluation in order to be eligible for inclusion as a valid patient. In actual practice, the patient might be in the study for only 1 hr 45 min since our general rule is to allow a plus or minus 15-min window around each hourly time point. We also invalidate the efficacy data for patients who remedicate with pain intensity less than moderate and/or relief greater than "a little." Inclusion of these patients would prevent getting a true picture of the time effect of the drug evaluated.

In cases where the patient remedicates before the end of the study period some researchers use the last rating prior to remedication as the rating for subsequent evaluations. For example, if a patient who had severe baseline pain remedicates at hour 4 of an 8-hr study while having moderate pain and a little relief, that patient will be considered as having moderate pain and a little relief for hours 5 to 8. This is difficult to understand since it assumes the patient would continue at the same level of pain and relief if untreated. A more conservative approach would be to assign a pain intensity score equal to the baseline or the last rating prior to remedication, whichever is more severe. The pain relief score would be considered none and the starting pain would not be considered half gone. This procedure might make the drug look less efficacious; however, clinical experience suggests this scoring method is more realistic. Left untreated, a patient's pain will usually stay the same or increase over the short run, and the patient will not likely have continued relief.

To standardize the evaluation interval and awaken a sleeping patient, all subjects in our studies are issued timers with a bell. Despite this precaution, some patients fall asleep during the evaluation period. The problem is potentially more aggravating when patients have surgery in the afternoon and medicate near their routine bedtime. In our 12-hr studies patients are not entered if surgery is not completed by 1 PM. In a 12-hr evaluation of diflunisal approximately 25% of the patients treated with diflunisal were asleep for one or more interval evaluations, compared to 11% in the placebo group (24).

It is tempting to consider the sleeping patient as being pain free; however, clinical trials with inpatients (25–27) having postoperative pain following general or orthopedic surgery suggest that is not necessarily the case. It was not uncommon for the nurse-observer to awaken a patient for an interval evaluation and have the patient report being in pain at that time. How then do we handle the situation where the outpatient, whom we cannot awaken, has indicated on the self-rating record that he or she was asleep for some portion of the study? We include any patient who has completed the first 2 hrs of the study prior to falling asleep; the ratings for the previous hour are carried over for the evaluations missed while sleeping.

STATISTICAL ANALYSIS

Even a cursory review of analgesic studies in the archival literature suggests that there is a difference of opinion concerning the level of measurement (nominal, ordinal, interval, ratio) of the scales employed to evaluate analgesic efficacy. Measures of pain and its relief, obtained from categorical or VAS scales, are analyzed by parametric analyses in some published studies and by nonparametric procedures in others. The selection of the method of analysis is based on the assumptions we are willing to make about the data we have collected. Are we willing to consider categorical ratings of pain relief as representing an interval scale, and meeting the formal properties of that level of measurement (28), or do we feel more comfortable considering these evaluations as satisfying the less stringent criteria of an ordinal measure? A comprehensive discussion of this issue is beyond the scope of this chapter and the author; however, it will be addressed in Chapter 29. In general, parametric analyses have more power, that is, the ability to detect a real difference between treatments, than nonparametric procedures if the data meet the necessary assumptions. On the other hand, nonparametric procedures generally give true α levels under very broad assumptions about the underlying variables.

We routinely analyze efficacy data using both parametric and nonparametric procedures. When 20 studies were reviewed there was 100% agreement between the results of a parametric analysis of variance (F) (29) and the Kruskal-Wallis analysis of variance by ranks (H) (28); however, there were marked differences between the results of multiple comparisons made by Duncan's new multiple range test (30) and those made by Dunn's distribution-free comparisons (31) in some studies. Across the 20 studies, only 67% of the statistically significant pairwise differences found by parametric analyses were detected by nonparametric multiple comparisons. Dunn's test is considered to be very conservative and there are other less stringent nonparametric methods of multiple comparisons.

The length of a study is also important since it can influence apparent analgesia. Total analgesic effect increases for placebo as the number of hours of evaluation increases; this appears to be true for all measures of total effect. This exaggerated placebo effect may obscure differences between placebo and weak analgesic standards, such as aspirin 650 mg or codeine 60 mg, in 8- or 12-hr studies. It is often necessary to analyze the data for 4 or 6 hrs in order to demonstrate statistically significant differences between placebo and a weak standard (16).

Interim Analysis of Efficacy Data

Modell and Houde (32) point out the need for conducting periodic analyses of data in order to monitor the "sensitivity of the method" employed in the clinical evaluation of a drug. This procedure is routine in basic science and is particularly important in the measurement of subjective phenomena. My associates and I agree with this point of view and until recently performed the calculations necessary to provide us with time-effect curves (TECs) for pain intensity differences, relief from starting pain, and the percentage of patients indicating their baseline pain was half gone. When a block, or several blocks, of patients had been completely evaluated and the case report forms for these patients had been received and accepted by the study sponsor, the medication codes for the patients would be forwarded to my office. My research assistant would enter the appropriate data in our computer and generate the aforementioned TECs. I then reviewed the TECs without looking at the data for specific patients; no other member of the research team was privy to this information. I took into consideration the relative performance of the study drugs in terms of onset, peak, and duration of effect, and compared the TECs with those for previous studies at that site. Particular attention was given to between-study differences in placebo response and response to standards or test medications previously evaluated. For example, the TEC for pain relief for patients treated with placebo should not differ substantially from previous TECs for placebo from the same analgesic unit being managed by the same nurse. Likewise, one would not expect substantial differences in the TECs for percentage of patients having 50% relief following treatment with ibuprofen 200 mg, if one compared studies or periods of time, for the same nurse-observer in the same unit.

These procedures allowed us to detect a variety of problems: an error in labeling the dosage of study medication; degradation of an aspirin standard packaged in envelopes that were not moisture-proof; poor bioavailability due to overcompaction of tablets; differences between manufacturing lots of investigational medication; and changes in procedures at the study site. Other investigators have also experienced similar problems. Interim analyses of efficacy data can tell us whether responses to the study medications are sensible; if not, we have an option of investigating.

Another less obvious reason for performing interim analyses is to monitor the system of measurement. We know changes can occur in the nurse-observer, office environment, and patient population. Our nurses use a clipboard with an attached outline to help standardize their "presentation" to patients. The outline is similar to the study consent form and indicates the study drugs, dosages, potential adverse effects, options if not participating in the study, and instructions for those who participate. Still, I find when monitoring the nurses' presentations to patients, that occasionally information may be omitted, added, or there is a change in emphasis. This is a potential source of variation in response to the drugs being evaluated. We have also discovered ancillary personnel, e.g., office receptionists, talking to patients about the research study and leaving the patient with some misunderstanding. Atypical TECs signal us to start looking at all parts of the measurement system.

When interim analyses were routinely performed the nurse-observers were well aware that periodic checks were being made and that the system was being monitored. Now the entire research team knows the study codes are not available until the end of the study; this may lead to a tendency to be less vigilant. If there is a problem with the system it may be months and hundreds of patients before we know about it. After interim analyses of a block of patients every member of the research team is still blinded with respect to the remainder of patients to be evaluated. Any interaction on my part with the nurse-observer, or office staff, as a result of reviewing interim TECs simply attempts to reinstitute, or put back into effect, the guidelines for standardizing the system. I strongly suggest that sponsors complete interim analyses at intervals specified in the study protocol using the investigator's scoring system. This data should be used to provide TECs for review by the study's principal investigator.

DEGREE OF TRAUMA AND EFFICACY

The 4 third molars are generally classified as: erupted (completely free of bone and soft tissue); tissue impacted (completely surrounded by the soft tissue of the gum); partially bony impacted (partially surrounded by bone of the mandible or maxilla as well as soft tissue); or completely bony impacted (the molar is completely surrounded by bone of the mandible or maxilla as well as tissue). Routinely, there are 4 third molars and it is highly unusual to find a supernumerary. The patient may have any combination of the above, e.g., 1 tissue impaction, 2 partial bony impactions, and 1 complete bony impaction. Since there are many possible combinations of impactions, it is impractical to stratify a study on this factor.

I am unaware of a controlled clinical trial demonstrating a significant relationship between the number and/or type of impactions and either baseline pain or analgesic efficacy. In fact, some oral surgeons indicate that the position of the tooth and the complexity of the root system can lead to more surgical trauma in removing an erupted third molar than one that is completely impacted by bone. It is very difficult to predict a patient's level of postoperative pain or the need for analgesics on the basis of the number or type of impactions. A patient with one tissue impaction and three erupted molars might have severe baseline pain and medicate for 4 or 5 days, whereas the next patient could have four complete bony impactions, no postoperative pain, and require no analgesic medication.

If one makes the assumption that pain increases as the degree of impaction increases, a pain or trauma index could be calculated to take into account the number and type of impactions. We have done this by assigning the following scores to the types of impactions: eruption (1); tissue impaction (2); partial bony impaction (3); and complete bony impaction (4). Supernumeraries were assigned the appropriate rating dependent upon the type of impaction; simple extractions that were concomitant with the impactions were assigned a score of 1. The trauma index was defined as the sum of scores for all the teeth removed. For example, a patient who had one tissue impaction, three partial bony impactions, and one simple extraction removed would have a trauma index of 12.

As indicated in Table 5, the trauma index was positively correlated with baseline pain intensity, and negatively correlated with total relief, peak relief, and the number of hours until remedication. Although these correlation coefficients are statistically significant they are very small and account for little variation. It is important to note, however, that they do make sense from the clinical point of view; that is, higher levels of trauma were associated with higher baseline pain and lower efficacy. It is worth repeating that baseline pain intensity (see Table 4) was related to higher values for SPID and peak PID, and lower values for the number of hours until remedication. If the magnitude of these correlations are indeed representative for this model, it seems likely that the number and/or type of impactions is of little practical importance in the conduct of clinical trials, but further work is needed to confirm these results.

Despite the aforementioned relationships *within* the third molar impaction model, the data suggest a hierarchy of pain between different types of dental surgery. I think it is generally accepted that simple extractions generate the least postoperative pain and the surgical removal of impacted third molars leads to the most severe pain (33). The degree of pain following periodontal surgery seems to be similar to or slightly less than that following removal of impactions; other procedures, e.g., multiple mandibular extractions, rate somewhere between the impaction model and simple extractions.

TABLE 5. *Correlation between measures of analgesic efficacy, demographic data, and data related to the surgical procedure*

	Baseline pain	SPID	Peak PID	Total relief	Peak relief	Hours of 50% relief	Patient's overall evaluation	Hours until remediation
Age	-0.08[a]	0.08[a]	0.05	0.08[a]	0.07[a]	0.08[a]	0.07[a]	0.12[b]
Sex	0.05	-0.03	0.001	-0.04	-0.03	-0.04	-0.05	-0.05
Height	-0.04	-0.002	-0.02	0.02	0.001	0.02	0.03	0.01
Weight	0.01	-0.01	-0.02	-0.03	-0.02	-0.02	-0.01	-0.004
Preoperative consultation[c]	-0.05	-0.02	-0.08[a]	0.01	-0.04	0.04	-0.01	-0.03
Patient's anxiety level[d]	0.04	-0.06	-0.04	-0.08[a]	-0.06	-0.05	-0.05	-0.10[b]
Number of impactions	0.11[b]	-0.06	-0.05	-0.09[a]	-0.09[a]	-0.07[a]	-0.06	-0.12[b]
Number of sutures	0.09[a]	-0.001	-0.001	-0.04	-0.05	-0.04	-0.03	-0.07
Trauma rating[e]	0.11[b]	0.01	-0.03	-0.04	-0.07	-0.03	-0.01	-0.09[d]
Length of surgery	0.03	-0.04	-0.03	-0.04	-0.07	-0.02	-0.02	-0.05
Trauma index[f]	0.16[b]	-0.01	0.04	-0.07[a]	-0.07[a]	-0.05	-0.05	-0.13[b]
Time until medicated[g]	-0.05	0.28[b]	0.17[b]	0.33[b]	0.24[b]	0.28[b]	0.28[b]	0.33[b]

[a] Statistically significant r: $p < 0.05$.
[b] Statistically significant r: $p < 0.01$.
[c] Preoperative consultation with nurse-observer: 0 = no, 1 = yes.
[d] Rated by nurse-observer using a 100-mm visual analogue scale.
[e] Rated by oral surgeon based upon amount of tissue damage, etc.: 1 = mild; 2 = moderate; 3 = severe.
[f] Sum of assigned ratings for impactions: 1 = erupted molar or simple extraction; 2 = tissue impaction; 3 = partial bony impaction; 4 = complete bony impaction.
[g] Time from end of surgery until taking the study medication.

We stratified for type of surgery and found patients with nonimpacted, multiple mandibular extractions had greater relief than patients who had impacted third molars removed (34). The relative efficacy of treatments remained the same; differences in efficacy between the two types of surgery was interpreted as indicating postoperative pain was less for mandibular extractions.

REPEAT-DOSE STUDIES IN THE ORAL SURGERY MODEL

Early studies of analgesics in oral surgery patients evaluated repeated doses of study medication and were crossover in design (2–4,6). These studies often measured the effect of drugs on swelling, pain, and patient drug preference using designs and procedures that were, in many respects, a closer approximation of actual treatment than the single-dose analgesic trials in vogue today. Despite the use of global measures of efficacy, investigators found differences between placebo and active medications as well as differences among active medications. It is unclear why study design switched from the repeat-dose, crossover design to single-dose, parallel-group trials. Certainly Cooper's work (1) stimulated interest in the oral surgery model among investigators in the United States and emphasized the use of periodic measures, e.g., hourly evaluations, of analgesia that could be used to plot TECs characterizing drugs. One could obtain very fine discrimination for one dose of medication; then patients continuing to have pain could be treated with a standard, marketed analgesic.

Patients having pathologic pain following oral surgery, or other surgery for that matter, almost always require multiple doses of medication. If differences demonstrated in single-dose studies correlated highly with response to treatment for the entire course of one's pain, there would be no problem. Unfortunately, repeat-dose data supporting the results of single-dose studies are lacking. In my opinion, many of the statistically significant differences my associates and I have found in our single-dose studies may be of little, if any, clinical significance in treating patients.

Two of our evaluations of oral ketorolac tromethamine in oral surgery outpatients employed a parallel-group design with repeated dosing (13,14). One study compared ketorolac 10 mg, aspirin 650 mg, a combination of acetaminophen 600 mg with codeine 60 mg, and placebo. The TECs for pain relief following dose 1 are presented in Fig. 5A. All active medications were statistically significantly superior to placebo, the codeine combination was superior to aspirin on some measures, and ketorolac was superior to both aspirin and the codeine combination on most measures of total and peak analgesia. The percent of patients taking medication (Fig. 5B) decreased from the day of surgery until postoperative day 6; the same was true for the mean number of doses taken and pain intensity. Relief from starting pain increased over time (Fig. 5C). Although both studies demonstrated good assay sensitivity for the first dose of medication, there were no statistically significant differences among the active treatments beyond the day of surgery.

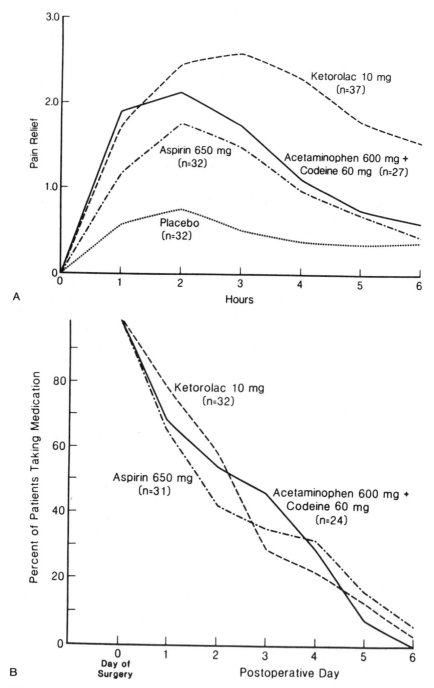

FIG. 5. A: Time-effect curves for dose 1 for ketorolac 10 mg, aspirin 650 mg, a combination of acetaminophen 600 mg with codeine 60 mg, and placebo. Pain relief on the ordinate is plotted against time in hours on the abscissa. **B:** Time-effect curves for ketorolac 10 mg, aspirin 650 mg, and a combination of acetaminophen 600 mg with codeine 60 mg. The percentage of patients taking medication on the ordinate is plotted against time in days on the abscissa. **C:** Time-effect curves for ketorolac 10 mg, aspirin 650 mg, and a combination of acetaminophen 600 mg with codeine 60 mg. Mean pain relief on the ordinate is plotted against time in days on the abscissa.

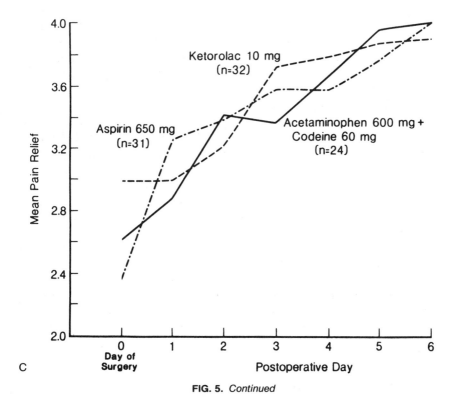

FIG. 5. *Continued*

These results could reflect a lack of sensitivity in this repeat-dose model or indicate that the treatments did not differ significantly after the day of surgery. We would anticipate that the usual decreasing need for analgesic medication in most patients, and concomitant variation in response, would decrease assay sensitivity, since assay sensitivity is less in milder pain states than in conditions of moderate to severe pain. In particular, the "upside" assay sensitivity of the study would be expected to suffer (35).

Although single-dose studies usually tell us little about the adverse-effect profile of a drug, daily evaluations of adverse effects, in our repeat-dose studies, provide more useful information. For example, the central nervous system (CNS) effects one usually sees with repeated dosing of narcotics and their combinations appear in the repeat-dose impaction model. This allows us to more accurately determine the efficacy/adverse-effect ratio for the study drugs (13).

ONSET AND DURATION OF ANALGESIA

Currently, there is much interest in the measurement of the onset and duration of analgesia. Laska and his associates (see Chapter 4) have had patients use a stopwatch to determine onset, and suggest this method provides excellent precision. We asked patients to use a stopwatch to determine the onset of "mean-ingful relief" and were surprised to find that many patients who had what my associates and I considered clinically significant relief from starting pain did not think their relief was "meaningful." We were not impressed with the use of a stopwatch and think adequate data could be obtained by simply asking the patient to record the time he or she first noticed *any* relief.

Alternatively, onset could be defined as the first interval evaluation at which pain intensity decreased, or relief occurred; duration would be the last interval before pain returned to baseline, or relief ceased. Similarly, one could calculate the onset and duration for 50% relief. The precision of this method is a function of the frequency of interval evaluations; however, the accuracy should be sufficient for orally administered medications. We have done this and find it interesting that onset occurs first with relief from starting pain, followed by pain intensity, and then 50% relief (17).

This issue can be illustrated by reviewing the TECs for 50% relief (Fig. 6) from a study evaluating aspirin 1,000 mg, effervescent aspirin 1,000 mg at two levels of acid neutralizing capacity (ANC 38 and ANC 56), effervescent placebo, and noneffervescent placebo. Effervescent aspirin 1,000 mg (ANC 56) was statistically significantly superior to noneffervescent placebo by hour $\frac{1}{4}$, indicating an onset of 15 min or less, and superior to effervescent placebo by hour $\frac{1}{2}$, suggesting an

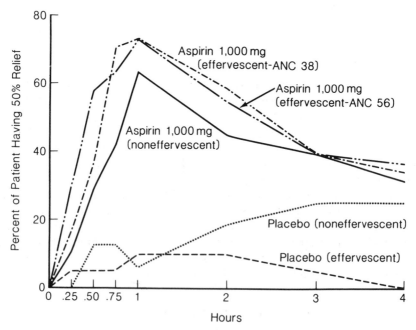

FIG. 6. Time-effect curves for aspirin 1,000 mg, effervescent (ANC 38 and 56) aspirin 1,000 mg, and placebo (effervescent and noneffervescent). The percentage of patients having 50% relief on the ordinate is plotted against time in hours on the abscissa.

onset between 15 and 30 min. Based upon the time until 50% relief first occurred for effervescent aspirin 1,000 mg (ANC 56), mean time of onset was 32 min; using a stopwatch, the time until "meaningful" pain relief was 25 min. The duration of effect was 4 hrs.

CONTROL: INPATIENT VERSUS OUTPATIENT STUDIES

There is a tendency for one to think that there is more control over an inpatient population (e.g., general or orthopedic surgery patients) than over outpatients (e.g., oral surgery patients), and that this control will allow one to conduct a better or more sensitive analgesic study. In my opinion, after having conducted many studies with inpatient and outpatient populations, the outpatient studies have greater sensitivity. Although the investigator or the nurse-observer will have greater control over certain aspects of the hospitalized patient's behavior, the behaviors controlled may have little to do with the successful outcome of an analgesic trial. The nurse-observer can administer the study medication and periodically evaluate the patient for efficacy and adverse effects; however, there may be little else that she can control that is germane to the problem of evaluating analgesic efficacy. In most cases the nurse-observer sees the patient at standard intervals and is not a watchdog during the entire study period. For example, it would be just as easy for the hospitalized patient to take additional, unauthorized medication during the study as it would be for the outpatient to do so. In addition, I think there are factors affecting the inpatient that may have a negative effect on an analgesic study.

In my opinion, patients who are hospitalized seem to have a higher level of state anxiety, that is, transient anxiety owing to their current situation, than patients who are in the natural surroundings of their home. Higher anxiety usually means higher levels of pain. In fact, one aspect of the primary ward nurse's job is to lower the patient's level of apprehension. When this coincides with analgesic administration, or administration of a dummy preparation, it often leads to an elevated placebo response.

A simplistic view of a patient's response to analgesic medication is that part is due to the chemical, i.e., the active medication, and the remainder of the response is due to the placebo effect. Most patients who participate in an analgesic study have taken some analgesic previously and have likely had a positive response; therefore, in a sense they are predisposed to think that they will have a positive response to the study medication despite being told that the study involves a placebo group. That is, taking a tablet, capsule, or receiving an injection in the past has lead to some response and there is no reason to think that this situation is any different. The situation is further complicated by the presence of the nurse, since nurses have a history of administering medication that works. The nurse is not present in the classic outpatient study and therefore there is less opportunity for a significant placebo effect.

In my opinion, the inpatient oral surgery analgesic model has even more potential for bias and methodologic problems than studies using hospitalized subjects, e.g., postoperative pain following orthopedic surgery. In the inpatient model, patients who have had surgery are asked to remain in the oral surgeon's office until they have at least moderate pain. Patients then medicate and remain in the office for a specified time period, e.g., 4 hrs, or until remediation is required. Clinical experience suggests that most patients who have oral surgery want to go home as soon as they are able to do so; therefore, patients might have a tendency to indicate pain and participate in the study in order get the study over and go home. Patients who remain in the office until remediation is required probably have a tendency to request medication earlier than necessary in order to complete the study and leave. If my associates and I are correct concerning this issue, the time from the end of surgery until taking study medication would be shorter in the inpatient setting and the duration of effect of a specific drug and dosage would be shorter than in the classic outpatient model. Unfortunately, there are too few published manuscripts for inpatient oral surgery studies that provide appropriate data (e.g., time from surgery until taking study medication), to adequately resolve this issue. It is my impression, however, based on discussions with other investigators, that inpatient oral surgery subjects medicate up to 1 hr sooner than outpatients, and overall the duration of analgesia is less for a given drug.

CONCLUSIONS

The single-dose oral surgery outpatient analgesic model as defined by Cooper and Beaver (1) is robust and very sensitive in detecting treatment differences. Numerous investigators have conducted assay-sensitive trials defining onset, peak, and duration of analgesia for investigational and marketed drugs. This chapter has discussed some of the issues one should consider when designing a single-dose study or interpreting the resultant data.

Unfortunately, the clinical significance of the statistically significant differences found in these trials, including those of the author and his associates, is not clear. Data from repeat-dose studies confirming the results of single-dose studies are, for the most part, not available. There is a great need for a repeat-dose analgesic model that would provide data highly correlated with treatment in actual clinical settings. Pharmaceutical company sponsors and regulatory agencies, such as the FDA, should encourage and support the research needed to develop this model.

ACKNOWLEDGMENTS

I am indebted to Dr. William T. Beaver for his encouragement and scientific support during the past 15 years, to the numerous pharmaceutical companies who sponsored my research, and to Alice L. Forbes for assistance in preparing this manuscript.

REFERENCES

1. Cooper SA, Beaver WT. A model to evaluate mild analgesics in oral surgery outpatients. *Clin Pharamacol Ther* 1976;20;241–250.
2. Lokken P, Olsen I, Bruaset I, Norman-Pedersen K. Bilateral surgical removal of impacted lower third molar teeth as a model for drug evaluation: a test with ibuprofen. *Eur J Clin Pharmacol* 1975;8:209–216.
3. Hepso HU, Lokken P, Bjornson J, Godal HC. Double-blind crossover study of the effect of acetylsalicylic acid on bleeding and post-operative course after bilateral oral surgery. *Eur J Clin Pharmacol* 1976;10:217–225.
4. Sveen K, Gilhuus-Moe O. Paracetamol/codeine in relieving pain following removal of impacted mandibular third molars. *Int J Oral Surg* 1975;4:258–266.
5. Ahlstrom U, Lantz B. A comparison between dextro propoxyphene hydrochloride and acetyl salicylic acid as analgesics after oral surgery. *Odent Rev (Malmo)* 1968;19:55–63.
6. Ruedy J, Bentley KC. Comparison of glaphenine and codeine in postoperative dental pain. *Clin Pharmacol Ther* 1969;11:718–723.
7. Cooper SA. *A new model to evaluate mild analgesics in oral surgery outpatients.* Doctoral Dissertation, Georgetown University, School of Dentistry, Washington, DC, March 19, 1975.
8. Cooper SA, Wagenberg B, Zissu J, Kruger GO, Reynolds DC, Gallegos LT, Allwein JB, Desjardins PJ, Friedmann N, Danna RP. The analgesic efficacy of suprofen in periodontal and oral surgical pain. *Pharmacotherapy* 1986;6:267–276.
9. Sunshine A, Marrero I, Olson NZ, Laska EM, McCormick N. Oral analgesic efficacy of suprofen compared to aspirin, aspirin plus codeine, and placebo in patients with postoperative dental pain. *Pharmacology* 1983;27(suppl 1):31–40.
10. Cooper SA. New peripherally acting analgesics. *Annu Rev Pharmacol Toxicol* 1983;23:617–647.
11. Cooper SA, Schachtel BP, Goldman E, Gelb S, Cohn P. Ibuprofen and acetaminophen in the relief of acute pain: a randomized, double-blind, placebo-controlled study. *J Clin Pharmacol* 1989;29:1026–1030.
12. Forbes JA, Butterworth GA, Burchfield WH, Yorio CC, Selinger LR, Rosenmertz SK, Beaver WT. Evaluation of flurbiprofen, acetaminophen, an acetaminophen-codeine combination, and placebo in postoperative oral surgery pain. *Pharmacotherapy* 1989;9:322–330.
13. Forbes JA, Butterworth GA, Burchfield WH, Beaver WT. An evaluation of ketorolac, aspirin, and an acetaminophen-codeine combination in postoperative oral surgery pain. *Pharmacotherapy* 1990;10.
14. Forbes JA, Kehm CJ, Grodin CD, Beaver WT. An evaluation of ketorolac, ibuprofen, acetaminophen, and an acetaminophen-codeine combination in postoperative oral surgery pain. *Pharmacotherapy* 1990;10.
15. Sidman M. *Tactics of scientific research.* New York: Basic Books, 1960.
16. Beaver WT, Forbes JA, Shackleford RW. A method for the 12-hour evaluation of analgesic efficacy in outpatients with postoperative oral surgery pain. *Pharmacotherapy* 1983;3(pt 2):23S–37S.
17. Beaver WT, Forbes JA, Jones KF, Moore EM, Byrd WG. An evaluation of effervescent and noneffervescent aspirin and acetaminophen in postoperative oral surgery pain. *Clin Pharmacol Ther* 1990;47:164.
18. Houde RW, Wallenstein SL, Beaver WT. Clinical measurement of pain. In: deStevens G, ed. *Analgetics.* New York: Academic Press, 1965;75–122.
19. Cooper SA, Needle SE, Kruger GO. Comparative analgesic potency of aspirin and ibuprofen. *J Oral Surg* 1977;35:898–903.
20. Wallenstein SL. Scaling clinical pain and pain relief. In:Bromm B, ed. *Pain measurement in man: neurophysiological correlates of pain.* Amsterdam: Elsevier, 1984;389–396.
21. Forbes JA, Jones KF, Smith WK, Gongloff CM. Analgesic effect of an aspirin-codeine-butalbital-caffeine combination and an acetaminophen-codeine combination in postoperative oral surgery pain. *Pharmacotherapy* 1986;6:240–247.

22. Rosenthal R. *Experimenter effects in behavioral research.* New York: Appleton-Century-Crofts, 1966.
23. Forbes JA, Barkaszi BA, Ragland RN, Hankle JJ. Analgesic effect of fendosal, ibuprofen and aspirin in postoperative oral surgery pain. *Pharmacotherapy* 1984;4:385–391.
24. Forbes JA, Foor VM, Bowser MW, Calderazzo JP, Shackleford RW, Beaver WT. A 12-hour evaluation of the analgesic efficacy of diflunisal, propoxyphene, a propoxyphene-acetaminophen combination, and placebo in postoperative oral surgery pain. *Pharmacotherapy* 1982;2:43–49.
25. Forbes JA, Kolodny AL, Beaver WT, Shackleford RW, Scarlett VR. A 12-hour evaluation of the analgesic efficacy of diflunisal, acetaminophen, an acetaminophen-codeine combination, and placebo in postoperative oral surgery pain. *Pharmacotherapy* 1983;3(2 pt 2):47S–54S.
26. Forbes JA, Kolodny AL, Chachich BM, Beaver WT. Nalbuphine, acetaminophen, and their combination in postoperative pain. *Clin Pharmacol Ther* 1984;35:843–851.
27. Bostrom A, Forbes JA, Sevelius H, Bynum L, Beaver WT. A repeat dose evaluation of naproxen sodium and a naproxen sodium-codeine combination in postoperative pain. *Clin Pharmacol Ther* 1987;41:228.
28. Siegel S. *Nonparametric statistics for the behavioral sciences.* New York: McGraw-Hill, 1959.
29. Winer BJ. *Statistical principles in experimental design.* New York: McGraw-Hill, 1962.
30. Kramer CY. Extension of multiple range tests to group means with unequal numbers of replications. *Biometrics* 1956;12:307–310.
31. Kirk RE. *Experimental design: procedures for the behavioral sciences.* Belmont, California: Brooks/Cole, 1968.
32. Modell W, Houde RW. Factors influencing clinical evaluation of drugs with special reference to the double-blind technique. *JAMA* 58;167;2190–2198.
33. Cooper SA. Five studies on ibuprofen in dental pain. *Compend Contin Educ Dent* 1986;7:578–597.
34. Forbes JA, Calderazzo JP, Bowser MW, Foor VM, Shackleford RW, Beaver WT. A 12-hour evaluation of the analgesic efficacy of diflunisal, aspirin, and placebo in postoperative dental pain. *J Clin Pharmacol* 1982;22:89–96.
35. Forbes JA, White RW, White EH, Hughes MK. An evaluation of the analgesic efficacy of proquazone and aspirin in postoperative dental pain. *J Clin Pharmacol* 1980;20:465–474.

Advances in Pain Research and Therapy, Vol. 18,
edited by M. Max, R. Portenoy, and E. Laska,
Raven Press, Ltd., New York © 1991.

16

Chronic Orofacial Pain

James R. Fricton

*TMJ and Craniofacial Pain Clinic, Department of Diagnostic and Surgical Sciences,
School of Dentistry, University of Minnesota, Minneapolis, Minnesota 55455*

Chronic pain is one of the most prevalent chronic illnesses, costing our country over $80 billion annually in lost work, health care, and medications with an untold cost in human suffering (1). Chronic pain syndromes can involve pain anywhere in the body, but the most frequent site of persistent pain is in the head. Headache, jaw pain, and other orofacial pains have their own individual characteristics and effect on the patient. A recent Louis Harris poll found more adults working full-time miss work from head and face pain than any other site of pain (2). In addition, temporomandibular joint disorders of all stages have been noted in over 40% of the population, with 10% of the population having a problem severe enough to warrant treatment (3). Because pain in the orofacial structures has close associations with functions of eating, communication, sight, and hearing, as well as forming a basis for appearance, self-esteem, and expression, pain of orofacial origin can deeply affect an individual (4). The pain can affect many areas of life, interfering with work and relationships, disturbing sleep and activity levels, and creating confusion and frustration. In addition, frustrating clinical situations result and may involve costly invasive treatments, long-term medications, continuous doctor shopping, and an ongoing dependency on the health care system.

Effective management of these problems is of paramount importance in preventing the devastating effect these problems can have on an individual. Yet, many of these patients are neglected, inadequately treated, or improperly managed. Patients are often passed from clinician to clinician with any form of new treatment attempted on them. Patients with mild problems can be overtreated in an effort to prevent further development of severe pain and dysfunction, whereas patients with complex problems are subjected to single-modality treatment approaches. There is an extensive list of treatments recommended for chronic orofacial pain including medication, splints, surgery, physical therapy, counseling, biofeedback, and others (5–8). Because of the lack of proper understanding of these disorders, as well as a lack of well-defined and tested meth-

TABLE 1. *Criteria for evaluating clinical trials testing the therapeutic efficacy of interventions for chronic orofacial pain*

A. Study design architecture
   Design in order of preference
   1. Randomized controlled trial
   2. Prospective cohort
   3. Retrospective cohort
   4. Case-control study
   5. Case series
   Specific aims and hypothesis stated
   Background to problem discussed
   Adequate review of literature
B. Interventions
   Described in detail with potential risks
   Standardized therapist, timing, and presentation
   Reproducible
   Patient blind to intervention
   Therapist blind to intervention
   Outcome rater blind to intervention
   Solitary versus multifaceted intervention
C. Population
   Generalizable to clinically relevant situation
   Groups matched for age, sex, ethnicity, duration, and severity
   Specific inclusion and exclusion criteria with rationale
   Homogeneous diagnostic group using tested diagnostic criteria
   Sample size calculated
   Heterogeneous distribution of severity
   Protection of human subjects described
   Selection process from sampling frame
D. Outcome Measures
   Clinically relevant
   Established reliability and validity
   Assessed by independent rater
   Subjective and objective components
   Multidimensional
   Taken at pretreatment and posttreatment
   Posttreatment of sufficient duration (>1 year)
   Follow-up is sufficiently complete (80%)
   Considers natural fluctuation in condition
   Worst case analysis considered
   Data collection procedures described
   Risk factors for treatment failure assessed
E. Statistics
   Appropriate test used
   Sample size calculated
   Possibility of type I or type II errors discussed
   Statistical power and confidence limits discussed

odology to study them, there is a wide disparity of opinions regarding which treatments are most effective for these disorders and when they should be used. Investigators designing clinical trials for orofacial pain conditions have confronted many problems, such as difficulty in obtaining control groups, lack of adequate sample size after fulfilling inclusion and exclusion criteria, ill-defined nonstandard interventions, untested measures of outcome, difficulty in randomization and blinding raters, and lack of knowledge of the natural course of these disorders.

However, in recent years, there have been many contributions to refining the methodology in studying orofacial pain disorders that enable researchers to improve the quality of clinical trials. This chapter discusses some of the problems that can exist in clinical trials for orofacial pain and presents recent advances that may improve the design quality of clinical trials for these disorders. Table 1 lists criteria that can be used to evaluate a clinical trial.

THE NEED FOR DIAGNOSTIC CRITERIA

The diagnosis is the identification of the pathophysiologic process that is responsible for presenting symptoms of a specific patient. It is commonly assumed that success in treatment depends directly on choosing the intervention that is specific to a diagnosis. Likewise, it is also assumed that an incorrect diagnosis is one of the most frequent causes of treatment failure. The most recent literature in the area of differential diagnosis of chronic orofacial pain has highlighted the importance of recognizing that multiple diagnoses do exist and treatment needs to be tailored to a specific diagnosis (9–12). However, in patients with chronic orofacial pain syndromes, it is difficult to establish the specific diagnosis because of the ill-defined nature of some diagnoses, the complex psychosocial and somatic interrelationships that exist, the many similarities between signs and symptoms of different diagnoses, and a high frequency of multiple overlying diagnoses. Because of this, the establishment of diagnostic criteria with acceptable sensitivity and specificity has yet to be done. This has lead to a major weakness of most studies in the area of chronic orofacial pain: using a heterogenous mix of diagnoses within the study sample. Patients with temporomandibular joint (TMJ) internal derangements are combined with patients with muscular pain disorders and treated as a single general category of chronic orofacial pain or temporomandibular (TM) disorder. This creates significant problems in interpretation and generalizability of the study. For example, if the study, designed to examine the efficacy of surgery for "TMJ disorders," includes subjects with preauricular pain from both intracapsular joint problems as well as muscular problems owing to bruxism, the success in alleviating the symptoms might be compromised for the subjects with a muscular pain disorder. This is true for other interventions including the use of analgesics, physical therapy, and splints. The intervention that is most successful for one affected tissue is usually different than that for another tissue. Joint disorders, muscle disorders, neurologic disorders, and vascular pain disorders each must be distinguished from the others. Disorders of orofacial structures such as teeth, salivary glands, or sinuses as well as intracranial disorders need to be ruled out. The possibility of multiple overlying disorders also needs to be considered, perhaps by adding mixed diagnostic groups.

In designing a clinical trial for orofacial pain, specific inclusion and exclusion criteria need to be defined to determine the overall population and specific diagnostic groups that the study sample will be chosen from. However, the lack of appropriately tested diagnostic criteria, the multiple overlapping diagnoses, and the similarities between signs and symptoms of different disorders make these tasks particularly difficult. For example, in a study by LeResche and associates (13), there were considerable differences among clinicians in diagnoses of the same patients with temporomandibular disorders.

Schiffman and associates (14) recently completed a study to determine how accurate specific diagnostic criteria were in diagnosing the presence and stage of TMJ internal derangements compared to arthrotomography as the gold standard. The criteria were comprised of items from the craniomandibular index (15,16) and included specific signs such as range of motion that were tested for reliability and validity (Table 2). These diagnostic criteria were compared in two samples. The overall percent agreement between the arthrogram and diagnostic criteria was 77.8%. The sensitivity and specificity without tomography was 88% and 75%, respectively, in diagnosing temporomandibular disorders. As part of these criteria, muscle disorders were separated from joint disorders and from mixed muscle-joint disorders (17). The authors recommend that the clinician first establish the presence or absence of a joint problem with appropriate diagnostic criteria or soft-tissue imaging and then establish diagnostic criteria for the subgroups that include joint with muscle problems and muscle problems alone. Masticatory muscle disorder criteria include (a) jaw and/or temporal pain, (b) tenderness in masticatory muscles, and (c) alteration of pain with specific muscle palpation.

TABLE 2. *Diagnostic criteria for intraarticular temporomandibular disorders*

	Normal	ID with reduction	ID without reduction/acute	ID without reduction/chronic
History:	None	None	Positive history of mandibular limitation	Positive history of TMJ noise
Exam:	No reciprocal click	Reproducible reciprocal click or popping present	No reciprocal click	No reciprocal click
	No coarse crepitus		No coarse crepitus	Coarse crepitus or joint sound other than reciprocal click
	Passive stretch ≥ 40 mm	No coarse crepitus	Maximum opening ≤ 35 mm	
	Lateral movements ≥ 7 mm	Passive stretch ≥ 35 mm	Passive stretch < 40 mm	
	If S-curve deviation is present, then joint must be silent		Contralateral movement < 7 mm	
			No S-curve deviation	
Tomography:	No decreased translation in ipsilateral condyle	None	Decreased translation of ipsilateral condyle	Ipsilateral condyle[a] has: Decreased translation, or Positive osseous changes
	No osseous changes			

[a] Disregard if coarse crepitus is present.
ID, Internal derangement; TMJ, temporomandibular joint.
(Reprinted with permission from ref. 14.)

In a recent study of the prevalence of muscle and joint disorders using these diagnostic criteria, Schiffman et al. (17) found that 23% of a general population had a muscle pain disorder alone, 27% had a combined muscle and joint disorder, 19% had a joint problem alone, and the remaining 31% were normal. These diagnostic criteria are also found to be accurate in clinical populations. In addition to using these tested diagnostic criteria for TMJ disorders, it is still recommended that soft-tissue imaging (either arthrography or magnetic resonance imaging) should be used to determine the presence of a TMJ internal derangement, because of the increased accuracy of these procedures. Untested criteria for exluding other orofacial pain disorders can be found in the International Headache Society Taxonomy (11).

USE OF MULTIDIMENSIONAL MEASURES OF OUTCOME

Most past studies examining orofacial pain have used single subjective measures of outcome and broad categories of objectively measured dysfunction. However, chronic pain problems are typically complex, vary significantly, and have symptoms that have many dimensions, including sensory and affective intensity, frequency and duration, and scope and tolerability of symptoms. The impact of these disorders can be quite profound with an effect on functional status, use of health care, mood, and other factors. Although a specific intervention such as an analgesic may have an effect on reducing sensory intensity, this effect may have little consequence on helping the patient restore normal function or reduce the frequency of pain. Furthermore, subjective impressions of the patient can be biased by numerous factors including attempting to please the clinician, lack of stability in the measures used, and problems in memory of subjective symptoms (18,19). For these reasons, an objective measure of pain and dysfunction is also required to establish validity of the changes in the subjective symptoms.

Both subjective and objective outcome measures need to be clinically relevant and readily identifiable by clinicians who will use the intervention. The instruments and administration need to be simple, relatively brief, and easy to read and comprehend. They should have sufficient sensitivity to detect differences among different treatments and have established reliability and validity over the natural course of the illness. For example, since chronic orofacial pain symptoms fluctuate greatly over a period of a month, the measure must be tested for stability over that same period of time.

Subjective components should be multidimensional in nature and include sensory and affective intensity, frequency and duration of symptoms, number of different symptoms, and tolerability of the symptoms. The Symptom Severity Index (16,20) is an example of a brief single-page instrument that measures these components with five visual analogue scales and a symptom checklist (Fig. 1). Both the McGill Pain Questionnaire (21) and Gracely's descriptor scales (22) measures pain severity and include sensory and affective aspects of pain using verbal descriptors.

The symptom severity index (SSI) is calculated by adding sensory intensity (SI), affective intensity (AI), tolerability (TO), frequency (FR), duration (DU), and scope of symptoms (symptom checklist) and dividing by 6. Each subscale has a 0 to 1 range.

SI:	How intense is your usual level of symptoms?	Zero	The most that can be imagined
AI:	How unpleasant or disturbing is your usual level of symptoms?	Zero	The most that can be imagined
TO:	How difficult is it to endure the problem over time?	No difficulty	The most that can be imagined

FR: How often do the symptoms generally occur?

Never   1/mo   1/day   1/hour   Constant

DU: When the symptoms occur, how long do the symptoms usually last?

Never   1/minute   1/hour   1/day   1week   Continuous

Have you had any of these symptoms in the past six months?

neck lumps or swelling	headaches
sore throat	hoarse voice
jaw shakes	tight throat
voice difficulties	constant need to clear throat
tongue pain	eye strain
double vision	blurred vision
seeing a halo	earaches
hearing difficulty	ringing in ears
itchy/plugged ears	vertigo (spinning)
loose teeth	locking or restricted jaws
noise in jaws	jaw or facial pain
taste changes	swelling in gums
soreness in teeth/gums	bite feels off
shortness of breath	congested nose or sneezing
cold hands	racing heart
frequent fever	swollen feet or ankles
chest pain	bleed easily
unusual sweating	swollen glands
hot flashes	weakness
fatigue	itching/burning skin
vomiting	constipation
nausea	kidney problems
arm pain/tingling	low back pain
neck/shoulder pain	hip pain
mid back pain	aching joints or muscles
painful feet	swollen joints
tendency to shake or tremble	convulsions
dizziness	numbness
speech difficulty	fainting/blackouts

FIG. 1. The Symptom Severity Index uses five visual analogue scales and a symptom checklist to provide a brief multidimensional measure of chronic pain. (Reprinted with permission from ref. 16.)

Objective components, particularly for temporomandibular disorders, should measure the degree of tenderness, dysfunction, and other objective characteristics such as decrease in sensation. These objective components should be clinically relevant measures that are characteristics of the disorder studied. For example, studies of patients with temporomandibular joint disorders need to use measures

CHECK IF EXAMINED

Pos. DYSFUNCTION INDEX (DI)

(1) Mandibular Movement (Normal Values in Parens)

- ☐ Maximum Opening (incisor to incisor) ☐☐ mm (40-60)
- ☐ Passive Stretch ☐☐ mm (42-62)
- ☐ Restriction
- ☐ Pain on Opening
- ☐ Jerky Opening
- ☐ S. Deviation on Opening (≤ 2mm)
- ☐ L. Deviation on Opening (≤ 2mm) To ______
- ☐ Protrusion - Pain
- ☐ Limitation ☐☐ mm (≥ 7mm)
- ☐ Right Laterotrusion - Pain
- ☐ Limitation ☐☐ mm (≥ 7mm)
- ☐ Left Laterotrusion - Pain
- ☐ Limitation ☐☐ mm (≥ 7mm)
- ☐ Clinically is or can lock open ____ R ____ L
- ☐ Clinically is or can lock closed ____ R ____ L
- ☐ Rigidity of Jaw Upon Manipulation

TOTALS

DI ☐ MI ☐ CMI ☐

Scoring

DI = (MM + TN + TP)/26

DI = (EM + IM + NM)/36

CMI = (DI + MI)/2

Opening Path

R 7mm — L 7mm

40mm

TMJ Noise TN (Check no more than 2 on each side)

(Right)		(Left)
☐	Reciprocal Click (Soft)	☐
☐	Popping (Loud)	☐
☐	Reproducible Opening Click	☐
☐	Reproducible Closing Click	☐
☐	Nonreproducible Opening Click	☐
☐	Nonreproducible Closing Click	☐
☐	Crepitus - Fine	☐
☐	Crepitus - Course	☐

(Right)	TMJ Palpation (TP)	(Left)
☐	Lateral Capsule ____	☐
☐	Post Capsule ____	☐
☐	Sup Capsule ____	☐

MUSCLE INDEX (MI)

	Muscle: Extraoral (IM)	
☐	Ant Temp. ____	☐
☐	Mid Temp. ____	☐
☐	Post Temp. ____	☐
☐	Deep Masseter ____	☐
☐	Ant Masseter ____	☐
☐	Inf Masseter ____	☐
☐	Post Digastric ____	☐
☐	Med Pterygoid ____	☐
☐	Vertex ____	☐

	Muscle: Intraoral (IM)	
☐	Lat Pterygoid ____	☐
☐	Med Pterygoid ____	☐
☐	Temp Insertion ____	☐

	Muscle: Neck (NM)	
☐	Sup Scm ____	☐
☐	Mid Scm ____	☐
☐	Inf Scm ____	☐
☐	Ins Trap ____	☐
☐	Upper Trap ____	☐
☐	Splenius Cap ____	☐

PALPATION

INDICATE REFERRAL PATTERNS

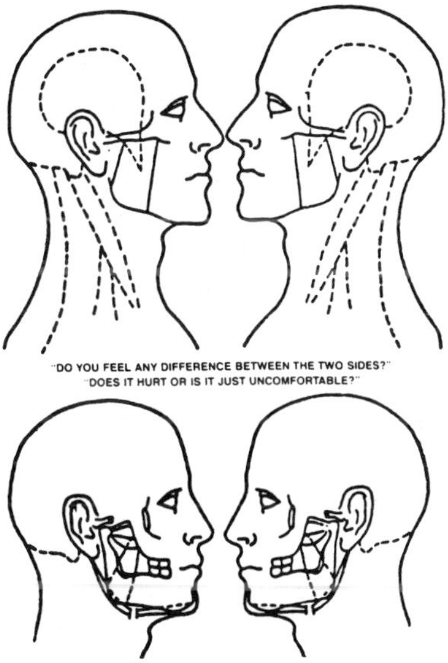

FIG. 2. The Craniomandibular Index includes a dysfunction index to evaluate joint dysfunction and a muscle index to evaluate muscle tenderness. (Reprinted with permission from ref. 16.)

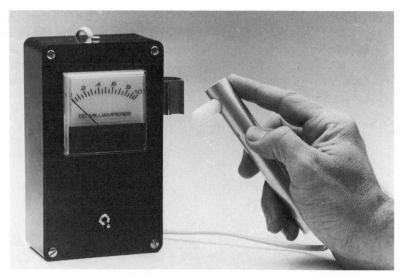

FIG. 3. A pressure algometer can be used to determine the pressure pain threshold in patients with muscle or joint disorders. (Reprinted with permission from ref. 26.)

for the degree of tenderness and noise within the joints, range of motion of the jaw, pain in movement, and deviation in movement. Two scales have been used in the literature and are similar. Helkimo's dysfunction index (23,24) includes these parameters and has been used in epidemiological studies. Some of its limitations have been addressed in the Craniomandibular Index (15,16). This recent instrument has operational definitions, has been tested for reliability and validity, and has been used in epidemiological studies (17) (Fig. 2).

In assessing outcome for myofascial pain, the degree of tenderness, determined by using pressure algometry (Fig. 3) to measure pressure pain threshold with individual muscles, and the scope of muscle tenderness (number of muscles tender) can be considered as outcome measures (16,25). Jensen (25) reviewed the use of pressure algometers and concluded they allow better scoring and scaling of tenderness than does finger palpation and they reduce observer and subject bias. Both finger pressure, measuring scope of tenderness, and pressure algometers, measuring pressure pain thresholds, have been tested for reliability and validity and are useful for outcome studies because of their high correlation with subjective symptom severity (26,27).

THE NATURAL VARIABILITY OF SIGNS AND SYMPTOMS

Studies of daily variation of different chronic orofacial pain conditions demonstrate their tendency to fluctuate greatly in terms of subjective symptoms. For example, patients may describe pain occurring approximately 2 to 3 times per week, but some weeks there is no pain and other weeks it is severe and occurs daily. Patients go through periods of remission where months may go by without pain whereas in other months the facial pain occurs on a daily basis. With this degree of natural variation in the symptoms, a measurement bias can occur if the measures do not reflect long-term changes in symptoms with sufficient reliability and stability. However, the severity of symptoms on any particular day is as important as the overall pattern of symptoms that a patient describes over a period of 6 months.

The lack of knowledge of long-term natural progression further complicates our understanding. Currently, there are no prospective epidemiologic studies that examine the natural progression of any specific chronic orofacial pain condition. There is some literature suggesting that TMJ internal derangements, for example, may progress from clicking to occasional locking to permanent locking and eventual degenerative changes within the joint (28). In cases of trigeminal neuralgia, it is not unusual to have some patients go through remission of 1 to 2 years and then have a significant increase in symptoms during a follow-up year. This lack of knowledge of the natural progression of these different orofacial pain disorders makes it difficult for researchers to determine whether the effects of an intervention may have occurred due to the intervention or due to the natural progression of the disorder. Although adequate sample sizes may help alleviate this problem, further research is needed on natural progression and the ability of scales to detect this progression before an adequate understanding of clinical outcome is achieved.

We recommend using a two-tier method for collecting posttreatment outcome measures. This involves collecting daily measures of signs and symptoms (intensity and hours with pain) for the one week prior to and following collection of a long-term measure of objective and subjective severity such as the Symptom Severity Index and the Craniomandibular Index for TM disorders. Since chronic pain rehabilitation often requires at least 6 months of intervention, these sets of measures can be administered pretreatment and then at 3 months, 6 months, 1 year, and 2 years. This schedule will help reduce bias, such as daily versus monthly fluctuation of signs and symptoms, memory bias, and poor long-term maintenance of improvement. In addition, daily measures can be aggregated and compared to long-term measures to support their validity.

UNDERSTANDING THE STUDY POPULATION

A clinical trial should usually try to achieve the widest potential for generalizability of the results. To do this, the study population needs to be examined to determine how well it represents the wider population to which the study might be generalized. Factors such as age, gender, socioeconomic status, employment status, duration of the problem, and severity each need to be examined within the comparison groups to ensure that there is a broad sampling. The inclusion of a wide distribution of patient demographic characteristics will ensure that no specific subgroup of subjects will bias the results. Duration of the problem needs to be considered because of the distinct differences between acute and chronic pain. The severity of the problem needs to be balanced in the sample because of the wide range of responses that can occur between patients with severe chronic orofacial pain versus mild orofacial pain. Obtaining an adequate sample size is the key to this generalizability, but is limited by pragmatic reasons.

Recruiting a sufficient number of patients is a difficult task that is complicated by the need for long-term follow-up, the high potential for dropouts, the difficulty in finding a homogeneous diagnostic study population, and the frequency of crossover to other treatment interventions. Changes in the study sample during a long-term study will cause significant problems in the interpretation of results. For example, it is possible that the patients who have been treated unsuccessfully with the proposed intervention will have a higher tendency to drop out or cross over to a different intervention. These factors need to be controlled within the analysis and reporting of results. Obtaining a large sample size while minimizing recidivism can be accomplished by integrating data collection procedures as part of the normal clinical protocol, and implementing a tight recall system involving letters, multiple phone calls, and incentives to return.

The subject selection process also needs to be carefully considered. There are subtle confounders associated with subject selection. For example, patients drawn from a tertiary referral center may be quite different from those found in a primary care facility. Patients drawn from a pool of patients suffering from orofacial pain at a certain instant in time (cross section) may overrepresent a chronic illness in terms of its incidence and prevalence. Although it is convenient and inexpensive to recruit patients from those attending a certain clinic, it is safer to identify a broad sampling frame of patients that includes both private practice and tertiary referral clinics. Ideally, the sampling frame could consist of all individuals living in a certain community or working in a certain institution who develop chronic orofacial pain. It is then possible to describe the general makeup of the population from which the study population originates. Once the sampling frame is defined, the researcher can decide on the sampling method to use that reflects the inclusion and exclusion criteria. Commonly, a researcher may select all eligible subjects using these criteria and if there are too many, select a random rather than arbitrary sample. In this way, the researcher starts with a sample whose only bias is determined by the characteristics of the sampling frame, which is as broad as possible.

As noted above, duration and severity of symptoms are major sources of variability and need to be considered in the distribution of the sample. Although an even distribution may minimize false negative or positive results, it also requires a large number of subjects in determination of sample size. For example, an intervention may appear to be unsuccessful with patients with severe symptoms, but may be quite effective for patients with mild to moderate symptoms.

In these situations, it may be useful to stratify the population for duration and severity of symptoms in assignment to experimental and control groups or simply in the analysis of the results.

STUDY DESIGN ARCHITECTURE

There are a variety of different study designs that have been used previously in clinical trials of chronic orofacial pain. A vast majority of articles on therapeutic efficacy are *case series,* which describe a group of patients treated a certain way (29,30). In this study design, there is no control group with which to compare results. A good case series follows sequential patients for an appropriate follow-up period, whereas lesser quality series are based only on an arbitrary selection of patients. A *case control series* analyzes treatment received by a group of patients who show different outcomes. For example, risk factors for treatment failure can be identified in a case control series by examining characteristics of those patients who succeeded compared to those who failed. *Cohort studies,* either prospective or retrospective, compare outcome of patients receiving different treatments (31,32), but the choice of specific treatments is not based on random allocation. Typically, a sequential group of patients is treated one way and a different sequential group serves as a control. A less revealing cohort study compares outcomes in two groups of patients individually chosen for one treatment or the other. In these studies, the exclusion and inclusion criteria and selection procedures need to be described carefully. The design that has the best potential for the most robust results is the *randomized double- or triple-blind clinical trial* (33,34). In the triple-blind design, neither the patient, therapist, nor the outcome rater knows the true treatment allocation. Although this design is ideal, it is rarely possible in its strictest form.

More conclusions can be drawn with more sophisticated study designs. Case reports can conclude only that the phenomenon described actually exists, whereas case series can indicate that the phenomenon is not uncommon. Cohort studies and case control studies suggest conclusions regarding one treatment over another. Randomized control trials allow a more reliable estimate for the soundness of a specific hypothesis regarding treatment effects.

Randomization needs to be used whenever possible because it can prevent recognizable bias and assignment of treatments and also balance treatment groups in terms of unrecognized prognostic factors. Nevertheless, there are three areas that can distort results and need to be addressed in clinical trials (35).

The first area includes "referral bias." Many clinicians who treat orofacial pain patients are unwilling to refer patients to an institution that is conducting a randomized trial. The general result of such bias is the selection of a relatively skewed subset of patients for randomization. The biased referring clinician is most likely to refer patients about whom he feels less strongly, thus maintaining his professional conscience and still facilitating adequate clinical trials. This type of bias is a problem particularly with comparison of unlike treatment interventions, such as surgery with analgesics or analgesics with physical therapy.

A second form of bias includes the "patient consent bias." Personality characteristics such as type A or other personalities may have a covariance with a number of orofacial pain disorders and thus may affect whether or not a patient consents to participate in the study. This may affect not only the dropout rate, but also the crossover rate in choosing a different treatment than the one that was assigned. This distribution of behavioral patterns will bias the results of any disease influenced by stress or psychosocial factors.

A "crossover bias" in the randomization occurs when patients cross over from one group to another as a result of ineffectiveness of one treatment. Although patients may agree to participate in a randomized clinical trial, a certain percentage of them will choose to cross over and be treated with the other treatment apart from the study. Although they may not be included in the results, there is the potential that the results of the treatment group may be biased. This occurs frequently in the comparison of surgical treatments to nonsurgical treatments where a nonsurgical treatment is initiated and then for whatever reason, the patient chooses to have surgery.

Another bias that can affect outcome of studies comparing similar treatments includes the "waiting-time bias." With some treatment, such as surgical treatment, there is a period of time between initial assignment into a study group and beginning of the intervention. If complications occur during that waiting period, or changes in the patient's attitude occurs, this may affect the outcome of the intervention or influence the dropout or crossover rate. Although this change in status cannot be controlled for, it makes the generalization of studies comparing unlike interventions using randomization difficult.

The long-term nature of many orofacial pain disorders makes the inclusion of a randomized no-treatment control group difficult and often ethically unsound. It is rare that a patient would consent to participate in a no-treatment study group over a period of 1 year or more. This reduces the sample size of the control group, often introduces a selection bias, and prevents adequate conclusions based on results. Other types of control groups have been suggested, including the use of waiting list controls or an alternative treatment control group. However, this can introduce a specific bias in subject selection and does not consider the possibility of fluctuation in symptoms owing to the natural variation of the disorder.

Since the purpose of randomization is to minimize this bias, studies that cannot be randomized for ethical or pragmatic reasons need to minimize biases in other ways. The most important goal of a nonrandomized trial is to match treatment and control groups for demographic characteristics, severity of illness, and prognostic factors. This can usually be done with large sample sizes using sequential consenting patients for treatment and control groups. Use of sequential patients often reduces patient consent bias, crossover bias, and waiting-time bias by including all patients who normally present to a clinic for treatment of a problem. However, referral bias will still exist.

THE NEED FOR STANDARDIZED INTERVENTIONS

A specific bias related to the intervention with chronic orofacial pain is the difficulty of maintaining patients on a single therapy. For example, with TM surgery patients it is common for a surgeon to recommend physical therapy and analgesics in addition to surgery. The frequent use of multiple interventions with chronic orofacial pain patients prevents the determination of whether one intervention by itself has an effect on the disorder. This is particularly true of surgery being compared to nonsurgical interventions such as analgesics or physical therapy where standardization of the additional treatments cannot be accomplished. Furthermore, studies of a single intervention such as a medication have low generalizability to a clinical setting because of the frequent use of multiple clinical modalities. If a specific intervention includes a multifaceted treatment plan, the experimental treatment needs to be different while maintaining the techniques, timing, and therapist involved in the remaining management program. For example, it is unusual to prescribe solely an analgesic for patients with myofascial pain. If the aim is to study the effects of a specific analgesic in the context of an overall management program, the analgesic may be provided in one group and a placebo medication provided in the other group while the other treatments such as a splint remain standardized between the two groups. However, the differential effects of the other treatments need to be considered as a potential confounder in discussing conclusions.

Basic rules regarding the standardization of one or more interventions need to be followed to allow for the maximum generalizability. Paramount to this is a clear description of the treatment modalities so that it can be reproduced at another investigator's facility. For example, if use of a splint is recommended, the description should include whether it provides full or partial coverage, how it is adjusted, whether it is adjusted in a sitting or reclining position, the type of guidance, the thickness, instructions on use and cleaning, and how often it is adjusted. This description should include not only the components of the intervention, but also the decision algorithms that must be used to complete the treatment. The timing of the intervention as well as the potential risks involved must also be articulated. Standardization of the therapist's explanation of the study and the interventions is required to allow for consistent reproducibility.

The patient characteristics that determine the choice of treatment must be stated clearly. In the ideal clinical design, the randomized double-blind clinical trial, allocation of subjects to treatment branches should be determined by chance alone. In addition, the patient, therapist, and the outcome rater need to be blind to the intervention by using a placebo intervention whenever possible. This is generally not possible with interventions such as surgery or splints because they are technique-specific and depend on the expertise of the clinician. However, it is still critical to blind the rater to the treatment status of the subject.

Unlike analgesics, the techniques involved with these interventions also vary and evolve over time. If a specific technique used in the study did not demonstrate sufficient efficacy, it is possible that the experiences that occur in using the technique during the study will be sufficient to revise it and correct the problems encountered and thus improve its efficacy. Readers of any study evaluating nonpharmacological treatments as the intervention or control may reject the results because it uses the old technique and a revised technique or procedure may prove to be better in their hands. This bias applies both to generalization of results to other studies as well as changes that inadvertently occur in surgical or nonsurgical treatment protocols during the course of the study.

CONCLUSIONS

This chapter discussed the problems that can occur in a clinical trial of analgesics as well as in other interventions in chronic orofacial pain. Recommendations are presented regarding decisions that need to be made in designing these clinical trials. However, there needs to be more research on methodologic issues in order to improve the quality of these studies. Future areas of study should include multicenter studies of diagnostic criteria, reliability and validity of examination items, and the development of new techniques to objectively measure orofacial pain disorders, as well as further basic research examining the mechanisms of pain and dysfunction of orofacial pain disorders.

REFERENCES

1. Bonica JJ. Preface. In: Bonica JJ, Liebeskind JC, Albe-Fessard, eds. *Advances in pain research and therapy,* vol 3. New York: Raven Press, 1985, v–viii.
2. Sternbach RA. Survey on pain in the United States: the Nuprin pain report. *Clin J Pain* 1986;2: 49–53.
3. Schiffman E, Fricton JR. Epidemiology of TMJ and craniofacial pain. In: Fricton JR, Kroening RJ, Hathaway KM, eds. *TMJ and craniofacial pain: diagnosis and management.* St. Louis: IEA Publishers, 1988;1–10.
4. Fricton JR, Kroening RJ, Hathaway KM. Preface. In: Fricton JR, Kroening RJ, Hathaway KM, eds. *TMJ and craniofacial pain: diagnosis and management.* St. Louis: IEA Publishers, 1988;iii.
5. Check R, et al. *Report of ad hoc committee on craniomandibular and temporomandibular joint disorders.* Minneapolis: Minnesota Dental Association, 1988.
6. McNeill C, Mohl ND, Rugh JD, Tanaka TT. Temporomandibular disorders: diagnosis, management, education, and research. *J Am Dent Assoc* 1990;120:253–263.
7. Griffiths RH. Report of the president's conference on examination, diagnosis and management of temporomandibular disorders. *J Am Dent Assoc* 1983;106:75–77.
8. Clark GT, Seligman DA, Solberg WK, et al. Guidelines for the examination and diagnosis of temporomandibular disorders. *J Cranio Dis Facial Oral Pain* 1989;3:6–14.
9. Eversole LR, Machado L. Temporomandibular joint internal derangements and associated neuromuscular disorders. *J Am Dent Assoc* 1985;110:69–79.
10. McNeill C, et al. Craniomandibular disorders: guidelines for the evaluation, diagnosis and management. *J Cranio Dis Facial Oral Pain* 1990; (in press).
11. International Headache Society classification and diagnostic criteria for headache disorders, cranial neuralgias and facial pain. *Cephalalgia* 1988; suppl 7.
12. Bell WE. *Orofacial pains: classification, diagnosis, management,* 4th ed. Chicago: Yearbook Medical Publishers, 1989.

13. LeResche L, Dworkin SF, et al. An epidemiologic evaluation of two diagnostic classification schemes for TMD. *J Dent Res* 1988;68:258(abstr).

14. Schiffman E, Anderson G, Fricton J, Burton K, Schellhas K. Diagnostic criteria for intraarticular TM Disorders. *Community Dent Oral Epidemiol* 1989;17:252–257.

15. Fricton JR, Schiffman ES. Reliability of a craniomandibular index. *J Dent Res* 1986;65:1359–1364.

16. Fricton J, Schiffman E. The craniomandibular index: validity. *J Prosthet Dent* 1987;58:221–228.

17. Schiffman E, Fricton JR, Haley D, Shapiro BL. The prevalence and treatment needs of subjects with temporomandibular disorders. *J Am Dent Assoc* 1990;120:295–303.

18. Friedman MH, Weisberg J. Pitfalls of muscle palpation in TMJ diagnosis. *J Prosth Dent* 1982;48:331.

19. Duinkerke A, Luteijn F, Bouman TK, deJong HP. Reproducibility of a palpation test for the stomatognathic system. *Community Dent Oral Epidemiol* 1986;14:80–85.

20. Fricton J, Nelson A, Monsein M, Davison, M. IMPATH: microcomputer assessment of behavioral and psychosocial factors. *Pain* (suppl) 1987;5(4):372–381.

21. Melzack R. The short form McGill Pain Questionnaire. *Pain* 1987;30:191–197.

22. Gracely RH. Pain language and ideal pain measurement. In:Melzack R, ed. *Pain measurement and assessment.* New York: Raven Press, 1983;71–78.

23. Helkimo M. Studies on function and dysfunction of the masticatory system. II. Index for anamnestic and clinical dysfunction and occlusal state. *Swed Dent J* 1974;67:101–121.

24. Helkimo, M. Studies on function and dysfunction of the masticatory system. III. Analysis of anamnestic and clinical recordings of dysfunction with the aid of indices. *Swed Dent J* 1974;67:165–182.

25. Jensen K. Quantification of tenderness in myofascial pain with pressure algometry. In: Fricton JR, Awad E, eds. *Myofascial pain and fibromyalgia.* New York: Raven Press, 1990;165–182.

26. Schiffman E, Fricton J, Haley D, Tylka D. A pressure algometer for myofascial pain syndrome: reliability and validity testing. In: Dubner R, et al., eds. *Proceedings of the Fifth World Congress on Pain.* Amsterdam: Elsevier, 1988;407–413.

27. Ohrbach R, Gale EN. Pressure pain thresholds, clinical assessment and differential diagnosis: reliability and validity in patients with myogenic pain. *Pain* 1989;39:157–170.

28. Rasmussen OC. Description of population and progress of symptoms in a longitudinal study of temporomandibular arthropathy. *Scand J Dent Res* 1981;89:196–208.

29. Okeson JP, Hayes DK. Longterm results of treatment for temporomandibular disorders: an evaluation by patients. *J Am Dent Assoc* 1986;112:473–478.

30. Mejersjo C, Carlsson GE. Longterm results of treatment for temporomandibular pain dysfunction. *J Prosth Dent* 1983;49:809–815.

31. Fricton J, Hathaway K, Bromaghim C. Interdisciplinary management of patients with TMJ and craniofacial pain: characteristics and outcome. *J Craniomandib Dis* 1987;1:115–122.

32. Pierce CJ, Gale EN. A comparison of different treatments for nocturnal bruxism. *J Dent Res* 1988;67:597–601.

33. Langemark M, Lodrup D, Bech P, Oleson J. Clomipramine and mianserin in treatment of chronic tension headache: a double blind controlled study. *Headache* 1990;30:118–121.

34. Jaeger B, Skootsky SA. Double blind controlled study of different myofascial trigger point injection techniques. *Pain* 1987;4(Suppl):560.

35. Byar DP, Simon RM, et al. Randomized clinical trials: perspectives on some recent ideas. *N Engl J Med* 1976;295:74.

36. Bonchek LI. The role of the randomized clinical trial in the evaluation of new operations. *Surg Clin North Am* 1982;64:761–769.

Advances in Pain Research and Therapy, Vol. 18,
edited by M. Max, R. Portenoy, and E. Laska,
Raven Press, Ltd., New York © 1991.

Commentary

Chronic Orofacial Pain

Glenn T. Clark

*UCLA Dental Research Institute, School of Dentistry, University of California
at Los Angeles, Los Angeles, California 90024-1762*

Dr. Fricton's chapter on chronic orofacial pain is lucid and timely. He identifies many of the flaws of prior clinical research on chronic orofacial pain disorders and makes numerous suggestions for designing improved clinical trials to look at the various treatments for chronic orofacial pain. Although he focuses more on nonpharmacologic treatment methods than on analgesic drugs, many of his comments could be generalized to analgesic drug trials, too.

Fricton discusses but does not strongly emphasize that chronic orofacial pain disorders should not be considered as a single disorder but rather as multiple conditions. These conditions include the anatomically distinct neurologic and neuropathic disorders, the cervical and temporomandibular arthritic disorders, the oral mucous membrane disorders, the musculoskeletal conditions, and the vascular conditions, as well as the atypical neuropathic pain disorders that occur in the orofacial region. It would be very logical to assume each of these conditions would have a different therapeutic approach and it is difficult, therefore, to talk about the overall set of conditions under the rubric of chronic orofacial pain. A clinical trial would never involve all of these disorders simultaneously and if it targeted any one of these disorders, it would need a definitive case definition that is valid and widely accepted. Rather than attempt to define each type of chronic orofacial pain, the chapter focuses on one of the most prevalent of these problems, myofascial and temporomandibular (TM) disorders. It should be noted that chronic painful TM disorders and craniomandibular myofascial pain have not traditionally been treated with analgesic drugs and, in fact, as with chronic back pain, analgesic medications are usually not prescribed for these patients.

Further, it is not infrequent that these patients are put in analgesic drug detoxification programs as a part of their chronic pain management program. Non-narcotic pharmacologic approaches, usually antidepressants, are used. These medications clearly need to be tested in this population using a controlled clinical trial. Other medications frequently utilized are the nonsteroidal antiinflammatory (NSAID) medications. It must be noted that long-term utilization of NSAID medication is quite different than the more typical short-term use of NSAIDs in acute pain. Medication side effects that are minor on a short-term basis become much more significant on a long-term basis. The usual design of a short-term (6- to 10-week) analgesic clinical trial should be extended to evaluate for the slowly developing medication side effects (e.g., aplastic anemic, ulcers).

In most chronic pain conditions, the possibility is strong that psychological factors influence the patient's pain level. This means that these patients are very susceptible to their environment and no clinical trial could be performed without assessing and dealing with the psychological status of the patient.

One major difficulty with clinical research that evaluates nonpharmacologic treatments for chronic orofacial pain is that it is difficult, if not impossible, to identify a therapeutic intervention that would be considered a true placebo or control "nontreatment" condition. Creation of a suitable nonpharmacologic control condition that is nontherapeutic and to which the subject is blind is a great challenge for the investigator. An alternative approach for a true no-treatment waiting list control condition would be a "rescue drug" paradigm.

Because of the long-standing nature of most of the chronic orofacial pain conditions, the treatments are also likely to be prolonged. This increases the duration of the clinical trial and the expense. Expense is probably the major reason that limited research has been conducted on these problems.

The question, "What is the appropriate duration of the study?" can only be answered based on knowledge regarding the natural history of the disease under study. False positive results could easily occur owing to the known tendency of these disorders to undergo spontaneous remissions. In other words, if you evaluate patients who attend for treatment at the height of their disease, they have a tendency (regardless of treatment interventions) toward reduced severity. Thus, it is essential to have a truly blind control or "no treatment" condition as stated earlier. It would also be wise to have multiple pretreatment data points to be assured of a stable disease state.

In summary, the task of conducting high-quality controlled clinical trials in chronic orofacial pain conditions is formidable. However, with adequate controls, proper design, good disease definitions, and appropriate outcome measures, it is likely that clinical trials can elucidate the mechanisms and guide treatment of the diverse orofacial pain syndromes.

Advances in Pain Research and Therapy, Vol. 18,
edited by M. Max, R. Portenoy, and E. Laska,
Raven Press, Ltd., New York © 1991.

17

Sore Throat Pain

Bernard P. Schachtel

*Medical Department, Whitehall Laboratories, Inc., New York, New York 10017;
and Clinical Epidemiology Unit, Yale University School of Medicine,
New Haven, Connecticut 06510*

A sore throat is a complaint well known to all persons from childhood through
adulthood. It is also the familiar condition for which physicians over the years
have been telling patients to "take two aspirin." Despite this clinical truism (for
aspirin does appear to "work"), no clinical trials had been published that demonstrated that aspirin 650 mg does provide effective relief of throat pain when
compared to placebo. In this chapter, I shall review the development and refinement of the sore throat pain model as a single-dose assay for analgesic agents.

Our first study directly addressed the question of whether aspirin 650 mg or
acetaminophen 650 mg is effective compared to placebo under double-blind
conditions (1). This clinical trial was conducted on 150 adults who presented to
their physician with the complaint of sore throat accompanied by other evidence
of upper respiratory infection (URI). To be certain of the condition causing sore
throat, tonsillopharyngitis, we identified specific features that any physician would
note in examining a patient with a sore throat. These findings (temperature,
oropharyngeal color and enanthems, anterior cervical adenopathy and adenitis)
were documented on an index similar to the Apgar score, with each feature being
rated 0, 1, or 2 (Table 1). By adding the scores for each feature, a tonsillopharyngitis score (TPS) was created that confirmed not only the condition but also
its severity (2).

At the same time, I had certain clinical hunches about other features of URI
that might confound the evaluation of sore throat. Because sore throat is just
one expression of upper respiratory tract illness, we examined these other features
of URI. In particular, I was concerned that mouth breathing, which can be
caused by the nasal congestion of URI, would dry the throat, thus exacerbating
the pain of tonsillopharyngitis and making it impossible to show that aspirin
was effective compared to placebo. Severe nasal congestion might also distract

TABLE 1. *Indices of tonsillopharyngitis*

	0 Points	1 Point	2 Points
Oral temperature (°C)	≤37.0	37.1–38.2	≥38.3
Oropharyngeal color	Pink	Red	Beefy red
Oropharyngeal enanthems (exudates, vesicles, or petechiae)	None	Some	Many
Cervical adenopathy (increased size or number)	None	Some	Marked
Cervical adenitis	None	Slight or moderate	Severe

From ref. 1, with permission.

the patient if there was relatively more discomfort from a stuffy nose: the patient might not be able to appreciate any analgesia of the throat. Therefore, we created a Nasal Congestion Evaluation on which the physician examined these features: nasal obstruction in each naris, total nasal secretions, hyponasality, and, in particular, mouth breathing. We identified these potentially confounding variables *a priori* so that we could determine from the study results if, in fact, they do have an influence on the patient's assessment of sore throat pain.

As a measurement instrument for sore throat pain intensity, we created a 100-mm visual analogue scale, the sore throat pain intensity scale (STPIS) (Fig. 1). We also used a categorical pain intensity scale at baseline to determine the relationship between pain intensity measured on a categorical scale and on a visual analogue scale. Patients with baseline scores that were 50 to 74 mm were con-

(a.)

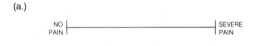

(b.)

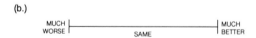

(c.)

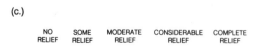

FIG. 1. Measurement instruments used in the assessment of sore throat pain. **A:** Sore Throat Pain Intensity Scale. **B:** Transitional Change-In-Pain Scale. **C:** Categorical Relief Scale.

sidered to represent moderate sore throat pain, and those that were in the 75- to 100-mm range were considered severe: these strata were created to determine if relatively severe sore throat pain enchanced the opportunity to show drug effect, and randomized allocation of treatment was stratified according to each patient's pain stratum.

After treatment, the patients completed the same sore throat pain intensity visual analogue scale at regular intervals. They were also administered a new scale, a transitional change-in-pain scale, on which they were asked to rate their pain "compared to the last time." This question is similar to what the doctor asks in his office, "How are you now (compared to the last time we spoke)?" This question requires a comparison directly to the last time or the last evaluation. Finally, we administered a five-category relief scale (no, some, moderate, considerable, complete relief) at the same posttreatment times over 3 hrs.

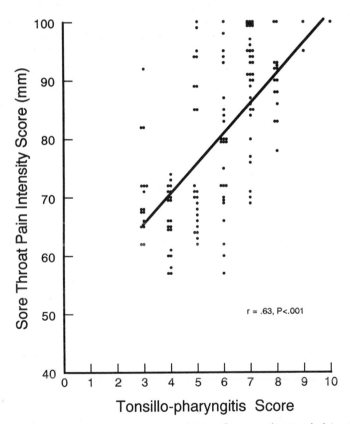

FIG. 2. Correlation of tonsillopharyngitis score with baseline sore throat pain intensity score. (From ref. 2, with permission.)

The results of the visual analogue STPIS that were ranked as moderate or severe correlated well with the actual moderate or severe ordinal scores ($\kappa = 0.96$). Thus, in terms of sore throat pain intensity, the visual analogue scale represented the same pain state as did the categorical pain intensity scale. We also had objective confirmation of the condition causing the pain, for the tonsillopharyngitis score correlated well ($r = 0.63$) with the baseline STPIS (Fig. 2).

If we had merely analyzed this study as a straightforward study of 150 patients with sore throat, the results would have been unconvincing (Fig. 3). Although there is a suggestion that reduction in pain intensity in the placebo group was slightly less than in the two active treatments, in fact these are three statistically indistinguishable treatment responses. However, when we examined the stratum of 75 patients with severe sore throat, we observed some separation between each active drug and placebo beginning at 2 hrs which was encouraging. Still, the results are not striking, hardly the degree of sore throat pain relief that is experienced by patients in actual practice.

Fortunately, all patients had been examined for their degree of nasal congestion. Approximately one-third, 51, were severely congested: if they had comprised our study sample by chance, results would have been very discouraging (Fig. 4). Because these patients were included in our total study sample, their responses were confounding the true assessment of the study medications. However, when we looked at the 42 patients who were *not* mouth breathing (i.e., who had mild or no nasal congestion) and who had severe sore throat (Fig. 5), significant dif-

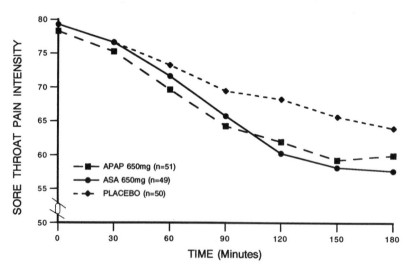

FIG. 3. Mean sore throat pain intensity scores in 150 patients with sore throat without regard for the severity of pain at baseline or degree of nasal congestion. APAP, acetaminophen; ASA, aspirin. (From ref. 1, with permission.)

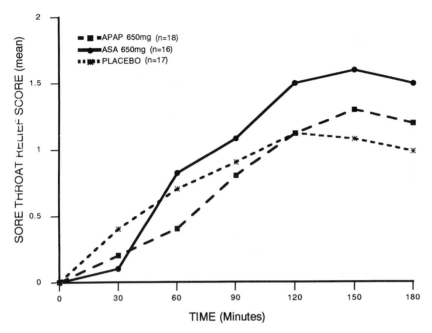

FIG. 4. Mean sore throat relief scores in the subset of 51 patients with severe nasal congestion. (From ref. 1, with permission.)

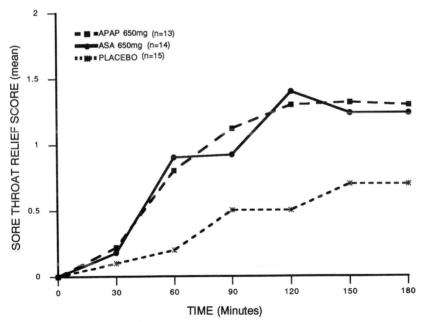

FIG. 5. Mean sore throat relief scores in the subset of 42 patients with severe sore throat at baseline and mild nasal congestion. (From ref. 1, with permission.)

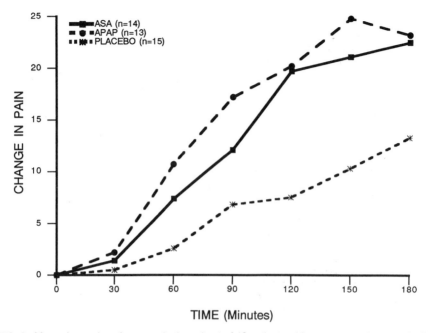

FIG. 6. Mean change-in-pain scores in the subset of 42 patients with severe sore throat and mild nasal congestion. (Adapted from ref. 1, with permission.)

ferentiation of each treatment group from placebo was detected from 1 to 3 hrs ($p < 0.05$). The same results were demonstrated on the pain intensity visual analogue scale and on the new transitional scale, the change-in-pain scale (Fig. 6).

From this study we concluded (a) that for a pain model to be effective in evaluating analgesic treatment for a sore throat, relatively severe baseline pain is advisable; (b) that the subjective pain state can be objectively confirmed using the tonsillopharyngitis score; and (c) that using one's clinical sense can help identify potentially confounding variables (e.g., mouth breathing) and add precision to the analgesic assay. We also were able to demonstrate for the first time that a transitional scale can be used successfully to measure change in pain and detect significant therapeutic effects.

During this first trial and in subsequent trials, we have asked patients to tell us in their own words what their pain feels like, to offer those terms or qualities of pain that they use in common parlance. Our next study represented our effort to reach the patient by using these same terms as indicators of therapeutic response. From these words (2), we discovered 15 qualities that were volunteered most frequently to describe throat pain (Table 2), of which ten are sensory terms,

TABLE 2. *Qualities of acute throat pain*

Sensory qualities	Affective qualities	Evaluative qualities
Raw	Irritating	Sore
Difficult to speak	Annoying	Painful
Hot		It hurts
Scratchy		
Tight		
Difficult to swallow		
Dry		
Burning		
Swollen		
Raspy		

From ref. 4, with permission.

two are affective, and three are evaluative (the same three clusters of pain qualities that Melzack and Torgerson (3) have in their McGill Pain Questionnaire). For each of these 15 words, we created a visual analogue scale; however, because completing all 15 assessments was cumbersome, these quality-of-pain scales were included in the trial at baseline and only 2 and 4 hrs after treatment. To test if these new scales could be used by patients to rate pain and analgesia, we compared the results from these scales to the results measured on a visual analogue sore throat pain intensity scale and a six-category sore throat relief rating in another

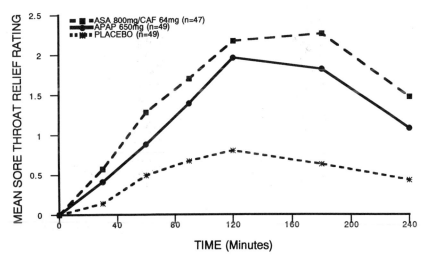

FIG. 7. Mean sore throat relief ratings in 145 patients with sore throat. (Adapted from ref. 4, with permission.)

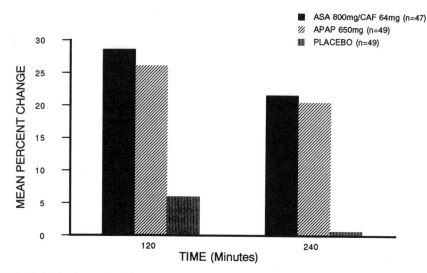

FIG. 8. Evaluative quality-of-pain scales: mean percent change from baseline in 145 patients with sore throat. (Adapted from ref. 4, with permission.)

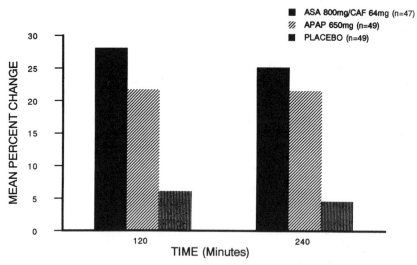

FIG. 9. Affective quality-of-pain scales: mean percent change from baseline in 145 patients with sore throat. (Adapted from ref. 4, with permission.)

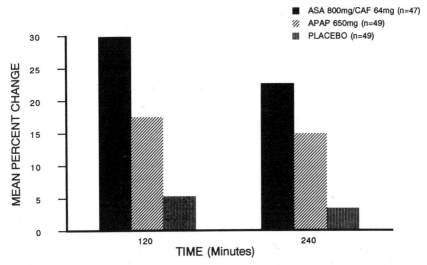

FIG. 10. Sensory quality-of-pain scales: mean percent change from baseline in 145 patients with sore throat. (Adapted from ref. 4, with permission.)

study of 150 patients with sore throat (4). In this clinical trial, all patients had moderately severe pain, objective evidence of tonsillopharyngitis, and no mouth breathing; aspirin 800 mg with caffeine 64 mg, acetaminophen 650 mg, or placebo were randomly administered under double-blind conditions, and treatment responses were assessed over 4 hrs.

The results were clear. As shown on the relief rating scale (Fig. 7), the drug responses for the aspirin-caffeine combination and for acetaminophen 650 mg were clearly distinguished from placebo ($p < 0.05$). When we analyzed the mean percent change from baseline for the quality-of-pain scales at 2 and 4 hrs, both active drugs were again significantly distinguished from placebo. The evaluative qualities of pain (Fig. 8) yielded results similar to the mean percent pain intensity differences ($p < 0.05$). For the percent change in the affective qualities of pain (Fig. 9), both active treatments also separated from placebo at 2 and 4 hrs in a statistically significant fashion. The most striking differences were detected on the sensory quality-of-pain scales (Fig. 10): both actives were significantly distinguished from placebo at 2 and 4 hrs, and we could see significant differences between the active drugs at 2 hrs ($p < 0.05$). This finding is not surprising, for Melzack and Torgerson (3) had discovered in their research that patients with acute pain tend to relate it more frequently with sensory qualities of pain. From this study, therefore, we concluded (a) that quality-of-pain scales can complement conventional pain rating scales to demonstrate the efficacy of analgesic agents compared with placebo, (b) that sensory qualities of pain are especially sensitive, and (c) that these scales can be used to differentiate between active drugs in patients with acute sore throat.

Our next task was to refine the model further and make it easier to implement. To achieve these objectives, we selected the two qualities of throat pain that appeared to provide the finest detection of treatment effect, difficulty swallowing and how swollen the throat felt. Thus we reduced our original 15 terms to two. At the same time, we wanted to determine if a patient could conduct this simplified study at home, as performed by patients following oral surgery. Therefore, in this clinical trial (5), the first 3 hrs were conducted in the physician's office (as in our original study), but the remaining 3 hrs were conducted at home. Efficacy measurements included the 100-mm visual analogue sore throat pain intensity scale and the six-category sore throat relief rating scale, a 200-mm visual analogue change-in-pain scale, and the two quality-of-pain scales, which were rated before treatment and at each posttreatment assessment time.

The 120 patients in this study were comparable before randomization to treatment with acetaminophen 1,000 mg, ibuprofen 400 mg, or placebo under double-blind conditions. They had sore throat of recent onset (on average, 2 days), objective evidence of tonsillopharyngitis (an average TPS around 7), sore throat

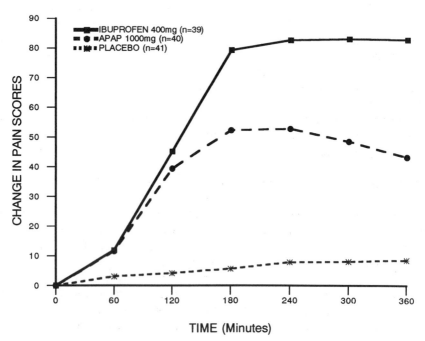

FIG. 11. Mean change-in-pain scores in 120 patients with sore throat. (Adapted from ref. 5, with permission.)

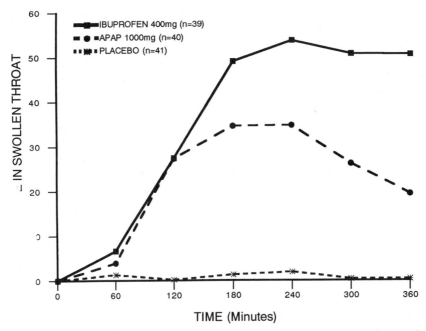

FIG. 12. Mean change from baseline on a 100-mm visual analogue scale measuring how swollen the throat feels in 120 patients with sore throat. (From ref. 5, with permission.)

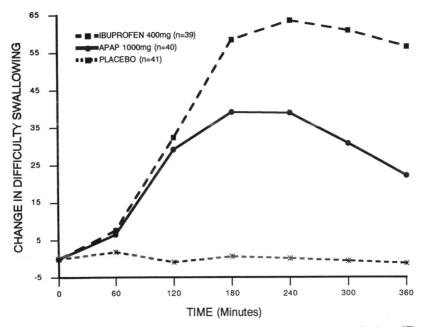

FIG. 13. Mean change from baseline on a 100-mm visual analogue scale measuring how difficult it is to swallow in 120 patients with sore throat. (From ref. 5, with permission.)

pain intensity averaging about 90 mm, and similar, though lower, baseline scores for the two qualities of pain (67–81 mm).

The results from this refined model were clinically convincing (Fig. 11). By one hour, acetaminophen 1,000 mg and ibuprofen 400 mg were clearly separated from placebo ($p < 0.01$), a finding that persisted over the 6-hr trial. There was also significant differentiation between the two actives from 3 hrs through 6 hrs ($p < 0.01$), which was confirmed on the quality-of-pain scales (Figs. 12 and 13). From this study, therefore, we concluded that the sore throat pain model can be successfully conducted on an ambulatory basis and that individual quality-of-pain scales yield the same results as obtained on other pain rating scales. Furthermore, we learned that these quality-of-pain scales enhance the assay sensitivity of the sore throat pain model; though lower than the baseline pain intensity scores, the quality-of-pain scales detected the same statistically significant treatment effects. The conventional requirement of relatively severe baseline intensity in order to demonstrate statistically significant drug-placebo or drug-drug differences did not restrict the sensitivity of these newer scales. A corollary to this observation was that when we applied this convention to these scales, the same statistically significant results still obtained, even though used by one-quarter fewer patients. We have observed the same need for a reduced sample size in other studies, suggesting that these quality-of-pain scales are very sensitive indicators of therapeutic response, perhaps because patients are using their own words.

We also discovered another interesting finding: the ability of the model to detect a dose-response relationship. Because the same investigator had studied

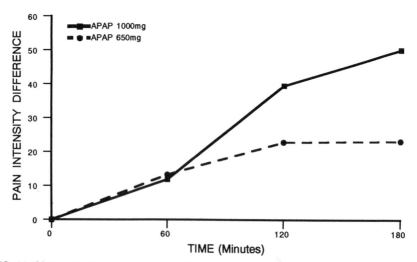

FIG. 14. Mean sore throat pain intensity differences from baseline for two different dose levels of acetaminophen (1,000 mg and 650 mg) discerning a dose-response relationship. (From ref. 5, with permission.)

the 1,000-mg dose of acetaminophen here and had used the same pain intensity scale to measure the treatment response of a 650-mg dose of acetaminophen in our initial study (1), we could compare the time-effect curves over 3 hrs, the common time interval of the two studies. As seen in Fig. 14, the model does discern a dose-response relationship for acetaminophen at 650 mg and 1,000 mg, thus fulfilling another desirable feature of a pain model.

The most recent refinement of the sore throat pain model I owe to the challenge presented by William Beaver when he referred to "the limited assay sensitivity [of analgesic assays], especially for combination analgesics" (6). Based on the steps we had already taken in developing this model, we concentrated now on the methodology necessary for evaluating a mild analgesic agent when combined with caffeine. In conceiving a trial (7) to compare aspirin 800 mg with caffeine 64 mg to aspirin 800 mg and placebo, we reasoned that if there is any adjuvant activity of caffeine, it would be seen early, when caffeine has been reported to have an effect on the absorption of the analgesic with which it is administered (8,9). Therefore, we designed a 2-hr study, with assessments 15, 30, 45, 60, 90, and 120 min after treatment. We employed the same rating scales we have just reported and adhered to the same admission criteria. As a result of maintaining these criteria, the clinical features of the patients were homogeneous among the three treatment groups, and treatment effects were readily apparent. There was differentiation of aspirin 800 mg with caffeine 64 mg from aspirin 800 mg and placebo ($p < 0.05$) on all rating scales, demonstrating the adjuvant role of caffeine 64 mg, beginning at 15 to 30 min and extending throughout the 2 hr trial. From this study, therefore, we appreciated the sensitivity of the sore throat pain model as an assay for adjuvant activity. Moreover, we had used the model successfully to detect the onset of action of an analgesic and at an earlier time point (15 min) than usually studied or demonstrable in other onset-of-action models.

In the way of summarization, I should like to refer to Dr. Stephen Cooper's recently described percentage of theoretical maximum total pain relief (TOT-PAR), or % TMT (10) as an indicator of the sensitivity of the sore throat pain model (see pp. 117–124). Even with its limitations, the % TMT is a useful paradigm for assessing the relative ability of different pain models to distinguish placebo from a common standard, such as aspirin or acetaminophen in the 600 to 1,000 mg range. Similar to the dental pain model (with its low placebo response and small variance), the sore throat pain model can readily differentiate between an active control and placebo. Moreover, as in the dental pain model, there is a very wide ceiling effect evident in the sore throat pain model in which to detect between-treatment differences, which can make for considerable upside assay sensitivity.

Beyond its use as a single-dose assay, the sore throat pain model has value in other clinical research settings. As a multiple-dose assay, for example, the model can be conducted over several days, during the course of tonsillopharyngitis as part of upper respiratory tract illness. For patients with oral and pharyngeal fungal overgrowth owing to chemotherapy or for patients with radiation-induced mucositis, the model has the requisite sensitivity to determine effective analgesic interventions. Finally, the model has been applied to the evaluation of topical therapy for pharyngeal pain, too, in order to demonstrate demulcent action (11).

In conclusion, the development and refinement of the sore throat pain model testify to the importance of the basic elements of clinical trial methodology. Having been implemented at several different investigative sites, capable of demonstrating the efficacy of different active agents compared with placebo and the differences between them, as well as a dose-response relationship, the sore throat pain model is a definitive and sensitive assay for analgesics.

ACKNOWLEDGMENT

I wish to acknowledge and thank Bill Thoden and Georgia Williams for their unfailing technical assistance in preparing this manuscript.

REFERENCES

1. Schachtel BP, Fillingim JM, Beiter DJ, Lane AC, Schwartz LA. Rating scales for analgesics in sore throat. *Clin Pharmacol Ther* 1984;36:151–156.
2. Schachtel BP, Fillingim JM, Beiter DJ, Lane AC, Schwartz LA. Subjective and objective features of sore throat. *Arch Intern Med* 1984;144:497–500.
3. Melzack R, Torgerson WS. On the language of pain. *Anesthesiology* 1971;34:50–59.
4. Schachtel BP, Paull B, Baybutt R. Qualities of pain as endpoints in the evaluation of combination analgesics (abstract). *Acta Pharmacol Toxicol* 1986;59:268.
5. Schachtel BP, Fillingim JM, Thoden WR, Lane AC, Baybutt RI. Sore throat pain in the evaluation of mild analgesics. *Clin Pharmacol Ther* 1988;44:707–711.
6. Beaver WB. Caffeine revisited (editorial). *JAMA* 1984;251:1732–1733.
7. Schachtel BP, Fillingim JM, Lane AC, Thoden WR, Baybutt RI. Caffeine as an analgesic adjuvant: a double-blind study comparing aspirin 800 mg with caffeine 64 mg to aspirin 800 mg and placebo in patients with sore throat. *Arch Intern Med* 1991; in press.
8. Dahanukar SA, Pohujani S, Sheth UK. Bioavailability of aspirin and interacting influence of caffeine. *Indian J Med Res* 1978;66:844–848.
9. Yoovathaworn KC, Sriwatanakul K, Thithapandha A. Influence of caffeine on aspirin pharmacokinetics. *Eur J Drug Metab Pharmacokinet* 1986;11:71–76.
10. Cooper SA, Strow L. Comparing assay sensitivity of pain models (abstract). *Clin Pharmacol Ther* 1990;47:189.
11. Schachtel BP, Fillingim JM. Demulcent action (abstract). *Clin Pharmacol Ther* 1984;35:273.

DISCUSSION

Dr. William Beaver: Dr. Schachtel has presented what amounts to a methodologic tour-de-force in this exposition of the development of the sore throat pain model for the evaluation of analgesic efficacy. The model has "downside" assay sensitivity as demonstrated by its ability to discriminate the prototypic oral analgesics, aspirin, acetaminophen, and ibuprofen, from placebo. In addition, the sore throat model has "upside" assay sensitivity as demonstrated by significant differences between acetaminophen 1,000 mg and ibuprofen 400 mg and between aspirin 800 mg and the combination of aspirin 800 mg with caffeine.

The relative efficacy of over-the-counter (OTC) analgesics is often established in models such as cancer pain, inpatient postoperative pain, and postpartum pain that do not constitute "OTC indications." Although there is no reason to think that the relative efficacy of OTC analgesics would be substantially different in the kinds of pain for which OTC analgesics are usually self-administered, it is comforting to have that opinion confirmed by studies such as these in sore throat pain, a typical OTC indication. I hope that other investigators will take advantage of this model in the evaluation of other NSAIDs that are used as prescription or OTC analgesics.

Of at least equal importance is that this series of studies serves as an elegant demonstration of the scientific logic that should underlie the effort to establish optimal methodology for and validate any new analgesic model. Early studies explored a number of possible inclusionary and exclusionary criteria to define those that would improve assay sensitivity and hence be incorporated in the later studies. In addition, asking patients to volunteer terms to describe their pain with the intention of selecting the most promising of these ("difficulty in swallowing" and "feeling swollen") to incorporate as scaling systems in later studies is likewise a fundamental strategy in the development of methodology.

Advances in Pain Research and Therapy, Vol. 18,
edited by M. Max, R. Portenoy, and E. Laska,
Raven Press, Ltd., New York © 1991.

18

Muscle-Contraction Headache

Bernard P. Schachtel

*Medical Department, Whitehall Laboratories, Inc., New York, New York 10017;
and Clinical Epidemiology Unit, Yale University School of Medicine,
New Haven, Connecticut 06510*

Headache is a common malady, a well-known affliction to people over several centuries. However, the pharmacologic agents used to treat muscle-contraction headache have undergone controlled clinical evaluation only recently. This chapter reviews the clinical research methods from peer-reviewed, placebo-controlled evaluations of single-ingredient analgesic drugs used to treat this condition.

Because of the striking need for control in conducting clinical trials on subjects with headache, several critical issues must be considered in designing, conducting, and interpreting these studies. As in other areas of clinical research, it is requisite to define the condition and to evaluate patients with the same condition in order to determine if changes after therapeutic intervention are, in fact, attributable to medication. Perhaps the most comprehensive delineation of the features of muscle-contraction headache is provided by Diamond (1), who defined it as a common, persistent headache that is nonspecific. He further characterizes the pain of muscle-contraction headaches as "usually bilateral and may be localized or generalized. Patients describe this pain as a tightness, squeezing, or soreness, or as the sensation of wearing a tight band or skull cap or of carrying a weight on the head . . . (often) associated with painful contractions of the skeletal muscles of the face, neck, and scalp." Diamond distinguishes chronic headaches (which are usually constant and occasionally unremitting for weeks) from episodic headaches (which may be triggered by such factors as fatigue, depression, or stress at work or home). These are also the criteria cited by the Ad Hoc Committee on Classification of Headache (2). Although other criteria have been discussed and proposed, these are useful to the clinical investigator and serve to screen subjects who are eligible for a clinical trial on muscle-contraction headache.

The inclusion criteria defining muscle-contraction headache are as important as the criteria used to exclude certain patients, such as those with classic migraine headaches. Like most investigators, von Graffenried and Nuesch (3), for example, used explicit criteria to exclude subjects with classical migraine from their studies and thus concentrate only on those with tension headache, or, as they termed it, "non-migrainous headache."

The significance of obtaining patients with as specific and appropriate diagnoses as possible is exemplified by the results of the study by Peters et al. (4). Despite attention to other pertinent features of headache, patients were admitted to the study with two diagnoses: tension headaches and tension-vascular headaches. According to the investigators, the former "usually occur in response to stress, are bilateral and steady in pain character," and the latter "share these characteristics, although persons with this type of headache also experience focal or throbbing pain, nausea, or anorexia, and pain at times when not experiencing obvious stress or fatigue. These tension-vascular headaches are considered more intense than standard tension (muscle-contraction) headaches." The results for each type of patient are interesting, for they reveal that tension headaches are indeed more amenable to the evaluation of mild analgesics (Fig. 1). In this study, Peters et al. could not clearly demonstrate that aspirin 650 mg or acetaminophen 1,000 mg was clinically active in the more intense category of headache, tension-vascular headache. Efficacy could be demonstrated, however, for patients with tension headache.

Having identified patients with these features of muscle-contraction headache, the next key step in identifying suitable subjects for a clinical trial on muscle-contraction headache is to match potential subjects to the specific analgesic agents being evaluated. For example, in their crossover study on two different formulations of aspirin compared to placebo, Langemark and Olesen (5) recruited 33 patients with "non-migrainous headache problems" from a private neurology clinic or neurological hospital department who reported 3 to 30 headache days per month (i.e., very frequent). The severity of these headaches was underscored by the necessity of advising patients not to evaluate any headache when they had taken either a prescription or a nonprescription medication within the last 12 hrs. Clearly, patients from a neurology clinic who use prescription medications for almost daily headaches are unsuitable for the evaluation of a mild analgesic agent. As commented by Langemark and Olesen, "patients were rather severely afflicted and had no confidence in the test medication, which was explained as similar to aspirin." As a result, there was relatively weak evidence in this study of the efficacy of either formulation of aspirin compared to placebo.

For this reason, Diamond (1) does not select many patients from his headache clinic for studies on mild analgesics because they usually have headaches that are more frequent and constant and require prescription medications for control. In his study on ibuprofen 800 mg, ibuprofen 400 mg, and aspirin 650 mg, however, patients with specific criteria for muscle-contraction headache had an average of 15.9 to 22.1 headaches per month, approximately 1 every other day. The frequency of these headaches and the possibility that they are more refractory to treatment may depreciate the sensitivity of this assay for the drugs being evaluated. In future studies, Diamond recommends the evaluation of patients

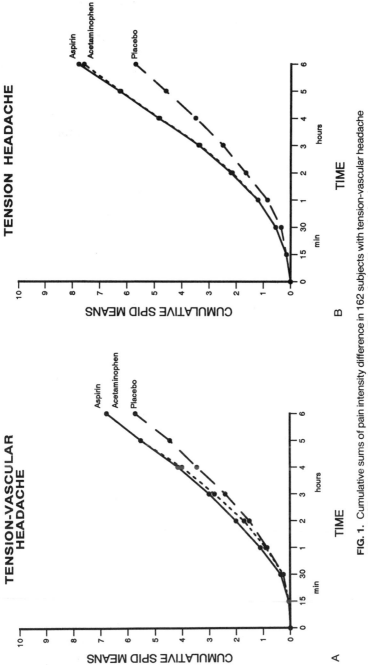

FIG. 1. Cumulative sums of pain intensity difference in 162 subjects with tension-vascular headache (**A**) and 107 subjects with tension headache (**B**). (From ref. 4, with permission.)

with less frequent headaches in order to better demonstrate the analgesic efficacy of study drugs. In von Graffenried and Nuesch's (3) studies, therefore, as in ours, subjects are eligible who have a history of headaches more than once per month, but not daily—thus providing a frequency of headaches that is not too frequent but often enough for the study of mild analgesic drugs.

Matching the usual severity of the subjects' headaches to the medication being tested makes sense, too. Most of Diamond's patients, for example, described their headaches as usually moderately severe. Similarly, Peters et al. (4) would not accept any patient whose "headache was considered clinically mild (that is, the headache was not intense enough to prompt taking medications) . . . or so clinically severe as to render them bedfast or unable to work. . . ." Instead, they admitted to their trial only patients whose headaches were by history "clinically considered to be moderately severe, that is, requiring, and having been responsive to, either or both aspirin or acetaminophen. . . ." One should note here another criterion that is particularly apt: patients should be included only if they give a history of responsiveness to aspirin or other mild analgesics. This feature is an obvious component of research on the efficacy of mild analgesics for muscle-contraction headache.

In addition to these historical features, the pretreatment status of the subject is critical to the success or failure of the headache trial. Headache pain that is too mild or too intense can have serious consequences on the outcomes measured for analgesics compared with placebo. It is for this reason that von Graffenried and Nuesch (3) required the assessment of headaches of only "moderate" or "severe" intensity—not "mild" or "unbearable." Patients with mild to moderate headache pain would experience relief from most agents (perhaps even including placebo), regardless of their inherent potency. Pretreatment pain levels in this range leave little room for the differentiation between analgesic agents or between dosages of these agents. At the other end of the spectrum, for incapacitating headaches, aspirin would constitute insufficient treatment: a baseline pain intensity that is too severe would make it very difficult to distinguish a nonprescription-strength analgesic from placebo.

Ryan's (6) placebo-controlled study on aspirin 650 mg and ibuprofen 400 mg provides a relevant example of unfortunately weakened assay sensitivity. In this early headache model, a double-blind, randomized crossover trial on 59 patients with muscle-contraction headache, there is no mention of the baseline severity of the headaches before treatment. The results of this study (Table 1) reveal that there were small pain intensity differences: perhaps because the subjects were instructed to treat each attack when it began, the baseline pain intensity was not sufficiently intense before treatment. Even so, the pain intensity differences were greater for the actives than for placebo, confirming the efficacy of these agents for this condition. Another consequence of this low pretreatment level, however, was that 18 (or 31%) of the 59 subjects, when treated with placebo, reported complete relief, similar to the rates of complete relief reported by the subjects when receiving ibuprofen and aspirin (Table 2). As a result, there was no differ-

TABLE 1. *Pain intensity differences from baseline in a study comparing aspirin 650 mg, ibuprofen 400 mg, and placebo*

Time	Aspirin 650 mg	Ibuprofen 400 mg	Placebo
1 Hr	0.37	0.35	0.28
2 Hrs	0.69	0.48	0.30
3 Hrs	0.74	0.59	0.31
Summary	1.80	1.43	0.89

From ref. 6, with permission.

entiation observed between the two active drugs, either in terms of pain intensity differences or the degree of relief.

The "unpredictable" and "erratic nature of headache" (3) makes it one of the more complicated pain conditions to study. Thus the need for a controlled clinical trial. In a classic study, William Murray (7) reported on 100 pharmacists and medical students with a history of "common headache." The subjects were told that the purpose of the study was to evaluate the effectiveness of aspirin in the treatment of headache and that several dosages of aspirin (163 mg, 325 mg, or 650 mg) would be employed. (A placebo was also included in the trial, but the subjects were not apprised of this feature of the study design.) Over a 12-week period, the subjects were able to treat headaches as they occurred with each of the four randomly assigned agents. Regardless of the severity of the headache at the time of treatment (Table 3), and with only one endpoint, approximately 81% of the headaches were rated as having some degree of relief within 1 hr. However, the placebo response (57%) is remarkably high in Murray's study, probably because all subjects believed that they were always receiving a dose of an active analgesic. Even though this aspect of the study design reduces its ability to distinguish active drug from placebo (downside assay sensitivity), this study is noteworthy in its ability to confirm the clinical efficacy of a 650-mg dose of aspirin.

In terms of the measurement instruments in clinical trials on headache, two types of rating scales have been employed predominantly, pain intensity and

TABLE 2. *Degree of relief in a study comparing aspirin 650 mg, ibuprofen 400 mg, and placebo*

	Aspirin 650 mg	Ibuprofen 400 mg	Placebo
Ineffective	18	24	31
Slight	4	4	2
Moderate	11	6	4
Almost complete	6	3	4
Complete	20	22	18
Total	59	59	59

From ref. 6, with permission.

TABLE 3. *Distribution of 322 headaches by treatment, severity and degree of relief*

Aspirin dose (mg)	Severity of headache	Degree of relief					Total	Percent improved[a]
		Worse	Unchanged	Slight	Moderate	Complete		
650	Mild	0	2	2	9	15	28	93 ⎫
650	Moderate	2	9	7	12	12	42	74 ⎬ 81[b]
650	Severe	0	2	4	4	0	10	80 ⎭
325	Mild	0	8	4	10	11	33	76 ⎫
325	Moderate	4	14	14	10	9	51	65 ⎬ 68
325	Severe	0	4	3	1	2	10	60 ⎭
163	Mild	2	11	5	3	7	28	54 ⎫
163	Moderate	2	16	8	11	6	43	58 ⎬ 57
163	Severe	0	1	3	3	1	8	88 ⎭
Placebo	Mild	2	5	5	7	6	25	72 ⎫
Placebo	Moderate	3	16	9	4	5	37	49 ⎬ 57
Placebo	Severe	1	3	1	2	0	7	43 ⎭

[a] Percent improved $= \dfrac{\text{number of cases reported slight, moderate, or complete relief}}{\text{total number of cases}} \times 100.$

[b] Statistically significantly different from placebo and other two dosages of aspirin, which do not significantly differ from placebo ($p < 0.005$).
From ref. 7, with permission.

relief. One basic example of a pain intensity scale used by the subject to indicate "headache pain now" is found in the study of Peters et al. (4), a categorical scale (none, slight, moderate). Diamond (1) uses a four-category pain intensity scale (by adding the extreme category "intense"), but, in contrast to posttreatment assessments at regular intervals, ratings on this scale are obtained at the onset of a headache and only 3 hrs after treatment for each headache episode. Both categorical pain intensity scales can impose limitations on investigators and their subjects. Although their simplicity may imply easier comprehension and use by a variety of subjects, there is little room on these scales to relate a therapeutic effect. Unless other features of a headache model are exceptionally well-controlled, this tightness of scores may indicate a lack of difference between an active agent and placebo or between active agents when true effects and differences actually exist.

Von Graffenried et al. (8), in fact, used two different types of pain intensity scales, a verbal rating scale with four categories (none, slight, moderate, severe) and a 100-mm horizontal visual analogue scale (with the left end marked "no pain" and the right end marked "unbearable pain"). He found that the categorical pain intensity difference scores were the less sensitive efficacy measure, since he could discern more statistically significant differences between active drug and placebo on the visual analogue pain intensity scale. Von Graffenried reported that the visual analogue scale was easier for his subjects to use, mainly because it afforded more than the limited number of choices "available on the verbal scale."

Langemark and Olesen (5) also used a 100-mm visual analogue scale for pain intensity, with "no pain" at the far left extreme, and "strongest imaginable pain" at the far right. We, too, have used a 100-mm visual analogue scale, but have avoided this far-right extreme (9). Instead, we used the anchor term "very severe pain," and, in an ordinal era where everything is familiarly ranked from 1 to 10, we employed numerical subheadings for this scale. Like von Graffenried, we have found that subjects can use visual analogue scales quite easily and meaningfully.

The categorical relief scale, such as Peters et al.'s (4) four-category relief scale, is the other mainstay of instruments used to measure efficacy. Langemark and Olesen (5) had an interesting seven-category relief scale, with ratings from much worse to no change and complete relief, but it failed to reveal any significant differences in their study. The six-category relief scale that we reported in our ibuprofen-placebo trial (9) is the same scale we have used in other studies on over-the-counter (OTC) agents. The results from this scale revealed significant treatment effects, complementing those from the pain intensity scale (Fig. 2).

Some of the other components that we take for granted in the design and conduct of a randomized controlled trial also bear mentioning, for any deviation from these general principles of clinical trial methodology can "sink the ship." How study treatments are, in fact, randomized is rarely mentioned in a study report. One assumes that the randomization code is computer-generated today

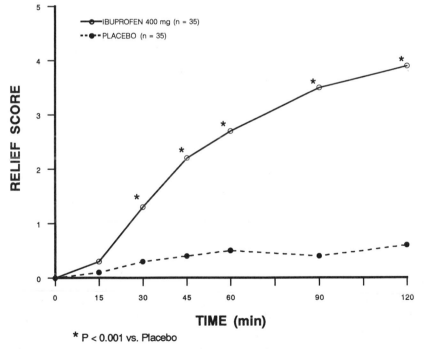

FIG. 2. Mean relief scores using a six-category relief scale comparing ibuprofen 400 mg and placebo in 70 subjects. (From ref. 9, with permission.)

and maintained by a third party, such as the biostatistics department, until all subjects have been evaluated by the investigator. One also assumes "double-blinding" by the employment of identical study medications. However, although a study may be called placebo-controlled and may also be described as "double-blind," as in Ryan's study (6), when tablets are used that "resemble each other in size, color, and shape," this may be inadequate. Subjects can taste the tablets and think that they recognize one agent, or a bitter taste may sour their appreciation of analgesia. This lack of total blinding can undermine an otherwise well-designed study.

Other important methodological decisions involve the number of test treatments each subject will evaluate and the number of headache episodes that will comprise the trial. Some investigators have successfully conducted complete crossover trials. For example, Murray (7) evaluated several headache episodes with four different treatments in a Latin square design. von Graffenried et al. (8) evaluated one headache episode for each of four different treatments in 33 patients (comparable to 132 patients per treatment group in a parallel study). The best differentiation of aspirin 1,000 mg from placebo, in fact, is derived from a summary of four of von Graffenried et al.'s (8) crossover studies (Fig. 3): in this pooled sample of 108 patients, there is very clear distinction between the 1,000-mg dose of aspirin and placebo.

A potential problem in crossover designs is the change in pretreatment status, particularly baseline pain intensity, that can occur from one period to another. The early crossover study by Vecchio (10) is illustrative. Although Vecchio was able to distinguish ibuprofen 200 mg from aspirin 650 mg and placebo in a statistically significant fashion on a global evaluation (Fig. 4), as well as on hourly pain relief and pain intensity difference scores, Vecchio was unable to detect statistically significant differences between aspirin and placebo. This occurred perhaps because of low pretreatment pain intensity levels, differences in baseline pain intensity for each headache episode, by chance, or because aspirin 650 mg was, in fact, not efficacious in these patients.

A parallel-group design randomly allocates patients to separate treatment groups. This may be for a single dose or for multiple treatments with the same medication. In the parallel-design studies conducted by Diamond, for example, four headache episodes are evaluated by each patient, who knows that he or she is receiving the same (though unknown) medication for all four headache episodes (1,11).

Regardless of the study design, headache trials are conducted by subjects in an ambulatory setting. To insure the success of a headache study, therefore, it is necessary to hold "an extensive prestudy instruction session" with the subjects, as von Graffenried et al. (8) advise. It is also important to note the usual headache course of potential subjects and incorporate it into the conduct of a headache trial. Thus, for example, Peters et al. (4) evaluated subjects when they felt they required treatment, matching the actual pattern of taking medication in a clinical trial to the patients' "therapeutic habits."

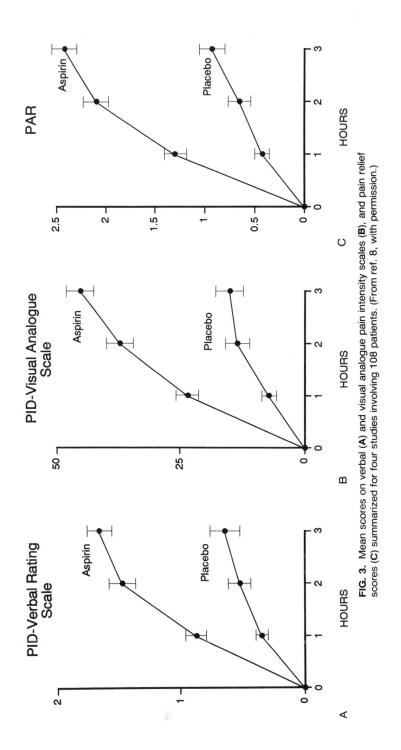

FIG. 3. Mean scores on verbal (**A**) and visual analogue pain intensity scales (**B**), and pain relief scores (**C**) summarized for four studies involving 108 patients. (From ref. 8, with permission.)

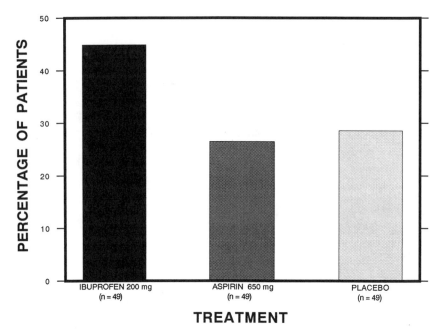

FIG. 4. "First in efficacy" ranking by 49 subjects in a crossover study comparing ibuprofen 200 mg, aspirin 650 mg, and placebo (10).

The timing, or frequency, of posttreatment assessments varies from study to study. Some headache trials, like Peters et al.'s (4) study on aspirin, or ours on ibuprofen (9), include early assessments, beginning at 15 min after treatment, with assessments at regular intervals, usually over 3 to 4 hrs. Individual time points can provide meaningful information, as in assays of onset of action: our study (9), for example, showed the differentiation of ibuprofen 400 mg from placebo by 30 min (Fig. 2). However, assessments need not be taken frequently. Diamond (1) and Diamond and Medina (11) make only one posttreatment evaluation, at 3 hrs, as we did in our study on aspirin with caffeine, acetaminophen, and placebo (12). Clearly, if analgesic medication has not worked by 3 hrs, it will not.

Summary measures, such as the summed pain intensity differences (SPID) or total pain relief (TOTPAR), provide other conventional expressions of the overall pharmacologic effect of a drug. An alternate to these conventions was used by Peters et al. (4) who produced what they termed "cumulative sums of pain intensity difference scores" and "cumulative pain relief scores" (Fig. 5): in the 107 subjects with tension headache, both aspirin and acetaminophen were distinguished from placebo at 1 hr and beyond.

Another summary measurement has been used effectively in headache trials: the global efficacy rating. In Langemark and Olesen's (5) crossover trial, positive

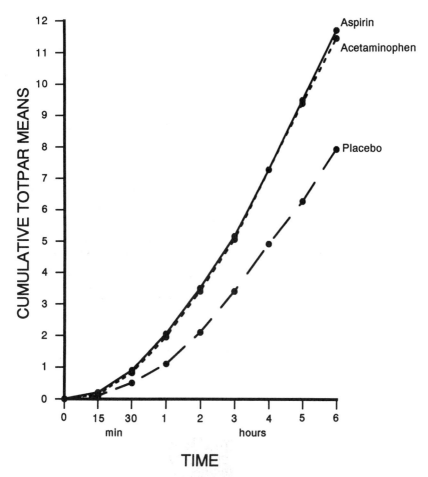

FIG. 5. Mean cumulative pain relief score in 107 subjects with tension headache. (From ref. 4, with permission.)

results were obtained on a five-category global rating, on which patients gave their overall opinion of the preparation (Fig. 6). The global scores showed that one formulation of aspirin was more effective than placebo, confirming the SPID scores at 2 and 3 hrs. We have used a ten-point ordinal global evaluation that was rated by the subject 3 hrs after taking a single dose of study medication (12). This global scale was also sensitive to drug effects (Fig. 7). Finally, a similar type of global rating has been used in Diamond's headache pain model (1,11). In this approach, the investigator appraises each subject's responses to the same medication taken to treat four headache episodes (as a physician in the office would), rating the overall efficacy of the medication. A corollary to the physician's global evaluation, patient preference, has also been used successfully as a measurement

What is your overall opinion of the preparation?

☐　　　　☐　　　　☐　　　　☐　　　　☐

worthless　　poor　　　fair　　　good　　excellent

FIG. 6. Five-category global rating scale used by Langemark and Olesen (5) on 33 patients with "non-migrainous headache." (Adapted from ref. 5, with permission.)

instrument. All other things being equal, in a crossover study on three successive headache episodes each treated with a different medication (6), patients probably can relate their preference among treatments.

One other summary endpoint comes close to describing the ultimate benefit of an analgesic to a person with a headache: the achievement of higher degrees of relief or complete relief. When Murray (7) examined only one endpoint, moderate or complete relief, regarding only these two categories as indicative of clinically significant improvement (Fig. 8), 65% of the 650-mg aspirin treatment

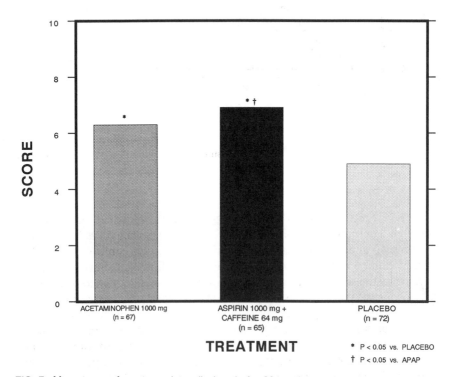

TREATMENT

* P < 0.05 vs. PLACEBO
† P < 0.05 vs. APAP

FIG. 7. Mean scores for a ten-point ordinal scale for 204 patients comparing acetaminophen 1,000 mg, aspirin 1,000 mg with caffeine 64 mg, and placebo (12).

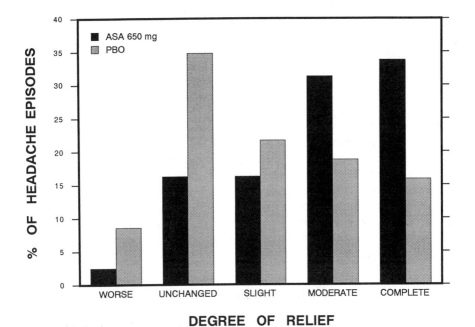

FIG. 8. Percent of headache episodes plotted against degree of relief. (Adapted from ref. 7, with permission.)

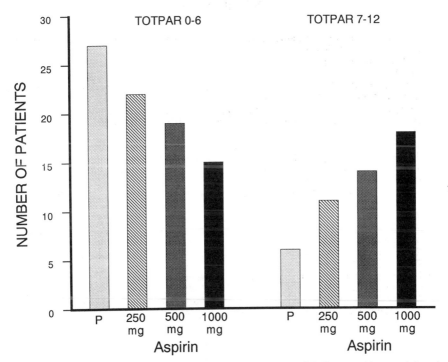

FIG. 9. Number of patients reporting poor to moderate pain relief (*left*) or good to complete pain relief (*right*) in 33 patients. (From ref. 8, with permission.)

group derived this degree of relief, in contrast to the placebo response (35%). In a different approach at defining this clinically relevant endpoint, von Graffenried et al. (8) dichotomized the TOTPAR responses into those that indicate "poor to moderate" pain relief (0 to 6) and scores representing "good to complete" pain relief (7 to 12). Expressed this way, there is an apparent dose-response pattern, from placebo ascending to 1,000 mg of aspirin (Fig. 9).

In conclusion, these are the research methods employed in the design and conduct of controlled clinical trials on muscle-contraction headache. By carefully defining muscle-contraction headache, the eligibility criteria, and the pretreatment status of the patients, by maintaining controlled study conditions during the conduct of the trial, and by selecting appropriate measurement instruments and clinically relevant endpoints, investigators should be able to conduct successful studies on this complex condition.

ACKNOWLEDGMENTS

I wish to thank Mike Minor and Georgia Williams for their dedicated technical assistance in preparing this manuscript.

REFERENCES

1. Diamond S. Ibuprofen versus aspirin and placebo in the treatment of muscle contraction headache. *Headache* 1983;23:206–210.
2. Ad Hoc Committee on Classification of Headache. Classification of headache. *JAMA* 1962;179: 717–718.
3. von Graffenried B, Nuesch E. Non-migrainous headache for the evaluation of oral analgesics. *Br J Clin Pharmacol* 1980;10:225S–231S.
4. Peters BH, Fraim CJ, Masel BE. Comparison of 650 mg aspirin and 1,000 mg acetaminophen with each other, and with placebo in moderately severe headache. *Am J Med* 1983;74(suppl 6A): 36–42.
5. Langemark M, Olesen J. Effervescent ASA versus solid ASA in the treatment of tension headache. A double-blind, placebo controlled study. *Headache* 1987;27:90–95.
6. Ryan RE. Motrin—a new agent for the symptomatic treatment of muscle contraction headache. *Headache* 1977;16:280–283.
7. Murray W. Evaluation of aspirin in treatment of headache. *Clin Pharmacol Ther* 1964;5:21–25.
8. von Graffenried B, Jill RC, Nuesch E. Headache as a model for assessing mild analgesic drugs. *J Clin Pharmacol* 1980;20:131–144.
9. Schachtel BP, Thoden WR. Onset of action of ibuprofen in the treatment of muscle contraction headache. *Headache* 1988;28:471–474.
10. Vecchio TJ. Efficacy of ibuprofen in muscle contraction headache (abstract). *Clin Pharmacol Ther* 1983;33:199.
11. Diamond S, Medina JL. A double-blind study of zomepirac sodium and placebo in the treatment of muscle contraction headache. *Headache* 1981;21:45–48.
12. Schachtel BP, Baybutt R, Schechter C. Gastric side effects of aspirin compared to acetaminophen and placebo in the treatment of headache (abstract). *Acta Pharmacol Toxicol* 1986;59:170.

Advances in Pain Research and Therapy, Vol. 18,
edited by M. Max, R. Portenoy, and E. Laska,
Raven Press, Ltd., New York © 1991.

Commentary
Crossover Design in Headache Studies

Joseph R. Migliardi* and Michael Friedman**

*Medical and Regulatory Affairs, **Statistical Services Department,
Bristol-Myers Products, Hillside, New Jersey 07205*

In planning our studies to demonstrate the contribution of caffeine as an analgesic adjuvant when it is combined with acetaminophen in the tension headache model, we were aware that in many previously reported studies the tension headache model had been plagued by a lack of upside sensitivity, mainly because of weaknesses in the study design (1–4) (see also Chapter 18). Since it was necessary to use a design that would provide upside sensitivity, we considered employing a crossover design for these studies, because with the crossover design each patient provides information for two or more treatments. The data permit assessment of treatment comparisons within the usually more sensitive framework of within-subject, as opposed to among-subject, variability (5; and see Chapter 4.)

The crossover design is appropriate for acute, repetitive conditions (5). For this reason, we believed that the crossover design could be appropriate for the tension headache model. Although the patient may have been suffering from tension headaches for years, if the individual headaches are acute or episodic, and not chronic, the repetitiveness of the condition and the independent but strikingly similar nature of each episode provide the potential advantage that the severity of pain at baseline may be similar for several episodes, thus permitting valid within-subject analyses. This commentary describes the specific methodology that we followed in conducting these crossover studies, thereby increasing the sensitivity of tension headache studies sufficiently to differentiate the analgesic effects of active drugs.

There are three components of crossover designs that require consideration (5): the number of treatment periods, the types of treatment sequences, and the number of patients for each sequence. The number of treatment periods is important because the effort and cost of maintaining data quality are directly related to the duration and complexity of the study; the probability of successfully completing the study is inversely related to the number of crossovers. On the other hand, by increasing the number of treatment periods we can obtain more information from each patient and improve the precision of our estimates.

The choice of treatment sequences is important because possible changes in the clinical condition may result in the appearance of carryover effects (5–7) that may then require additional adjustments in order to avoid bias. Obviously, it is important that whatever types of sequences are selected, they should be randomized as to the order of administration.

The number of patients who participate is important because insufficient numbers will decrease the sensitivity of the study and make it difficult to pick up real differences when they exist. This has been a major problem in previously reported studies and often accounts for a lack of sensitivity of the studies (1,2,8).

We have recently completed two multicenter studies of tension headache in which a crossover design was successfully employed. We compared two active agents and a placebo control. As previously stated, the purpose of the studies was to determine the adjuvant effects of caffeine when it is combined with acetaminophen. The active drugs tested were acetaminophen 1,000 mg alone (APAP) or in combination with 130 mg of caffeine (APAP/CAFF). Because the actives have shallow dose-response curves (8–10) and because we wanted to determine the extent of any differences between the actives while, at the same time, limit the number of patients required to participate in the studies, it was necessary to maximize the precision of the comparison of the actives. These considerations led us to the choice of the specific crossover design to be described.

In the classical design of a crossover study that involves three treatments, A, B, and P, there would be three treatment periods for each patient and six sequences would be involved: A/B/P, B/A/P, A/P/B, P/A/B, B/P/A, and P/B/A. This design obviously requires that each patient be exposed to each of the three treatments, and problems in analysis arise if significant numbers of patients skip or miss one of the treatments. A way to address this is to increase the number of times a patient is administered a specific treatment, for example, by treating two headache episodes in each period. A patient can then be considered analyzable as long as valid data are provided for at least one treated headache for each of the assigned treatments.

STUDY DESIGN

We believed that it would not be feasible to modify the classical design by treating two headaches in each of the three periods because the patients would lose interest in continuing their participation after three or four treatments. Therefore, a modified two-period crossover design was employed with the following sequences: A/B, B/A, A/P, P/A, B/P, and P/B, each period of which represents treatment of two headaches with the same medication. These six treatment sequences also allow the estimation of period effects, treatment effects, and carryover effects (5).

However, since the difference between the two actives was of primary interest and this difference was expected to be smaller than the expected differences between the actives and placebo, the randomization was weighted with three times as many patients randomly assigned to each of the two active drug treatment sequences (A/B and B/A) as to the four treatment sequences of active drug with placebo in order to avoid overpowering the placebo comparisons and to reduce the total number of patients that would be required to participate in the study. Successive blocks of ten patients were randomly assigned to the following ten treatment sequences: A/B, A/B, A/B, B/A, B/A, B/A, A/P, P/A, B/P, P/B, where A equals APAP 1,000 mg combined with 130 mg CAFF, B equals 1,000 mg APAP, and P equals placebo.

It should be pointed out that alternative crossover designs are available for comparing three treatments in four headache episodes, so that a design can be chosen according to the specific requirements of the study. One design with some attractive properties uses the following sequences with equal frequency: A/B/P/P, B/A/P/P, A/P/B/B, P/A/B/B, B/P/A/A, and P/B/A/A. However, in this design, all three paired comparisons would be estimated with equal precision. Koch et al. (11) discuss additional designs that can be used for comparing three treatments in four headache episodes, including designs that are weighted in favor of the two active treatments.

Based on the results of previous, parallel-group relative potency studies in postoperative patients (8,12), it was anticipated that the summed pain intensity differences (SPID) would differ between the actives by about 0.35 and that each active would have a SPID greater than 0.80 over placebo over a 4-hr period. These differences were considered to be clinically meaningful because in those relative potency studies a SPID of 0.35 represented the difference between a two-tablet (1,000 mg) dose of APAP and a dose that contains 41% more APAP (i.e., 1,410 mg). The other assumption made was that the within-patient variance would be about 7.25. On the basis of these assumptions, we decided to enroll 420 patients in each study. (Because the difference between actives turned out to be larger than anticipated, a smaller sample size would have sufficed.)

The population studied was adult males or females with a history of an average of from four to ten tension headache attacks per month during the previous year that were usually successfully treated with over-the-counter analgesic medications. In order to be admitted into the study, subjects had to meet the criteria for tension headaches as defined by the Ad Hoc Committee on the Classification of Headache (13). There was no major change in the revised definitions of tension-type headache which were published in 1988 (14). Therefore, the population conforms to the current definition of tension-type headache. The inclusion and exclusion criteria of the protocol for the study clearly defined for inclusion only patients with acute tension headaches.

Since the nature of tension headache studies requires that the patients self-evaluate on an outpatient basis, the patients were carefully instructed by the study personnel both orally and in writing to evaluate their headache pain intensity as well as relief of pain following treatment with the blinded medication. Pain intensity was assessed at baseline and at $\frac{1}{2}$ hr, 1 hr, and 2, 3, and 4 hrs after

TABLE 1. *Instructions to patients*

The headache pain must be of at least moderate severity.
They must not have ingested any analgesic during the previous 8 hrs.
They must not have ingested any alcoholic beverages during the previous 6 hrs.
At least 48 hrs must have elapsed before a subsequent trial with test drug could be undertaken.

ingestion of study medication. Pain relief was assessed at the same time intervals following ingestion of study medication. The patients were also instructed how to complete the diary for each headache treated, and to take the study medication only when specific conditions were met (Table 1).

RESULTS

The results of the studies show that the crossover design is indeed an appropriate one for the headache model. The baseline pain intensity values (Tables 2 and 3) indicate that severity of pain for the various episodes was quite similar across treatments. SPIDs between the actives were 0.52 and 0.57 respectively, rather than the assumed difference of 0.35. Total pain relief (TOTPAR) differences between the actives were 1.05 and 0.98, respectively. These differences were all highly statistically significant. All the SPID and TOTPAR active versus placebo differences were statistically significant, with the exception of the B versus P differences in study 1, which were smaller in size than expected. (The small B versus P differences are not due to attenuation of effect over the course of the crossover; it is already apparent in the first headache episode.) The within-subject variance was even lower than we had assumed, 7.0 for SPID in study 1 and 6.6 in study 2. Tests for carryover effects indicated that this was not a problem in these studies. For instance, the difference in estimated carryover effect between

TABLE 2. *Mean pain intensity differences, summary measures, and treatment comparisons (study 1)[a]*

	Treatment			Treatment comparisons		
	A	B	P	A vs B	A vs P	B vs P
Baseline pain						
intensity—Mean (S.E.)	2.31 (.02)	2.31 (.02)	2.33 (.03)	.513	.398	.699
PID $\frac{1}{2}$ Hr	0.35 (.03)	0.27 (.03)	0.18 (.03)	.016 (A)[b]	<.001 (A)	.059
1 Hr	0.90 (.04)	0.70 (.03)	0.67 (0.5)	<.001 (A)	<.001 (A)	.763
2 Hrs	1.33 (.04)	1.19 (.04)	1.10 (.06)	.007 (A)	.002 (A)	.216
3 Hrs	1.61 (.04)	1.49 (.04)	1.40 (.06)	.019 (A)	.002 (A)	.154
4 Hrs	1.74 (.04)	1.63 (.04)	1.52 (.06)	.043 (A)	<.001 (A)	.029 (B)
SPID	5.32 (.13)	4.80 (.13)	4.45 (.20)	.002 (A)	<.001 (A)	.104
TOTPAR	10.45 (.20)	9.40 (.21)	8.82 (.30)	<.001 (A)	<.001 (A)	.080

[a] All *p* values based on adjusted means from crossover model.

[b] Indicates favored treatment: A = APAP/CAFF, B = APAP, P = placebo.

PID, pain intensity difference; SPID, sum of pain intensity differences; TOTPAR, total pain relief.

TABLE 3. *Mean pain intensity differences, summary measures, and treatment comparisons (study 2)[a]*

	Treatment			Treatment comparisons		
	A	B	P	A vs B	A vs P	B vs P
Baseline pain intensity—Mean (S.E.)	2.26 (.02)	2.26 (.02)	2.28 (.02)	.853	.427	.356
PID $\frac{1}{2}$ Hr	0.33 (.02)	0.26 (.02)	0.17 (.03)	.005 (A)[b]	<.001 (A)	.025 (B)
1 Hr	0.83 (.03)	0.71 (.03)	0.50 (.04)	.001 (A)	<.001 (A)	<.001 (B)
2 Hrs	1.33 (.04)	1.17 (.04)	0.92 (.05)	<.001 (A)	<.001 (A)	<.001 (B)
3 Hrs	1.63 (.04)	1.48 (.04)	1.22 (.06)	<.001 (A)	<.001 (A)	<.001 (B)
4 Hrs	1.79 (.04)	1.62 (.04)	1.34 (.06)	<.001 (A)	<.001 (A)	<.001 (B)
SPID	5.33 (.12)	4.76 (.13)	3.82 (.91)	<.001 (A)	<.001 (A)	<.001 (B)
TOTPAR	10.54 (.19)	9.56 (.20)	7.86 (.32)	<.001 (A)	<.001 (A)	<.001 (B)

[a] All p values based on adjusted means from crossover model.
[b] ( ) indicates favored treatment: A = APAP/CAFF, B = APAP, P = placebo.
PID, pain intensity difference; SPID, sum of pain intensity differences; TOTPAR, total pain relief.

the actives and placebo averaged over the two studies was 0.43 for SPID; this difference was statistically insignificant, and also considerably smaller than the typical active versus placebo direct effect. The detailed data that resulted from these studies are being submitted for publication in the near future.

Additional analyses demonstrate that the crossover design is very cost-effective relative to the parallel design. We analyzed the data for the first headache only; these data are precisely what would be obtained if a parallel design had been employed. Because of our weighting of the treatment sequences, the treatments A, B, and P occurred in the first headache in the ratio of 2:2:1. Based on the standard errors obtained for the A versus B difference, we calculated the number of patients in the parallel design that would be needed to yield the same precision as 100 patients in the crossover design. As Table 4 shows, about four times as many patients would be needed in the parallel design as in the crossover design. Thus the crossover design yields considerable savings, because it is much more costly to enroll a new patient in a study than to observe additional headache episodes in a patient who has already been enrolled.

TABLE 4. *Relative efficiency of crossover and parallel designs[a]*

	SPID	TOTPAR
Study 1	393	439
Study 2	375	412

[a] Estimated number of patients needed in a parallel-design study to achieve same precision of A vs B comparison as 100 patients in the crossover design.
SPID, sum of pain intensity differences; TOTPAR, total pain relief.

Since the possibility of a higher dropout rate is of concern in crossover designs, we examined this phenomenon in our studies and found that dropouts and other nonanalyzable patients did not constitute a problem. Out of all the patients who were administered treatment for the first headache, 1% failed to provide analyzable data, and 5% did not provide efficacy analyzable data for the actual crossover trial (by having at least one analyzable headache for each of the two treatments). Thus, although the incidence of nonanalyzable patients in our crossover study was, as expected, somewhat higher than it might have been in a parallel design, this incidence was so low that it did not diminish the advantage of the crossover design over the parallel design.

In summary, although one must be cautious about the use of the crossover design in clinical studies of analgesics, the acute tension-type headache model lends itself to this design provided that one is aware of the potential problems and takes precautions to minimize them. The population to be studied must be carefully defined, there must be a sufficient time lapse between treatments, and, because the patient serves as the rater and the ratings are done in an outpatient situation, the study population must be carefully and thoroughly instructed both orally and in writing in the completion of the rating instruments.

REFERENCES

1. Peters BH, Fraim CJ, Masel BE. Comparison of 650 mg aspirin and 1,000 mg acetaminophen with each other, and with placebo in moderately severe headache. *Am J Med* 1983;74(6A):36–42.
2. Ryan RE. Motrin—a new agent for the symptomatic treatment of muscle contraction headache. *Headache* 1977;16:280–283.
3. Clough C. Non-migrainous headaches. *Classification and Management Brit Med J* 1989;299: 70–72.
4. Diamond S, Dalessio DJ. The practicing physician's approach to headache. In: *Muscle contraction headache,* 3rd ed. Baltimore: Williams and Wilkins, 1982;99–108.
5. Koch GG, Amara IA, Brown BW, et al. A two-period crossover design for the comparison of two active treatments and placebo. *Stat Med* 1989;8:487–504.
6. Laska E, Meisner M, Kushner M. Optimal crossover designs in the presence of carryover effects. *Biometrics* 1985;39:1087–1091.
7. Matthews JNS. Optimal crossover for the comparison of the two treatments in the presence of carryover effects and autocorrelated errors. *Biometrika* 1987;74:311–320.
8. Laska EM, Sunshine A, Mueller F, et al. Caffeine as an analgesic adjuvant. *JAMA* 1984;251: 1711–1718.
9. Fingl E. Drug dosage, time of observation and duration of medication as factors in drug evaluation. In: Tedeschi DH, Tedeschi RE, eds. *Importance of fundamental principles in drug evaluation.* New York: Raven Press, 1968;33–51.
10. Beaver WT. Caffeine revisted—editorial. *JAMA* 1987;251:1732–1734.
11. Koch GG, Amara IA, Simmons PD. Multi-period crossover designs for the comparison of two or more active treatments and placebo. *Proceedings of the Biopharmaceutical Section of the ASA.* 1988;69–78.
12. Laska EM, Sunshine A, Zighelboim I, et al. Effect of caffeine on acetaminophen analgesia. *Clin Pharmacol Ther* 1983;33:498–509.
13. Ad Hoc Committee on Classification of Headache. Classification of headache. *JAMA* 1962;179: 717–718.
14. Headache Classification Committee of the International Headache Society. Classification and diagnostic criteria for headache disorders, cranial neuralgias and facial pain. *Cephalalgia* 1988; 8(suppl 7):9–96.

Advances in Pain Research and Therapy, Vol. 18,
edited by M. Max, R. Portenoy, and E. Laska,
Raven Press, Ltd., New York © 1991.

19

Dysmenorrhea

M. Yusoff Dawood

*Division of Reproductive Endocrinology, Department of Obstetrics, Gynecology,
and Reproductive Sciences, University of Texas Health Science Center
at Houston, Houston, Texas 77030*

Dysmenorrhea, or painful menstruation, is one of the most frequently encountered gynecologic disorders. There are two types of dysmenorrhea, primary and secondary (1,2). In primary dysmenorrhea, the patient experiences painful menstrual cramps but no visible disease is present to account for it. In secondary dysmenorrhea, the painful menstrual period is secondary to an identifiable pelvic lesion. Primary dysmenorrhea is estimated to affect more than 50% of menstruating women, 10% of whom have pain severe enough to cause absenteeism for 1 to 3 days each month. It is estimated that about 600 million working hours and at least $2 billion are lost annually because of incapacitating dysmenorrhea (3). Furthermore, dysmenorrhea appears most commonly between the ages of 20 and 24, as well as in the late teens, and affects the quality of life and work and educational performance (4,5). Although primary dysmenorrhea does not give rise to any documented mortality, the combined economic, personal, and interpersonal disruption resulting from the pain makes it imperative to obtain the optimum pain relief possible in the management of these patients.

The contemporary approach to the management of dysmenorrhea depends on whether it is primary or secondary (6,7). Causes of secondary dysmenorrhea include the use of the intrauterine device, endometriosis, pelvic adhesions, ovarian cysts, pelvic inflammatory disease, congenital malformation of the uterus (bicornuate uterus, uterus didelphys, subseptate uterus, blind uterine horn), uterine myomas, uterine polyps, uterine synechiae (Asherman's syndrome), adenomyosis, cervical strictures or stenosis, transverse vaginal septum, imperforate hymen, Allen-Master's syndrome (tears in the ligament), and pelvic congestion syndrome. If pain is related to one of these syndromes, the therapeutic approach is to remove the offending pelvic lesion. Although surgery is the principal approach for the management of secondary dysmenorrhea, some of the responsible disorders, such as the intrauterine device or endometriosis, may respond to medical management equally well.

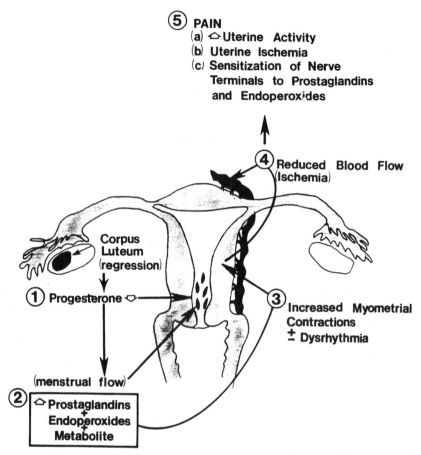

FIG. 1. Postulated mechanisms in the pathogenesis of primary dysmenorrhea as the cramps start in the pelvis. (Reproduced from ref. 10, with permission.)

In primary dysmenorrhea, medical management is effective and should be directed at correcting the biochemical abnormality that underlies the condition (8–13). In most women with primary dysmenorrhea, there is increased endometrial production and release of prostaglandins (Fig. 1). This process leads to increased, abnormal uterine activity (Fig. 2); reduced uterine blood flow, with resultant uterine hypoxia; and sensitization of nociceptive sensory fibers in the pelvis to the action of noxious stimuli. Since these mechanisms are cumulatively responsible for the pain and associated symptoms in primary dysmenorrhea, inhibition of endometrial prostaglandins with the nonsteroidal antiinflammatory drugs (NSAIDs) is the most effective and rational treatment of primary dysmenorrhea for most women (1,2,10). Furthermore, it has been convincingly shown that inhibition of menstrual fluid prostaglandin levels to normal or below normal range is accompanied by relief of primary dysmenorrhea (Fig. 3).

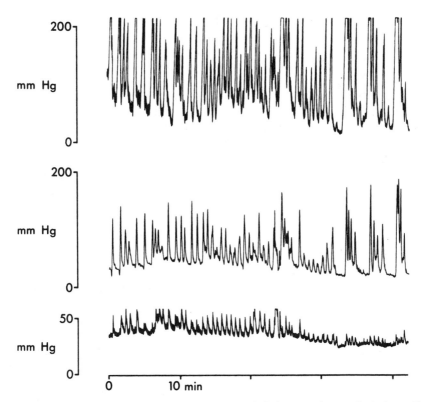

FIG. 2. Intrauterine pressure recorded by a three-channeled microtransducer catheter in a patient with severe primary dysmenorrhea. The frequency of contractions, contraction amplitude, and resting pressure are increased. (Reproduced from ref. 28, with permission.)

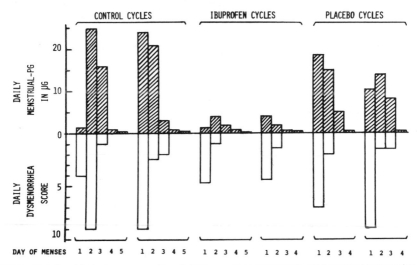

FIG. 3. Relationship between severity of dysmenorrhea and levels of menstrual prostaglandin released without treatment and with placebo or ibuprofen treatment of a patient with severe primary dysmenorrhea. The daily dysmenorrhea score employed a ten-point scale visual analogue method. There is a significant reduction of menstrual prostaglandin released and dysmenorrhea score when the patient is treated with ibuprofen. (Reproduced from ref. 8, with permission.)

CLINICAL NEEDS AND OPPORTUNITIES

Primary dysmenorrhea is a unique, acute, and cyclically repetitive pain model that readily lends itself to clinical trials of analgesics. As noted, the treatment of primary dysmenorrhea is usually accomplished with medications, and there are several approaches to the medical ablation of the pain. Although current understanding of the pathophysiology of primary dysmenorrhea (*vide supra*) indicates that the most logical approach is correction of excessive endometrial prostaglandin production and release with NSAIDs, other approaches may involve the use of centrally acting analgesics or oral contraceptives. Despite the advent of these drugs, about 20 to 30% of patients with primary dysmenorrhea either do not respond or obtain insufficient relief (6,7). Combined with the high prevalence rate of primary dysmenorrhea, this inadequate response to current treatment clearly indicates the need to carry out better studies to further define the pathophysiology of primary dysmenorrhea and more analgesic trials to expand the alternatives available to treat this condition.

The pain syndrome in dysmenorrhea is unique. In many ways, the pain in primary dysmenorrhea is akin to a chronic pain model because it cannot be eradicated completely in a single treatment and will continue to occur for a long period of time. Yet it is short-lived, lasting for 2 to 3 days, and recurs on a regular, cyclical basis. This latter feature, together with the fact that primary dysmenorrhea occurs only in ovulatory cycles and begins usually at or after the onset of menstrual flow, provides a very predictable, repeatable, and definable pain model for the evaluation of analgesics. Because the pain in primary dysmenorrhea recurs, it is a potentially useful model for testing analgesics, since each patient can be her own control in randomized, double-blind, crossover studies (8).

The finding that primary dysmenorrhea is owing to increased abnormal endometrial production and release of prostaglandins, which leads to abnormal uterine hypercontractility and decreased uterine blood flow (8–14), has suggested the use of objective measures of therapeutic response, including measurement of menstrual fluid prostaglandin levels (8–12) and uterine contractility (15,16). The ability to monitor or evaluate the response to treatment with a biochemical or biophysical marker adds to the uniqueness of primary dysmenorrhea as a pain model.

Because dysmenorrhea is a disorder occurring in young women who are otherwise basically healthy, the evaluation of medications or analgesics poses very little risk of significant side effects. Also, patients need to take the medication for only a couple of days, thus reducing chronic exposure to the drug with consequent potential chronic toxicity. The brief exposure to the drug also eliminates much of the potential pharmacological carryover effect from one cycle to the next in crossover trials.

CURRENT APPROACHES

Until the early 1970s, there were few controlled or double-blind analgesic studies in primary dysmenorrhea. Since that time, many analgesic studies have been performed, most of which evaluated NSAIDs (1–3,6–9,11–13,16,17). A few studies have examined other treatments including the Progestasert (progesterone-medicated intrauterine device) in dysmenorrhea (18), acupuncture, and transcutaneous electrical nerve stimulation in primary dysmenorrhea (19), and hormonal (danazol, gonadotropin-releasing hormone agonist and progestins) therapy in women with secondary dysmenorrhea related to endometriosis (20,21).

The analgesic studies that evaluated NSAIDs were initially carried out often without a placebo control; some were not blinded (6,7). More recently, most studies have a placebo control and have employed one of four basic study designs;

1. Single cycle, parallel study.
2. Multiple cycle, parallel study.
3. Multiple cycle, two-way crossover (A to B and B to A) study.
4. Multiple cycle, randomized, crossover study.

SINGLE CYCLE, PARALLEL STUDY

In this study design, each subject is studied for only one cycle of exposure to the medication tested. Several arms of the study involving either one test medication or more and a placebo are run parallel in a randomized fashion. Thus, if only one medication is being evaluated, there are two arms in the study (a medication and a placebo arm) and if *n* medications are evaluated, there are *n* + 1 arms in the study.

The potential advantages of this study design are the rapidity with which it can theoretically be accomplished (more patients can be recruited quickly and each patient requires a study duration of only slightly more than a month), and the likelihood of lower patient dropout rates and better compliance.

Because there is no second treatment, this design has no carryover effect and is strongly advocated by some statisticians who are concerned about the possibility of carryover effect but fail to understand the true nature of the short-lived cyclical pain model in dysmenorrhea and the relevance of the carryover effect from cycle to cycle in such a model (*vide infra*).

The disadvantage of this design is that each subject does not act as her own control and therefore the intersubject variability in pain reporting and pain intensity potentially gives rise to a poorer or less sensitive discrimination between the placebo-treated group and the medication group. One possible way to overcome this is to use a larger number of subjects. In studies with more than two arms, the number of subjects required to obtain adequate sensitivity can become very large. Another disadvantage of this design is that it does not take into account the variability of dysmenorrhea from cycle to cycle; thus, it is possible that more severe or only moderate or mild dysmenorrhea may be represented in one treatment arm more than in another, and this may skew results. Although it may be argued that randomization and blinding may take care of this, or alternatively that treatment could be initiated only when the pain is moderate or more intense, these approaches may still not eliminate the differences in initial pain intensity.

MULTIPLE CYCLE PARALLEL STUDY

This design is similar to the single cycle, parallel design except more than one cycle is studied in each of the arms. Designed to overcome the inherent problem of variability between cycles, and reduce the number of subjects needed, it suffers from additional disadvantages that are somewhat different from the single cycle, parallel design. If each subject is studied for two or more cycles for each treatment, then the bias is magnified by the number of cycles studied. For example, if there is poor response to the first cycle of treatment, there is every likelihood that the subject will anticipate, and therefore report, a similar response in the subsequent cycle since the informed consent must disclose that the medication (placebo or active compound) is similar for all cycles studied. Additionally, if a patient has poor or no response to the first cycle of treatment, there may be a higher probability of dropout since the patient knows she will be receiving the same ineffective treatment. Consequently, patients receiving placebo treatment may demonstrate a particularly high dropout rate after the first cycle of treatment. In one such study we performed, uneven dropout rates prevented us from obtaining dependable, meaningful data analysis.

MULTIPLE CYCLE, TWO-WAY CROSSOVER STUDY

Several unpublished and published studies on the analgesic efficacy of NSAIDs have been carried out using a two-way crossover technique (22). In a study design involving a comparison between a study medication A and a placebo B, the patients either receive A first and crossover to B, or receive B first and crossover to A. Either one cycle of each treatment is employed or the patient may receive two or more cycles of each treatment before crossing over to a similar number of cycles with the alternative treatment. The use of each patient as her own control may increase the sensitivity of the study, and is an advantage of the crossover design.

Notwithstanding the potential benefits of the crossover, this approach may yield a high likelihood of bias. If the response in the initial treatment is poor, then the patient may anticipate improvement with subsequent treatments, and this may alter her response. This element of bias is further accentuated when more than one cycle is tested before crossing over. For example, if the patient receives three cycles of A before crossing over to three cycles of B or vice versa, the patient, as well as the investigator, can anticipate a response in the second and third cycle similar to the first cycle and a response in the fifth and sixth cycle similar to the fourth cycle. Thus, two-thirds of the cycles may be prejudiced in terms of patient response because of the lack of true complete blinding. In some unpublished studies, this design has caused contradictory results.

MULTIPLE CYCLE RANDOMIZED CROSSOVER STUDY

In these study designs, each of the treatments is given more than once to each patient, but not in the easily predictable patterns described above. Given a particular number of treatments and treatment periods, biostatisticians can construct an optimal set of treatment sequences, and patients are randomly assigned one of the sequences. (The statistical criterion for optimality is that the crossover design provides minimum-variance unbiased estimators of the treatment and carryover effects.) For example, in a six-cycle randomized crossover design involving a study medication A and a placebo B, an optimal design is comprised by the four sequences A-B-B-A-A-B, B-A-A-B-B-A, A-A-B-A-A-B, and B-B-A-A-A-B (23).

The use of multiple crossovers and optimal sets of sequences offers unique advantages over the two-way crossover design or the parallel-cycle studies. With the above designs, the chances of bias are markedly reduced, the patient acts as her own control, and concern about the intercycle variability of dysmenorrhea intensity is readily addressed by having more than one cycle for each type of treatment tested. In contrast to the standard two-treatment, two-period crossover, the effects of random cycle-to-cycle variability in pain can be readily estimated and distinguished from period and carryover effects. Although some patients may not complete all of the intended treatments, there are statistical methods to handle incomplete data sets.

PATIENT SELECTION

Studies that include patients with primary and secondary dysmenorrhea are poor because the two conditions are owing to different etiologies and the responses to an analgesic may differ as a result. It is, therefore, imperative that selection criteria are rigid and clearly defined. Primary dysmenorrhea can be reliably diagnosed only from its clinical history. The two cardinal features in the history include onset of dysmenorrhea dating to shortly after the menarche (usually within a year) and the experience of painful cramps that begin just a few hours before or with menstrual flow and continue for two to three days. Pelvic examination should reveal no detectable pathology that could account for the menstrual cramps. In most women with primary dysmenorrhea, the cramps are recurrent with each menstrual flow; the subject should have sufficiently painful menstrual cramps in 75 to 80% of her cycles to be eligible for inclusion in the study.

Only patients with moderate to severe menstrual cramps should be studied, and medications or contraceptive practices that could improve or worsen the primary dysmenorrhea should not be allowed for the duration of the study. Specifically, patients on oral contraceptives who were permitted in some early studies of dysmenorrhea (24) should not be eligible for studying the analgesic effects of other compounds in primary dysmenorrhea. Oral contraceptives are not only effective in the relief of primary dysmenorrhea, but also reduce menstrual fluid prostaglandin output through inhibition of endometrial tissue development (10–12). Patients using the intrauterine device should also be excluded from analgesic studies unless the study is specifically designed to evaluate the analgesic affects of a particular compound on the relief of intrauterine device–related dysmenorrhea (25,26). The presence of the intrauterine device leads to increased menstrual prostaglandins and this is probably the basis of the resulting dysmenorrhea (27). Finally, patients should not be allowed to consume any alcohol-containing drinks for at least 24 hrs before the onset of menstrual flow and throughout the menstrual period under study. The consumption of alcohol can interfere with the assessment of the study drug because it has a direct smooth-muscle relaxing effect, inhibits vasopressin release, and may alter the response to painful stimuli.

TIMING OF MEDICATION

In most analgesic studies, the medication is taken at the time when the pain intensity exceeds a certain defined threshold (usually moderate or severe pain). However, in studies involving primary dysmenorrhea, the timing of medication depends on the specific questions asked and the objectives of the study. If the study is designed purely to assess the analgesic effect of a medication, it is best for medication to be administered when pain has occurred and exceeded a certain defined threshold, usually moderate or severe pain. This kind of medication timing allows for evaluation of the initial effects of the medication, as well as the overall effect produced throughout that menstrual period (17). Thus, the time to onset of relief, the duration of relief, the sum of the pain intensity differences (SPID), and total pain relief (TOTPAR) can be derived (*vide infra*) (17). In addition, administration of medication after the pain reaches a specific intensity will obviate the inadvertent inclusion of cycles that may have minimal or even no pain.

If the objective of the study is to evaluate the analgesic affect of the medication through its specific modulation of prostanoid release by the endometrium, then the medication should be started with the onset of menstrual flow irrespective of whether a certain level of pain intensity has been attained (6–8,11). In this model, remediation is also given on a continuing basis for at least 48 hrs and usually 72 hrs, which coincides with the time of maximum prostaglandin release in the menstrual flow. The frequency of remediation is defined by the half-life and pharmacokinetics of the study drug. Although this model does not allow for evaluation of single-dose efficacy, daily pain measurements can be compared with control or placebo-treated cycles (8,11). Remediation is either given regularly for the next two to three days, based on the pharmacokinetics of the medication, or intermittently on an as-needed basis (that is, only when pain recurs). If the goal of the study is to obtain information about both single-dose analgesic efficacy and effects on menstrual fluid prostaglandin, a combination of these two approaches can be used.

To avoid exposure of an undiagnosed early pregnancy to the effects of the study drug, it is prudent to withhold medication until the onset of menstrual flow even if pain is present. Should there be a need to evaluate the analgesic effect of medication prior to the onset of menstrual flow, pregnancy testing using a highly sensitive serum human chorionic gonadotropin assay should be carried out, preferably one day before, or at least within three days of starting medication. Additionally, the study could be confined to women who have had bilateral tubal ligation, are sexually abstinent, or are absolutely reliable in the use of barrier contraception.

PLACEBO AND REFERENCE MEDICATION

The need for a placebo in any analgesic study performed in patients with primary dysmenorrhea cannot be overemphasized. Pain relief is obtained in 20 to 50% (average 30%) of placebo-treated cycles in these studies (6,7) and the true efficacy of an active compound cannot be determined with such a control. However, it has become difficult to include control, untreated cycles, in present day trials because of the availability of proven, effective, and safe medications for the relief of primary dysmenorrhea, such as ibuprofen. The availability of these drugs has enabled a new approach to analgesic studies, in which the effects of the treatment under study is compared to the efficacy of ibuprofen. Indeed, in many studies, the study medication is compared to ibuprofen as well as a placebo. In this way, the medication can be evaluated for both its analgesic effects above that of a placebo and its comparative analgesic potential compared to that of a "gold standard" such as ibuprofen. This is a useful and very frequently employed approach in many recent trials.

RESCUE MEDICATION

Like many other pain models, there are effective analgesics for the relief of primary dysmenorrhea. This gives rise to both ethical and methodological difficulties when studying a new medication for primary dysmenorrhea. Institutional review boards will often insist on the availability of a rescue medication for patients who do not obtain relief with the study medication. The use of a standardized, single rescue medication that is also blinded can provide another quantitative measure in these pain studies. Specifically, we have employed the use of ibuprofen, labeled as rescue medication and given at the same time as the blinded study medications. In this way, the analgesic efficacy, or lack of efficacy of the study medications can be measured by the total dose of rescue medication (ibuprofen) required during the study period. We have also found such an approach useful when conducting nonpharmacologic modalities of treatment for primary dysmenorrhea, such as transcutaneous electrical nerve stimulation (16).

INDICES OF EVALUATION

Analgesic Effects

Two types of analgesic effect are usually monitored in dysmenorrhea studies. They are the *acute analgesic effect* of a single-dose medication and the *daily global analgesic effect* for each day (usually the first two or three days) of the menstrual flow. In addition, most studies assess the overall analgesic experience of the subject during that particular menstrual period. This is usually a less sensitive index than the acute and the daily global effect.

As mentioned above, the acute analgesic effect allows evaluation of the efficacy of a single dose (usually the first dose) of the study medication. The method employed for such an evaluation is similar as for most other analgesic models (see Chapter 4.) Briefly, the patient takes the first dose of the medication with the onset of a certain level of pain intensity, usually moderate to severe pain in primary dysmenorrhea. Thereafter, the patient evaluates the intensity of her pain at 30 min and at 1, 2, 3, 4, 5, and 6 hrs. The responses are then analyzed to obtain the time to onset of pain relief, the duration of pain relief, and the SPID and TOTPAR scores. This information is important, since the rapidity of onset of analgesic effect and the duration of pain relief are both important in the selection of analgesic agents for the treatment of primary dysmenorrhea. Newer techniques for obtaining estimates and duration have been proposed (see Chapter 4). Subtle differences in these acute analgesic effects among the different NSAIDs may encourage better clinical choices.

The daily analgesic effect is evaluated in a manner similar to the acute analgesic effect except that a single assessment of the pain intensity is made at the beginning and at the end of each day when menstrual flow is occurring. This daily global analgesic effect is preferable to that of a global cycle effect, since significant differences obtained during the first two or three days of the cycle could be blunted by the global effect during the whole menstrual period.

Biochemical Markers

As indicated previously, there is a large subset of women with primary dys-menorrhea who have elevated levels of menstrual fluid prostaglandins that can be directly correlated to their menstrual pain scores (10,11). Therefore, menstrual fluid prostaglandin levels may be measured and used as an objective biochemical marker of drug effects. A change in this biochemical marker may also indicate the likely mechanism by which analgesic effects are brought about.

The measurement of menstrual fluid prostaglandin levels can be carried out separately on a smaller number of patients; 10 to 12 women studied for one cycle per medication in a randomized crossover design are sufficient. Alterna-tively, in a larger clinical trial, a smaller subgroup of patients may be examined for their menstrual fluid prostaglandins at the same time the study is proceeding. Details of the study design involving the measurements of menstrual fluid pros-tanoids have been previously described by us (8,11). When such a study is per-formed, it is imperative that the patients do not consume alcohol or alcohol-containing beverages for at least 24 hrs, and preferably 72 hrs, before the onset of menstruation and throughout menstruation. The subjects should also either refrain from intercourse or condoms should be used by the male partners for at least 72 hrs before the onset of menstrual flow and throughout the menstrual phase of the cycle; this eliminates the risk of identifying spurious levels of pros-taglandins owing to prostanoids present in seminal fluid.

RECOMMENDED APPROACH

Based on the above considerations and our own experience in conducting clinical trials of therapy in primary dysmenorrhea, there are essentially two pre-ferred pragmatic approaches to study design in this population. These approaches are complementary. For large-scale pivotal studies that are designed to dem-onstrate the efficacy and safety of a medication in the relief of primary dysmen-orrhea, a multiple cycle, randomized, placebo-controlled, crossover study in-volving the test compound, a placebo, and a "gold standard" or reference preparation, such as ibuprofen, should be performed. In this design, a three-cycle crossover study involving one cycle of treatment with the medication, one cycle with ibuprofen, and one cycle with placebo should be sufficient. In mul-ticenter studies, the risk of significant dropout limits the more preferred approach of using a six-cycle crossover study, with each medication given for two cycles. However, if only one center is involved, a six-cycle crossover study with two cycles of treatment for each medication is preferred, or a compromise approach using four cycles (two cycles of study medication, one cycle of placebo, and one cycle of ibuprofen) can be adopted.

In any of these pivotal studies, strict selection of patients, as discussed above, is needed so that the patients belong to a homogeneous group. Medication should be given only with the establishment of moderate to severe pain and only after the onset of menstrual flow. The medication should also be given on a continuing, rather than on an as-needed basis, and it should be continued for the first 3 days of menstrual flow. Analgesic efficacy, such as time to onset of relief, duration of relief, and time to maximum relief, can all be obtained from analysis of the patient responses at regular intervals after the administration of the first dose of medication for each cycle tested. Categorical pain scores such as none, mild, moderate, or severe, rather than the visual analogue scale score, are preferred. Both pain intensity and pain relief should be reported so that the SPID and TOTPAR scores can be calculated. The daily global response in terms of pain intensity and pain relief should also be obtained for the first, second, and third day of the menstrual flow. This should provide the daily global effect of the treatment. Patients should be allowed to take rescue medication, but this is preferably discouraged during the first 2 hrs after taking the study medication so that a sufficient time has been given for any potential efficacy of the study medication to become manifest. Again, one type of blinded rescue medication, such as ibuprofen, should be provided by the study. The amount of such rescue medication used by the patient in any particular cycle can be calculated to provide another quantitative assessment of the efficacy of the study medication.

The second approach complements the first. A smaller number of patients with severe dysmenorrhea can be studied in a similar multiple cycle, randomized, placebo-controlled crossover study, as described above, but additionally menstrual fluid is collected for measurements of prostaglandin levels. With this approach, any rescue medication should not be an NSAID or other medication likely to inhibit prostaglandin biosynthesis.

SECONDARY DYSMENORRHEA

Intrauterine Device–Related Dysmenorrhea

Analgesic trials in dysmenorrhea due to the presence of an intrauterine device can be performed using designs similar to those employed in primary dysmenorrhea. One difference, however, may be the need to give the medication throughout the menstrual flow. Another essential is the need to wait until pain begins prior to the administration of medication because not all patients and not all cycles with the intrauterine device in place are painful.

Endometriosis

When conducting analgesic trials for dysmenorrhea due to endometriosis, it is essential that pelvic pain and dysmenorrhea are not mixed together. These are two different kinds of pain and probably arise from different mechanisms. The study design can be similar to that for primary dysmenorrhea, and it is probably best to evaluate both acute analgesic efficacy (single-dose efficacy) and the global efficacy. Because onset of the pain may not have a precise relationship to onset of menstrual flow, it is necessary that medication be initiated only after a defined pain intensity threshold level is exceeded. Caution against pregnancy or measures to prevent pregnancy must be advised in such trials because the medication may have to be given prior to menstruation. The multifactorial nature of the pelvic pain and dysmenorrhea in patients with endometriosis increases the heterogeneity of the study population and may therefore necessitate larger number of patients. Indeed, acute exacerbations of chronic pelvic pain, or the occurrence of dysmenorrhea during a period of chronic pelvic pain, can thoroughly confound the pain evaluation. Thus, the pain associated with pelvic endometriosis is probably better studied as a chronic pain model in analgesic trials. In this setting, a crossover design is less desirable than the parallel-study design.

FUTURE RESEARCH

Future research in analgesic studies for dysmenorrhea should focus on more precise quantification of pain assessment, the use of objective markers that can be correlated with the intensity of the clinical pain, elucidation and measurement of new or biochemical mediators of pain, better understanding of the interactive biochemical mechanisms bringing about pain in primary dysmenorrhea, and the use of less invasive methods of continuously measuring uterine blood flow to determine the role of uterine vascularity and hypoxia in the etiology of primary dysmenorrhea. Currently, two objective markers, menstrual fluid prostaglandin output and uterine contractility, have been used in conjunction with the assessment of pain in studies examining analgesic effects of medications in primary dysmenorrhea (8,11–13,15,16). With menstrual fluid prostaglandins, particularly PGF_{2a}, there is excellent correlation between the amount of PGF_{2a} released by the uterus and the intensity of pain experienced by the patient at different times throughout the menstrual flow (10,11). Although quantification of uterine contractility does not always readily lend itself to correlation with intensity of clinical pain, objective changes can be correlated with pain relief over short time periods during the menstrual flow. In the absence of a less invasive method of measuring uterine contractility, however, the latter index is more limited in application for clinical trials than the measurement of menstrual fluid PGF_{2a}.

Future research needs to address the relative imbalance between the different types of prostanoids, such as prostacyclins (potent vasodilators) versus PGF_{2a} and thromboxanes (potent vasoconstrictors). The ratios between uterine-stimulating and vasoconstricting prostanoids, and uterine-relaxing and vasodilating prostanoids may prove to be useful correlates with clinical pain. The influence of leukotrienes must also be evaluated. Determination of the endogenous opiate β-endorphin levels may also be helpful in understanding the mechanism of pain relief. The effect of naloxone on pain may be a useful method of assessing the role of endorphinergic systems. Again, this can be tested in a small subset in any large clinical trial.

Finally, two other clinical entities, endometriosis and pelvic pain, warrant carefully conducted research into the pathophysiology and methods for relieving the pain. It is very likely that the mechanisms responsible for pain in these two conditions are multifactorial.

REFERENCES

1. Dawood MY. Dysmenorrhea. *J Reprod Med* 1985;30:154–167.
2. Dawood MY. Dysmenorrhea. *Clin Obstet Gynecol* 1990;33:168–178.
3. Dawood MY. Ibuprofen and dysmenorrhea. *Am J Med* 1984;77(1A):87–94.
4. Svennerud S. Dysmenorrhea and absenteeism. *Acta Obstet Gynecol Scand* 1959;38(Suppl 12): 1–116.
5. Bergsjo P. Socioeconomic implications of dysmenorrhea. *Acta Obstet Gynecol Scand Suppl* 1979;87:67–68.
6. Dawood MY. Overall approach to the management of dysmenorrhea. In: Dawood MY, ed. *Dysmenorrhea.* Baltimore: Williams and Wilkins, 1981;261–279.
7. Dawood MY. Overall approach to the management of dysmenorrhea. In: Dawood MY, McGuire JL, Demers LM, eds. *Premenstrual syndrome and dysmenorrhea.* Baltimore: Urban and Schwarzenberg, 1985;177–204.
8. Chan WY, Dawood MY, Fuchs F. Relief of dysmenorrhea with the prostaglandin synthetase inhibitor ibuprofen: effect on prostaglandin levels in menstrual fluid. *Am J Obstet Gynecol* 1979;135:102–108.
9. Dawood MY. Dysmenorrhea and prostaglandins: pharmacological and therapeutic considerations. *Drugs* 1981;22:42–56.
10. Dawood MY. Hormones, prostaglandins and dysmenorrhea. In: Dawood MY, ed. *Dysmenorrhea.* Baltimore: Williams and Wilkins, 1981;21–52.
11. Chan WY, Dawood MY, Fuchs F. Prostaglandin in primary dysmenorrhea: comparison of prophylactic and nonprophylactic treatment with ibuprofen and use of oral contraceptive. *Am J Med* 1981;70:535–541.
12. Chan WY, Dawood MY. Prostaglandin levels in menstrual fluid of nondysmenorrheic and of dysmenorrheic subjects with and without oral contraceptive or ibuprofen therapy. *Adv Prostaglandin Thromboxane Leukotriene Res* 1980;8:1443–1447.
13. Chan WY, Fuchs F, Powell AM. Effects of naproxen sodium on menstrual prostaglandins and primary dysmenorrhea. *Obstet Gynecol* 1983;61:285–291.
14. Chan WY, Hill JC. Determination of menstrual prostaglandin levels in non-dysmenorrheic and dysmenorrheic subjects. *Prostaglandins* 1978;15:365–375.
15. Smith RP, Powell JR. Spontaneous objective and subjective evaluation of meclofenamate sodium in the treatment of primary dysmenorrhea. *Am J Obstet Gynecol* 1987;157:611–616.
16. Milsom I, Andersch B. Effect of ibuprofen, naproxen sodium and paracetamol on intrauterine pressure and menstrual pain in dysmenorrhea. *Br J Obstet Gynaecol* 1984;91:1129–1135.
17. Dawood MY. Efficacy and safety of subprofen in the treatment of primary dysmenorrhea: a multicenter, randomized, double-blind study. *Curr Ther Res* 1988;44:257–266.
18. Trobough G, Guderian AM, Erickson RR, et al. The effect of exogenous intrauterine progesterone on the amount of prostaglandin F_{2a} content of menstrual blood in dysmenorrheic women. *J Reprod Med* 1978;21:153–158.
19. Dawood MY, Ramos J. Transcutaneous electrical nerve stimulation (TENS) for the treatment of primary dysmenorrhea: a randomized cross-over comparison with placebo TENS and ibuprofen. *Obstet Gynecol* 1990;75:656–660.
20. Henzl MR, Corson SL, Moghissi K, et al. Administration of nasal nafarelin as compared with oral danazol for endometriosis. *N Engl J Med* 1988;318:485–489.
21. Dawood MY, Spellacy WN, Dmowski WP, et al. A comparison of the efficacy and safety of buserelin vs. danazol in the treatment of endometriosis. In: Chadha DR, Buttram VC Jr, ed. *Current Concepts in Endometriosis.* New York: Alan R. Liss, 1990;253–267.

22. Budoff PW. Use of mefenamic acid in the treatment of primary dysmenorrhea. *JAMA* 1979;241: 2713-2716.
23. Jones B, Kenward MG. *Design and analysis of cross-over trials.* London: Chapman and Hall, 1989;140-188.
24. Henzl MR, Buttram V, Segre EJ, et al. The treatment of dysmenorrhea with naproxen sodium: a report of two independent double-blind trials. *Am J Obstet Gynecol* 1977;127:818-823.
25. Anderson ABM, Gillebaud J, Haynes PJ, et al. Reduction of menstrual blood-loss by prostaglandin synthetase inhibitors. *Lancet* 1976;1:774-776.
26. Roy S, Shaw ST. Role of prostaglandins in IUD-associated uterine bleeding—effect of a pros- taglandin synthetase inhibitor (ibuprofen). *Obstet Gynecol* 1981;58:101-106.
27. Hillier K, Kasonde JM. Prostaglandin E and F concentrations in human endometrium after insertion of intrauterine contraceptive device. *Lancet* 1976;1:15-16.
28. Ulmsten U. Uterine activity and blood flow. In: Dawood MY, Demers LM, McGuire JL, eds. *Premenstrual syndrome and dysmenorrhea.* Baltimore: Urban and Schwarzenberg, 1985;103- 124.

Advances in Pain Research and Therapy, Vol. 18.
edited by M. Max, R. Portenoy, and E. Laska,
Raven Press, Ltd., New York © 1991.

20

Pediatric Analgesic Trials

Charles B. Berde

*Pain Treatment Service, Children's Hospital, Boston, Massachusetts 02115;
and Departments of Anaesthesia and Pediatrics, Harvard Medical School,
Boston, Massachusetts 02115*

Surveys indicate that infants and children frequently receive inadequate analgesia following surgery or trauma (1–3). A contributing factor is the paucity of controlled trials of analgesic agents in children until the last 5 years. Analgesic trials in children pose a distinct set of difficulties (Table 1). Each of these difficulties is, in principle, surmountable, but requires specific modifications of design and practice relative to trials employed for adults.

INFORMED CONSENT

Most adults are capable of understanding the risks and benefits of an analgesic trial and can give informed consent for clinical trials. For minors, parental informed consent is required. It remains important that children receive age-appropriate instruction regarding what will occur during the study. Most children ages 2 to 3 and older benefit from simple explanation of medical procedures, and most children ages 7 and above appear to understand basic concepts related to clinical trials.

In general, although parents give "consent" for clinical trials, it is strongly encouraged that pediatric patients give "assent," that is, that they be willing participants whenever possible.

For studies that involve some risk, it is generally required that both parents provide consent. Situations involving parental disagreement can be problematic, and often the advice of clinical investigation committees or legal counsel may be helpful.

Because of these problems with consent and age-related pharmacologic differences (see below), new analgesic agents are generally tested in children only after assessment of safety and efficacy has been performed in adults.

TABLE 1. *Problems with pediatric analgesic trials*

Problem	Possible solutions
Difficulties with informed consent	1. Parental informed consent (patient assent whenever possible) 2. Age-appropriate explanations
Age-related differences in pharmacokinetics and pharmacodynamics	1. Studies stratified for different age groups 2. Newborn animal testing for new drug classes to detect specific toxicities
Difficulties with pain assessment	1. VAS for ages 7 and above 2. Novel self-report scales for ages 3–7 (Faces, ACCS, Oucher, Poker Chip) 3. Behavioral scales for ages 3 and under 4. Correlation of behavioral and self-report measures in the 3–9-year-old age groups
Small population sizes	1. Multicenter trials 2. Initial studies on relatively large and uniform postoperative patients
Rapidly changing intensity of cancer pain	1. Study designs with short time courses 2. Multicenter trials

Difficulty with blood sampling
  Distress with venipuncture
  Small blood volume
  Difficulty finding veins
  Difficulty with repeated sampling from peripheral "heparin-locks"
	1. Enrollment among patients with central lines required for surgery, cancer therapy, or intensive care
	2. Placement of venous or arterial lines while patients are receiving general anethesia
	3. Development of micromethods for plasma drug assay

AGE-RELATED PHARMACOLOGIC DIFFERENCES (4,5)

Pharmacokinetics (6)

For all of the opioids studied [including morphine (7–9), fentanyl (10–12), sufentanil (13), methadone (14), and alfentanil (15)], age-related differences in pharmacokinetics have been minor beyond the first 6 months of life. Toddlers and younger children generally clear opioids slightly faster than young adults.

Opioid clearance is variably diminished in the first weeks of life, owing to immaturity of either hepatic metabolism or renal clearance. For example, studies of morphine, fentanyl, and sufentanil kinetics in newborns show a diminished clearance and a prolonged elimination half-life. The immaturity of the blood-brain barrier may lead to increased entry of morphine into the brain in the first week of life (15). Immaturity of hepatic metabolism in infants may actually increase the therapeutic ratio for acetaminophen, since the production of a toxic metabolite is decreased. Rectal absorption of acetaminophen in infants is inconsistent, and doses of up to 20 mg/kg result in plasma levels below those regarded as therapeutic for adults.

Plasma elimination half-lives of the local anesthetics lidocaine and bupivacaine are prolonged in neonates. This effect is counterbalanced by larger volumes of distribution for local anesthetics in newborns.

Pharmacodynamics

Hemodynamic effects of opioids in newborns and young infants receiving assisted ventilation are mild or even beneficial (16,17). Opioids may be beneficial for critically ill newborns or newborns with cyanotic congenital heart disease, because they blunt harmful pulmonary vasoconstriction in response to noxious stimulation. Thus, infants receiving prolonged mechanical ventilation may receive opioids with a wide margin of safety, and (except in the case of uncontrolled hemorrhage or difficulty with establishing an airway) it is a rare critically ill infant who is "too sick" to receive opioids.

Opioids alter ventilatory responses to hypoxia and hypercarbia to some degree in patients of all ages (18). Newborns are commonly stated to be more "sensitive" to opioid-induced respiratory depression than older patients, and clinical experience would support this statement. Unmedicated newborns exhibit diminished ventilatory responses to hypoxemia and hypercarbia, and opioids appear to blunt these responses even further (19,20). Based on both kinetic and dynamic considerations, recommended morphine infusion rates (normalized for weight) for newborns following surgery are about $\frac{1}{4}$ those for older infants (8).

A study by Hertzka and coworkers (21) examined ventilatory depression (measured by incremental increases in transcutaneous carbon dioxide levels) as a function of plasma fentanyl level in infants, children, and adults following hernia repair. Infants above age 6 months showed no greater ventilatory depression than adults at any given plasma fentanyl level. In general, nonintubated infants under age 6 months should receive opioids with caution and only in circumstances that permit close observation and skilled intervention and airway management if needed. Beyond age 6 months, the average infant is probably able to tolerate opioids with infusion rates per kg similar to adults. Further studies are needed to establish population data on minimal effective analgesic concentrations for opioids in infants and children.

Epidural and subarachnoid opioids appear to be well tolerated and effective in infants and children (22–24). Clinical experience at a number of locations, including children's hospitals in Seattle, Philadelphia, Denver, Boston, and Milwaukee suggests that significant respiratory depression from epidural opioids is quite rare in children (25).

Nonsteroidal antiinflammatory drugs (26) have been used effectively for analgesia in children following surgery. Maunuksela and coworkers (27) showed that intravenous infusion of indomethacin reduced but did not eliminate the need for opioid analgesics postoperatively in children undergoing major surgery.

Local anesthetic pharmacodynamic studies in infants suggest that intermediate concentrations (e.g., bupivacaine 0.25%) may provide more intense surgical anesthesia and motor blockade in infants than in older patients. The duration of analgesia following caudal epidural blockade or peripheral nerve blockade with bupivacaine in young infants may be longer than in older children and adults (28,29). Prolonged epidural infusion of local anesthetics in children is an extremely effective and safe modality for major thoracoabdominal, pelvic, or lower extremity surgery (30,31). Hemodynamic effects tend to be extremely mild, and the technique is especially useful for children with respiratory insufficiency (31). Spinal anesthesia in neonates requires much larger doses than for older children and adults, e.g., for tetracaine, 0.8 mg/kg versus 0.25 mg/kg for hernia repair. In addition, the duration of spinal anesthesia is much shorter in infants than in adults (32,33).

Major peripheral nerve blocks or plexus blocks can be performed safely in anesthetized children with the aid of a peripheral nerve stimulator (33,34). For newborn circumcision, penile blockade has been shown to diminish behavioral, autonomic, and endocrine indices of nociception (35,36).

For children undergoing brief painful procedures, such as bone marrow aspiration, local anesthetic infiltration diminishes the pain of the procedure, but there is enormous anxiety and some discomfort related to the needle for skin infiltration. The topical/transdermal use of a eutectic mixture of local anesthetics (EMLA) lidocaine and prilocaine has been shown to be an extremely safe and effective method for skin or mucosal analgesia (37,38). Currently, this product is not available in the United States.

Developmental Toxicology (39)

Historically, several drugs that appeared safe for adults were associated with unforeseen toxicities in infants and children related to critical phases in organ development. For example, tetracyline, which is quite benign for most adults, alters the progression of mineral deposition in tooth development, leading to discoloration and abnormal growth. There is inevitably a concern when new drugs are advanced that they will produce toxicities not apparent from adult testing. There is therefore a need for (a) careful testing in realistic young animal models, (b) judicious application of new drugs for children, and (c) careful record keeping and recording of adverse outcomes.

Concerns regarding toxicities are particularly important in evaluation of the long-term administration of analgesics for chronic nonmalignant pain syndromes. For example, in weighing the risks and benefits of prophylactic medications for migraine, such as anticonvulsants, there needs to be evaluation of the chronic toxicities of these agents, including subtle neurobehavioral effects. These factors can be difficult to assess in individual patients, since there may certainly be behavioral consequences of long-term untreated pain as well.

ASSESSMENT OF PAIN AND RELATED SYMPTOMS (40–52)

In any analgesic trial, assessment of endpoints, including pain intensity, patient satisfaction, and side effects are crucial factors. Pain intensity is routinely assessed in adults using self-report measures, such as visual analogue scales (VAS).

Experience in children suggests that children ages 7 and above can routinely perform VAS ratings, and some investigators have used VAS ratings from ages 5 to 6 and above (40). Other self-report scales based on pictures or drawings of faces, a color intensity slide rule, poker chips, etc., have been investigated and found to be useful for children ages 3 to 7. Nevertheless, some of these scales require some training to administer, and have significant problems with some 3- and 4-year-olds. Because of their fear of hospital experience in general and of injections in particular, it is important that the child's scores not be linked (either in fact or in the child's mind) to receiving intramuscular injections.

Behavioral measures have been widely advocated to permit pain assessment in younger children. Certain scales have been developed specifically for painful procedures, and others are commonly employed for postoperative pain assessment. Advantages of behavioral scales include: (a) applicability to all ages, including infants, (b) lack of dependence on patient cooperation, and (c) good inter-rater reliability.

Behavioral scales nevertheless have several problems. Most importantly, despite efforts to discriminate pain from fear or anxiety, many of these scales score fear and anxiety as well as pain. (That is to say, if points are scored for "crying behavior," crying owing to fear will be rated along with crying owing to pain.) For this reason, some of the scales are called "distress" scales. This has important ramifications for analgesic studies, however. For example, administration of a benzodiazepine such as midazolam prior to a procedure [e.g., a lumbar puncture or computed tomography (CT) scan] will diminish distress scores, although there is little basis to regard midazolam as an analgesic. In addition, although some children react to acute pain with behavioral arousal including crying and writhing, in other circumstances, children respond to acute or chronic pain by withdrawal and behavioral inhibition. Stated another way, a child may lie motionless in bed because it hurts to move, and "tuning out" is his way of reacting to pain. In a recent analgesic trial with children ages 3 to 7 undergoing major surgery, Beyer et al. (53) found very little correlation between CHEOPS (45) scores and two self-report measures, the Oucher (41,42) and the ACCS (44). Conversely, the two self-report measures correlated with each other very well. In particular, it was common for patients to have CHEOPS scores interpreted as very low pain intensity with patients reporting moderate pain. In a recent trial of epidural analgesic regimens in children, there was a lesser degree of disparity between a different combined behavioral-physiologic measure (the "Objective Pain Scale" developed by Hannallah, Rice, and Broadman [49]) and the Oucher (manuscript in preparation). Again, behavioral scores rated lower pain intensities than self-report measures.

Other scales applied to young infants involve precise observation of facial expression (50) using videotapes and spectral analysis of crying (51). These methods are promising, though they require sophisticated techniques that are not as easily applied in routine daily practice.

Behavioral responses to pain may also vary considerably with age. For example, it is a common pattern for very young infants postoperatively to lie relatively immobile with a stiff posture, elbow flexion, and clenched fists.

Physiologic measures of pain intensity have been used most prominantly to assess the responses of newborns (and subsequently, older children) to surgery under general or regional anesthesia (35,36,52). Although useful for showing trends in highly structured situations, it is apparent that parameters such as heart rate and blood pressure can be influenced by an enormous variety of conditions in addition to pain. Hormonal and metabolic measures of stress, including plasma catecholamines, cortisol, and beta-endorphin–like immunoreactivity, have been used to assess the responses of infants and older children undergoing major surgery.

Assessment of associated symptoms such as nausea and pruritus can also be difficult in younger children. The usual approach is to have observers rate episodes of emesis or frequency of scratching behaviors.

DIFFICULTIES RELATED TO BLOOD SAMPLING

Whereas adults usually mildly dislike venipuncture for blood sampling, for many children the procedure can be profoundly distressing. Venous access can be difficult, particularly in younger children and children with chronic illnesses. Although an antecubital vein or a forearm vein can often permit repeated blood sampling via a heparin-locked cannula in older children and adults, it is often difficult to draw blood from a heparin lock in infants with small veins.

The small blood volume of infants also constrains blood sampling for analgesic trials. Commonly, it is required that clinical investigations remove no more than 5% of the estimated blood volume over a period of hours to days. For a 2 kg premature newborn, estimated blood volume is 95 cc/kg $\times$ 2 kg = about 190 cc. (Blood volume per kg decreases with advancing age to reach the adult value of 70 cc/kg by about 10 years of age.) Thus a total of 9.5 cc would be permitted for a complete study. For studies to determine pharmacokinetic parameters related to distribution and elimination phases, 15 or more plasma samples are usually required, and thus each sample would be constrained to be no more than about 0.6 cc. Thus, it becomes important for pediatric studies to employ micromethods for measurement of drug concentrations.

For these reasons, it is common to perform pharmacokinetic studies in children who require central venous or arterial catheters for reasons related to anesthesia, surgery, cancer therapy, and intensive care. Since anesthesia and abdominal surgery may transiently alter hepatic and renal blood flow, pharmacokinetic estimates for drugs whose clearances are flow limited may be erroneous unless care is taken to avoid these perturbations.

Similarly, obtaining renal clearances of drugs becomes more difficult in children who are not yet toilet trained or who have no medical indication for bladder catheterization; "urine bags" frequently become dislodged. "Spot" clearances using drug/creatinine ratios are often convenient approximations in clinical practice.

PROBLEMS RELATED TO POPULATION SIZES
AND ENROLLMENT

Although pain is common in childhood cancer (54), cancer is much less common in children than in adults. For major pediatric oncology centers, it is typical to have serious disease-related pain problems occurring for only about 10 to 40 patients each year. These patients are distributed over a broad range of ages, and have widely differing diagnoses and pain mechanisms. In experience in our pain clinic, although leukemia is the commonest cancer, the major population of pediatric oncology patients referred for difficult pain problems are the patients with sarcomas, especially osteosarcoma. Thus, it appears likely that clinical trials of analgesics, adjuvants, or other techniques in pediatric cancer disease-related pain may require multicenter trials.

Brief painful and/or terrifying medical procedures are a major part of the therapy of many childhood illnesses. In therapy of malignancies, especially leukemias, children receive repeated lumbar punctures and bone marrow aspirations and biopsies. A number of sedative and analgesic regimens have been effective in reducing the distress of these procedures (55). Further research should examine the relative safety and efficacy of different regimens. Assessment of efficacy should be multifaceted, and might include (a) degree of distress and "operating conditions" during the procedure; (b) measurement of parameters pertaining to respiration, such as oxygen saturation or respiratory rate; (c) speed of wake up and duration of loss of protective reflexes; (d) incidence of side effects including nausea and dysphoria; and (e) psychological assessments related to subsequent anxiety over procedures.

Although dental pain models have become standard in adults undergoing extraction of molars, advances in pediatric dentistry have made painful extractions a less common occurrence among younger children, and there is no analogous painful dental procedure commonly required for children that can serve as an equivalent model.

Enrollment of pediatric patients in postoperative analgesic trials is somewhat easier, particularly at children's hospitals with busy surgical services. Postoperative pain in children is probably the most versatile model for study of analgesic medications, since it is feasible to identify populations with relatively uniform types of tissue injury and a predictable time course of acute pain (56). The most commonly studied patients for pediatric postoperative trials have traditionally been children undergoing orthopedic operations (posterior spine fusion and instrumentation for scoliosis, hip and femur osteotomies, club foot repairs, etc.) and urologic operations (hypospadius repair, ureteral reimplantation, orchidopexy). Orthopedic and urologic trials have several advantages: (a) much of the surgery is painful and extensive but nonemergent, and is performed on otherwise healthy children; (b) children of broad age ranges come for these operations; (c) since the gastrointestinal tract is not involved, surgical influences on emesis and ileus postoperatively are minor; (d) most patients can take oral analgesics by the first postoperative day, when pain is still substantial; and (e) many patients need to remain hospitalized for surgical reasons for several days, so that prolonged studies can be accomplished in the hospital. Inguinal hernia repair is probably the most feasible general surgical procedure to study, although methods of assessing pain in outpatients are more cumbersome. Lateral thoracotomies and abdominal explorations in children are often performed in the setting of significant systemic disease. Pectus excavatum repairs are painful and have been used recently in a trial of patient-controlled analgesia. Tonsillectomies are commonly performed and could be a useful model for the study of oral analgesics postoperatively.

TIME COURSE OF PAIN IN CHILDHOOD CANCER

It is common for adults with metastatic cancer and pain to have relatively slow progression of disease and slowly varying degrees of nociceptive input for periods of months. Childhood cancer generally has a different natural history than adult cancer. Primary cancer therapy, especially chemotherapy and radiation therapy, serves as a major pain treatment modality. Thus, for many children, cancer pain varies rapidly in intensity. It may improve rapidly with effective chemotherapy or it may progress exponentially with untreatable end-stage disease. The practical implication of this is that it may be more difficult to perform trials with crossover designs or that require prolonged periods of drug administration. Most analgesic trials in disease-related pediatric cancer pain have not employed double-blind, randomized, or crossover assignments. Open trials have suggested that oral opioids can be used for children with cancer with good success and a low side effect profile (57) in most circumstances.

CONCLUSIONS

Although there are certain age-related differences and difficulties in the conduct of pediatric analgesic trials, these problems are not insurmountable. There is a need for increased funding of pediatric trials and for greater effort in this area.

REFERENCES

1. Beyer J, DeGood DE, Ashley LC, Russell GA. Patterns of postoperative analgesic use with adults and children following cardiac surgery. *Pain* 1983;17:71–81.
2. Eland JM, Anderson JE. The experience of pain in children. In: Jacox AK, ed. *Pain—a source book for nurses.* Boston: Little, Brown, 1977;453–473.
3. Schechter NL, Allen DA, Hanson K. The status of pediatric pain control: a comparison of hospital analgesic use in children and adults. *Pediatrics* 1986;77:11–15.
4. Shannon M, Berde CB. Pharmacologic management of pain in children and adolescents. *Pediatr Clin North Am* 1989;36:855–871.
5. Roberts RJ. *Drug therapy in infants.* Philadelphia: WB Saunders, 1984.
6. Morselli PL, Franco-Morselli R, Bossi L. Clinical pharmacokinetics in newborns and infants: age-related differences and therapeutic implications. *Clin Pharmacokinet* 1980;5:485–527.

7. Dahlstrom B, Bolme P, Feychting H, Noack G, Paalzow L. Morphine kinetics in children. *Clin Pharmacol Ther* 1979;453:365.
8. Koren G, Butt W, Chinyanga H, Soldin S, Tan YK, Pape K. Postoperative morphine infusion in newborn infants: assessment of disposition characteristics and safety. *J Pediatr* 1985;107:963–967.
9. Lynn AM, Slattery JT. Morphine pharmacokinetics in early infancy. *Anesthesiology* 1987;66: 136–139.
10. Johnson KL, Erickson JP, Halley FD, Scott JC. Pharmacokinetics of fentanyl in the pediatric population. *Anesthesiology* 1984;61:1441.
11. Koehntop D, Rodman J, Brundage D, Hegland M, Buckley J. Pharmacokinetics of fentanyl in neonates. *Anesthesiology* 1984;61(3A):A449.
12. Collins C, Koren G, Crean P, et al. Fentanyl pharmacokinetics and hemodynamic effects in preterm infants during ligation of patent ductus arteriosus. *Anesth Analg* 1985;64:1078–1080.
13. Greeley WJ, de Bruijn NP, David DP. Sufentanil pharmacokinetics in pediatric cardiovascular patients. *Anesth Analg* 1987;66:1067–1072.
14. Berde CB, Sethna NF, Holzman RS, Reidy P, Gondek E. Pharmacokinetics of methadone in children and adolescents in the perioperative period. *Anesthesiology* 1987;67:A519.
15. Meistelman C, St-Maurice C, Loose JP, Levron JC. Pharmacokinetics of alfentanil in children. *Anesthesiology* 1984;61(3A):A443.
16. Hickey PR, Hansen DD, Wessel DL, Lange P, Jonas RA, Elixson EM. Blunting of stress responses in the pulmonary circulation of infants by fentanyl. *Anesth Analg* 1985;64:1137–1142.
17. Anand KJS, Hickey PR. Pain and its effects on the human neonate and fetus. *N Engl J Med* 1987;317:1321–1329.
18. Weil JV, McCullough RE, Kline JS, Sodal IF. Diminished ventilatory response to hypoxia and hypercarbia after morphine in normal man. *N Engl J Med* 1975;292:1103–1106.
19. Way WL, Costley EC, Way EL. Respiratory sensitivity of the newborn infant to meperidine and morphine. *Clin Pharmacol Ther* 1965;6:454–461.
20. Mitchell AA, Louik C, Lacouture PG, Slone D, Goldman P, Shapiro S. Risks to children from computed tomographic scan premedication. *JAMA* 1982;247:2385–2388.
21. Hertzka RE, Gauntlett IS, Fisher DM, Spellman MJ. Fentanyl-induced ventilatory depression: effects of age. *Anesthesiology* 1989;70:213–218.
22. Attia J, Ecoffey C, Sandouk P, et al. Epidural morphine in children: pharmacokinetics and CO_2 sensitivity. *Anesthesiology* 1986;65:590–594.
23. Benlabed M, Ecoffey C, Levron JC, et al. Analgesia and ventilatory response to CO_2 following epidural sufentanyl in children. *Anesthesiology* 1987;67:948–951.
24. Glenski JA, Warner MA, Dawson B, Kaufman B. Postoperative use of epidurally administered morphine in children and adolescents. *Mayo Clin Proc* 1984;59:530–533.
25. Berde CB, Sethna NF, Levin L, Retik A, Millis M, Lillehei C, Micheli L. Regional analgesia on pediatric medical and surgical wards. *Intensive Care Med* 1989;15:S40–S43.
26. Brewer EJ, Arrovo I. Use of non-steroidal anti-inflammatory drugs in children. *Pediatr Ann* 1986;15:575–581.
27. Maunuksela EL, Olkkola KT, Korpela R. Does prophylactic intravenous infusion of indomethacin improve the management of postoperative pain in children? *Can J Anesth* 1988;35(2):123–127.
28. Warner MA, Kunkel SE, Atchison SR, Dawson B. The effects of age, epinephrine, and operative site on duration of caudal analgesia in pediatric patients. *Anesth Analg* 1988;66:995–998.
29. Blaise G, Roy WL. Postoperative pain relief after hypospadias repair in pediatric patients: regional analgesia versus systemic analgesics. *Anesthesiology* 1986;65:84–86.
30. Desparmet J, Meistelman C, Barre J, Saint-Maurice C. Continuous epidural infusion of bupivacaine for postoperative pain relief in children. *Anesthesiology* 1987;67:108–110.
31. Meignier M, Souron R, Leneel J. Postoperative dorsal epidural analgesia in the child with respiratory disabilities. *Anesthesiology* 1983;59(5):473–475.
32. Abajian JC, Mellish RWP, Browne AF, Perkins FM, Lambert DH, Mazuzan JE Jr. Spinal anesthesia for surgery in the high-risk infant. *Anesth Analg* 1984;63:359–362.
33. Sethna NF, Berde CB. Pediatric regional anesthesia. In: Gregory G, ed. *Pediatric anesthesia.* New York: Churchill-Livingstone, 1989;647–678.
34. Dalens B. Regional anesthesia in children. *Anesth Analg* 1989;68:654–720.
35. Stang HJ, Gunnar RM, Snellman L, Condon LM, Kestenbaum R. Local anesthesia for neonatal circumcision. Effects on distress and cortisol response. *JAMA* 1988;259(10):1507–1511.

36. Williamson PS, Williamson ML. Physiologic stress reduction by a local anesthetic during newborn circumcision. *Pediatrics* 1973;71:36–40.
37. Maunuksela EL, Korpela R. Double-blind evaluation of a lignocaine-prilocaine cream (EMLA) in children. Effect on the pain associated with cenous cannulation. *Br J Anaesth* 1986;58:1242–1245.
38. Halperin DL, Koren G, Attias D, Pellegrini E, Greenberg ML, Wyss M. Topical skin anesthesia for venous, subcutaneous drug reservoir and lumbar punctures in children. *Pediatrics* 1989;84:281–284.
39. Blumer JL, Reed MD. *Pediatric toxicology. Pediatr Clin North Am,* Vol. 33(2). Philadelphia: WB Saunders, 1986.
40. McGrath PA. An assessment of children's pain: a review of behavioral, physiological and direct scaling techniques. *Pain* 1989;31:147–176.
41. Beyer JE. *The Oucher: a user's manual and technical report.* Evanston, Illinois: The Hospital Play Equipment Co., 1984.
42. Beyer JE, Aradine CR. Content validity of an instrument to measure young children's perceptions of the intensity of their pain. *J Pediatr Nurse* 1986;1:386–395.
43. Maunuksela EL, Olkkola KT, Korpela R. Measurement of pain in children with self-reporting and behavioral assessment. *Clin Pharmacol Ther* 1987;37:589–596.
44. Grossi E, Borghi C, Cerchiari EL, et al. Analogue chromatic continuous scale [ACCS]: a new method for pain assessment. *Clin Exp Rheumatol* 1983;1:337–340.
45. McGrath PJ, Johnson G, Goodman JT, Schillinger J, Dunn J, Chapman J. The CHEOPS: a behavioral scale to measure postoperative pain in children. In: Fields HL, Dubner R, Cervero F, eds. *Advances in pain research and therapy.* New York: Raven Press, 1985:395–402.
46. Hester N. The pre-operational child's reaction to immunization. *Nurs Res* 1979;28:250–255.
47. Attia J, Amiel-Tison C, Mayer MN, Barrier G. Measurement of postoperative pain and narcotic administration in infants using a new clinical scoring system. *Anesthesiology* 1987;66:A532.
48. Ross DM, Ross SA. The importance of type of question, psychological climate and subject set in interviewing children about pain. *Pain* 1984;19:71–79.
49. Broadman LM, Rice LJ, Hannallah RS. Testing the validity of an objective pain scale for infants and children. *Anesthesiology* 1988;69:A770.
50. Grunau RVE, Craig KD. Pain expression in neonates: facial action and cry. *Pain* 1987;28:395–410.
51. Johnston CC, O'Shaughnessy D. Acoustical attributes of infant pain cries: discriminating features. In: *Proceedings of the Vth World Congress on Pain.* Elsevier Science Publisher, 1988;336–340.
52. Anand KJS, Sippell WG, Aynsley-Green A. A randomised trial of fentanyl anaesthesia in preterm neonates undergoing surgery: effects on the stress response. *Lancet* 1987;1:243–248.
53. Beyer JE, McGrath PJ, Berde CB. Behavioral responses to postoperative pain in 3–7 year olds. *Pain Supplement* 1990;5:S33.
54. Miser AW, Dothage JA, Wesley M, Miser JS. The prevalence of pain in a pediatric and young adult cancer population. *Pain* 1987;29:73–83.
55. Zeltzer L, Jay S, Fisher D. The management of pain associated with pediatric procedures. *Pediatr Clin North Am* 1989;36:4.
56. Berde CB. Pediatric postoperative pain management. *Pediatr Clin North Am* 1989;36:921–940.
57. Pichard-Leandri E, Poulain PH, Gauvain-Piquard A. Evaluation of the side effects related to long term opioid treatment in cancer pain children. *Pain Supplement* 1990;5:S8.

DISCUSSION

Ada Rogers: I agree with Dr. Charles Berde's assessment of the problems in conducting clinical analgesic trials. His recommendations and possible solutions as outlined in Table 1 are excellent guidelines. However, I would like to add a few recommendations.

In designing studies in children, placebo should be avoided. Parents will not agree for their children to participate in analgesic studies if a placebo is one of the test medications. Instead of the placebo, a lower and upper dosage of the test and standard medication may be used. Every effort should be made to use double-blind, randomized, and crossover design in analgesic trials. In this way, the patient serves as his own control. Even in postoperative analgesic studies, a 2-day study could be done by selecting those children undergoing surgical procedures where pain will persist for at least 2 days. We should discourage the use of intramuscular or subcutaneously administered analgesics either clinically or in studies, thus diminishing one of the fears children experience.

Very few studies have been done in children to determine relative potencies of nonopioid and opioid analgesics and the safety of intravenously administered opioid analgesics. Until this is done, clinicians will continue to undermedicate the pediatric patient.

Advances in Pain Research and Therapy, Vol. 18,
edited by M. Max, R. Portenoy, and E. Laska,
Raven Press, Ltd., New York © 1991.

21

Spinal Opioids
in Acute and Chronic Pain

Michael J. Cousins and John L. Plummer

*Department of Anaesthesia and Intensive Care, Flinders University of South Australia,
Flinders Medical Centre, Bedford Park, South Australia 5042*

DESIGN OF STUDIES OF OPIOIDS

Clinical Background

Most rigorously controlled studies to date have been carried out in *postoperative patients.* Presently there is almost a total lack of definitive evidence in *cancer patients* of comparative efficacy, side effects, and other information fundamental to rational clinical use (1). A few preliminary descriptive studies in cancer pain (2) and chronic noncancer pain (3) have raised the possibility that spinal opioids can be used to diagnose etiology (3) and guide subsequent treatment. In postoperative patients, there is the problem of decreasing pain over time, whereas in cancer the disease process and the pain may increase in severity over time.

Study Designs: General Considerations

Placebo Controls

Use of a placebo-only treatment is inappropriate in most spinal opioid studies. Ample evidence exists for the efficacy of spinal opioids, and hence comparative studies should aim to demonstrate relative efficacy compared to some alternative treatment.

Outcome Measures

Outcome measures suitable for analgesic studies have been discussed by Max and Laska (Chapter 4). As spinal analgesia is associated with many outcomes (e.g., maximum pain relief, duration of relief, side effects, patient satisfaction), it usually will be necessary to make a number of measurements to assess the overall treatment effects.

Crossover Versus Parallel-Group Designs

Some relative merits and drawbacks of crossover compared to parallel-group studies have been discussed by Max and Laska (Chapter 4). In crossover studies, each patient receives each treatment under study on different occasions. Statistical tests of treatment effects are then based on the within-subject variation, rather than on the among-subject variation as in parallel-group (completely randomized) designs (4). The large among-subject variability in pain reporting and response to opioids provides a strong motivation for use of crossover designs in analgesic studies. However, there are many circumstances in which crossover designs are inappropriate; these designs have often been used without proper consideration being given to their drawbacks (5–8). These drawbacks include the changing state of the subjects between treatment periods, the necessity for a washout interval between treatments, and the possibility of carryover effects, that is, the effects of a treatment being influenced by previous treatments. Furthermore, the power of a completely randomized design can be greatly increased by using baseline data, e.g., baseline pain score, as a covariate; this has the effect of removing some of the among-patient variability. Baseline data cannot be used in the same way in a crossover design.

The changing state of subjects in the study has different implications for postoperative and cancer pain. It is important to distinguish between "randomly" changing state and change that follows some fixed pattern. The former might occur over a relatively short period (e.g., several days) in cancer patients; that is, their pain or responsiveness to opioids may fluctuate without following any obvious pattern. This reduces the power of the crossover design, as within-subject variation is increased, but does not introduce bias. In contrast, postoperative pain has a larger component of change following a pattern. James et al. (4) found that pain relief due to analgesics increased with time since surgery, and suggested that this was because of diminution of the underlying pain. This again does not necessarily introduce bias, though it is of course necessary that subjects have sufficient pain to assess analgesic effects. The effects of such trends, averaged over patients, may be separated in the analysis and are usually known as period effects.

Determination of a suitable washout interval in spinal opiate studies poses major problems. To minimize carryover effects, we wish to make the washout interval as long as possible. However, this would leave the subjects in pain, as well as increasing the likelihood of changes in the level of pain. In the case of systemic opioids, known pharmacokinetic data can be used to estimate the minimum time that should be allowed between treatments; however, there is little data available regarding kinetics of spinal analgesics. Often the second treatment is given when the pain score returns to the baseline value. However, in some patients, especially in the postoperative setting, pain may not return to that level. This is particularly likely if a score with a high level of discrimination, such as a visual analogue pain score, is used. An alternative is to take as a criterion, after an interval sufficient to allow onset of treatment effect, two consecutive scores within, say, 15% of the baseline separated by 15 min.

In determining a washout interval, the likelihood and consequences of carryover effects should be taken into consideration. If carryover effects are likely to lead to bias in estimation of treatment effects, a long washout interval is preferable. However, in some cases carryover effects do not introduce bias (see below) and a lengthy washout is not necessary. The problems caused by carryover effects depend on whether two or more than two treatments are being compared.

Two-Period Crossover Design

In a two-period crossover design, usually, half the subjects receive two treatments (A and B) in one sequence (e.g., AB), and the other half receive them in the reverse sequence (BA). This allows estimation of treatment effects (mean difference in effect of treatments A and B), as well as period effects (difference in effect of receiving a treatment first or second). If both treatments have the same carryover effects, then these effects are absorbed into the period effects and do not bias estimation of treatment effects (8). In some spinal analgesia studies, it might be reasonable to assume this is the case. For example, if two opioids of similar duration of action are being compared, it is likely that any carryover effects will be similar. However, if a long-acting and a short-acting opioid (e.g., morphine and fentanyl), or two different dose levels of the same opioid, are being compared, carryover effects are likely to differ. Grizzle (9) showed that a test of equality of carryover effects could be made. If these are found to be unequal, then data from only the first period can be analyzed as a completely randomized design. However, Brown (8) showed that the test of equality of carryover effects does not have sufficient power to reliably detect differences large enough to lead to substantial bias. This has led to a number of authors recommending that two-period crossover designs be employed only when it is reasonable to assume the absence, or at least equality, of carryover effects (7,8). In some cases, particularly in cancer pain, equality of carryover effects can be assured by allowing a lengthy washout period, but providing bridging analgesia. The carryover effects of the treatment would then be negligible; effects of the bridging analgesia may carry over into the second treatment period but, being the same for all patients, would not lead to bias in estimation of treatment effects.

The two-period crossover design thus appears useful in assessment of spinal analgesia in cancer pain, but careful consideration should be given to the likelihood of unequal carryover effects before applying it to studies in postoperative pain.

Crossover Designs for More than Two Treatments

Crossover designs for more than two treatments differ from the two-period design in an important aspect. Designs in which each treatment follows each of the others the same number of times allow unbiased estimation of treatment effects even when carryover effects of the treatments differ (10). Carryover effects of any particular treatment are assumed to be independent of which treatment follows it, and considered to persist only into the immediately following period. Dropout rates tend to be high in multiple treatment crossover analgesic studies (4,11) but this is more than offset by the precision offered by these designs where they are appropriate. These designs appear especially suited to studies in cancer patients, but may also have application in postoperative pain studies when treatment effects do not have a long duration.

Study of "Selectivity" of Spinal Opioids

The spinal route would seem to offer little to patients unless it can be shown that it is more efficacious and at least as safe, but preferably safer, than existing and other recently developed methods [e.g., patient-controlled analgesia (PCA)]. In our opinion, this hinges on obtaining various types of data that combine to address the question of "selectivity" of the analgesia of spinal opiates alone, or in combination with agents that have additive or supraadditive effects with spinal opioids (1). Too few studies are designed on the basis of this question: Is this method of spinal opiate administration more selective than the "standard" method used for comparison? How can "selectivity" be studied in the clinical setting?

Selectivity of Blockade of Pain Compared to Sensory, Motor, and Sympathetic Neural Function

This form of selectivity is probably least in question when spinal opiates are used alone; however, tests of selectivity become important when nonopioid drugs are combined with opioids. Clinical tests that are reasonably simple include tests of sensory function (pin prick, etc.), motor function (e.g., Bromage scale), sympathetic function (skin temperature, laser-doppler, sympathogalvanic response, ice response, plethysmography, cobalt blue sweat tests, etc.) (12), blood pressure and heart rate responses to pressor stimuli, and postural changes (1). Motor function can be studied in a more sophisticated manner by objective testing of force of muscle contraction by variations of the force transducer concept. Motor function can also be studied by measuring monosynaptic stretch reflexes (opioids had no effect in one study) and polysynaptic flexion reflexes (suppression) (13,14). Sensitive tests of effects of "toxic doses of opiates" on motor function are needed, e.g., early indices of motor rigidity and localized seizures.

Selectivity of Blockade of Pain with Respect to Effects on Other Systems

Cardiovascular System

Few studies have investigated effects of pain relief by spinal opioids on the high levels of sympathetic activity that may exist prior to pain relief; this is likely to explain some anecdotal reports that blood pressure is sometimes reduced following spinal opiates (15). In the absence of pain, "analgetic" doses of opiate given spinally do not result in cardiovascular depression (16), so this apparent paradox needs to be resolved.

It is possible that, as with local anesthetic epidural blockade, cardiac vagal activity may increase following administration of spinal opioids. Cardiac vagal activity has been studied in dogs but not in humans (17).

When alpha-adrenergic agonists are added to spinal opioids, studies of cardiac function and peripheral resistance become critical, since such effects may limit the dose of the alpha-adrenergic agonist. Investigations should include blood pressure responses to posture, to Valsalva, and to cold pressor.

Gastrointestinal System

Gastric emptying (paracetamol absorption), volume of gastric aspirate (direct measurement), and gut motility (electroenterography) are all adversely affected by systemic opiates (16). Too little attention has been given to comparative studies of spinal opiates and alternative analgesic measures in fasted and fed patients. Such studies are important both for patients following surgery and for cancer patients, since interference with gut function as a result of systemic opioids is a problem in both situations.

Respiration

Such effects appear to be of minor concern in cancer pain. In postoperative pain, both *early* and *delayed* respiratory depression need to be studied under carefully controlled conditions:

1. Optimized doses of spinal opioids (see below).
2. Comparisons with optimized doses of other techniques (e.g., IM, IV, PCA, etc).
3. Measurements over a time course that includes the daytime and sleep periods, following multiple doses.

It seems likely that continuous recording of oxygenation (pulse oximetry), carbon dioxide (end tidal or transcutaneous CO_2), respiratory rate interval, and/ or other measures may be needed in combination rather than singly to give a reliable picture. Combining measurements of respiration with other indices, such as pupil size and level of consciousness, may be helpful. Such studies are among the most important in deciding the relative safety of spinal opioid (and possibly nonopioid) drugs.

Bladder Function

Volume-evoked micturition reflex, detrusor muscle tone, and bladder capacity are all reported to be diminished by spinal morphine, whereas urethral sphincter tone is increased. Such effects are proposed, but not proven, to be owing to vesicosphincter dysynergia, possibly by inhibition at a spinal level of postganglionic nerves to the urinary bladder (1).

It is puzzling that bladder effects of morphine are reported not to be dose related (18), but to be antagonized by naloxone (1). One study reported a hierarchy of bladder effects produced by various opioid ligands (1), but this has not been tested rigorously in a clinical setting. Such information is critical, since a major drawback of spinal opioids (and local anesthetics) in postoperative pain is urinary retention. This is viewed as a *contraindication* to their use by some surgeons, e.g., hip replacement surgery where bladder catheterization may result in infection. In cancer pain, the time course of development of tolerance to urinary bladder effects of spinal opiate has not been studied.

Anecdotal reports of a lesser incidence of bladder dysfunction following lipid soluble opioids [e.g., methadone, sufentanil, and fentanyl (19,20)] need to be rigorously investigated with randomized prospective controlled studies. Objective evaluation is also needed to confirm the efficacy of spinal opiates for bladder spasm (21) and for enuresis (22).

Nausea and Vomiting, and Pruritus

For postoperative pain, these "minor" side effects of spinal opiates have not been adequately studied with respect to their severity and frequency in comparison to other pain relief techniques. Also, the frequency and severity of such effects for different opiate drugs need to be studied.

Selectivity with Respect to Delivery of Drug to Cerebrospinal Fluid and Thence to Spinal Cord in Close Proximity to Site of Injection

Investigation of this aspect requires integrated studies of cerebrospinal fluid (CSF) concentrations of opioid at different levels of neuraxis, blood pharmacokinetics, and studies of opioid effects (1). Only a small number of studies have provided parallel pharmacokinetic and drug effect data (1) and very few studies have used such a design to compare different opiate drugs (Table 1).

TABLE 1. *Unanswered key issues in spinal opioids—pharmacodynamics*

Confirmation of predominant spinal site of action in humans after intrathecal and epidural administration of newly developed opioids.
Selection of opioid with best duration and efficacy/safety ratio for spinal administration.
Do subtherapeutic doses of nonopioid and opioid drugs have synergistic effects?
Role of peptides in selective spinal analgesia.
Role of nonopioid drugs in selective spinal analgesia.
Method of alternation of spinal opioid and nonopioid drugs to avoid tolerance.
Relationship between epidural-intrathecal opioid dose and oral-intramuscular dose after chronic treatment.
Rates of development of tolerance to opioids with chronic "top-ups" compared with continuous infusion of epidural-intrathecal opioids.
Efficacy of lumbar compared with thoracic injection of lipid-soluble opioids for pain originating above the lumbar region.
Efficacy, safety, and neuropathology of chronic intrathecal versus epidural administration.
Optimum volume and concentration of injectate.
Comparison of spinal opioids with current options, for example, with "on-demand" intravenous opioids, "continuous" opioid infusion, epidural local anesthetic infusion, transdermal opioid, and patient-controlled oral opioids in postoperative pain and cancer pain and subcutaneous opioid infusion in cancer pain.
Significance of multiplicative analgesic interaction between intraventricular and intrathecal morphine.

Indirect evidence indicates that truly "segmental analgesia" may be obtained by placing the epidural catheter close to the area of noxious input and injecting small doses of lipid soluble agents, e.g., fentanyl (23). In patients with chronic pain, lumbar epidural administration of fentanyl 1 μg/kg body weight was studied with respect to blood and CSF pharmacokinetics. CSF samples were obtained close to the site of injection and also far removed, at the C7-T1 level. Fentanyl appeared rapidly in lumbar CSF in high concentrations but was barely detectable in cervical CSF. Blood concentrations of fentanyl were low or undetectable when a sensitive and specific gas-liquid chromatography (GLC) assay was used. The CSF pharmacokinetic data are in keeping with prior animal data using the lipid soluble opioid methadone (24). They are in contrast to studies using hydrophilic (morphine, hydromorphone) and moderately lipophilic (meperidine) opioids; these drugs rapidly diffuse from the lumbar to cervical regions and achieve high concentrations far removed from the site of injection (25–27).

Further clinical studies of lipid soluble opioids are needed. For example, lumbar and thoracic level catheters could be compared for thoracotomy pain or for thoracic cancer pain with the thoracic catheter tip placed precisely in the center of the spinal cord segments associated with the painful area. Doses for both levels of administration could then be optimized and comparisons made of CSF opioid concentration at operative level, dose requirements, analgesic efficacy, and side effects. A double-blind randomized design would be most desirable.

A complex relationship between lipid solubility and CSF pharmacokinetics is emerging (28). Moderately high (but not very high) lipid solubility may favor spinal cord uptake at the expense of vascular uptake. A challenge here lies in the development of sensitive and selective assays for the potent opioids, such as fentanyl and sufentanil, thereby permitting measurement of low concentrations in blood and CSF.

In short, all comparative studies of opioid administration by various routes would benefit from pharmacokinetic data. Such data may help answer the question: Are the analgetic and other effects likely to be produced by drug borne to brain (in blood or CSF) or by drug acting predominantly at a spinal level?

Postoperative Pain: Critique of Current Approaches and Design Recommendations

Dose Variability

Because of the variability in dosage that has been documented in the clinical use of opiates by IM, IV, and PCA (29) methods, such variability should be investigated among and within patients following spinal opioid administration. Such studies should select a particular type of operation, e.g., thoracotomy or lower abdominal surgery, and standardize the "conditions of the study" as far as possible, including the surgeon, "anesthetic regimen," length of surgery, patient factors, etc. These data on "effective doses" will help to impress clinicians with the need to titrate doses in individual patients by careful observation of effects and side effects.

Dose-Response Relationships

A small number of studies have shown a rather gross dose-response relationship for morphine analgesia after either intrathecal or epidural administration (30–32). However, the methodology was crude, employing a range of "best guess" dosages; usually there was no analgesia at low doses and analgesia at several high doses, which showed little dependence on dose. Certainly, no rigorous attempt has been made to determine ED_{50} or ED_{99} for satisfactory pain relief. This could be attempted with the shorter acting drugs, such as fentanyl, by using step increments and decrements among a patient population in infusion rate. Also the statistical method of "up-down" described by Dixon (33) could be employed to help determine the ED_{50} and its confidence interval.

It should be acknowledged that current data in humans point to a rather steep dose-response curve followed by a plateau with respect to analgesic *efficacy* (30,31). The aim, therefore, should be to define minimum effective analgesic dose (MEAD) in nontolerant patients as a reference point among opioids.

In contrast, the relationship between dose and duration of analgesia seems easier to define (34,35). However, the increasing emphasis on infusion techniques and concerns that large bolus doses increase side effects suggest that information relating dose increments with duration of effect is irrelevant once a minimum effective dose has been defined.

Margin of Safety

Margin of safety in nontolerant patients between MEAD and the dose associated with defined toxic effects requires clear definition for spinal opiates compared to other routes of administration (36). Methodological problems have previously prevented a rigorous approach to this issue. For example, there are currently no clear data about the incidence and severity of adverse respiratory effects associated with intramuscular opioids. As indicated previously, continuous monitoring over 24-hr periods is now possible using measurements relevant to clinical management.

Methods to assess *neuropsychological sequelae* have also been developed to help document neurotoxicity in association with opioid administration by various routes (37). Such tests can detect the following:

1. *Changes in processing of information.* "Choice reaction time" may reflect CNS impairment whereas "simple reaction time" may indicate either slowed neural transmission of information or impaired attention (37).
2. *Sustained attention and memory.* The "trail-making test" is probably an indicator of impaired brain function, but is a nonspecific measure, whereas the "Paced Auditory Serial Addition Task" (PASAT) is a sensitive indicator of sustained attention and memory (38).
3. *Discrete tests of memory,* e.g., immediate memory for digits and reversed digits (37).

In any attempts to document neuropsychological sequelae a range of tests should be used, particularly when the mechanism is unknown. Also, tests should be employed that permit repeated evaluation during multiple-dose studies, thereby documenting the time course of effects (37). Randomized, prospective controlled design is important in these assessments. Finally, neuropsychological effect and in particular effect of the underlying medical condition or treatment (e.g., those associated with cardiac surgery or cancer) must also be evaluated as an independent factor that may influence outcome. Unfortunately, the few studies reported to date have suffered from at least some design problems (39,40).

Some attempts to document neuropsychological sequelae have been crude and have contributed little to defining the "margin of safety." Such methods have included visual analogue and other scales of "sedation," "confusion," etc. All relied on the patients assessment of their own state and lacked evidence of sensitivity and construct validity. Other validated tests are required, such as those described above. Another possibility is the use of standardized conditions for measurement of pupil size and pupil reaction to light stimulus. This shows promise of giving an indication of significant opiate effects on brain.

Comparison of Spinal Route and Systemic Route

Currently available studies can be largely described as comparisons between a defined technique of spinal opioid and an ill-defined and often suboptimal systemic opioid method (e.g., IM, IV). Studies can be improved by the use of double-blind design, crossover, and a "double dummy" approach, e.g., simultaneous epidural and IV, IM (41), or subcutaneous routes so that the patient always receives treatment by both routes and is unaware which route is active (Fig. 1).

The key to comparative studies is the use of "optimally effective" regimens for the spinal and systemic methods. Thus a vigorous "optimization period" is required for both methods prior to the study period. Although optimization can be guided by data on the safety margin, it relies on titration, probably using

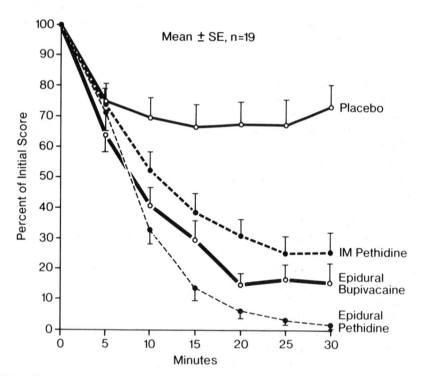

FIG. 1. Example of double-blind, within-patient "double dummy" crossover study of epidural (EPI) and intramuscular (IM) administration of the opioid drug meperidine. Control injections of saline and bupivacaine were also made. Each patient had an epidural catheter as well as an intramuscular butterfly insert. Each patient received four treatment regimens: (1) IM saline + EPI saline; (2) IM meperidine + EPI saline; (3) EPI bupivacaine + IM saline; and (4) EPI meperidine + IM saline. In this example of the data from the study, the mean pain scores are expressed as a percentage of pretreatment scores over the first 30 min. Each treatment is labeled according to the active ingredient, e.g., "placebo" = IM saline + EPI saline; IM meperidine (pethidine) = IM meperidine + EPI saline. (Reproduced with permission from ref 41.)

infusion and a predetermined rationale for increases and decreases in rate of infusion. A problem lies in providing convincing data that optimization did indeed occur. For example, if analgesia was suboptimal, should dosage be pushed until documented side effects occur (e.g., signs of neuropsychological impairment, increased CO_2, increased respiratory rate interval, etc.)?

Comparison of "analgesic efficacy" of spinal and systemic routes should utilize criteria in addition to visual analogue scale for pain. Such criteria should include:

1. patient preference (41)
2. patient expectation/patient satisfaction
3. indirect indices such as ease of mobilization, timing of discharge from hospital, and perhaps nursing time required.

Relative Potency Studies Using "Classic" Four-point Design

Virtually no studies of spinal opiates have employed the classic four-point crossover design, using two doses of a new spinal opiate and two doses of a "standard" spinal opiate. It is usual to use a twofold range of dosage and this poses a risk of respiratory depression, making it necessary to monitor respiration. In postoperative patients, the obvious problem with such four-point studies is the time available to obtain complete four-point crossover and the need to contend with the problem of decreasing pain stimulus. Nonetheless, there would appear to be a defect in current data, since such studies may give the following information:

1. With a significant slope and no significant deviation from parallelism, relative potency could be estimated, e.g., for spinal opiate A versus B or IM versus epidural. At present this is only "estimated" for the various opiates used via the spinal route.
2. The dose-response curve for analgesia can be compared to that for various side effects (e.g., respiratory rate depression) to obtain an indication of relative safety.
3. Analgesic time-effect curves can be obtained for different doses over an appropriate time course, based upon previously obtained pharmacokinetic data (Fig. 1); this has been found to be of utmost importance, for example, in the case of morphine, where pharmacokinetic studies pointed to a slow onset but a long duration of analgesia (1).

Analgesic Combinations

Studies are needed of combinations of spinally administered drugs (42), and of spinally and systemically administered drugs. Time-effect curves and dose-response curves would be valuable to help determine if there are advantages in terms of increased intensity and duration of analgesia from such combinations.

As noted above, the dose-response curves for individual opiates given spinally have not been defined. However, it is likely that the curves are steep and have an early plateau similar to systemic administration. It has indeed been found clinically that doubling the dose of spinal opiates does not give a doubling of effect (1). Dose is ultimately limited by side effects. Therefore, it appears attractive to combine subtoxic doses of opioids with nonopioids in the hope of achieving adequate analgesia without serious side effects.

However, there are substantial design problems in the clinical evaluation of such combinations. The classic "isobologram" method is impractical clinically. An alternative approach was used to assess the effects of combining intrathecal morphine and intrathecal clonidine in rats (43). Rats were given 2 mcg morphine, one of a number of dose levels of clonidine, and a combination of 1 mcg morphine plus half the dose of clonidine in random sequence at intervals of 2 to 3 days. Responses in the hot plate and tail-flick tests were measured at intervals after dosing. If antinociceptive effects of clonidine and morphine are synergistic, response to the combination will at some dose level exceed responses to both morphine and clonidine alone (Fig. 2). Evidence of synergism was found in the tail-flick test over much of the dose range (Fig. 3). Clinically, it would be important to also examine side effects of the combination; additivity of analgesia with subadditivity of side effects would be a desirable aim, whereas synergism of analgesic effects may be of little benefit if side effects are also synergistic.

Some Challenging Areas of Further Study in Postoperative Patients

Neuroendocrine Response to Surgery/Trauma

In postoperative pain, studies by Kehlet (44) indicate that currently available spinally administered opioids are not very effective in modifying the neurohu-

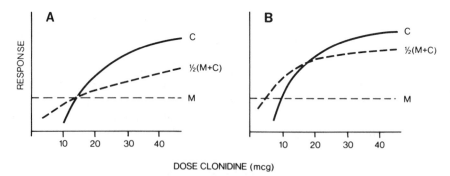

FIG. 2. Hypothetical dose-response curves for intrathecal morphine, intrathecal clonidine, and a combination of these treatments. The solid line (C) shows the dose-response relationship for clonidine at the dose level given on the horizontal axis. The horizontal line (M) represents response to a fixed dose of morphine, and the dashed line $[\frac{1}{2}(M + C)]$ represents response to a combination of half the fixed dose of morphine plus half the dose of clonidine shown on the horizontal axis. If drug effects are additive, the response to $\frac{1}{2}(M + C)$ will always be between responses to C and M (**A**); if response to $\frac{1}{2}(M + C)$ at any dose level exceeds responses to both M and C, drug effects are synergistic (**B**).

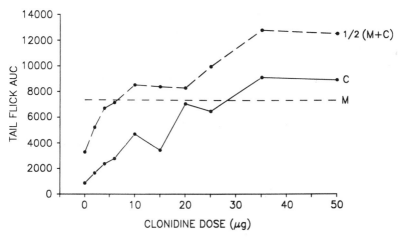

FIG. 3. Response of rats in the tail-flick test to a fixed dose (2 mcg) of morphine (M), clonidine (C), or a combination of 1 mcg morphine plus half the dose of clonidine [$\frac{1}{2}$(M + C)], given intrathecally. The vertical axis shows the area under the tail-flick latency (converted to percent maximum possible effect) × time curve. Each point represents the mean response of five to seven rats. Where drug effects are synergistic, the response to the combination is greater than that to either drug given alone.

moral responses to surgery and trauma. Indeed, even highly effective analgesia with a combination of local anesthetic, opioid, and nonsteroidal antiinflammatory agents is still ineffective in modifying neurohumoral responses (45). Analgesia appears to be an insensitive indicator of agents that may help to prevent the "stress response." Furthermore, it is possible that a spinal route of administration may be irrelevant for such effects. A new strategy of investigation is required. An intriguing possibility is that fast-conducting afferent nerve fibers need to be effectively blocked in spinal cord during surgery (46). If so, assessment may need to include neurophysiological monitoring of spinal cord.

Prevention of Postoperative Pain and Its Sequelae

The value of commencing analgetic regimens prior to surgery has been suggested by animal data, which indicate that this is a more effective and economical use of dose than starting pain relief after surgery (47). "Preemptive" use of spinally administered opioids and nonopioids needs to be compared with appropriate control regimens with respect to:

1. postoperative pain intensity and analgesic requirements
2. subsequent development of "subacute" and chronic pain states, e.g., phantom limb pain, causalgias, reflex sympathetic dystrophies, etc. (47).

Cancer Pain: Critique of Current Approaches and Design Recommendations

Studies of spinal opioids in cancer pain have been, to date, largely limited to prospective case series and uncontrolled retrospective reports of pain relief and side effects. In one study, spinal opioids were used subsequent to oral opioids: no significant difference in analgesia or neurotoxicity was reported (39). However, this study had major design problems and was an example of "failure to find difference does not equate with absence of difference" (37). There is also a requirement for studies comparing spinal opioids to alternative treatments, such as neurolytic blocks and percutaneous cordotomy.

In general, it has been accepted that the more simple approach of oral opioids and adjuvants should be used before spinal administration of drugs. Certainly, this is noninvasive, cheap, and simple. It is also widely applicable. But is it as effective, and does it have similar side effects as spinal opioids? Would some or many patients prefer spinal opioids, even at an early stage because of fewer side effects? Alternatively, is it of any use to follow oral opioids with spinal opioids? If so, in which patients and how should spinal opioids be used? How do spinal opioids compare with subcutaneous opioid infusion in terms of efficacy and side effects?

A logical approach to providing a rationale for use of spinal opioids in cancer pain include the following:

1. *Studies performed in a setting where oral opioids and adjuvants are carefully optimized and reevaluated.* Optimization should use a generally agreed upon approach to adjusting doses and adding adjuvants.

2. *Studies in which failure of oral opioids is carefully documented.* "Failure" is demonstrated by increasing dosage until pain relief can only be obtained when side effects are unacceptable.

3. *Data to be obtained, for each opiate, of relative oral to epidural doses, and oral to intrathecal doses for effective analgesia.* At this effective dose, relative side effects need to be documented. At present, only very broad guidelines are available for intrathecal and epidural doses after oral opioids.

4. *Studies of optimal spinal therapy.* These studies can use a rapid optimization method. For spinal opioids, infusion can be used, with rate rapidly adjusted based on analgesic and side effect responses. For example, we have used an *adaptive, stepwise decreasing* morphine infusion. A scaling factor, M, takes an initial value as follows, depending upon oral morphine requirements per day: if less than 100 mg/day, M = 0.75; if 100 to 200 mg/day, M = 1; if over 200 mg/day M = 1.4. Then, stabilization is performed as follows: 0 to 2 hrs, 5 × M mg morphine/hr is infused, after which 2.5 × M mg morphine/hr is infused over 2 to 4 hrs, and 0.75 × M mg morphine/hr is infused over 4 to 24 hrs. At intervals of not less than 6 hrs, the value of M is halved if the patient suffers troublesome side effects, or multiplied by 1.5 if the patient suffers unacceptable pain. The efficacy of such regimens of opioid optimization needs to be tested and the most favorable methods documented.

When Patients Report Increased Pain During the Course of Cancer

"Reoptimization" should be done to ensure adequate treatment is provided. A prospective study, using this approach, should document the *rate of escalation,* or otherwise, of spinal opioids by either intrathecal or epidural routes. A retrospective study reported that most patients show only modest increases in dose, with only a minority requiring very large dose increases (48). This is contrary to anecdotal claims and points to the need for a careful prospective study, along the lines indicated above. In such a study, rigorous attempts to document disease progression should be made in patients whose dose increases markedly, in an attempt to attribute such changes to tolerance or disease progression or other factors (e.g., technical problems with the spinal opioid system).

Randomized Prospective Studies are Required of Epidural Compared to Intrathecal Opioids

Both analgetic efficacy and side effects must be evaluated in clinical trials comparing epidural and intrathecal opioid administration.

Randomized Prospective Studies are Required for Epidural "Top-up" Techniques Compared to Continuous Infusion with Respect to Efficacy and Side Effects, Including Potential for Infection

Currently, many clinics use nurse or patient administered "top-ups" via a portal or externalized catheter (e.g., Hickman-Broviac) (48–50). Other clinics use only infusion techniques via the external catheter or via a right-angled needle or "gripper" placed through the skin into the portal. The efficacy of these techniques in the treatment of cancer pain is similar (51), but it is not known whether patient acceptance or potential for infection or side effects differs. Also, the costs of equipment, nursing time, and other costs should be documented.

Comparison of Systemic and Spinal Opioids

Having determined the "route" of spinal administration (epidural or intrathecal) and the regimen (top-up or infusion), this "ideal" combination can then be compared with other methods. Also, the availability of starting doses relative to oral opioids, rapid optimization methods, and other fundamental data, such as onset and duration of analgesia and CSF pharmacokinetics, will permit the most efficient use of spinal opioids. In our view, the most logical comparison is that of continuous epidural opioid infusion (CEPI) and continuous subcutaneous infusion (CSI). Currently many palliative care units, oncologists, and others use CSI as a standard second line of defense when oral opioids fail. Only very limited data support an advantage of CSI over "reoptimized" oral opioids; however, there is no argument that CSI is useful in patients who are no longer able to take oral opioids because of gastrointestinal tract problems.

On the other hand many neurosurgeons and pain clinics have treated many thousands of patients with cancer pain with spinal opioids and have provided anecdotal reports of efficacy (1). However, there are no randomized prospective controlled studies that definitively guide clinicians as to the relative efficacy of CSI and CEPI and possible patient populations that may benefit from one or the other. Suggested design features for such studies could include:

1. *Entry criteria:* "failed Step 3 WHO Ladder."
2. *Primary response measure:* patient preference (crossover studies) or patient satisfaction (parallel-group studies).
3. *Secondary response measures:* (a) pain relief as reported by the patient, (b) side effects as reported by the patients and/or observer.
4. *Pharmacokinetic studies* to determine a possible relationship between blood morphine concentration and severity of side effects during the two treatments.
5. *Study design.* Within patient, randomized prospective double-blind crossover study of CSI and CEPI, using the "double dummy." Thus, all patients who complete such a study would receive CSI and CEPI, with the order of treatment randomly allocated. An epidural portal and a subcutaneous needle would be placed and connected to identical external pumps. At the first study phase, one pump would contain active (opioid) and the other placebo (saline). At the second stage this arrangement would be reversed.
6. *An "optimization" phase* would be used for *each stage* prior to documenting response variables during a subsequent *evaluation phase.*
7. At the conclusion of the two evaluation phases, patient preference would be determined.

Problems in Such a Design

1. As in any studies of cancer pain, stability of the "conditions of the experiment" is impossible to guarantee. However, the randomization and crossover design helps to address this issue. Also, prior stability of oral dose and stability of clinical and laboratory data prior to study entry will increase the chances of stability during the study. Patients who develop a sudden requirement for increased dosage or who have new symptoms during the study should be reassessed, and if disease progression is documented, should be withdrawn.

2. Some clinics may object to using CEPI *prior to* CSI. However, at present, CEPI and CSI have to be regarded as equivalently efficacious until proven otherwise. Also, the epidural portal may prove valuable in a percentage of patients for subsequent local anesthetic or other nonopioid drugs.

3. Patients admitted at a late stage of their disease, at Step 3 WHO Ladder, may be rapidly deteriorating and not complete the study. It thus may be necessary to relax the criteria for "failed oral opioids" to permit earlier entry into the study. This would ideally be done by a prior study of adverse neuropsychological sequelae of oral opioids, which aimed to develop precise criteria for unacceptable side effects associated with oral opioids (see above). For example, patients with progressive impairment of memory, inability to concentrate, etc. during oral

opioid therapy could be offered entry into the study of CSI and CEPI, even if their period of oral opioid treatment was brief.

Prospective Study of Different Spinal Catheter Systems

Animal and clinical data indicate that fibrous sheath reaction may "wall off" epidural catheters (and possibly intrathecal catheters). Anecdotal clinical reports document pain and difficult injection in some patients and some pathology data report a "fibrous mass" in a small number of cases. More inert catheter materials have now been developed to address this issue. Prospective controlled studies of "standard" compared to new catheters are required. Such studies should include the following design features.

1. A standardized method of catheter insertion and level of catheter tip location in epidural or subarachnoid space.
2. Documentation of successful catheter placement by image intensifier screening and injection of contrast medium to verify adequate delivery of material to epidural or subarachnoid space; notation must be made of any "leakage" out of epidural or intrathecal space.
3. Comparison of analgesic efficacy and side effects.
4. Reexamination under image intensifier if problems ensue with catheters, including pain on injection, difficult injection, and sudden increase in dose. Again, examination for "leakage" should be made.
5. Where possible, postmortem neuropathology studies should be performed, using an agreed upon protocol for documentation of abnormalities.

"Walling off" of the epidural catheter may explain the observed "tracking back" of injected fluid along the catheter to subcutaneous tissues (52). We have recently obtained evidence of leakage from the epidural space in an animal model (53).

Approaches to Studying Novel Classes of Opioid and Nonopioid Drugs Given by Spinal Administration

As discussed previously, the question of selectivity in all its aspects is critical in studying novel opioid and nonopioid drugs, and tests are available to determine the effects of spinal opioids on neural function and other body systems.

Important contributions that may be made by novel drugs include:

1. *Synergism with mu receptor opioids, e.g., morphine.* Study design is critical to detect such effects as discussed above.

2. *Lack of cross-tolerance with mu receptor agonists.* Study design requirements are similar to those described above. In particular, a crossover "within-patient" design is essential, together with randomization of order of treatment. Although

preliminary data point toward incomplete cross-tolerance between delta receptor agonists and mu agonists, more definitive studies are required.

3. *Efficacy in cancer pain refractory to spinal mu receptor agonists.* Preliminary data indicate that neuropathic pain may respond to spinally administered alpha-2 agonists but not to opioids (1). However, anecdotal data indicate that high doses of lipid soluble opioids given *intrathecally,* at the appropriate spinal segmental level, do relieve neuropathic pain. It is known clinically that pain of plexopathies is relieved by epidural and also intrathecal local anesthetics. However, controlled studies are required to document efficacy in different pain states for different agents, including mu, delta, and kappa opioid receptor agonists, nonopioids, etc.

A particular problem in this area of study is the difficulty in assigning weight to nociceptive, neuropathic, and other etiologic factors in cancer patients. For example, a myelogram may reveal pathology consistent with neuropathic pain and some clinical signs may support this, but the clinical picture is rarely purely neuropathic.

Design of Pharmacokinetic Studies of Spinal Opioids

Although often appearing simple, such studies are inherently difficult. Cerebrospinal fluid circulation in the spinal region is quite slow, depending upon bulk flow, transmitted vascular pulsations, and effects of intrathoracic pressure changes. Drugs injected directly into the CSF are not instantly and homogeneously distributed in the CSF. This problem is further increased with epidural injection, since there is a delay as drugs are absorbed from the epidural space to the intrathecal space (54). Thus, presentation of data from CSF pharmacokinetic studies after intrathecal and epidural injection should be limited to a description of the time course of CSF opioid concentrations. It is not appropriate to attempt to calculate classic pharmacokinetic parameters, such as half-life, clearance, etc. Another problem lies in interpretation of the relevance of CSF concentrations: do they correlate with analgetic effects and side effects? Particularly in the case of epidural injection, absorption into CSF and blood continues for a long time after injection. Thus, the absorption phase overlaps with the distribution and clearance phases, making it difficult or impossible to clearly define these phases and to characterize their parameters (54). Despite the above problems, studies of CSF and blood concentrations of opioids following spinal administration can be valuable (54).

A number of principles are important:

1. Parallel studies of pharmacokinetics and pharmacodynamics are desirable (54).

2. Sampling should be performed in a manner that avoids contamination of the sampling site by the injected bolus of opioid.

3. A reliable method should be used to confirm that the injection is made entirely into the intended site (viz., intrathecal or epidural). In the case of intrathecal injection, CSF aspiration prior to injection and at the end of injection is one method. In the case of epidural injection, prior "testing" of the catheter with local anesthetic is helpful, but image intensifier screening after injection of contrast medium is a more objective test.

4. Blood concentration data are more useful if the same dose of opioid is given spinally (e.g., epidural) and intravenously on separate occasions, on a within-patient basis. This permits calculation of absorption of opioid from the epidural space. Also, after the IV dose, analgesic blood concentration can be determined, in individual patients, and this can be related to the blood concentration achieved after spinal administration (23).

5. CSF migration of opioids of varying physicochemical properties can be studied by sampling near the site of injection and also distal from that site. We have found the C7-T1 interspace to be a convenient site, where it is easy to enter the CSF with a low complication rate in experienced hands.

Pharmacokinetic studies can assist in addressing some of the unanswered "key issues" in the use of spinal opioids (Table 2). We have attempted to compare the cephalad migration in CSF of lipophilic and more hydrophilic drugs. An initial study compared the moderately lipid soluble drug, meperidine, with the poorly lipid soluble drug, morphine, sampling CSF at the C7-T1 level (Fig. 4). The raw CSF concentration/time data showed clear evidence of rapid migration of meperidine to brain stem region but a relatively rapid decline to low concentrations. Such data were in keeping with early, rather than delayed, respiratory depression reported in association with meperidine (26). In contrast, cervical CSF concentrations of morphine peaked later and were sustained at relatively higher levels (26). Such data were in keeping with reports of delayed and sustained respiratory depression in some patients following spinal morphine. In a similar study, comparison of hydromorphone to morphine revealed that these two drugs, with similar lipid partition coefficients, had similar CSF time profiles (27).

A study that exemplifies most of the principles noted above compared lumbar epidural and intravenous administration of fentanyl in the same subjects on different occasions (23). On each study day samples were obtained for opioid

TABLE 2. *Unanswered key issues in spinal opioids—pharmacokinetics*

Factors determining clearance of opioids from CSF and residual CSF concentrations in brain stem region after injection, at different neuraxial levels, of various opioids.
Time course of CSF-borne drug migration and penetration of neuraxis for the various opioid and nonopioid drugs.
Comparative rates of systemic bioavailability of water-soluble (e.g., morphine) and lipid-soluble (e.g., fentanyl) opioids and nonopioid drugs.
Effects of CSF and blood pH changes on CSF and blood concentrations of opioids.
Relationships between endogenous opioids and exogenous spinal opioid administration.
Ease of antagonism of various opioid drugs after spinal use in humans.

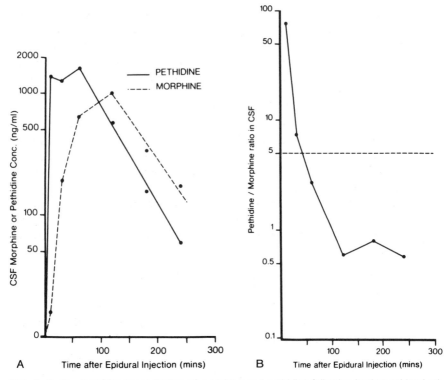

FIG. 4. A: Cervical CSF concentration of morphine and pethidine following lumbar epidural administration of 10 mg morphine and 50 mg pethidine. **B:** Pethidine/morphine ratio in CSF as a function of time. The dashed line shows the ratio expected if both drugs behaved the same. (Reproduced with permission from ref. 26.)

analysis from blood and CSF at both lumbar and C7-T1 levels. Parallel studies of analgetic and side effects were performed (Fig. 5). This study confirmed the very rapid absorption of fentanyl from epidural space into CSF and also documented the minimal cephalad migration in CSF of this highly lipid soluble drug, at the low dose of 1 mcg/kg employed. Also, the specific GLC assay confirmed minimal vascular absorption (23).

CONCLUSION

Clinical use of spinal opioids is currently based largely on empirical observation and anecdotal report, the validity of which must be challenged by carefully designed prospective studies. Such studies are difficult; they will require development of new techniques and use of innovative designs to overcome ethical limitations. However, the major advances already made over the last decade demonstrate that these problems can be overcome.

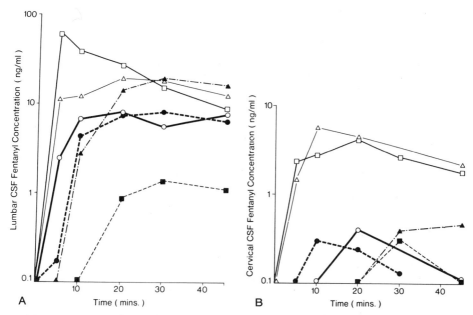

FIG. 5. Lumbar (**A**) and cervical (**B**) CSF concentrations of fentanyl in six patients following lumbar epidural administration of fentanyl, 1 mcg/kg bodyweight in 10 ml saline. (Reproduced with permission from ref. 23.)

REFERENCES

1. Cousins MJ, Cherry DA, Gourlay GK. Acute and chronic pain: use of spinal opioids. In: Cousins MJ, Bridenbaugh PO, eds. *Neural blockade in clinical anesthesia and management of pain,* 2nd ed. Philadelphia: JB Lippincott, 1988;955–1029.
2. Yablonski-Peretz T, Klin B, Beilin Y, Warner E, Baron S, Olshwang D, Catane R. Continuous epidural narcotic analgesia for intractable pain due to malignancy. *J Surg Oncol* 1985;29:28.
3. Cherry DA, Gourlay GK, McLachlan M, Cousins MJ. Diagnostic epidural opioid blockade and chronic pain: preliminary report. *Pain* 1985;21:143.
4. James KE, Forrest WH, Rose RL. Crossover and noncrossover designs in four-point parallel line analgesic assays. *Clin Pharmacol Ther* 1985;37:242–252.
5. Fliess JL. *The design and analysis of clinical experiments.* New York: John Wiley and Sons, 1986;263.
6. Fisher AC, Wallenstein S. Crossover designs in medical research. In: Buncher CR, Tsay J-Y, eds., *Statistics in the pharmaceutical industry.* New York: Marcel Dekker, 1981;139–156.
7. Hills M, Armitage P. The two-period crossover clinical trial. *Br J Clin Pharmacol* 1979;8:7–20.
8. Brown BW Jr. The crossover experiment for clinical trials. *Biometrics* 1980;36:69–79.
9. Grizzle JE. The two period change-over design and its use in clinical trials. *Biometrics* 1965;21:467–480.
10. Cochran WG, Cox GM. *Experimental designs,* 2nd ed. New York: John Wiley and Sons, 1957;133–139.
11. Wang RIH, Waite E. Crossover and parallel study of oral analgesics. *J Clin Pharmacol* 1981;21:162–168.
12. Lofstrom JB, Cousins MJ. Sympathetic neural blockade of upper and lower extremity. In: Cousins MJ, Bridenbaugh PO, eds. *Neural blockade in clinical anesthesia and management of pain,* 2nd ed. Philadelphia: JB Lippincott, 1988;461–500.

13. Willer JC, Bergeret S, Gaudy JH. Epidural morphine strongly depresses nociceptive flexion reflexes in patients with postoperative pain. *Anesthesiology* 1985;63:675.
14. Willer JC, Bussel B. Evidence for a direct spinal mechanism in morphine-induced inhibition of nociceptive reflexes in humans. *Brain Res* 1980;187:212.
15. Boas RA. Hazards of epidural morphine. *Anaesth Intensive Care* 1986;8:377.
16. Yaksh TL, Noueihed R. The physiology and pharmacology of spinal opiates. *Annu Rev Pharmacol Toxicol* 1985;25:443.
17. Hotvedt R, Refsum H. Cardiac effects of thoracic epidural morphine caused by increased vagal activity in the dog. *Acta Anaesthesiol Scand* 1986;30:76.
18. Rawal N, Mollefors K, Axelsson K, Lingardh G, Widman B. An experimental study of urodynamic effects of epidural morphine and of naloxone reversal. *Anesth Analg* 1983;62:641.
19. Naulty JS, Johnson M, Burger GA, et al. Epidural fentanyl for post cesarean delivery pain management. *Anesthesiology* 1983;59:A415.
20. Evron S, Samueloff A, Simon A, Drenger B, Magora F. Urinary function during epidural analgesia with methadone and morphine in post-cesarean section patients. *Pain* 1985;23:135.
21. Baxter AD, Kiruluta G. Detrusor tone after epidural morphine. *Anesth Analg* 1984;63:464.
22. Cardan E. Spinal morphine in enuresis. *Br J Anaesth* 1985;57:354.
23. Gourlay GK, Murphy TM, Plummer JL, Kowalski SR, Cherry DA, Cousins MJ. Pharmacokinetics of fentanyl in lumbar and cervical CSF following lumbar epidural and intravenous administration. *Pain* 1989;38:253.
24. Payne R, Inturrisi CE. CSF distribution of morphine, methadone and sucrose after intrathecal injection. *Life Sci* 1985;37:1137–1144.
25. Gourlay GK, Cherry DA, Cousins MJ. Cephalad migration of morphine in CSF following lumbar epidural administration in patients with cancer pain. *Pain* 1985;23:317–326.
26. Gourlay GK, Cherry DA, Plummer JL, Armstrong PJ, Cousins MJ. The influence of drug polarity on the absorption of opioid drugs into CSF and subsequent cephalad migration following lumbar epidural administration: application to morphine and pethidine. *Pain* 1987;31:297–305.
27. Brose WG, Tanelian D, Brodsky JB, Cousins MJ, Mark JB. CSF and blood pharmacokinetics of hydromorphone compared to morphine following lumbar epidural administration. (abstract) *Pain* 1990;(Suppl 5):S118.
28. Plummer JL, Cmielewski PL, Reynolds GD, Gourlay GK, Cherry DA. Influence of polarity on dose-response relationships of intrathecal opioids in rats. *Pain* 1990;40:339–347.
29. Gourlay GK, Kowalski SR, Plummer JL, Cousins MJ, Armstrong PJ. Fentanyl blood concentration—analgesic response relationship in the treatment of postoperative pain. *Anesth Analg* 1988;67:329–337.
30. Martin R, Salbaing J, Blaise G, Tetrault JP, Tetrault L. Epidural morphine for post-operative pain relief. A dose-response curve. *Anesthesiology* 1982;56:423.
31. Crawford RD, Batra MS, Fox F. Epidural morphine dose response for postoperative analgesia. *Anesthesiology* 1981;55:A150.
32. Hughes SC, Rosen MA, Shnider SM, Norton M, Curtis JD. Epidural morphine for the relief of postoperative pain after cesarean section. *Anesth Analg* 1982;61:190.
33. Dixon WJ. The up-and-down method for small samples. *J Am Statist Assoc* 1965;60:967–978.
34. Pybus DA, Torda TA. Dose-effect relationships of extradural morphine. *Br J Anaesth* 1982;54:1259.
35. Nordberg G. Pharmacokinetic aspects of spinal morphine analgesia. *Acta Anaesthesiol Scand* 1984;79:1.
36. Cousins MJ, Mather LE. Spinal and intrathecal administration of opioids. *Anesthesiology,* 1984;61:276–310.
37. Wood MM, Cousins MJ. Iatrogenic neurotoxicity in cancer patients. *Pain* 1989;39:1–12.
38. Mather LE, Seow LT, Roberts JG, Cousins MJ. Development of a model for integrated pharmacokinetics and pharmacodynamic studies of intravenous anaesthetic agents. *Eur J Clin Pharmacol* 1981;19:371–381.
39. Sjogren P, Banning A. Pain, sedation and reaction time during long-term treatment of cancer patients with oral and epidural opioids. *Pain* 1989;39:5–12.
40. Bruera E, Macmillan K, Janson J, MacDonald RN. The cognitive effects of the administration of narcotic analgesics in patients with cancer pain. *Pain* 1989;39:13–16.
41. Brownridge P, Frewin DB. A comparative study of techniques of postoperative analgesia following cesarean section and lower abdominal surgery. *Anaesth Intensive Care* 1985;13:123.

42. Brownridge P. Epidural bupivacaine-pethidine mixture. Clinical experience using a low-dose combination in labour. *Aust NZ J Obstet Gynaecol* 1988;28:17–24.
43. Plummer JL, Cmieleswki PL, Gourlay GK, Owen H, Cousins MJ. Lack of supraadditivity of antinociceptive effects of intrathecal morphine and intrathecal clonidine in rats (abstract). *Pain* 1990;(Suppl 5):S125.
44. Kehlet H. Modification of responses to surgery by neural blockade: clinical implications. In: Cousins MJ, Bridenbaugh PO, eds. *Neural blockade in clinical anesthesia and management of pain,* 2nd ed. Philadelphia: JB Lippincott, 1988;145–188.
45. Schulze S, Roikjaer O, Hasselstrom L, Jensen N, Kehlet H. Epidural bupivacaine and morphine plus systemic indomethacin eliminates pain but not systemic response to convalescence after cholecystectomy. *Surgery* 1988;103:321–327.
46. Kehlet H. The stress response to surgery: release mechanisms and the modifying effect of pain relief. *Acta Chir Scand* 1988;Suppl 550:22–28.
47. Cousins MJ, John J. Bonica Distinguished Lecture. Acute pain and the injury response: immediate and prolonged effects. *Reg Anaesth* 1989;14:162–179.
48. Cousins MJ, Plummer JL, Cherry DA, Gourlay GK, Onley MM, Evans KH. Use of implanted Port-A-Caths for epidural administration of morphine in the control of cancer pain (abstract) *Pain* 1990;(Suppl 5):S116.
49. Cherry DA, Gourlay GK, Cousins MJ, Gannon B!. A technique for the insertion of an implantable portal system for the long term epidural administration of opioids in the treatment of cancer pain. *Anaesth Intensive Care* 1985;13:145.
50. Dupen SL, Peterson DG, Bogosian AC, Ramsey DH, et al. A new permanent externalized epidural catheter for narcotic self-administration to control cancer pain. *Cancer* 1987;59:986–993.
51. Cherry DA, Plummer JL, Wood MM, Gourlay GK, Onley MM, Cousins MJ. Comparison of intermittent bolus with continuous infusion of epidural morphine in the treatment of cancer pain (abstract). *Pain* 1990;(Suppl 5):S115.
52. Driessen JJ, de Mulder PHM, Claessen JJL, van Diejen D, Wobbes TL. Epidural administration of morphine for control of cancer pain: long-term efficacy and complications. *Clin J Pain* 1989;5:217–222.
53. Plummer JL, Cmielewski PL, Gourlay GK, Cherry DA, Cousins MJ, Szep PF, Davis RP. Leakage of fluid administered epidurally to rats into subcutaneous tissue. *Pain* 1990;42:121–124.
54. Cousins MJ. Editorial: Comparative pharmacokinetics of spinal opioids in humans: a step towards determination of relative safety. *Anesthesiology* 1987;67:875–876.

Advances in Pain Research and Therapy, Vol. 18,
edited by M. Max, R. Portenoy, and E. Laska,
Raven Press, Ltd., New York © 1991.

22

Patient-Controlled Intravenous Analgesia for Postoperative Pain Relief

Klaus A. Lehmann

*Institute of Anesthesiology, University of Cologne Medical School,
Cologne, Federal Republic of Germany*

There are many reasons for the inadequate treatment of postoperative pain. Doctors generally delegate pain relief to the nursing staff, who are overloaded with work. As a consequence, rigid intramuscular doses are administered in fixed intervals or only at (urgent) request, without adapting the types of analgesic or application modes to the patients' individual requirements. Feedback, essential in the control of any medical therapy, is too seldom applied despite the unpredictability of individual pain intensity and tolerance (1). So far it has been virtually impossible to establish the role played by age, sex, anesthetic technique, and type or duration of surgery, probably because psychological factors, such as previous experience, anxiety, depression, neuroticism, and self-discipline on the part of the patient, can seldom be satisfactorily standardized or recorded in an objective manner (2).

The therapeutic concept of intravenous patient-controlled analgesia (PCA) is considered an attempt to solve many of the above-mentioned problems at once. If only the patient can decide how much pain he or she is suffering or is prepared to suffer, self-administration of potent analgesics should satisfy the need for analgesia and reduce the nursing staff workload. In this way, the *dynamic* process of analgesia *titration,* with its optimistic aim of complete pain relief (a determination that the patient can make better than any technique that relies on attempts to quantify pain intensity) can be added to the *static* methods so far used in pain measurement.

It is now commonly believed that pain measurement can be accomplished by assessing drug intake during PCA. This chapter reviews PCA studies that aimed to determine predictors of postoperative pain, influence of anesthetic and surgical techniques, equipotency of analgesic agents, types of analgesic drug interactions, minimum analgesic plasma concentrations, and therapeutic outcome of non-

PCA pain treatment. These data indicate that the amount of underlying pain and the pain relief achieved during PCA are more variable than generally believed, and that additional variables should be determined for proper interpretation (e.g., the classical verbal or visual analogue pain and psychological ratings, side effects, measures of patient acceptance). Patients' selection, as well as pump settings, should be carefully controlled. PCA demonstrates that clinical *pain measurement* cannot be separated from patients' individual *pain behavior.*

First attempts to establish intravenous PCA were made in the late 1960s; early devices, which simply allowed patients in labor to adjust flow rates of analgesic dilutions, were followed by electronically controlled pumps that could be activated by the patient, thus releasing small preprogrammed analgesic doses into the infusion. Initially, it was considered a particular advantage that such systems not only helped improve the quality of analgesia, but also reduced total dosage when compared with conventional regimens. This later proved too rash a conclusion.

The incessant admonitions of the Canadian anesthetist M. Keeri-Szanto, who stressed the need to individualize acute pain therapy, helped to spread the idea of PCA. At present, more than 300 papers and reviews (3–12), and even a handbook (13) have been published on the uses and problems of analgesic self-administration.

PCA DEVICES

Except for technical details, most available PCA machines differ only slightly in concept and handling. They consist of electronically controlled infusion pumps supervised by microprocessors (7,9,13). Whenever the patient feels that pain

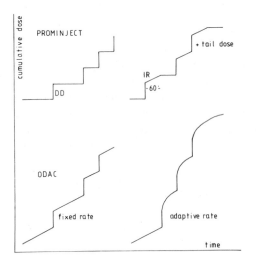

FIG. 1. Idealized cumulative dose-time curves for different infusion strategies.

relief is necessary, he or she can activate the system by pressing a button. The unit dispenses an amount of analgesic, which has been programmed by the physician. The device can be used to deliver drug into a running intravenous infusion, the epidural space, or even intramuscularly. Unauthorized alteration of dosing parameters is excluded by a number of safety factors. After a demand dose has been administered, the next request will only be executed at the end of a freely programmable lockout time in order to prevent overdosage; thus, the next bolus is only administered after enough time has elapsed for the previous one to achieve a significant pharmacological effect. With some devices, additional control mechanisms are provided, such as integrated reaction time tests or hourly maximum dosages. Small printers or displays are generally available for programming and documentation of application patterns or cumulated dosage.

There are, however, some differences between the systems regarding the use of concurrent infusions along with the bolus demand dosages (Fig. 1, Table 1). In some, there is no demand-independent infusion available, whereas in others continuous, adaptive rates or tail dosages can be programmed. For example, Fig. 1 displays idealized cumulative dose-time plots that reflect commonly used strategies. A tail dose (as delivered by Prominject) can be considered a fixed-rate

TABLE 1. *Patient-controlled analgesia pump comparisons[a]*

	(a) Gynecological patients, fentanyl				
	$ODAC_f$	$ODAC_a$	$Prom_n$	$Prom_t$	CODIC
n	20	20	20	20	24
Demand dose (μg)	34.5	34.5	34.0	34.0	(var)[b]
Infusion rate (μg/h)	4	$(4.0)^c$	0	$(17.0)^d$	(var)[b]
PCA duration (hrs)	17.2	17.8	17.0	14.8	16.4
Demands/patient	17.6	11.8	14.6	14.6	19.5
μg/kg/h	0.62	0.72	0.57	0.93	0.31
Retrospective painscore[e]	2.2	1.7	1.8	1.9	2.1

	(b) General surgical patients, morphine		
	$ODAC_f$	$ODAC_f$	Lifecare
n	40	20	21
Demand dose (mg)	1.92	3.0	1.7–2.5
Infusion rate (mg/h)	0.23	0.36	0
PCA duration (hrs)	20.3	18.7	18.1
Demands/patient	18.3	9.7	15.3
μg/kg/h	29.6	28.0	27.5
Retrospective painscore[e]	1.52	1.04	1.67

$ODAC_f$: fixed rate; $ODAC_a$: adaptive rate; $Prom_n$: Prominject without concurrent infusion; $Prom_t$: with tail dose.
[a] Data are arithmetic means.
[b] Variable according to patients' characteristics.
[c] Starting value for adaptive infusion.
[d] Tail dose infusion rate for 60 min following a demand.
[e] See Table 3.
From refs. 14, 16, 17, and author's unpublished results.

infusion for a certain period of time following a patient demand. In contrast, the on-demand analgesia computer (ODAC) allows a baseline infusion, either as a fixed or a so-called adaptive rate. In the latter the actual infusion is calculated from the dose administered during the respective last 60-min interval, i.e., high analgesic consumption as expressed by high demand frequencies increases the baseline infusion. As can be seen from Table 1a, this application mode finally leads to a significant reduction of total demands, which is appreciated by many patients. The CODIC (Table 1) is a system that is primarily aimed at pharmacokinetically designed infusion regimes. Using weight, height, and age, it calculates a 5-min loading infusion, which is followed by a small individualized maintenance infusion. Infusion rates are increased for a 2-min period whenever the patient presses the button, but the amount of drug delivered is reduced each time depending on the inherent pharmacokinetic model (14). An even more sophisticated delivery strategy was proposed by Bullingham et al. (15).

It appears from Table 1, therefore, that the use of a particular PCA pump, i.e., the infusion strategy it employs, must not be considered unimportant if different PCA studies are compared. On the whole, however, the differences seem to be of less importance than the variability caused by patient characteristics (9,18,19).

CLINICAL EXPERIENCE

Among possible areas for PCA use, postoperative pain treatment remains the most frequently reported. PCA during labor or for the treatment of cancer pain has so far been published only sporadically (3,7,9,13). Most papers describe *intravenous* self-administration; *intramuscular* PCA has been reported seldomly. Even *epidural* PCA has been tried. This chapter will concentrate only on intravenous application within the early postoperative period.

Almost every opiate analgesic has been administered by PCA in the postoperative period (7). The common concepts of these investigations are exemplified by the author's own results. In comparative series, groups of 40 patients recovering from elective major abdominal or orthopedic surgery were treated with different analgesics for about 24 hrs after extubation. Dosing parameters can be seen from Table 2; lockout time was 1 min. Demand rate and analgesic consumption were documented, as were retrospective verbal pain scores obtained in standardized interviews on the following day (Table 3). Although the patients had virtually free access to the dose, the therapeutic outcome was often different. From these data, mean opioid consumption (μg/kg/h) and mean retrospective pain score were used for equipotency comparisons (Table 2).

As can be seen in Figs. 2 and 3, individual variability in analgesic requirement was extremely high for all drugs. It is evident, too, that the self-administered dosage was hardly correlated with overall efficacy. There were patients who requested rather low dosages, even after upper abdominal interventions, and felt

TABLE 2. *Equipotency studies*[a]

Analgesic	Demand dose (μg)	Hourly maximum dose (mg/h)	Consumption (μg/kg/h)	Retrospective pain score (0–5)	Relative equipotent dose (product)
Sufentanil[b]	6	0.04	0.10	1.85	0.004
Fentanyl	34	0.25	0.46	1.07	0.01
Buprenorphine	40	0.32	0.63	1.57	0.02
Alfentanil	212	1.5	4.96	1.37	0.15
1-Methadone	1,145	5.95	14.20	1.60	0.50
Piritramide	1,990	15.0	30.44	1.42	0.96
Morphine	1,920	14.8	29.60	1.52	1
Nalbuphine	3,846	28.5	117.52	1.82	4.75
Pentazocine	7,980	60.0	135.57	1.60	4.82
Nefopam	3,846	28.5	132.75	2.90	8.56
Pethidine	9,615	100.0	175.10	2.22	8.63
Tramadol	9,615	100.0	203.12	2.27	10.24
Metamizol	50,000	500.0	1,804.21	3.02	121.09

[a] Results are arithmetic means; relative equipotent dose was calculated from the product of consumption and retrospective pain score (7).

[b] Sufentanil: 40 patients recovering from major gynecological surgery. Other drugs: patients after major abdominal and orthopedic surgery.

quite comfortable, whereas others recovering from minor surgery, such as meniscectomy, experienced comparatively little pain relief despite high analgesic consumption (Fig. 3). Grouping patients by gender or type of surgery did not yield significant differences for cumulative dosage.

Contrary to our expectation, even strict standardization (for sex, type of intervention, anesthesia, etc.) led to only minor reductions of variability, which confirms observations made by McQuay et al. (21). Data from three fentanyl studies demonstrate that the coefficients of variations (CV) for demands, analgesic consumption, and overall efficacy (retrospective pain scores) are rather comparable, regardless of efforts to reduce patient heterogeneity (Table 4). The CV for group A patients (both sexes recovering from abdominal or orthopedic surgery performed without standardization of anesthetic technique) were similar to group B (male and female patients undergoing thoracotomy in which anesthesia was well controlled) and group C patients (women undergoing hysterectomy performed by the same surgical and anesthesiological team under strictly standardized neuroleptanalgesia).

TABLE 3. *Retrospective pain scores*

0	No pain at all during the PCA period
1	Sometimes moderate pain
2	Always moderate pain
3	Sometimes severe pain
4	Always moderate, sometimes severe pain
5	Discontinuation due to inefficacy

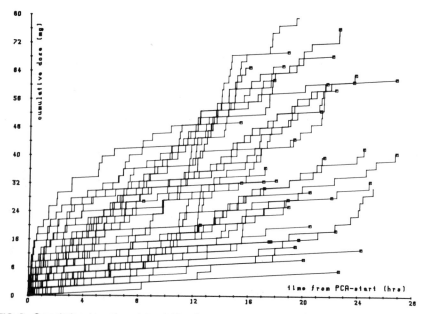

FIG. 2. Cumulative dose-time plots of 40 patients recovering from major abdominal or orthopedic surgery who were allowed to self-administer morphine (ODAC_{fixed rate}, cf. Table 2). Each step is indicative of a valid demand (16).

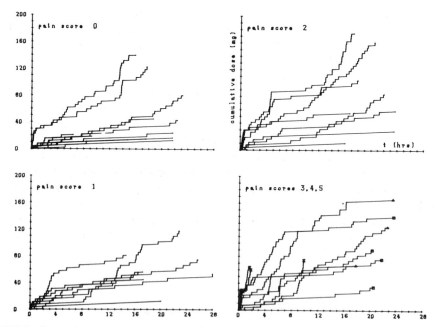

FIG. 3. Cumulative dose-time plots of 40 patients recovering from major abdominal or orthopedic surgery who were allowed to self-administer nalbuphine (ODAC_{fixed rate}, cf. Table 2). Curves are grouped according to the retrospective pain scores achieved (Table 3). In some patients, very low doses were needed to become virtually pain-free (score 0), whereas extremely high doses were sometimes associated with poor pain relief (20).

TABLE 4. *Effects of standardization*

	Abdominal/orthopedic surgery	Thoracotomies	Hysterectomies
n (male/female)	40 (15/25)	19 (13/6)	92 (0/92)
Age (yrs)	54.9 ± 16.6	60.2 ± 11.3	44.5 ± 8.2
Weight (kg)	70.1 ± 14.4	70.8 ± 11.8	66.4 ± 14.9
Anesthesia (min)	165.2 ± 65.3	266.8 ± 228.2	151.5 ± 45.8
PCA (hrs)	20.2 ± 4.3	23.8 ± 5.3	18.8 ± 3.9
Demands/patient (CV)	15.5 ± 12.9 (83.2%)	28.3 ± 15.2 (53.7%)	20.4 ± 11.8 (57.7%)
μg/kg/h (CV)	0.5 ± 0.4 (76.1%)	0.7 ± 0.4 (57.4%)	0.7 ± 0.4 (53.8%)
Retrospective score (CV)	1.1 ± 0.9 (82.2%)	0.8 ± 0.8 (98.8%)	2.2 ± 1.3 (59.3%)

ODAC$_{fixed\ rate}$, fentanyl, demand dose 34.5 μg, infusion rate 4 μg/h.
From ref. 22 and author's unpublished results.
CV, coefficient of variation.

Altogether, patients' acceptance proved to be excellent. Of the 1,334 patients treated so far by the author's team in controlled studies using different analgesics, 74.4% preferred PCA to previously experienced conventional pain therapy; 56.0% wished to remain connected to the PCA pump at the end of the observation period. Only 9.8% would have preferred personal treatment by the nursing staff. Difficulties in handling the device were reported in 13.8% of the cases; these comprised mostly elderly patients.

Table 5 compares patient acceptance with retrospective pain scores and the incidence of side effects. It is reasonable to assume that such results are correlated, and this must be studied systematically in the future. It is worth mentioning that in the author's own studies, clinically relevant respiratory depression never occurred, which corresponds with the great majority of published PCA work.

Which analgesics are particularly useful for PCA? The ideal drug should have an immediate onset and medium duration of effect, and be potent (i.e., not exert an early ceiling effect, which limits efficacy at higher dosages). Side effects should be minor or even absent, and abuse potential minimal. Although these options exclude, in the opinion of some authors, all agonist-antagonistic opiates and both extremely short-acting (e.g., alfentanil) and extremely long-acting (e.g., buprenorphine) analgesics from use in PCA systems, the author's results (Table 5) suggest that the best guideline is that the staff is comfortable using the drug.

An important factor that may influence PCA efficacy, and that so far has been underestimated in the literature, is the size of the demand dose. It is easily understandable that the patient will trust the concept of self-application only if he or she notices a direct connection between demand and effect. Of course, this will not be the case if too small a demand dose is chosen. It was thought for a long time that high demand frequencies would obviate this problem and finally result in a sufficient cumulative effect. Investigations on tramadol showed, however, that doubling the demand dose resulted in significantly higher efficacy without doubling analgesic intake (23,24). From such observations, it can be concluded that, on the one hand, patients are able to *reduce* their demand fre-

TABLE 5. *Side effects and patient acceptance*

Analgesic	n	(Male/female)	Side effects (%)								
			NAU	EM	H	SE	EU	DYS	PR	SW
Alfentanil	40	(21/19)	30	15	0	30	13	5	0	20
Buprenorphine	139	(67/72)	42	17	0	0	4	6	11	37
Fentanyl	295	(28/267)	47	37	6	1	3	2	4	23
Metamizol	40	(16/24)	35	30	0	3	0	0	0	73
1-Methadone	120	(22/98)	38	22	0	0	2	0	3	16
Morphine	141	(47/94)	26	11	0	5	4	4	3	18
Nalbuphine	40	(19/21)	18	8	0	0	3	8	0	13
Nefopam	40	(20/20)	3	3	0	0	0	0	0	0
Pentazocine	40	(19/21)	20	15	0	0	5	5	3	35
Pethidine	40	(20/20)	8	5	0	13	0	0	0	8
Piritramide	160	(73/87)	26	12	0	12	1	3	2	14
Sufentanil	40	(0/40)	50	33	3	3	5	8	0	40
Tramadol	199	(61/138)	41	16	2	2	0	0	0	6
Σ	1,334	(413/921)	35	20	2	3	3	3	3	21

Analgesic	Psc	Patient acceptance (%)						Preferred nurse	Difficult to handle
		Comparison of PCA with earlier conventional pain treatment			Continuation of present treatment desired				
		+	=	−	+	=	−		
Alfentanil	1.37	80.0	13.3	6.7	67.5	25.0	7.5	15.0	2.5
Buprenorphine	1.37	87.8	10.8	1.3	67.6	19.4	12.9	3.6	13.7
Fentanyl	1.84	80.1	9.9	9.9	68.1	13.6	18.3	7.5	11.2
1-Methadone	1.49	91.1	4.5	4.5	45.0	24.2	30.8	6.7	11.7
Metamizol	3.02	11.1	37.0	51.9	20.0	37.5	22.5	22.5	37.5
Morphine	1.36	76.3	17.5	6.3	34.0	31.9	34.0	7.1	9.2
Nalbuphine	1.82	56.5	26.1	17.4	37.5	27.5	35.0	7.5	5.0
Nefopam	2.90	46.2	7.7	46.2	27.5	15.0	57.5	15.0	7.5
Pentazocine	1.60	68.4	15.8	15.8	40.0	35.0	25.0	5.0	7.5
Pethidine	2.22	47.1	35.3	17.6	52.5	30.0	17.5	5.0	30.0
Piritramide	1.51	82.2	9.6	8.2	65.0	21.9	52.5	11.3	17.2
Sufentanil	1.85	57.5	27.3	15.2	75.0	10.0	15.0	55.0	7.5
Tramadol	1.25	70.1	12.6	17.2	58.8	29.1	12.1	8.5	19.1
Σ	1.64	74.4	13.5	12.1	55.9	22.9	25.3	9.8	13.8

NAU, nausea; EM, emesis; H, headache; SE, heavy sedation; EU, euphoria; DYS, dysphoria; PR, pruritus; SW, sweating.

PSc, mean retrospective pain score; +, better/positive; =, comparable/uncertain; −, worse/negative.

quency as soon as they feel comfortable, but on the other, they are not willing to approach the permitted maximal doses by *raising* the demand frequency. Similar results were reported by Tamsen and his colleagues (25) from PCA studies with ketobemidone (25), and a comparable experience was described with 1-methadone (demand doses 0.58 or 1.1 mg) (26) and buprenorphine (demand doses 40 or 80 µg), although in the latter case the increase in analgesic efficacy was comparably small (27,28). Gibbs et al. (29) studied buprenorphine demand doses of 100 or 200 µg, and found no further differences. The reasons for this behavior remain to be clarified, but the phenomenon suggests that there are *optimum demand doses* for all analgesics, which have not been systematically evaluated up to now (8,9). Some authors feel that demand doses should be adjusted to patients' weight (30–32), whereas others deem body surface more appropriate (30,33–35) or suggest that they should be adjusted according to therapeutic efficacy (35–37). In a controlled study, Owen et al. (38) found that a demand dose of 0.5 mg morphine often proved ineffective, whereas 2 mg sometimes resulted in mild respiratory depression; these authors recommended 1 mg as an optimum demand. Graves et al. (39) demonstrated in a case report that in some patients demand doses up to 8 mg morphine can be necessary. It seems that more systematic studies on optimum demand doses are required before conclusive recommendations can be made.

Another, now widely accepted strategy to improve the efficacy of PCA is an *intravenous loading dose,* which is increased stepwise until the patient reports sufficient pain relief. With this approach, PCA itself is used only to *maintain* analgesia rather than to *establish* it (as was proposed in earlier studies). Although this concept is appealing, comparative investigations are still missing (24,40). The excellent effect of loading dosages confirms the general observation that analgesic intake is highest during the first few hours after an operation and then tends to decrease slowly (see below). The latter, in turn, suggests caution in the use of analgesic intake as a measure of pain. Adequate standardization would require a well-controlled time period between the end of surgery and PCA start, as well as a comparable duration of PCA treatment in all patients under study. Because there are some hints for circadian rhythms in pain intensity, and thus for time-dependent analgesic intake (41–44), the author's studies were always done for about 24 hrs after surgery, and weight- and time-adjusted analgesic consumption (µg/kg/h) was used for comparisons. Whether it is useful or even necessary to extend the observation period to the second or third postoperative day remains to be clarified.

There has been little concern so far regarding the duration of the *lockout time period,* i.e., the time interval required between drug administrations. Most modern PCA devices now restrict lockout time to a minimum of 5 min. It was the author's clinical impression in early studies that did not use loading doses that some patients needed shorter refractory times, and that programming the lockout time to 1 min did not prove particularly dangerous. If initial loading doses are titrated to a sufficient primary pain relief, however, lockout times in the range of 5 to 10 min should be appropriate in most cases, as long as optimum demand doses are prescribed. Table 6 displays PCA settings reviewed from the literature. To the author's knowledge, there have been no controlled studies to define optimum lockout periods, although some conclusions were tried from the frequency ratio of valid and invalid demands (45).

Successful use of PCA requires that the concept is understood and accepted by patient, nursing staff, and physician (10,32). Pre- and postoperative infor-

TABLE 6. *PCA settings for some frequently used postoperative opiates*[a]

Analgesic	Demand dose		Lockout time (min)	
	Mean	Median	Mean	Median
Morphine (mg)	1.6	1.4	7.9	6.0
Pethidine (mg)	20.2	17.5	11.1	10.0
Nalbuphine (mg)	4.0	3.9	5.5	5.0
Fentanyl (μg)	23.7	20.0	3.5	5.0
Alfentanil (μg)	116.5	100.0	3.3	1.0
Sufentanil (μg)	5.2	6.0	8.0	8.0
Buprenorphine (μg)	62.5	60.0	3.0	3.0

[a] Averaged from 70 studies reviewed.

mation should not only address appropriate handling of the device, but also predict that partial *relief,* rather than complete *freedom* of pain, can be expected.

USES OF PCA FOR PAIN MEASUREMENT

It is quite obvious that both the subjective description of pain intensity and the objective documentation of analgesic consumption under PCA conditions can be analyzed in relation to various perioperative factors. Hence, studies on the painfulness of surgical procedures, on the effectiveness of non-PCA treatment, on predictors of postoperative pain, on analgesic equipotency, and on drug interactions are possible, and have all been performed. Since repetitive demand dosages are applied at a point of time defined by clinical-pharmacodynamic parameters, i.e., at the individual pain tolerance threshold, pharmacokinetic predictions are verifiable and threshold concentrations or therapeutic windows can be defined.

Pain after Various Types of Surgery

Supposing that postoperative analgesic consumption reflects pain intensities after surgical operations, a rank order of painfulness can be established on that basis (46). It has been shown several times, however, that physicians' prescribing practices and nursing staff's application of physicians' orders are greatly influenced by tradition and fears of side effects, rather than by individual needs. Thus, retrospective analyses of analgesic dosages are more likely to indicate what patients received than what they needed (1,47–49). For this reason only complete independence of patients from normal drug administration procedures would justify the above assumptions (44,50,51). Unfortunately, only a few PCA studies have addressed this question systematically. Table 7 demonstrates the author's results with fentanyl. Although all patients had virtually free access to the fentanyl dosage, drug intake as well as retrospective pain judgment varied significantly. Thus, it must be concluded that even under PCA conditions, drug consumption

TABLE 7. *Postoperative fentanyl consumption following various types of surgery*

	n	(m/f)	μg/kg/h[a]	Retrospective pain score[b]	Product
Abdominal surgery	20	(10/10)	0.39 ± 0.31	1.25 ± 1.11	0.488
Orthopedics	20	(5/15)	0.53 ± 0.39	0.89 ± 0.55	0.472
Hysterectomies	92	(0/92)	0.65 ± 0.35	2.16 ± 1.28	1.404
Thoracotomies	19	(13/6)	0.68 ± 0.39	0.84 ± 0.83	0.571

[a] abd/orth and abd/thor: $p \le 0.05$.
[b] abd/hyst, orth/hyst and thor/hyst: $p \le 0.05$.
ODAC$_{fixed\ rate}$, demand dose 34.5 μg, infusion rate 4 μg/h, lockout time 1 min, hourly maximum dose 0.25 mg/h; results as arithmetic mean ± standard deviation.
From ref. 22 and unpublished results.

alone does not allow a valid comparison of the painfulness of various operations. Additional classical pain measurement must be performed. Whether the concept proposed by the author (i.e., calculation of the product of analgesic intake and retrospective verbal pain ratings) is valid for comparing painfulness (as well as equipotency ratios) remains to be proven. Although it corresponds to clinical experience (see Table 2), the data in Table 7 raise doubts: it is difficult to believe that pain following hysterectomy should be stronger than that following major abdominal surgery or thoracotomies. Obviously, more subjective parameters are needed; for example, it was the author's impression in the hysterectomy patients that the meaning of the operation to the patient (e.g., loss of an aspect of womanhood) was of utmost importance in the judgment of postoperative well-being, which is certainly reflected in the retrospective pain classification and possibly in analgesic consumption.

Differences in analgesic consumption following orthopedic and abdominal surgery were hardly distinguishable for most drugs, although they were obvious for some (20,52). It should be kept in mind, however, that interpretation of such results is always complicated by considerable individual variations that render statistical comparisons difficult.

Influence of Anesthetic Technique

Slowey et al. (53) observed that premedication with controlled release oral morphine 90 mg reduced postoperative pethidine PCA consumption in comparison with premedication using intramuscular morphine 15 mg. Judkins and Harmer (54) failed to demonstrate any analgesic interaction of the antiemetic haloperidol in 34 patients recovering from upper abdominal surgery under standardized neuroleptanalgesia; during the 24-hr observation period, pethidine consumption by PCA did not differ significantly whether the patients had been premedicated with 5 to 10 mg haloperidol or placebo, although antiemetic effects were evident after haloperidol. Owen et al. (55) investigated morphine and ketamine as intraoperative bolus and postoperative infusion in 60 patients whose postoperative analgesia was provided by morphine PCA. Postoperative pain scores and additional morphine consumption were comparable for both groups. Sjöström et al. (56) did not find any significant difference in postoperative pethidine consumption in 14 patients recovering from either balanced anesthesia or isoflurane inhalation. These studies suggest that PCA can be used to assess the analgesic consequences of different anesthetic techniques. Obviously, more are required.

Other Predictors of Postoperative Pain

Personality, age, and drug history are additional factors that presumably predict postoperative pain. Conclusive PCA studies of these questions are still lacking (57). Some particularly interesting investigations by Tamsen and his group (56,58,59) demonstrated a close correlation between postoperative analgesic consumption and preoperative neurotransmitter concentrations (endorphins, substance P) in CSF; women after cesarean section who had higher intrathecal enkephalin concentrations than a comparable group of patients undergoing elective gynecologic surgery self-administered significantly less postoperative morphine (60).

Bullingham et al. (61) and Watson et al. (62) found that male patients recovering from orthopedic surgery demanded more buprenorphine than female patients. Burns et al. (41) came to similar conclusions for morphine, as did Gourlay et al. (63) for fentanyl. Tamsen et al. (25) and Dahlström (64), on the other hand, did not observe any differences in morphine or pethidine demands between the sexes, nor did Keeri-Szanto (65) in studies with hydrocodone or Bennett et al. (35) with morphine.

It is generally accepted that analgesic demand decreases with age. Figure 4 shows unpublished data demonstrating in a group of 120 patients that cumulative morphine dosage was significantly correlated with age, and that retrospective pain scores were not. Similar results were obtained by Burns et al. (41). Tamsen et al. (66) on the contrary, did not find any influence of age on pethidine consumption and/or analgesic plasma concentrations, nor did Keeri-Szanto (65) for analgesic plasma concentrations during PCA with hydrocodone.

Gourlay et al. (63) assessed some psychologic variables in 30 patients prior to abdominal surgery; there was no important correlation with fentanyl consumption, plasma levels, and/or pain ratings during postoperative PCA. Similar conclusions with respect to the complexity and/or uncertainty of psychological predictors can be derived from studies with pethidine (67,68).

PCA for the Assessment of Non-PCA Pain Treatment

Many studies have used PCA to assess the efficacy of non-PCA pain treatment. Watson et al. (69) monitored postoperative fentanyl consumption to compare

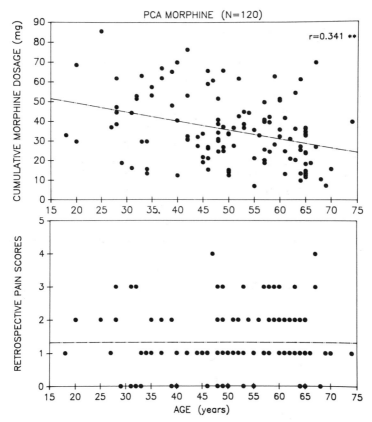

FIG. 4. Influence of age on morphine requirements (cumulative dose) and on retrospective pain scores during postoperative PCA (mean PCA duration 22 hrs, demand dose 2–3 mg, lockout time 1–2 min; author's unpublished results).

the effectiveness of epidural morphine and heroin, which had been administered during nucleotomy, and found no significant differences. Self-administered fentanyl was used in a similar study by McQuay et al. (70) to assess the efficacy of epidural heroin and fentanyl against placebo; a clear-cut difference in efficacy and duration of effect could be shown. Phillips et al. (71), using heroin as an intravenous PCA agent, could not demonstrate any difference in analgesic efficacy provided by 2 mg of thoracic epidural heroin or morphine, and Cohen et al. (72) found PCA with sufentanil suitable to evaluate the duration and quality of epidural versus intravenous sufentanil after cesarean section. The latter study demonstrated that the epidural group had a longer duration of analgesia, but similar analgesic efficacy (72). Coombs et al. (73) were unable to show a positive effect of adding small amounts of clonidine to intrathecal morphine for postoperative analgesia, which employed intravenous morphine PCA. Transdermal clonidine, however, reduced postoperative morphine PCA requirements (74).

Watson et al. (62) used PCA with heroin to test the analgesic effects of single postoperative buprenorphine doses (0.3 vs. 0.6 mg); the time until the fifth demand, the demands during 15 min intervals, and the mean cumulative heroin consumption all demonstrated a clear dose-effect relationship. These authors also reported the successful use of PCA with heroin or methadone to measure the effects of intra- and postoperative methadone or buprenorphine (61,75). Tamsen et al. (25) could not verify the influence of a spasmolytic on postoperative ketobemidone consumption or analgesic efficacy.

Transdermal fentanyl is a newer approach for continuous noninvasive delivery of narcotic analgesics. It could be shown in the author's double-blind investigations that fentanyl patches with a delivery rate of 75 μg/h, applied 8 hrs prior to urologic surgery, significantly reduced postoperative pain intensity and analgesic consumption, as determined with fentanyl PCA (Fig. 5) (76). Similar results were obtained by Rowbotham et al. (77), who studied 40 patients after upper abdominal surgery and tried fentanyl patches with a 100 μg/h delivery rate.

Alston et al. (78) assessed the efficacy of intraperitoneal bupivacaine versus placebo in a group of abdominal surgery patients who could self-administer

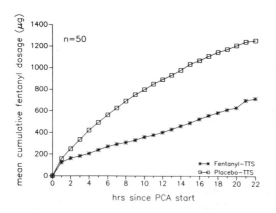

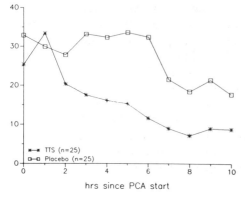

FIG. 5. Mean cumulative postoperative fentanyl consumption (demand dose 34 μg, lockout time 5 min) and mean visual analogue scale (VAS) in a group of 50 urologic patients with fentanyl (75 μg/h) or placebo transdermal application 8 hrs prior to surgery (76).

morphine postoperatively. Younger patients, but not older ones, had significantly less demands in the active treatment group during the 24-hr observation period.

McCallum et al. (79) used postoperative morphine PCA to evaluate transcutaneous electrical nerve stimulation (TENS). It was without effect in 20 patients recovering from nucleotomy; specifically, there were no statistically significant differences in number of demands, 24-hr morphine consumption, or morphine plasma levels between the active and sham group. Christensen et al. (80), studying pethidine PCA following gynecologic operations, found significantly less pethidine consumption only during the first 2 hrs after extubation when patients had been treated intraoperatively with electroacupuncture.

PCA for the Assessment of Analgesic Drug Interactions

Drug combinations are often used in clinical practice to reduce opiate doses. In most cases, however, objective evidence of potentiation is not available. PCA studies may be able to answer such questions. Jones et al. (81) determined the effectiveness of acetylsalicylic acid infusions in postthoracotomy patients who were allowed to self-administer papaveretum. In a similar investigation, Owen et al. (82) demonstrated a 20% reduction of morphine demand by the addition of ibuprofen to the postoperative regimen. Comparably positive interactions were reported by Gillies et al. (83), who evaluated the efficacy of postoperative ketorolac and placebo infusions in 71 abdominal surgery patients receiving morphine PCA. Rectal diclofenac, however, failed to augment postoperative analgesia after cholecystectomy in a placebo-controlled study that used PCA morphine consumption to evaluate effects (84). In a similar study by Goucke et al. (85), intramuscular diclofenac or nefopam failed to decrease postoperative morphine consumption. In the author's studies with 1-methadone, the antipyretic analgesic metamizol was found to increase the analgesic efficacy of methadone PCA and to decrease the 24-hr methadone consumption, although the differences were not statistically significant (26).

In 1985, von Bormann et al. (86) reported that the calcium channel blocker nimodipine reduced intraoperative fentanyl requirements in patients undergoing cardiovascular surgery, a finding that was discussed as analgesic potentiation. This conclusion was confirmed in animal experiments (87). In contrast, postoperative pain scores and on-demand fentanyl consumption in hysterectomy patients were comparable in patients receiving either placebo or 1 to 2 mg/kg/h nimodipine infusions (88).

Cholecystokinin and related peptides are not only effective as gastroenteral hormones, but are also thought to play an important role as neurotransmitters in the brain. There are good reasons to suggest that cholecystokinin acts as a physiological endorphin antagonist. Proglumide, a drug prescribed for the prevention and treatment of peptic ulcers, is a cholecystokinin antagonist and therefore believed to potentiate physiological endorphin effects. This assumption was verified by Watkins et al. (89) in animal experiments and by Price et al. (90)

with human volunteers, where morphine analgesia was intensified by some (not all) proglumide concentrations studied. On the other hand, patients recovering from elective abdominal surgery who were randomly assigned to self-administer morphine (3-mg demand doses) with either placebo, 50 μg, 100 μg, or 50 mg proglumide per demand, did not differ significantly with respect to morphine consumption or retrospective pain scores (Fig. 6) (17).

Positive interactions were found in the author's investigations on buprenorphine-naloxone combinations. A mixture of buprenorphine and 60% naloxone, which was thought to prevent misuse by drug addicts, proved to be significantly less analgesic and respiratory depressant than buprenorphine alone, although global efficacy was still comparable with morphine under PCA conditions (28). In a similar study performed by Clyburn and Rosen (91), the interactions between pethidine and the respiratory stimulant doxapram in cholecystectomy patients were evaluated, using the Cardiff Palliator. Although the duration of the few reported apnea periods was slightly shorter with doxapram, there was no statistically significant difference with respect to spontaneous respiration or analgesic consumption.

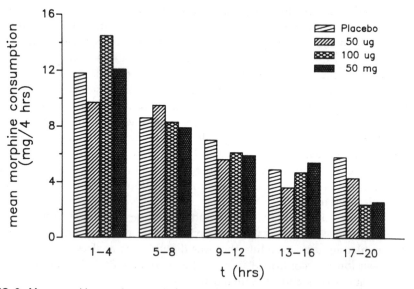

FIG. 6. Mean morphine requirements in four hourly observation periods in groups of 20 patients who were allowed to self-administer morphine (demand dose 3 mg, lockout time 2 min) with additional placebo or proglumide 50 μg, 100 μg, or 50 mg along with each demand (17).

Equipotency of Analgesic Drugs

Estimation of relative potency should be possible when analgesic consumption using PCA is analyzed in comparable groups of patients (6,23,92–95,97–100).

It was of particular interest, however, that comparative studies often revealed differences in overall therapeutic outcome, depending on the analgesic studied, despite the fact that maximum doses were virtually unlimited. Thus, it does not seem justified merely to compare drug consumption without taking into account efficacy. For this reason, in the author's studies the *product* of mean analgesic consumption (μg/kg/h) and mean retrospective pain score was calculated (Tables 2,3, and 7). The resulting figures take into account both intensity and duration of effect. It should be stressed that this attempt must be preliminary as long as nonoptimum demand doses are used (see above), that simply multiplying the variables (cumulative dose, dose/time, dose/weight/time?, actual or retrospective pain scores?) may be questionable, and that the approach is possibly not valid for agonist-antagonist opiates, for which analgesic ceiling effects limit an increase of efficacy with increasing doses. Nevertheless, the reported figures seem to reflect clinical experience and confirm data published by other authors. Chakravarty et al. (93) found a pethidine/buprenorphine consumption ratio of 1:600. The ratio for pentazocine/buprenorphine reported by Harmer et al. (101) was 1:233. Comparing fentanyl and alfentanil, Kay (95) differentiated between analgesic potency and duration of action and calculated a global ratio of 1:12, which fits well with the author's results (102). Sinatra et al. (97), studying morphine, pethidine, and oxymorphone, found relative equipotent dosages of 1, 9.1, and 0.16, respectively, based on either mean cumulative dose or mg/h. Further controlled investigations on this subject are highly desirable and obviously essential for drug comparisons.

"Analgesic" Plasma Concentrations

The most important goal of pharmacokinetics is to measure the time course of drug concentrations in blood or other body compartments, to describe them mathematically and to predict them from suitable models. It is evident that concentrations alone are of only minor value unless the correlation between concentration and pharmacodynamic effects are also known. Comprehensive studies have now been done for most analgesics (103,104). Unfortunately, their value for clinical practice is rather controversial because the concentration/effect relationship is extremely variable among patients (22,105–107). PCA is regarded as a suitable therapeutic regimen not only because it overcomes such individual differences, but also because it allows them to be measured.

Several studies have compared opiate blood concentrations measured under PCA with underlying pharmacokinetic models, as well as with pain relief achieved. Using pethidine during labor, Hogg and Rosen (31) found a rather bad correlation between predicted and measured blood levels. Tamsen and his colleagues (25,57,64,66,108), on the other hand, reported on a close correlation only if individual pharmacokinetic parameters derived from intraoperative analysis were used for comparison with postoperative data from the same patient;

intersubject variability, however, was found to be very high for all analgesics studied.

Much time was spent in the author's own experiments to determine analgesic "threshold" concentrations (minimum effective concentrations, MEC) for some opiates. For this reason, venous blood samples were taken immediately before a patient demand, i.e., at a point in time at which the patient was just becoming dissatisfied with analgesia (6,22,102,109,110). Figure 7 displays alfentanil results (40 ASA I-III patients recovering from abdominal or orthopedic surgery, Tables 2 and 5). It is evident that a generizable threshold concentration does not exist. In similar studies with fentanyl some patients had intraindividual stable MECs, which were different from other subjects, whereas some patients also showed remarkable intraindividual variation (Fig. 8).

Results from the literature underscore that MECs are usually log-normally distributed, and that the range is very broad. Studying hydrocodone, Keeri-Szanto (65) came to similar conclusions, as did Hackl et al. (94) with fentanyl and tramadol and Gourlay et al. (63) with fentanyl. Following proposals by Gourlay et al. (111), it could be shown for our own data that intraindividual variability in MEC was consistently lower than the interindividual one (Table 8); individual regression analyses (MEC vs time of MEC) as proposed by Tamsen et al. (66) never gave an indication of accumulation.

Gourlay et al. (63) found a mean postoperative fentanyl MEC of 0.63 ng/ml with an intraindividual variability of 30%. Mean fentanyl MEC in the study by

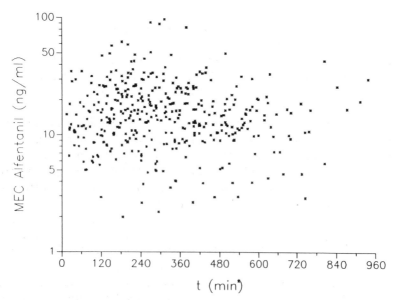

FIG. 7. Minimum effective alfentanil plasma concentrations during postoperative PCA (40 patients, 381 samples), plotted against duration of treatment (102).

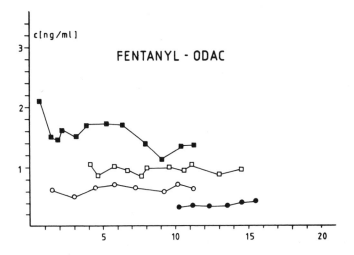

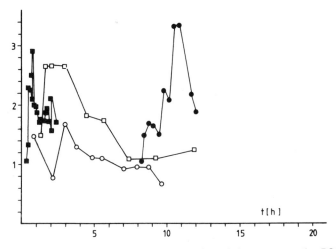

FIG. 8. Minimum effective fentanyl plasma concentrations during postoperative PCA (ODAC$_{fixed\ rate}$, cf. Tables 2 and 5 for dosing parameters and therapeutic outcome). Venous samples were taken just before a demand dose. Inter- and intraindividual variations in analgesic "threshold" are clearly shown for eight different patients (22).

Hackl et al. (94) was 1.54 ng/ml, and mean tramadol MEC was 915.5 ng/ml. Hydrocodone MEC, as reported by Keeri-Szanto (65), was 6 ng/ml. Morphine MEC was 16 ng/ml (64) and pethidine MEC was 455 ng/ml in studies by Tamsen and his colleagues (66). These results are compared in Table 9. They show a trend toward equipotency similar to that demonstrated in Table 2, although some differences are obvious. It is self-evident, however, that more data are necessary to render such conclusions reliable.

TABLE 8. *Minimum effective concentrations (MEC) during postoperative PCA*

Analgesic	Median (ng/ml)	Min	Max	Variability (%) Intrasubject	Intersubject
Sufentanil	0.04	0.01	0.56	80.0	81.0
Buprenorphine	0.38	0.01	6.56	67.9	107.3
Fentanyl	1.16	0.18	8.01	27.2	63.9
Alfentanil	14.87	0.57	99.20	37.0	62.5
Tramadol	289.40	20.20	1,358.90	41.7	55.9

From refs. 22, 28, 102, and author's unpublished results.

In summary, therefore, PCA investigations do not establish analgesic threshold concentrations that are valid for all patients and make a pharmacokinetic "design" of analgesia realistic. In view of the available data, it seems wiser to use the term "therapeutic window" instead of "threshold," and it should not be forgotten that the window is rather broad. For pain measurement, this conclusion implies that determining serum or plasma concentrations of narcotic analgesics can give only a vague impression of the pain intensity actually experienced by an individual patient.

RECOMMENDATIONS FOR THE USE OF PCA IN ANALGESIC STUDIES

As far as we know today, it is impossible to accurately predict how much pain a patient will experience after an operation, or what analgesic dosage will be required to provide adequate pain relief. Although suitable methods of clinical algesiometry are available, they are seldom used in everyday practice (1). The introduction of PCA has opened up new possibilities in the study of pain and analgesics. Since the patients have virtually free access to the dose, different agents or strategies can be compared more or less objectively. In principle, the

TABLE 9. *Opiate potency derived from minimum effective concentrations (MEC) during postoperative PCA*

Analgesic	Mean MEC	Relative potency (morphine = 1)
Sufentanil	0.04	400
Buprenorphine	0.38	42
Fentanyl	0.63	25
	1.16	14
	1.54	10
Hydrocodone	6	3
Alfentanil	15	1
Morphine	16	1
Ketobemidone	28	0.6
Tramadol	289	0.05
	915	0.02
Pethidine	455	0.04

For references, see text.

demand rate may be used as a measure of pain, but there is still no agreement on optimum demand dosage for the various analgesics. Cumulative dosage over a well-defined period of time may be used alternatively. It has to be kept in mind that all PCA studies have so far demonstrated that pain intensity and analgesic consumption decrease with time, and there are, as of now, no conclusive studies that indicate what time period is most suitable. The potential benefits obtained by adjusting cumulative dosage by weight and/or duration of treatment also remain to be clarified. All these variables, however, must be interpreted with caution. Patients usually control their analgesic demand within the limits available to them, and they seem to strike a balance between the desirable analgesic effect of the drug and undesirable effects such as nausea, sedation, or dysphoria. In other words, the demand rate is determined not only by the drug's analgesic properties but also by its overall acceptability. This finding includes the observation, although still not very well understood, that some patients are prepared to tolerate a certain amount of pain, whereas others are not. In short, analgesic demands do not reflect pain intensity alone. The influence of psychological variables (and thus patient selection) on pain behavior during PCA should be better defined before conclusive comparisons are possible. Because individual variability is so important in the study of acute pain, it seems that large numbers of patients are necessary for statistical conclusions; there is, however, still no objective evidence as to how large these numbers should be.

In view of the data presented in this review, it is the author's personal opinion that groups of at least 30 to 40 patients, matched as closely as possible for demographic variables, the anesthetic technique, and type of surgical operation are necessary for reliable comparisons. Patients should be well informed about objectives and handling of PCA on the day prior to PCA. The duration of PCA treatment should be in the range of 24 hrs. Analgesic consumption, adjusted to weight and duration of treatment, should be monitored, along with hourly pain scores, and a retrospective evaluation of overall effectiveness, side effects, and patient acceptance should be performed.

Finally, PCA researchers have the strong impression that most patients seem to use PCA to get *comfortable* rather than *pain free*. Interpretation of PCA results should therefore be particularly critical with respect to pain measurement experimental algesiometry. Nevertheless, results available so far suggest that PCA is not only efficacious and well accepted by the patients, but can also improve conventional postoperative pain therapy. Objective documentation of individual variability in analgesic demand, which is often much higher than anticipated from clinical "experience," must consequently lead to a greater confidence in patients' opinions.

REFERENCES

1. Lehmann KA, Henn C. Zur Lage der postoperativen schmerztherapie in der Bundesrepublik Deutschland. Ergebnisse einer Repräsentativumfrage. *Anaesthesist* 1987;36:400–406.
2. Bonica JJ. Current status of postoperative pain therapy. In: Yokota T, Dubner R, eds. *Current topics in pain research and therapy.* Amsterdam: Excerpta Medica, 1983;169–189.

3. Bennett RL, Griffen WO. Patient-controlled analgesia (PCA): optimization of in-hospital narcotic analgesia therapy. *Contemp Surg* 1983;23:75–89.
4. Dubois M. Patient-controlled analgesia for acute pain. *Clin J Pain* 1989;5(Suppl 1):S8–S15.
5. Graves DA, Foster TS, Batenhorst RL, Bennett RL, Baumann TJ. Patient-controlled analgesia. *Ann Intern Med* 1983;99:360–366.
6. Lehmann KA. On-demand analgesie: neue möglichkeiten zur behandlung akuter schmerzen. *Arzneimittelforschung* 1984;34:1108–1114.
7. Lehmann KA. Patient-controlled analgesia for postoperative pain. In:Benedetti C, Chapman R, Giron G, eds. Opioid analgesia: recent advances in systemic administration. *Advances in Pain Research and Therapy* 1990;297–324.
8. Mather LE, Owen H. The scientific basis of patient-controlled analgesia. *Anaesth Intensive Care* 1988;16:427–436.
9. Owen H, Mather LE, Rowley K. The development and clinical use of patient-controlled analgesia. *Anaesth Intensive Care* 1988;16:437–447.
10. White PF. Patient-controlled analgesia: a new approach to the management of postoperative pain. *Semin Anesth* 1985;4:255–266.
11. White PF. Postoperative pain management with patient-controlled analgesia. *Semin Anesth* 1986;5:116–122.
12. White PF. Use of patient-controlled analgesia for management of acute pain. *JAMA* 1988;259:243–247.
13. Harmer M, Rosen M, Vickers MD, eds. *Patient-controlled analgesia.* Oxford: Blackwell Scientific Publications, 1985.
14. Lehmann KA, Mehler O. Postoperative on-demand analgesie mit fentanyl unter verwendung des infusionssystems CODIC: erste klinische erfahrungen. *Anaesthesist* 1987;36:595–598.
15. Bullingham RES, Jacobs OLR, McQuay HJ, Moore RA. The Oxford system of patient-controlled analgesia. *Advances in Pain Research and Therapy* 1986;9:319–324.
16. Lehmann KA, Gördes B, Hoeckle W. Postoperative on-demand analgesie mit morphin. *Anaesthesist* 1985;34:494–501.
17. Lehmann KA, Schlüsener M, Arabatsis P. Failure of proglumide, a cholecystokinin antagonist, to potentiate clinical morphine analgesia. A randomized double-blind postoperative study using patient-controlled analgesia (PCA). *Anesth Analg* 1989;68:51–56.
18. Owen H, Szekely SM, Plummer JL, Cushnie JM, Mather LE. Variables of patient-controlled analgesia. 2. Concurrent infusion. *Anaesthesia* 1989;44:11–13.
19. Vickers AP, Derbyshire DR, Burt DR, Bagshaw PF, Pearson H, Smith G. Comparison of the Leicester micropalliator and the Cardiff palliator in the relief of postoperative pain. *Br J Anaesth* 1987;59:503–509.
20. Lehmann KA, Tenbuhs B. Patient-controlled analgesia with nalbuphine, a new narcotic agonist-antagonist, for the treatment of postoperative pain. *Eur J Clin Pharmacol* 1986;31:267–276.
21. McQuay HJ, Moore RA, Lloyd JW, Bullingham RES, Evans PJD. Some patients don't need analgesics after surgery. *J R Soc Med* 1982;75:705–708.
22. Lehmann KA, Heinrich C, van Heiss R. Balanced anaesthesia and patient-controlled postoperative analgesia with fentanyl: minimum effective concentrations, accumulation and acute tolerance. *Acta Anaesthesiol Belg* 1988;39:11–23.
23. Lehmann KA, Jung C, Hoeckle W. Tramadol und pethidin zur postoperativen schmerztherapie: eine randomisierte doppelblindstudie unter den bedingungen der intravenösen on-demand analgesie. *Schmerz-Pain-Douleur* 1985;6:88–100.
24. Lehmann KA, Brand-Stavroulaki A, Dworzak H. The influence of demand and loading dose on the efficacy of postoperative patient-controlled analgesia with tramadol. A randomized double-blind study. *Schmerz-Pain-Douleur* 1986;7:146–152.
25. Tamsen A, Bondesson U, Dahlström B, Hartvig P. Patient-controlled analgesic therapy, part III: pharmacokinetics and analgesic plasma concentrations of ketobemidone. *Clin Pharmacokinet* 1982;7:252–265.
26. Lehmann KA, Abu-Shibika M, Horrichs-Haermeyer G. Postoperative schmerztherapie mit l-methadon und metamizol. Eine randomisierte untersuchung im rahmen der intravenösen on-demand analgesie. *Anaesth Intensivther Notfallmed* 1990;25:152–159.
27. Lehmann KA, Gördes B. Postoperative on-demand analgesie mit buprenorphin. *Anaesthesist* 1988;37:65–70.
28. Lehmann KA, Reichling U, Wirtz R. Influence of naloxone on the postoperative analgesic and respiratory effects of buprenorphine. *Eur J Clin Pharmacol* 1988;34:343–352.

29. Gibbs JM, Johnson HD, Davis FM. Patient administration of i.v. buprenorphine for postoperative pain relief using the "Cardiff" demand analgesia computer. *Br J Anaesth* 1982;54:279–284.
30. Bennett RL, Batenhorst RL, Bivins BA, et al. Patient-controlled analgesia. A new concept of postoperative pain relief. *Ann Surg* 1982;195:700–705.
31. Hogg MIJ, Rosen M. Self-administered analgesia—pharmacokinetic limitations. In:Stoeckel H, ed. *Quantitation, modelling and control in anaesthesia.* Stuttgart: Thieme, 1985;291–301.
32. Rosenberg PH, Heino A, Scheinin B. Comparison of intramuscular analgesia, intercostal block, epidural morphine and on-demand-i.v. fentanyl in the control of pain after upper abdominal surgery. *Acta Anaesthesiol Scand* 1984;28:603–607.
33. Atwell JR, Flanigan RC, Bennett RL, Allen DC, Lucas BA, McRoberts JW. The efficacy of patient-controlled analgesia in patients recovering from flank incisions. *J Urol* 1984;132:701–703.
34. Bennett RL, Batenhorst R, Graves D, Foster TS, Baumann T, Griffen WO, Wright BD. Morphine titration in postoperative laparatomy patients using patient-controlled analgesia. *Curr Ther Res* 1982;32:45–52.
35. Bennett RL, Batenhorst R, Graves DA, Foster TS, Griffen WO, Wright BD. Variation in postoperative analgesic requirements in the morbidly obese following gastric bypass surgery. *Pharmacotherapy* 1982;2:50–53.
36. Brown RE, Broadman LM. Patient-controlled analgesia for postoperative pain control in adolescents. *Anesth Analg* 1987;66:S22.
37. Urquhart ML, Klapp K, White PF. Patient-controlled analgesia: a comparison of intravenous versus subcutaneous hydromorphone. *Anesthesiology* 1988;69:428–432.
38. Owen H, Plummer JL, Armstrong I, Mather LE, Cousins MJ. Variables of patient-controlled analgesia. 1. Bolus size. *Anaesthesia* 1989;44:7–10.
39. Graves DA, Baumann TH, Bennett RL, et al. Extraordinary analgesic requirement in a patient previously unexposed to narcotics. *Drug Intell Clin Pharm* 1984;18:598–600.
40. Ved SA, Dubois M, Carron H, Lea D. Sufentanil and alfentanil pattern of consumption during patient-controlled analgesia: a comparison with morphine. *Clin J Pain* 1989;5(Suppl 1):S63–S70.
41. Burns JW, Hodsman NBA, McLintock TTC, Gillies GWA, Kenny GNC, McArdle CS. The influence of patient characteristics on the requirements for postoperative analgesia. A reassessment using patient-controlled analgesia. *Anaesthesia* 1989;44:2–6.
42. Ferrante RM, Orav EJ, Rocco AG, Gallo J. A statistical model for pain in patient-controlled analgesia and conventional intramuscular opioid regimes. *Anesth Analg* 1988;67:457–461.
43. Graves DA, Batenhorst RL, Bennett RL, et al. Morphine requirements using patient-controlled analgesia: influence of diurnal variation and morbid obesity. *Clin Pharm* 1983;2:49–53.
44. Sechzer PH. Objective measurement of pain. *Anesthesiology* 1968;29:209–210.
45. Serrao J, Rosen M. Postoperative patient-controlled analgesia (PCA): a method of comparing intermittent demands with and without background infusion. *Br J Anaesth* 1986;58:812P–813P.
46. Parkhouse J, Lambrechts W, Simpson BRJ. The incidence of postoperative pain. *Br J Anaesth* 1961;33:345–353.
47. Cartwright PD. Pain control after surgery: a survey of current practice. *Ann R Coll Surg Engl* 1985;67:13–16.
48. Mather L, Mackie J. The incidence of postoperative pain in children. *Pain* 1983;15:271–282.
49. Weis OF, Sriwatanakul K, Alloza JL, Weintraub M, Lasagna L. Attitudes of patients, housestaff, and nurses toward postoperative analgesic care. *Anesth Analg* 1983;62:70–74.
50. Rosen M. The measurement of pain. In: Harcus AW, Smith R, Whittle B, eds. *Perspectives in measurement and management.* London: Churchill Livingstone, 1977;13–20.
51. Sechzer PH. Studies in pain with the analgesic-demand system. *Anesth Analg* 1971;50:1–10.
52. Lehmann KA, Tenbuhs B, Hoeckle W. Patient-controlled analgesia with piritramid for the treatment of postoperative pain. *Acta Anaesthesiol Belg* 1986;37:247–257.
53. Slowey HF, Reynolds AD, Mapleson WW, Vickers MD. Effect of premedication with controlled-release oral morphine on postoperative pain. A comparison with intramuscular morphine. *Anaesthesia* 1985;40:438–440.
54. Judkins KC, Harmer M. Haloperidol as an adjunct analgesic in the management of postoperative pain. *Anaesthesia* 1982;37:1118–1120.
55. Owen H, Reekie RM, Clements JA, Watson R, Nimmo WS. Analgesia from morphine and ketamine. A comparison of infusions of morphine and ketamine for postoperative analgesia. *Anaesthesia* 1987;42:1051–1056.

56. Sjöström S, Tamsen A, Hartvig P, Folkesson R, Terenius L. Cerebrospinal fluid concentrations of substance P and (Met)enkephalin-Arg6-Phe7 during surgery and patient-controlled analgesia. *Anesth Analg* 1988;67:976–981.
57. Tamsen A. Facteurs affectant l'analgésie. L'autoadministration d'analgésiques. *Cah Anesthesiol* 1985;33:115–118.
58. Tamsen A, Sakurada T, Wahlström A, Terenius L, Hartvig P. Postoperative demand for analgesics in relation to individual levels of endorphins and substance P in cerebrospinal fluid. *Pain* 1982;13: 171–183.
59. Terenius L, Tamsen A. Endorphins and the modulation of acute pain. *Acta Anaesthesiol Scand* 1982;Suppl 74:21–24.
60. Eisenach JC, Dobson CE, Inturrisi CE, Hood DD. Do spinal enkephalins mediate analgesia during pregnancy? *Anesth Analg* 1989;68:S78.
61. Bullingham RES, McQuay HJ, Dwyer D, Allen MC, Moore RA. Sublingual buprenorphine used postoperatively: clinical observations and preliminary pharmacokinetic analysis. *Br J Clin Pharmacol* 1981;12:117–122.
62. Watson PJQ, McQuay HJ, Bullingham RES, Allen MC, Moore RA. Single-dose comparison of buprenorphine 0.3 and 0.6 mg i.v. given after operation: clinical effects and plasma concentrations. *Br J Anaesth* 1982;54:37–43.
63. Gourlay GK, Kowalski SR, Plummer JL, Cousins MJ, Armstrong PJ. Fentanyl blood concentration–analgesic response relationship in the treatment of postoperative pain. *Anesth Analg* 1988;67:329–337.
64. Dahlström B, Tamsen A, Paalzow L, Hartvig P. Patient-controlled analgesic therapy, part IV: pharmacokinetics and analgesic plasma concentrations of morphine. *Clin Pharmacokinet* 1982;7: 266–279.
65. Keeri-Szanto M. The kinetics of postoperative analgesia. *Clin Pharmacol Ther* 1980;27:263.
66. Tamsen A, Hartvig P, Fagerlund C, Dahlström B. Patient-controlled analgesic therapy, part II: individual analgesic demand and plasma concentrations of pethidine in postoperative pain. *Clin Pharmacokinet* 1982;7:164–175.
67. Johnson LR, Ferrante FM, Magnani BJ, Rocco AG. Psychological modifiers of PCA efficacy. *Reg Anaesth* 1988;13(Suppl 1):52.
68. McGrath D, Thurston N, Wright D, Preshaw R, Fermin P. Comparison of one technique of patient-controlled postoperative analgesia with intramuscular meperidine. *Pain* 1989;37:265–270.
69. Watson J, Moore A, McQuay H, Teddy P, Baldwin D, Allen M, Bullingham R. Plasma morphine concentrations and analgesic effects of lumbar extradural morphine and heroin. *Anesth Analg* 1984;63:629–634.
70. McQuay HJ, Bullingham RES, Evans PJD, Lloyd JW, Moore RA. Demand analgesia to assess pain relief from epidural opiates. *Lancet* 1980;1:768–769.
71. Phillips DM, Moore RA, Bullingham RES, et al. Plasma morphine concentrations and clinical effects after thoracic extradural morphine or diamorphine. *Br J Anaesth* 1984;56:829–836.
72. Cohen SE, Tan S, White PF. Sufentanil analgesia following cesarean section: epidural versus intravenous administration. *Anesthesiology* 1988;68:129–134.
73. Coombs DW, Jensen LB, Murphy C. Microdose intrathecal clonidine and morphine for postoperative analgesia. *Anesthesiology* 1987;67:A238.
74. Segal IS, Jarvis DA, Duncan SR, White PF, Maze M. Perioperative use of transdermal clonidine as an adjunctive agent. *Anesth Analg* 1989;68:S250.
75. Porter EBJ, McQuay HJ, Bullingham RES, Weir L, Allen MC, Moore RA. Comparison of effects of intraoperative and postoperative methadone: acute tolerance to the postoperative dose? *Br J Anaesth* 1983;55:325–332.
76. Einnolf C, Eberlein HJ, Nagel R, Lehmann KA. Transdermal appliziertes fentanyl in der postoperativen schmerztherapie. Untersuchungen mit hilfe der on-demand analgesie. *Anaesthesist* 1989;38(Suppl 1):556.
77. Rowbotham DJ, Wyld R, Peackock JE, Duthie DJR, Nimmo WS. Transdermal fentanyl for the relief of pain after upper abdominal surgery. *Br J Anaesth* 1989;63:56–59.
78. Alston RP, Owen H, Bell M, Burns H. Analgesic effects of bupivacaine i.p. *Br J Anaesth* 1987;59: 1326P.
79. McCallum MID, Glynn CJ, Moore RA, Lammer P, Phillips AM. Transcutaneous electrical nerve stimulation in the management of acute postoperative pain. *Br J Anaesth* 1988;61:308–312.

80. Christensen PA, Noreng M, Andersen PE, Nielsen JW. Electroacupuncture and postoperative pain. *Br J Anaesth* 1989;62:258–262.
81. Jones RM, Cashman JN, Foster JMG, Wedley JR, Adams AP. Comparison of infusions of morphine and lysine acetyl salicylate for the relief of pain following thoracic surgery. *Br J Anaesth* 1985;57:259–263.
82. Owen H, Glavin RJ, Shaw NA. Ibuprofen in the management of postoperative pain. *Br J Anaesth* 1986;58:1371–1375.
83. Gillies GWA, Kenny GNC, Bullingham RES, McArdle CS. The morphine sparing effect of ketorolac tromethamine. A study of a new, parenteral non-steroidal anti-inflammatory agent after abdominal surgery. *Anaesthesia* 1987;42:727–731.
84. Colquhoun AD, Fell D. Failure of rectal diclofenac to augment opioid analgesia after cholecystectomy. *Anaesthesia* 1989;44:57–60.
85. Goucke CR, Eadsforth P, Kay B, Healy TEJ. Effect of diclofenac and nefopam on the postoperative morphine demand from a patient controlled analgesia apparatus. *Br J Anaesth* 1988;60: 333P.
86. von Bormann B, Boldt J, Sturm G, et al. Calciumantagonisten in der anaesthesie. Additive analgesie durch nimodipin während cardiochirurgischer eingriffe. *Anaesthesist* 1985;34:429–434.
87. Hoffmeister F, Tettenborn D. Calcium agonists and antagonists of the dihydropyridine type: antinociceptive effects, interference with opiate-μ-receptor agonists and neuropharmacological actions in rodents. *Psychopharmacology* 1986;90:299–307.
88. Lehmann KA, Kriegel R, Ueki M. Zur klinischen bedeutung von arzneimittelinteraktionen zwischen opiaten und kalziumantagonisten. Eine randomisierte doppelblindstudie mit fentanyl und nimodipin im rahmen der postoperativen intravenösen on-demand analgesie. *Anaesthesist* 1989;38:110–115.
89. Watkins LR, Kinschek IB, Mayer DJ. Potentiation of opiate analgesia and apparent reversal of morphine tolerance by proglumide. *Science* 1984;224:395–396.
90. Price DD, von der Gruen A, Miller J, Rafii A, Price C. Potentiation of systemic morphine analgesia in humans by proglumide, a cholecystokinine antagonist. *Anesth Analg* 1985;64:801–806.
91. Clyburn PA, Rosen M. Patient-controlled analgesia with a mixture of pethidine and doxapram hydrochloride. A comparison of the incidence of respiratory dysrhythmias with pethidine alone. *Anaesthesia* 1988;43:190–193.
92. Bahar M, Rosen M, Vickers MD. Self-administered nalbuphine, morphine and pethidine. Comparison, by intravenous route, following cholecystectomy. *Anaesthesia* 1985;40:529–532.
93. Chakravarty K, Tucker W, Rosen M, Vickers MD. Comparison of buprenorphine and pethidine given intravenously on demand to relieve postoperative pain. *Br Med J* 1979;2:895–897.
94. Hackl W, Fitzal S, Lackner F, Weindlmayr-Goettel M. Vergleich von fentanyl und tramadol zur schmerzbehandlung mittels on-demand-analgesie-computer in der frühen postoperativen phase. *Anaesthesist* 1986;35:665–671.
95. Kay B. Postoperative pain relief. Use of an on-demand analgesia computer (ODAC) and a comparison of the rate of use of fentanyl and alfentanyl. *Anaesthesia* 1981;36:949–951.
96. Lehmann KA. Practical experience with demand analgesia for postoperative pain. In: Harmer M, Rosen M, Vickers MD, eds. *Patient-controlled analgesia.* Oxford: Blackwell Scientific Publications, 1985;134–139.
97. Sinatra RS, Lodge K, Sibert K, et al. A comparison of morphine, meperidine, and oxymorphone as utilized in patient-controlled analgesia following cesarean delivery. *Anesthesiology* 1989;70: 585–590.
98. Slattery PJ, Harmer M, Rosen M, Vickers MD. Comparison of meptazinol and pethidine given i.v. on demand in the management of postoperative pain. *Br J Anaesth* 1981;53:927–931.
99. Sprigge JS, Otton PE. Nalbuphine versus meperidine for postoperative analgesia: a double-blind comparison using the patient controlled analgesic technique. *Can Anaesth Soc J* 1983;30: 517–521.
100. Welchew EA, Hosking J. Patient-controlled postoperative analgesia with alfentanil. Adaptive, on-demand intravenous alfentanil or pethidine compared double-blind for postoperative pain. *Anaesthesia* 1985;40:1172–1177.
101. Harmer M, Slattery PJ, Rosen M, Vickers MD. Comparison between buprenorphine and pentazocine given i.v. on demand in the control of postoperative pain. *Br J Anaesth* 1983;55:21–25.

102. Lehmann K. Relative wirkstärke von alfentanil bei postoperativer on-demand zufuhr. In:Zindler M, Hartung E, eds. *Alfentanil. Ein neues, ultrakurzwirkendes opioid.* München: Urban & Schwarzenberg, 1985;33–37.
103. Mather LE. Clinical pharmacokinetics of fentanyl and its newer derivatives. *Clin Pharmacokinet* 1983;8:422–426.
104. Mather LE. Pharmacokinetic and pharmacodynamic factors influencing the choice, dose and route of administration of opiates for acute pain. In:Bullingham RES, ed. *Opiate analgesia.* London: Saunders, 1983;17–40.
105. Austin KL, Stapleton JV, Mather LE. Multiple intramuscular injections: a major source of variability in analgesic response to meperidine. *Pain* 1980;8:47–62.
106. Austin KL, Stapleton JV, Mather LE. Relationship between blood meperidine concentrations and analgesic response: a preliminary report. *Anesthesiology* 1980;53:460–466.
107. Lehmann KA, Tenbuhs B, Hoeckle W. Postoperative on-demand analgesie mit pentazocin (fortral). *Langenbecks Arch Chir* 1985;367:27–40.
108. Tamsen A, Sjöström S, Hartvig P. The Uppsala experience of patient-controlled analgesia. *Advances in Pain Research and Therapy,* 1986;8:325–332.
109. Lehmann KA. Discussion. In: Harmer M, Rosen M, Vickers MD, eds. *Patient-controlled analgesia.* Oxford: Blackwell Scientific Publications, 1985;18–29.
110. Lehmann KA. Pharmakokinetik: gibt es analgetische blutkonzentrationen? In: Kettler D, Croizier T, Metzler H, eds. *Analgesie in der anästhesie.* München: Urban & Schwarzenberg, 1986;28–39.
111. Gourlay GK, Willis RJ, Wilson PR. Postoperative pain control with methadone: influence of supplementary methadone doses and blood concentration-response relationships. *Anesthesiology* 1984;61:19–26.

Advances in Pain Research and Therapy, Vol. 18,
edited by M. Max, R. Portenoy, and E. Laska,
Raven Press, Ltd., New York © 1991.

23

Patient-Controlled Analgesic Infusion

Harlan F. Hill, Adam M. Mackie, and Barbara A. Coda

*Clinical Research Division, Pain and Toxicity Research Program, Fred Hutchinson
Cancer Research Center, Seattle, Washington 98104; and Multidisciplinary
Pain Center, University of Washington, Seattle, Washington 98195*

Instrumentation and techniques for self-administration of opioid analgesics by
patients in pain (patient-controlled analgesia), have matured substantially over
the past 5 years. A wide variety of patient-controlled analgesia (PCA) systems
are now available that allow patients to self-administer opioids as bolus doses
alone or in combination with a continuous opioid infusion, in hospital or outpatient settings. PCA is an effective means of managing postoperative pain in
either mode of operation and may have significant advantages in longer-term
management of the pain of cancer or cancer treatment.

The impressive success of PCA is due in large part to two important pain
management considerations. First, it is extremely difficult for anyone besides
the patient with pain to judge accurately the magnitude of pain or the adequacy
of pain relief. Treatment of moderate and severe pain practically always involves
a compromise between incomplete but acceptable degrees of pain relief and side
effects of the analgesic. Only the patient can judge precisely when the optimal
balance between those two endpoints has been reached. Second, any attempt to
fix analgesic dosing on a basis other than patient-determined need (e.g., body
weight, fixed interval, etc.) is bound to lead to an unacceptably high incidence
of over- and underdosing due to the large (four- to tenfold) interpatient variability
in pharmacokinetics of opioid analgesics. Self-administration of opioid according
to patient need circumvents many uncertainties about pharmacokinetic variability. Of course, pharmacodynamic variability still remains, but patients may
adjust their drug intake accordingly.

The PCA technique has added a valuable dimension to our ability to compare
analgesic efficacy and potency of the wide variety of opioid analgesics available
for clinical use. By allowing the patient to determine how much and how often

drug is needed to maintain optimal pain relief, we gain the advantage of using total opioid intake over time, in addition to gradations in amount of pain relief produced by fixed doses of opioids, as a measure of both efficacy and potency. In a well-designed study, the PCA method allows accurate assessment of both potency and duration of effectiveness of analgesics based principally on the single parameter of frequency of self-administration of small fixed doses of a particular analgesic.

In this chapter, we review the development of PCA as a valuable clinical method and research tool, consider the potential of PCA in management of cancer-related pain, and describe our recent work with a novel approach to PCA that may have important applications in clinical pain management and the design of clinical trials of analgesic drugs.

DEVELOPMENT OF PCA

Drug Delivery Systems

Intravenous demand analgesia was first achieved by the straightforward method of having a nurse continuously at the patient's bedside deliver a small IV bolus of analgesic when requested (1). The success of this approach led to the development of patient-activated timing devices controlling regular IV infusion pumps or syringe drivers (2,3). On-line analogue recorders kept track of the delivery of drug and could provide research data. The Cardiff Palliator was the first commercial, dedicated device for PCA (4). It is loaded with a syringe filled with the desired drug; the drug dilution, incremental bolus, and lockout interval can each be selected, making the system flexible enough to be used with any drug. The pump displays the total dose delivered; an on-line analogue recorder can be used to chart demands and delivery of drug. Another early PCA device, the On-Demand Analgesia Computer (ODAC), included the capacity to give a continuous infusion at either a fixed rate or a fixed proportion of the last few hours total delivery in addition to bolus doses requested by the patient; this modification facilitates the use of analgesics with shorter elimination half-lives (5).

Improved microprocessor technology led to the current generation of pumps that have adequate memory to store several hours' worth of "events" (drug delivery, alarm conditions, pump settings, etc.) and the ability to monitor pump function and activate alarms. The memory can periodically be printed to provide permanent records for study use. Routinely required information (total dose delivered, pump settings) is also displayed on an LCD. Pumps such as the Abbott 4100 PCA Infuser and the Bard Harvard PCA can deliver bolus PCA, a fixed-rate continuous infusion, or a combination of both. Features desired in a PCA pump for analgesic drug research include a memory for at least 24 hrs of events (permitting daily printout), and the program capability to accurately deliver different opioids that vary widely in potency. The memory should be preserved if the pump is turned off or disconnected from power.

The devices described above are not portable and so are unsuitable for ambulatory patients. Miniaturization permits similar delivery modes (PCA, continuous infusion, or both) while sacrificing detailed event memory. For example, the Parker Micropump (Parker Biomedical, Irvine, California) is the size of a travel alarm clock and at 70 g is truly portable. It delivers drug from a separate collapsible medication reservoir. Much weight and size is saved by using a separate programmer, which is connected only when changes are needed. Such devices make PCA feasible away from the bedside, and may therefore be particularly suitable for long-term use in patients with chronic cancer pain.

Simple mechanical devices can replace electronic PCA pumps, with some loss of versatility, but significant gains in simplicity, cost, and portability. The Travenol Infusor with PCA Module (Travenol Laboratories, Deerfield, Illinois) delivers drug from a balloon reservoir at a rate determined by the fixed resistance at its outlet; this fills a 0.5 ml bladder in a wrist-strap module. Depressing a button on the wrist strap delivers the 0.5 ml bolus into the patient's IV line (6).

Opioids themselves need not be self-administered intravenously; subcutaneous administration can be used successfully, and has the advantage that the patient or his family can easily be trained to maintain and change the parenteral site as necessary (7). Patient-controlled epidural opioid administration has also been reported, although here a suitably long lockout interval must be chosen to allow for the slower onset and prolonged duration of effect when morphine is employed (8).

Effectiveness of PCA in Postoperative Pain

Conventional intramuscular regimens for administration of analgesics to patients after surgery leave many patients unsatisfied. Donovan (9) found 30% of 200 patients interviewed reported significant unrelieved pain when morphine or meperidine was prescribed on a 4-hr as-needed schedule. Keeri-Szanto and Heaman (2) found 40% of patients with extensive surgery were dissatisfied with their pain relief. In this context, they introduced a patient demand system that was used for 5 to 90 hrs after surgery in 60 patients; all but three of them were pain free. The patients then returned to conventional analgesia, and 30% found it unsatisfactory. Some patients self-administered more drug than a conventional regimen would have permitted; accommodating their needs contributed to the good results, according to Keeri-Szanto.

Further studies confirmed that there is wide interindividual dose variation in patients using PCA, with a mean dose that is of the same order as that conventionally administered. Using meperidine PCA, Tamsen et al. (10) found a dose range in 20 postoperative patients of 12 to 50 mg/hr (mean and SD 26 ± 10 mg/hr). By performing pharmacokinetic studies on each subject, then sampling blood during PCA therapy and relating the plasma drug concentration to the bolus delivery times, it was possible to estimate the plasma concentration at which patients made a demand. This "minimum effective concentration" (MEC) had a mean value of 455 ± 174 ng/ml for meperidine. Nineteen of 20 patients reported satisfactory analgesia; like most PCA studies, this was uncontrolled, and comparison must be made with retrospective reports such as Donovan's (9) or Keeri-Szanto and Heaman's (2). A similar study was performed in 10 adult surgical patients with morphine (11). The dose range was 1.1 to 4.0 mg/hr in the first 18 hrs, and MEC was estimated as 16 ± 9 ng/ml. All patients were satisfied with the analgesia.

Several studies have compared PCA with conventional intramuscular analgesia in a controlled design. In a crossover study (12), ten patients received PCA for 24 hrs, then IM analgesia for 24 hrs, and ten patients had IM then PCA. No difference between therapies was observed for pain report, side effects, or total morphine dose; however, most patients indicated a preference for PCA for future surgery. In a comparison with "conventional treatment" (13), 36 patients were randomly assigned to receive PCA or IM morphine; the IM morphine group could also receive an IV bolus of 2.5 mg on demand from the nursing staff. Both groups were cared for by recovery room staff for the 16 hrs of the study. No differences were observed between the groups for analogue pain score or total dose of morphine, but as noted the "conventional treatment" regimen included contingencies for patients not adequately relieved by IM drugs alone.

In a controlled trial of IM versus PCA meperidine in 89 parturients (14), no difference in pain score was found, but the PCA group used less drug. The difference was not large. McGrath et al. (15) reported similar results with meperidine (IM versus PCA) in patients after cholecystectomy. These studies suggest that intramuscular regimens, with a contingency for breakthrough pain, can be very effective under the care of well-trained personnel with the time to deliver it (16). Since it is probably impossible to replicate the deficiencies of conventional analgesia conventionally administered (smaller doses than prescribed at longer intervals than prescribed) in a controlled trial, these studies do not conflict with the clinical observation that PCA yields better results than standard treatment. In fact, the results of Hecker and Albert (17) indicate that PCA can produce *more* complete pain relief with *less* total analgesic than conventional postoperative pain management (IM or IV morphine at the discretion of house staff).

An imaginative application of PCA is its use to establish the relative analgesic potency of different drugs (see Chapter 22). A homogeneous population is randomized to receive different drugs in a double-blind fashion, and the mean cumulative doses for each group are taken to be equivalent. Thus, in the first 24 hrs after cholecystectomy, 13 patients used a mean of 1.9 mg/hr morphine, 15 used 25.6 mg/hr meperidine, and 14 used 2.9 mg/hr nalbuphine (18). The interindividual dose range for all three drugs was just over fourfold, as found in other PCA studies. No significant difference in analogue pain score was found between the drugs. Such studies require a valid pain measure to avoid the pitfall of labeling an aversive drug (of which little is self-administered) as potent.

Minimum Effective Analgesic Concentrations

Failure to administer IM analgesics by a patient's attendants is just one of the barriers to effective use of drugs by this route. The plasma concentration achieved after injection of meperidine is highly variable, both among patients and among administrations to the same patient (19). Austin et al. (19) gave 100 mg meperidine IM every 4 hrs to women having abdominal surgery. They found that the mean minimum plasma concentration in patients achieving freedom from pain was about 500 ng/ml (19). A pain score was derived from a two-part question: Do you have pain? No, score 0; yes, then ask: Do you think you need more medicine for pain? No, score 1; yes, score 2. The scores were then interpreted and graphically represented as 0 = no pain, 1 = moderate pain, and 2 = severe pain. In retrospect, scores of 1 and 2 probably represent the whole spectrum of mild to severe pain, equivalent to 10 to 100 on a typical 100-mm visual analogue scale. The same pain rating method was used in a subsequent study (20) that examined the dose-response curve more closely. Transition from a score of 0 to 1 to 2 was found to occur over a narrow plasma meperidine concentration range in any individual. Despite limitations in this study (since no score greater than 2 was available, the dose-response curve was flat at this end, and since more drug was usually given if requested, "severe pain" may not have been the invariable correlate of score 2), the results do suggest that a postsurgical patient will request additional analgesia at a consistent (for him or her) plasma concentration threshold, whether that request is expressed verbally or by activating a PCA device. This is consistent with findings by other groups (10,11).

The shape of the opioid plasma concentration-effect curve for clinical analgesia (postoperative or other) has not been thoroughly defined outside this threshold area of requesting or not requesting more drug. It is important to know whether opioid analgesia is a graded phenomenon or an on/off, all-or-nothing response, particularly when treating pain that may not be entirely responsive to opioids (some cancer and nerve injury–related pain, chronic nonmalignant pain, and the oropharyngeal mucositis of ablative chemoradiotherapy, for example). However, in the absence of intolerable or dangerous side effects, the adequate/inadequate analgesia threshold concentration is the most important to the patient. Establishing it and a drug's elimination half-life in an individual can permit sophisticated tailoring of oral drug administration schemes (21). Inturrisi and colleagues have taken a novel approach to quantifying the relationship between plasma opioid concentration and clinical analgesia using continuous intravenous opioid infusions. They have found that the concentration-effect curves are quite steep for hydromorphone (22), methadone, and morphine (23). These results demonstrate that pain relief is linearly related to plasma opioid concentration for mu selective opioid agonists. The clear relationship between plasma opioid concentration and analgesic effect provides the basic rationale for systems developed to maintain a constant plasma concentration of opioid in a patient once it has been adjusted to a level of comfort, as described below.

PCA IN CHILDREN

Relief of pain by conventional methods in children can be complicated by the opinions of a third party (usually a parent). Difficult as it is for medical staff to judge pain and its relief by analgesics, these difficulties are compounded by a parent reinforcing or denying pain reports, or requesting or discouraging the administration of analgesics. Adolescents (12 to 18 years) are able to understand the concept of pain, its causes, and its relief by analgesics. Autonomy is important to this age group, and although control of much of their life is surrendered to others when sick, they can be given the opportunity to exercise some control over their analgesic regimen. Adolescents are not usually prejudiced against or afraid of opioids, or electronic devices, and accept the principle of PCA readily. Children under 12 years vary in their understanding of abstract concepts, and can often but not invariably use PCA to good effect. As in adults, the patient must activate the device himself, and this must be clearly understood by the parents.

Brown and Broadman (24) administered morphine by PCA to 10 patients (age 11 to 19) postoperatively. All had previously experienced prn intramuscular analgesics. One 18-year-old was unable to use PCA effectively. The remainder were successful and preferred PCA to their prior experience with intramuscular analgesics. The dose range was 0.29 to 0.7 mg/kg/24 hr, and therapy continued up to 19 days. No pain measure was reported. Tyler (25) reviewed his experience with PCA morphine in 25 patients (age 13 and up), all but one with postoperative pain. Again, those who had previous surgery expressed a preference for PCA. The mean bolus dose established was 0.017 mg/kg, and the mean total dose on day 1 was 0.72 mg/kg/24 hr (range 0.24–1.92). Dodd et al. (26) used the Bard device to administer continuous infusion morphine at 0.015 mg/hr with concurrent PCA to eight postoperative patients (age 6 to 16 years). The PCA bolus dose range was 0.01 to 0.03 mg/kg. Again, no formal pain measure or controls were reported, but all patients (four of them under 12 years) used PCA successfully. PCA has also been used for the pain of sickle cell crisis (27): three patients (age 11 to 17 years) used PCA for 2 to 4 days, spontaneously reducing their daily dose as their condition improved. The same authors document the resistance they experienced from their peers when attempting to introduce PCA for this age/disease group (27).

The primary problem in nearly all analgesic studies using PCA is the lack of an adequate control group. Preliminary results of a controlled comparison of

PCA with continuous infusion (CI) morphine in 15 adolescents with pain due to chemoradiotherapy-induced mucositis (Mackie AM, Hill HF, *unpublished data*) show that, as in adults (28), adolescents achieve equivalent analgesia [determined by daily visual analogue scale (VAS)] with the two administration modes but use substantially less drug by PCA. Mean peak dose delivered on days 9 to 10 of treatment was 1.8 mg/kg/24 hr in the CI group, and 0.7 mg/kg/24 hr in the PCA group. Adolescents used PCA for an average of 15 days and spontaneously reduced their utilization when analgesia was no longer required. One 15-year-old was unable to rate pain on a VAS, but none of the eight patients randomized so far to PCA was unable to use it. We are not aware of any studies of PCA use in adolescents or younger children with cancer (as opposed to treatment-related) pain. But every indication is that adolescents are at least as successful using PCA to control pain as adults, and that PCA may be a practical option for management of pain uncontrolled by oral drugs.

PCA IN CANCER PAIN

Effective pharmacologic management of cancer-related pain requires an understanding of the types and pathophysiologic mechanisms of pain syndromes that these patients experience as well as the various drugs and methods of administration available.

About 40% of all cancer patients with active disease and up to 80% of patients with advanced cancer experience moderate to severe pain (29,30). Cancer patients may have pain related to direct tumor involvement, pain related to diagnostic procedures and treatment of cancer, pain indirectly related to cancer or its treatment, or pain owing to other factors. Within these categories, patients may experience acute or chronic pain, and may experience pain of multiple types at multiple sites (31,32). Finally, patients with preexisting chronic pain or a history of drug addiction may develop acute or chronic cancer-related pain (30). Although patients in this last group have traditionally been considered inappropriate candidates for PCA, this assumption has not been systematically examined. Perhaps cancer pain management could even be improved for this group using PCA with close monitoring and appropriate patient and staff education.

The common pain syndromes related to cancer and cancer treatment have been categorized as somatic, visceral, or deafferentation pain (33). Somatic pain arises from activation of nociceptors in cutaneous and deep tissues, e.g., bone pain due to metastatic disease. Visceral pain is described as the poorly localized pain due to stretching of viscera, and deafferentation pain results from nerve injury due to tumor infiltration, surgery, or chemotherapy.

Opioids continue to be the mainstay of treatment of moderate to severe cancer-related pain. Because of simplicity, safety, and cost, oral administration remains the preferred route of administration in most cases; and fixed-schedule dosing rather than "as needed" is able to provide more consistent analgesia (30). Parenteral administration is useful for breakthrough pain and for patients with dysphagia, nausea and vomiting, and absorption abnormalities.

Continuous intravenous and subcutaneous opioid infusions are generally effective and safe for acute and long-term use in cancer patients (34–37) but these techniques have some limitations. Continuous infusions do not allow for varying analgesic needs due to circadian effects (38,39) or increases in activity, and dose titration is slow. PCA allows rapid dose adjustment for varying analgesic need and also allows the patient to balance acceptable analgesia against unwanted side effects. PCA also allows the patient to exercise some control over his care and may reduce fear about inability to control cancer pain.

Although there have been very few trials using PCA for cancer-related pain, reports from those studies do support the theoretical advantages of PCA in cancer patients. In general, patients using PCA characteristically settle for less than total pain relief (40) and achieve equivalent (28) or better (41) analgesia using less drug, compared to other methods of administration. Patients benefit psychologically (41) and may experience significant lifestyle improvement with PCA (42). Anecdotal reports and prospective studies indicate that PCA is safe and effective in achieving pain relief acutely in cancer patients (41,43). Citron et al. (44) and Kerr et al. (42) reported that PCA is safe and effective treatment for cancer pain via both intravenous and subcutaneous routes on a long-term basis (up to 225 days) and for outpatients (42).

The utility of PCA in studies of cancer pain management extends beyond providing a safe, effective method of drug delivery. PCA can be used to assist in designing oral or other parenteral analgesic regimens for cancer patients. In an acute study, Bauman et al. (45) used PCA to determine analgesic requirements in patients with suboptimal pain control on oral analgesics. They were then able to convert some of these patients to oral regimens based on PCA results.

PCA has been used to compare effectiveness and side effects of self-administered opioids to other methods of delivery for an analgesic. Hill et al. (28) compared effects of morphine delivered by continuous infusion versus PCA for relief of mucositis pain over several weeks, and found that patients using PCA achieved equivalent analgesia using less drug per day and required opioids for fewer days than those receiving continuous infusion of morphine; side effects did not differ between the groups. PCA can also be used to compare subcutaneous versus intravenous drug delivery. In a postoperative study of intravenous PCA versus subcutaneous PCA in noncancer patients, Urquhart et al. (46) reported equivalent analgesia but greater hydromorphone requirement with subcutaneous administration. Another potential use for PCA is in epidural administration of short-acting lipophilic opioids, such as fentanyl and sufentanil (47,48). This technique has the theoretic advantage of providing an analgesic with rapid onset and relatively long duration, and possibly with fewer side effects than systemic administration.

PCA allows comparisons of properties such as relative potencies, side effects, and duration of analgesia among drugs used in acute and chronic cancer pain management. In a recent study, Grochow et al. (49) compared duration of analgesia of intravenous morphine and methadone. Over five days of administration using a modified PCA technique, patients initiated intravenous doses that were administered over 15 min/dose. The interval between doses, reflecting duration of analgesia, was about 4 hrs for both drugs. Since the duration of analgesia with methadone is significantly shorter than the drug's elimination half-life, the investigators concluded that intravenous methadone offers no advantage over other opioids. It would have been interesting to see this PCA study carried out beyond 5 days to determine whether methadone accumulates and causes adverse effects or whether patients increase the interval between doses and thus prevent drug accumulation to toxic levels. When comparing different drugs, it is important to remember that the amount of drug consumed reflects not only relative potency, but also a balance between acceptable analgesia and unacceptable side effects. Sensitivity to opioid analgesia and side effects varies greatly among patients, and dominant side effects that limit drug dosage may vary across drugs. Therefore, it is imperative to determine subjective analgesia and side effect ratings in addition to measuring drug intake as a dependent variable.

PCA does have limitations, particularly in chronic treatment of cancer pain. These include cost, potentially cumbersome equipment, and the requirement that the patient remains alert and understands how to operate the PCA pump. Furthermore, use of relatively small doses and brief lockout intervals as in acute postoperative studies could become bothersome and could result in periods of inadequate analgesia while the patient is asleep. Several approaches can circumvent these difficulties. Kerr et al. (42) combined a continuous infusion of morphine or hydromorphone with PCA delivery of a bolus dose equivalent to the hourly infusion dose. Citron et al. (44) used larger bolus doses (mean = 10 mg morphine) and a longer lockout interval (mean = 45 min). Grochow et al. (49) used an even larger bolus dose, predicted as $\frac{1}{8}$ the total daily drug requirement, and delivered each dose over 15 min. In this report, we describe a patient-controlled variable infusion rate opioid infusion system designed to rapidly achieve and maintain constant plasma concentration plateaus, and thus provide continuous analgesia in response to varying needs.

For long-term cancer pain management, especially for outpatients, the drug delivery equipment must be simple, portable, and cost-effective. In a retrospective analysis of cost-effectiveness of PCA in postoperative patients, Ross and Perumbeti (50) reported a decrease in hospitalization cost by as much as $1,700 and length of hospital stay by as much as 4.5 days in patients who used PCA. The portable PCA delivery systems described above allow continuous and intermittent drug administration; whether these are cost-effective for chronic use remains to be seen.

Two final issues are the development of opioid tolerance and dependence, and the risk of addiction. Although tolerance and dependence may occur, psychologic dependence (addiction) is rare in patients receiving opioids for cancer control (30). We have seen a preterminal phenomenon in which patients require rapidly increasing analgesic dose escalation; this has been reported during pain management with opioids administered by continuous intravenous infusion (37), subcutaneous infusion (36), and PCA (42). Whether this represents tolerance or another phenomenon is unclear, but it appears to be independent of the method of drug delivery. In the few clinical trials of chronic PCA use in cancer patients, tolerance has not been reported. Furthermore, Hill et al. (28) and Chapman and Hill (51) reported that tolerance did not occur during periods of up to 3 weeks of morphine administration using PCA for mucositis pain. This issue awaits systematic clinical evaluation. When interpreting increasing opioid requirements during long-term pain management, one must consider the contributing factors of disease progression and possible alterations in drug elimination as well as the possible development of opioid tolerance (52).

PATIENT-CONTROLLED OPIOID INFUSIONS

With PCA, patients can exert some control over drug concentration at central opioid receptor sites by self-administration of intravenous bolus doses of an opioid. This is a rapid means of changing plasma opioid concentration, but the relationship between plasma concentration, brain concentration, and analgesia after bolus doses of opioids is often obscured by the finite time required for opioid to diffuse from plasma to brain. Immediately after an intravenous bolus dose, opioid concentration in brain will increase as plasma concentration declines rapidly. As a consequence, brain opioid concentration and analgesic effect lag behind the changing plasma concentration. This disequilibrium adds an element of uncertainty to any patient-controlled analgesia system based on bolus dosing. Another difficulty with self-administered bolus doses is that either the bolus size must be increased at night or the patient must risk interruption of sleep by the need for additional analgesic. Alternatively a continuous infusion of opioid can be used at night to facilitate uninterrupted sleep, but this strategy removes control from the patient.

The rapid, uncontrolled changes in plasma and brain opioid concentrations following bolus doses complicate the direct comparison of analgesic effectiveness and relative potencies of opioid analgesics. One possibility for improvement of patient-controlled analgesia and comparative studies of analgesics is to develop infusion-based systems that would allow patients to adjust plasma opioid concentration around an initially effective (target) value. Appropriately designed continuous infusions have the potential to minimize the disequilibrium between blood and CNS opioid concentrations that are inherent to bolus doses. Prolonged pain is, characteristically, relatively constant but has periods of intensification as the patient moves about or encounters stressful situations. In these cases, a patient-controllable system for maintaining a steady plasma opioid concentration at most times with the ability to increase or decrease plasma concentration of analgesic in accord with variable need is a theoretically attractive approach to further improvement in pain management.

Using microprocessor-controlled infusion pumps, it is possible to rapidly reach and maintain preselected target plasma concentrations of opioids (53–55). Opioid analgesics exhibit "multicompartment" pharmacokinetics; plasma concentrations decline exponentially after a bolus dose. The requirements for rapidly producing stable plasma concentrations of such drugs have been described by others (56–58). The method involves administration of a bolus dose to immediately fill the central compartment to a preselected concentration, followed by a constant rate infusion to compensate for drug loss by elimination, plus an exponentially declining infusion to balance drug transfer from the central compartment to deep tissues. When plasma opioid concentration is held constant in this manner, there will be a direct relationship between drug concentration in plasma and at opioid receptors in the central nervous system; drug effect (e.g., analgesia) will therefore be proportional to plasma concentration.

We have used this technique of controlling plasma opioid concentrations at target values in normal volunteers (59,60) to study relationships between plasma concentration and analgesic effect for alfentanil, fentanyl, and morphine. By evaluating side effects as well as pain reduction under conditions of steady plasma opioid concentrations, the therapeutic windows of these three drugs were found to be very similar. We compared the opioids on the basis of effects on respiration (basal and CO_2 rebreathing) and subjective reports of nausea, alertness, mood, and itching produced by equally analgesic steady plasma concentrations of each drug. Based on these results, neither alfentanil nor fentanyl offer any major advantages over morphine on the basis of pharmacodynamics (61). However, the pharmacokinetics of alfentanil make it an attractive drug for conditions that require rapid changes in opioid effects. Its relatively low volume of distribution allows alfentanil to equilibrate rapidly between blood and brain and its short elimination half-life permits rapid decreases or increases in plasma and brain concentrations of opioid.

Application of steady-state infusion technology to control of pain requires knowledge of effective plasma concentrations for the opioids to be used. According to Hull (62), an optimal infusion strategy would be to define an effective plasma concentration of the chosen opioid and to then achieve an infusional steady state as soon as possible. Austin et al. (20) have shown that the effective plasma meperidine concentration varied substantially between patients but was relatively constant for each individual. They also reported that the minimum effective analgesic concentration (MEC) for meperidine was 460 ng/ml; however, the minimal effective concentration varied between 240 and 760 ng/ml, so a target concentration cannot be defined very precisely. PCA has also been employed to determine minimal effective analgesic concentrations for morphine, 16 ng/ml (11), fentanyl, 0.63 ng/ml (63), and alfentanil, 10 ng/ml (64). In each case, these MEC values are group averages and do not reflect characteristically large interindividual differences. Nonetheless, a pragmatic approach to infusion-based pain control would be to accept these values as initial estimates of target concentrations and then allow the patient to adjust plasma opioid concentration to achieve maximal benefit (62).

In previous work with bolus-dose PCA in bone marrow transplant patients, we found that patients self-administered morphine for up to 3 weeks for oral mucositis pain control without dose escalation (28,51). However, pain relief was never complete with either PCA or continuous infusion. As an attempt to improve pain control, we have developed an approach to patient-controlled analgesia that directly accounts for individual differences in pharmacokinetics. This approach is based on steady-state infusion of opioids and allows patients to regulate the concentration of opioid in plasma, using a computer-controlled infusion pump that accepts individual pharmacokinetic parameters.

To determine individual parameters, each patient receives a tailoring bolus of morphine or alfentanil on a day prior to marrow transplantation. A series of venous blood samples are drawn over the following 8 hrs and these are assayed for plasma opioid concentration. We then fit the concentration versus time data to bi- and triexponential functions by the nonlinear least squares program of MLAB (65). The function providing the best fit is selected for each patient:

$$Cp = Ae^{-\alpha t} + Be^{-\beta t}$$

and

$$Cp = Pe^{-\pi t} + Ae^{-\alpha t} + Be^{-\beta t}$$

The computer-pump system consists of a Toshiba 1100 microcomputer connected to the RS-485 communications port of an Abbott Model 4 infusion pump. The computer is programmed to use the constants and exponents from the exponential fit for that patient for calculations of loading dose size and the time-variant infusion rates needed to reach a preselected target plasma concentration and to hold the target concentration constant. Design of the delivery system is described elsewhere (66).

After the initial target plasma concentration (e.g., 20 ng/ml for morphine) has been maintained for an hour, patients can activate a hand-held switch to obtain small step increases or decreases in plasma opioid concentration in line with need for more analgesia or decreased side effects. The program also provides the ability to unhook the patient from the pump for brief periods with automatic restoration of target plasma concentration when reattached. The option for a fixed-rate infusion to maintain the current plasma opioid concentration is provided for nighttime use.

Results with this system have shown that pharmacokinetically based patient-controlled analgesic (PKPCA) infusion is an effective means of providing long-term pain control. Average plasma concentrations of morphine required for pain control by this method are shown in Fig. 1. Daily visual analogue scores of oral mucositis pain intensity from patients using PKPCA or conventional PCA are displayed in Fig. 2. Although PKPCA patients used more morphine than PCA

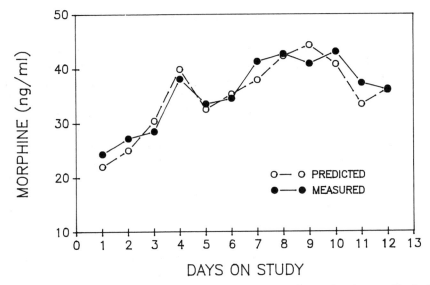

FIG. 1. Plasma morphine concentrations in marrow transplant patients using pharmacokinetically based patient-controlled analgesic (PKPCA) for oral mucositis pain control. Data shown are means of predicted and measured morphine concentrations in plasma of seven patients using the PKPCA infusion system. Daily blood samples were drawn for assay at 1500 to 1700 hrs daily.

patients, the former achieved more pain control. Side effect scores did not differ between the two groups of patients.

The utility of this approach is that it provides stable plasma concentrations of opioid analgesic and avoids the fluctuations in concentration and drug effect inherent in bolus dose approaches; it allows the patient to control drug effect precisely by altering plasma concentration; it advances our knowledge of relationships between plasma opioid concentration and analgesia in humans.

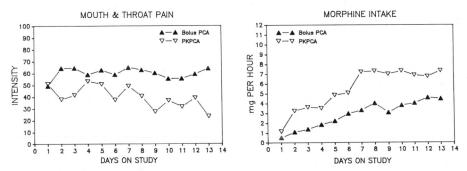

FIG. 2. Pain intensity reported by marrow transplant patients using morphine by PKPCA or patient-controlled analgesia (PCA) for oral mucositis pain control. Values are group means (PKPCA, N = 7; PCA, N = 14) of visual analogue scale ratings of pain intensity. The pain intensity scale (0–100 mm) has anchors of 0 = no pain at all to 100 = worst possible pain.

CONCLUSIONS

The bottom line in analgesia studies is the maximal relief of pain with minimal side effects. Furthermore, pain relief should not come at the expense of a return to normal function for the patient. The long-term potential consequences of use of even high doses of opioids for pain control (e.g., dependence and addiction) are grossly overrated. The amount of opioid used by patients to relieve pain should not be a primary concern; it may however be employed usefully as a secondary measure of the adequacy or effectiveness of pain control.

Sole dependence on this measure (opioid intake) can produce misleading results. Did the patient use less opioid because the pain was unrelieved by the drug, because of intolerable side effects, because of fear of "addiction," or for other reasons not related to pain relief? The key questions are what magnitude of pain relief was achieved, with what intensity and incidence of side effects, and only then how much opioid was required.

An important issue involving quantity of opioid required is that of tolerance development. Tolerance to analgesic effects develops more rapidly when high doses of opioid are used. But even then, we must recall that (a) tolerance develops to most side effects of opioids as rapidly and to a similar extent as to analgesia, and (b) opioid tolerance is relative, not absolute or complete. Development of tolerance merely means that more opioid should be administered to control the pain. And this is the final difficulty with use of opioid intake as the primary index of adequacy of pain control in analgesic studies. Pain relief may remain unchanged if tolerance development is matched by the ability of the patient (or others) to increase opioid intake to offset it.

We believe that PCA has great potential in management of the pains of cancer and its treatment. PCA can be used successfully for prolonged periods by cancer patients for sustained pain control (44). One of the main justifications given for not allowing PCA to be employed more widely by cancer patients and others on an outpatient basis is the fear of tolerance and physical dependence. Our experience and that of many other investigators argues strongly that such fears are unfounded and counterproductive (67). In children and in adults, morphine and probably other opioids can be used effectively for long-term pain relief without problems of inappropriate dosing. These qualities make the method uniquely valuable for analgesic studies, especially in the area of cancer pain and other prolonged pain states.

PCA is a valuable research tool for clinical analgesic studies. It is a precise means of measuring just how much and how often analgesic is required for pain control. It can be used for comparative analgesic studies (potency, efficacy, duration). It can also be used to compare the "painfulness" of different pain states and to study temporal variations in pain intensity and analgesic needs (38). PCA may further provide the means to study the efficacy of behavioral interventions for pain control and the utility of nonopioid analgesic enhancers by measuring the reduction in analgesic need when the interventions are co-administered with opioids. PCA may also have a place in clinical analgesic studies with chronic pain patients since opioids may be useful in selected chronic pain states (68).

Finally, PKPCA promises to assist advances in our knowledge of opioid pharmacodynamics in clinical pain states through studies in which plasma opioid concentration is held steady at preselected targets (obviating pharmacokinetic variability) whereas magnitude of pain relief is measured in individual patients with a common pain problem. PKPCA can also be used to ramp plasma opioid concentrations up or down in a controlled pattern so that plasma concentration–effect relationships, maximum effectiveness, and tolerance development can be assessed directly in individual patients. It is our opinion that the utility of PCA, especially PKPCA methods, in improved clinical studies of analgesia is just beginning to be appreciated.

ACKNOWLEDGMENTS

This research was supported by grants from the National Institute on Drug Abuse (DA 05513) and the National Cancer Institute (CA 38552 and CA 18029).

REFERENCES

1. Sechzer P. Objective measurement of pain. *Anesthesiology* 1968;29:209–210.
2. Keeri-Szanto M, Heaman S. Postoperative demand analgesia. *Surg Gynecol Obstet* 1972;134: 647–651.
3. Sechzer P. Studies in pain with the analgesic demand system. *Anesth Analg* 1971;50:1–10.
4. Evans JM, McCarthy JP, Rosen M, Hogg MIJ. Apparatus for patient-controlled administration of intravenous narcotics during labour. *Lancet* 1976;1:17–18.
5. Hull CJ. An on-demand analgesia computer. In:Harmer M, Rosen M, Vickers MD, eds. *Patient-controlled analgesia.* Oxford: Blackwell Scientific Publications, 1985;83–86.
6. Wermeling DP, Foster TS, Rapp RP, Kenady DE. Evaluation of a disposable non-electronic patient-controlled analgesia device for postoperative pain. *Clin Pharm* 1987;6:307–314.
7. Bruera E, Brenneis V, Michaud M, Macmillan K, Hanson J, MacDonald RN. Patient-controlled subcutaneous hydromorphone versus continuous subcutaneous infusion for the treatment of cancer pain. *J Natl Cancer Inst* 1988;80:1152–1154.
8. Marlowe S, Engstrom R, White PF. Epidural patient-controlled analgesia: An alternative to continuous epidural infusions. *Pain* 1989;37:97–101.
9. Donovan BD. Patient attitudes to postoperative pain relief. *Anaesth Intensive Care* 1983;11: 125–129.
10. Tamsen A, Hartvig P, Fagerlund C, Dahlstrom B. Patient-controlled analgesic therapy, Part II: Individual analgesic demand and analgesic plasma concentrations of pethidine in postoperative pain. *Clin Pharmacokinet* 1982;7:164–175.
11. Dahlstrom B, Tamsen A, Paalzow L, Hartvig P. Patient-controlled analgesic therapy, Part IV: Pharmacokinetics and analgesic plasma concentrations of morphine. *Clin Pharmacokinet* 1982;7: 266–279.
12. Bollish SJ, Collins CL, Kirking DM, Bartlett RH. Efficacy of patient-controlled versus conventional analgesia for postoperative pain. *Clin Pharm* 1985;4:48–52.
13. Dahl JB, Daugaard JJ, Larsen HV, Mouridsen P, Nielsen TH, Kristoffersen E. Patient-controlled analgesia: a controlled trial. *Acta Anaesthesiol Scand* 1987;31:744–747.
14. Robinson JO, Rosen M, Evans JM, Revill SI, David H, Rees GAD. Self-administered intravenous and intramuscular pethidine. *Anaesthesia* 1980;35:763–770.
15. McGrath D, Thurston N, Wright D, Preshaw R, Fermin P. Comparison of one technique of patient-controlled postoperative analgesia with intramuscular meperidine. *Pain* 1989;37:265–270.

16. Kleinman RL, Lipman AG, Hare BD, MacDonald SD. A comparison of morphine administered by patient-controlled analgesia and regularly scheduled intramuscular injection in severe, postoperative pain. *J Pain Symptom Manag* 1988;3:15–22.
17. Hecker BR, Albert L. Patient-controlled analgesia: a randomized, prospective comparison between two commercially available PCA pumps and conventional analgesic therapy for postoperative pain. *Pain* 1988;35:115–120.
18. Bahar M, Rosen M, Vickers MD. Self-administered nalbuphine, morphine, and pethidine. *Anaesthesia* 1985;40:529–532.
19. Austin KL, Stapleton JV, Mather LE. Multiple intramuscular injections: a major source of variability in analgesic response to meperidine. *Pain* 1980;8:47–62.
20. Austin KL, Stapleton JV, Mather LE. Relationship between blood meperidine and analgesic response: a preliminary report. *Anesthesiology* 1980;53:460–466.
21. Gourlay GK, Cherry DA, Cousins MJ. A comparative study of the efficacy and pharmacokinetics of oral methadone and morphine in the treatment of severe pain in patients with cancer. *Pain* 1986;25:297–312.
22. Inturrisi C, Portenoy R, Stillman M, Colburn W, Foley K. Hydromorphone bioavailability and pharmacokinetic-pharmacodynamic (PK-PD) relationships. *Am Soc Clin Pharmacol Ther* 1988;43:162.
23. Inturrisi CE, Colburn WA. Application of pharmacokinetic-pharmacodynamic modeling to analgesia. In: Foley KM, Inturrisi CE, eds. *Advances in pain research and therapy,* vol 8. New York: Raven Press, 1986;441–452.
24. Brown RE, Broadman LM. Patient-controlled analgesia for postoperative pain control in adolescents. *Anesth Analg* 1987;66:S22.
25. Tyler DC. Patient-controlled analgesia in adolescents. *Pain* 1987;4:S236.
26. Dodd E, Wang JM, Rauck RL. Patient-controlled analgesia for postsurgical pediatric patients ages 6–16 years. *Anesthesiology* 1988;69:A372.
27. Schecter NL, Berrien FB, Katz SM. The use of patient-controlled analgesia in adolescents with sickle cell pain crisis: a preliminary report. *J Pain Symptom Manag* 1988;3:109–113.
28. Hill HF, Chapman CR, Kornell J, Sullivan K, Saeger L, Benedetti C. Self-administration of morphine in bone marrow transplant patients reduces drug requirement. *Pain* 1990;40:121–129.
29. Deschamps M, Band PR, Coldman AJ. Assessment of adult cancer pain. Shortcomings of current methods. *Pain* 1988;32:133–139.
30. Foley KM. The treatment of cancer pain. *N Engl J Med* 1985;313:84–95.
31. Tanelian DL, Cousins MJ. Failure of epidural opioid to control cancer pain in a patient previously treated with massive doses of intravenous opioid. *Pain* 1989;36:359–362.
32. Twycross RG, Fairfield S. Pain in far-advanced cancer. *Pain* 1982;14:303–310.
33. Coyle N, Foley K. Prevalence and profile of pain syndromes in cancer patients. In:McGuire DB, Yarbro CH, eds. *Cancer pain management.* Orlando: Grune & Stratton, 1987;21–46.
34. Campbell CF, Mason JB, Weiler MD. Continuous subcutaneous infusion of morphine for the pain of terminal malignancy. *Ann Intern Med* 1983;98:51–52.
35. Citron M, Johnston-Early A, Fossieck BE, et al. Safety and efficacy of continuous intravenous morphine for severe cancer pain. *Am J Med* 1984;77:199–204.
36. Coyle N, Mauskop A, Maggard J, Foley KM. Continuous subcutaneous infusions of opiates in cancer patients with pain. *Oncol Nurs Forum* 1986;13:53–57.
37. Portenoy RK, Moulin DE, Rogers A, Inturrisi CE, Foley KM. IV infusion of opioids for cancer pain: clinical review and guidelines for use. *Cancer Treat Rep* 1986;70:575–581.
38. Burns JW, Hodsman NBA, McLintock TTC, Gillies GWA, Kenny GNC, McArdle CS. The influence of patient characteristics on the requirements for postoperative analgesia. *Anaesthesia* 1989;44:2–6.
39. Graves DA, Batenhorst RL, Bennett RL, et al. Morphine requirements using patient-controlled analgesia: influence of diurnal variation and morbid obesity. *Clin Pharm* 1983;2:49–53.
40. Vickers MD. Clinical trials of analgesic drugs. In:Harmer M, Rosen M, Vickers MD, eds. *Patient-controlled analgesia.* Oxford: Blackwell Scientific Publications, 1985;42–54.
41. Keeri-Szanto M. Demand analgesia for the relief of pain problems in "terminal" illness. *Anesth Rev* 1976;Feb:19–21.
42. Kerr IG, Sone M, DeAngelis C, Iscoe N, MacKenzie R, Schueller T. Continuous narcotic infusion with patient-controlled analgesia for chronic cancer pain in outpatients. *Ann Intern Med* 1988;108:554–557.
43. Citron M, Johnston-Early A, Boyer M, Krasnow SH, Hood M, Cohen MH. Patient-controlled analgesia for severe cancer pain. *Arch Intern Med* 1986;146:734–736.

44. Citron M, Walczak M, Seltzer V, et al. The safety and efficacy of patient-controlled analgesia (PCA) for severe cancer pain: a long-term study of inpatient and outpatient use. *Proc Am Soc Clin Onc* 1986;5:A260.
45. Bauman TJ, Batenhorst RL, Graves DA, Foster TS, Bennett RL. Patient-controlled analgesia in the terminally ill cancer patient. *Drug Intell Clin Pharm* 1986;20:297–301.
46. Urquhart ML, Klapp K, White PF. Patient-controlled analgesia: a comparison of intravenous versus subcutaneous hydromorphone. *Anesthesiology* 1988;69:428–432.
47. Lysak SZ, Eisenach JC, Dodson CE. Patient-controlled epidural analgesia during labor: a comparison of three solutions with continuous epidural infusion control. *Anesthesiology* 1990;72: 44–49.
48. White PF. Current and future trends in acute pain management. *Clin J Pain* 1989;5:S51–S58.
49. Grochow L, Sheidler V, Grossman S, Green L, Enterline J. Does intravenous methadone provide longer lasting analgesia than intravenous morphine? A randomized, double-blind study. *Pain* 1989;38:151–157.
50. Ross EL, Perumbeti P. PCA: is it cost effective when used for postoperative pain management? *Anesthesiology* 1988;69:A710.
51. Chapman CR, Hill HF. Prolonged morphine self-administration and addiction liability: evaluation of two theories in a bone marrow transplant unit. *Cancer* 1989;63:1636–1655.
52. Kanner RB, Foley KM. Use and abuse of narcotic analgesics in a cancer pain clinic. *Proc Am Assoc Cancer Res* 1986;21:381a.
53. Alvis MJ, Reves JG, Govier AV, et al. Computer-assisted continuous infusions of fentanyl during cardiac anesthesia: comparison to a manual method. *Anesthesiology* 1985;63:41–49.
54. Ausems ME, Stanski DR, Hug CC. An evaluation of the accuracy of pharmacokinetic data for the computer-assisted infusion of alfentanil. *Br J Anaesth* 1985;57:1217–1225.
55. Martin RW, Hill HF, Yee HC, Saeger LC, Walter MH, Chapman CR. An open-loop computer-based infusion system. *IEEE Trans Biomed Eng* 1987;BME-34:642–649.
56. Kruger-Theimer E. Continuous intravenous infusion and multicompartment accumulation. *Eur J Pharmacol* 1968;4:317–324.
57. Schwilden H, Schuttler J, Stoekel H. Pharmacokinetics as applied to total intravenous anaesthesia: theoretical considerations. *Anaesthesia* 1983;38:51–52.
58. Vaughan DP, Tucker GT. General derivation of the ideal intravenous drug input required to achieve and maintain a constant plasma drug concentration. *Eur J Clin Pharmacol* 1976;10: 433–440.
59. Hill HF. Pharmacokinetic tailoring of computer-controlled alfentanil infusions. In: Kroboth PD, Smith RB, Juhl RP, eds. *Pharmacodynamic research: current problems, potential solutions.* Cincinnati: Harvey Whitney Books, 1988;158–166.
60. Hill HF, Saeger L, Bjurstrom R, Donaldson G, Chapman CR, Jacobson R. Steady-state infusions of opioids in human: I. Pharmacokinetic tailoring. *Pain* (in press).
61. Hill HF, Chapman CR, Saeger L, Bjurstrom R, Walter MH, Kippes M. Steady-state infusions of opioids in human: II. Concentration-effect relationships and therapeutic margins. *Pain* (in press).
62. Hull CJ. Opioid infusions for the management of postoperative pain. In: Smith G, Covino BG, eds. *Acute pain.* London: Butterworths, 1985;155–179.
63. Gourlay GK, Kowalski SR, Plummer JL, Cousins MJ, Armstrong PJ. Fentanyl blood concentration-analgesic response relationship in the treatment of postoperative pain. *Anesth Analg* 1988;67:329–337.
64. Lehmann KA. Practical experience with demand analgesia for postoperative pain. In: Harmer M, Rosen M, Vickers MD, eds. *Patient-controlled analgesia.* Oxford: Blackwell Scientific Publications, 1985;134–139.
65. Knott GD. MLAB—a mathematical modeling tool. *Comput Programs Biomed* 1979;10:271–280.
66. Hill HF, Mackie AM, Jacobson R. Infusion-based patient-controlled analgesia systems. In:Ferrante FM, Ostheimer GW, Covino BG, eds. *Recent advances in patient-controlled analgesia.* Oxford: Blackwell Scientific Publications, 1990;214–222.
67. Hill HF, Chapman CR. Clinical effectiveness of analgesics in chronic pain states. *NIDA Res Monogr* 1990;231–247.
68. Portenoy RK, Foley KM. Chronic use of opioid analgesics in nonmalignant pain: report of 38 cases. *Pain* 1986;25:171–186.

Advances in Pain Research and Therapy, Vol. 18,
edited by M. Max, R. Portenoy, and E. Laska,
Raven Press, Ltd., New York © 1991.

Commentary

Patient-Controlled Analgesia

F. Michael Ferrante

*Pain Treatment Service, Department of Anaesthesia, Brigham and Women's Hospital,
Harvard Medical School, Boston, Massachusetts 02115*

Patient-controlled analgesia (PCA) is a superior analgesic modality as compared
to scheduled, around-the-clock, intramuscular injections of opioid, not because
of inherent superiority as an analgesic technique (1), but because of greater patient
satisfaction with this modality (2–4). Indeed, with attentive nursing care, routine
intramuscular therapy can become "on demand" and as effective as PCA (5).

Dr. Klaus Lehmann very eloquently discussed the role of various predictors
of the intensity and severity of postoperative pain, as well as the influence of
anesthetic techniques, type of surgical procedure, and choice of opioid on the
efficacy of PCA. As Dr. Lehmann so cogently states: "PCA is a good example
to demonstrate that clinical pain measurement (efficacy) cannot be separated
from patients' individual pain behavior." Irrespective of pharmacokinetic and
pharmacodynamic considerations, as well as the role of age, gender, anesthetic
technique, and type of surgery, an individual's "decision" to press or not to
press the patient demand button ultimately determines the effectiveness of PCA.
Thus, "illness" or "pain" behaviors may override other considerations so that
patients may accept higher levels of pain (1,6) or be unable to gain maximum
benefit from PCA (6,7).

Thus, the elucidation of factors determining patients' ability or inability to
most optimally activate the PCA infuser is (whether consciously or unconsciously)
the fundamental goal of most research with PCA. Let us examine our present
understanding of how an individual "decides" to activate or not to activate the
demand button.

THE PCA PARADIGM

The relation among opioid concentration, analgesic effect, and dosing interval defines the therapeutic effectiveness of a particular method of opioid administration (Fig. 1). After administration of an intramuscular depot, the attendant opioid plasma concentrations are unpredictable. Peak concentrations with multiple injections can vary twofold, whereas time to peak concentrations can vary threefold in any particular patient (8). At the same time, the plasma concentration of an opioid will fluctuate in phase with the dosing interval (Fig. 1) (1,9). It has been calculated that opioid concentrations are in excess of the minimum effective analgesic concentration (MEAC) only 35% of the time during any 4-hr dosing interval (8).

Originally, PCA was thought to be a superior analgesic modality as compared to scheduled or prn intramuscular administration of opioids because of the direct delivery of opioid into the venous compartment, thus avoiding variable absorption phenomena. When the patient's opioid concentration fell below MEAC, the patient could rapidly appreciate pain [steep concentration–analgesic response relation (10)] and would activate the demand button. Thus, an individual could "titrate" his plasma concentration of opioid around MEAC, providing more constant plasma levels of opioid (11–13) and more consistent analgesia (1). Unfortunately, such arguments ignore the influence of pain behaviors and the individual psychology of patients using PCA.

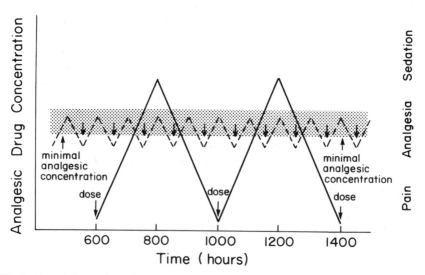

FIG. 1. The relation among plasma opioid concentration (ordinate), dosing interval (abscissa), and analgesic effect (z axis) defining therapeutic effectiveness. (Reprinted with permission from ref. 1.)

As Dr. Lehmann states: "It is now commonly believed that the main variable with respect to pain measurement is the amount of drug intake during PCA . . ." or stated otherwise, the individual analgesic requirement. Historically, then, a search was undertaken to determine the factors underlying the wide variability in individual analgesic requirements with use of PCA.

PHARMACOKINETIC FACTORS

In what is now a classic series of studies, Tamsen and colleagues studied the relative contribution of opioid pharmacokinetics upon analgesic requirements in patients using PCA (11–13). Meperidine (11), ketobemidone (12), and morphine (13) were studied in three separate groups of patients undergoing laparotomy. The volume of distribution, distribution rate constant, and elimination rate constant for a particular opioid were calculated and found to bear no relation to the individual patient's hourly analgesic requirement of the particular opioid. Tamsen and colleagues concluded that a patient's hourly use of PCA was not dictated by pharmacokinetic variations among individuals. However, individual hourly opioid use was significantly correlated with the mean plasma opioid concentration and MEAC. Thus, patients would activate the demand button to maintain plasma concentrations of opioid in the range of MEAC (Fig. 1) and thereby obtain adequate analgesia.

PHARMACODYNAMIC FACTORS

If patients use PCA to "titrate" their plasma opioid concentrations around MEAC, the next obvious question arises: What determines MEAC? Tamsen attempted to answer this question in patients receiving meperidine by PCA for pain relief after laparotomy (14). Prior to surgery, a sample of cerebrospinal fluid (CSF) was obtained. Another sample of CSF, as well as a sample of central venous blood, was obtained 24 hrs later while patients used PCA. Endogenous opioid content in CSF was assayed using a radioreceptor assay (14).

There was a significant inverse linear relation between individual preoperative CSF endogenous opioid concentrations and individual postoperative concentrations of meperidine in plasma ($r^2 = 0.29$, $p < 0.05$) and in CSF ($r^2 = 0.43$, $p < 0.02$) (Fig. 2). Tamsen concluded that patients with low preoperative endogenous opioid content in CSF administered more opioids postoperatively by PCA in order to maintain higher drug concentrations in the plasma. Likewise, the converse was true.

According to the results of this study, individual analgesic demand is dictated by individual CSF endogenous opioid content. Therefore, only the patient should determine when and how much analgesic is required. According to this argument, PCA is inherently superior to other forms of parenteral opioid administration:

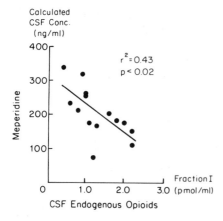

FIG. 2. The inverse linear relation between preoperative CSF levels of endogenous opioids (Fraction I) and postoperative analgesic demand (CSF concentration of meperidine) while using PCA. (Reprinted with permission from ref. 21.)

". . . PCA works so well because the patient is able to read the status of his endogenous analgesia system . . ." (15). In other words, PCA is "physiologic."

PSYCHOLOGIC FACTORS

If patients simply use PCA to "titrate" their postoperative plasma and CSF opioid concentrations according to their individual preoperative endogenous opioid content in the CSF, then PCA should be flawlessly efficacious in all patients. Unfortunately, this is not so. Some patients seem to be unable to effectively or optimally use PCA (1,6,7). Similarly, if PCA is "physiologic," it should uniformly provide superior analgesia as compared to other forms of parenteral opioid administration (excluding epidural or subarachnoid opioid). This, too, is not always the case (1,2,4).

Irrespective of pharmacokinetic and pharmacodynamic considerations, the patient's "decision" to press or not to press the demand button remains paramount. Is the administered quantity of analgesic purely the result of an appropriate response to pain or do other factors determine analgesic consumption?

A basic tenet of PCA is that analgesia is better with the patient in control. Indeed, the uniformly high patient satisfaction with PCA probably stems from affording patients a sense of control over their postoperative pain and its relief (16).

The psychologic construct of "locus of control" refers to a set of beliefs about the relation between personal behavior and reinforcement (17–19). If reinforcement is perceived by individuals to be the result of their own actions, then the individual is said to have an internal locus of control. If an individual perceives that luck, chance, fate, or the intervention of powerful people are more responsible for what happens to him than the results of his own actions, he is said to have an external locus of control. A psychometric test for locus of control focusing upon health, the Multidimensional Health Locus of Control (MHLC), has been developed (19).

With respect to PCA, an internal locus of control would imply that an individual adopts a more active or controlling posture toward his or her environment and would push the demand button when experiencing pain. An external locus of control could lead to a paralysis of response. These individuals may not optimally press the demand button, as they feel they have little control over their environment. In other words, patients with an internal locus of control may be innately better able to effectively use PCA.

Johnson and colleagues (7) used the MHLC and a number of other psychometric tests to correlate satisfaction with PCA and the degree of pain with the results of psychometric testing. They demonstrated that an "external" locus of control is predictive of higher pain scores and dissatisfaction with use of PCA. An "internal" locus of control was predictive of lower pain scores and greater satisfaction with PCA.

Although illness and pain behaviors have previously been hypothesized to be important in how patients use PCA, the work of Johnson et al. (7) is the first real definition of their effect. Psychologic factors exist that affect patients' ability to derive maximum benefit from PCA or make patients unable to effectively use PCA.

CONCLUSION

Heretofore, research with PCA has viewed patients rather deterministically, mechanically responding to the fluctuating plasma opioid concentrations of the PCA paradigm. However, recent evidence is accumulating that patients' use of PCA is a rather dynamic and fluid process and really the synthesis of several pharmacodynamic and psychologic factors.

The combined work of several authors (1,9,11–13) has shown that the PCA paradigm should probably no longer be referred to as "theoretical." However, we cannot ascribe any inherent analgesic superiority to PCA over intramuscular opioid simply on the basis of more constant plasma levels of opioid or more consistent pain scores. Indeed, several authors have failed to demonstrate the superiority of PCA over intramuscular opioid with respect to pain scores (1,2,4).

As Dr. Lehmann points out in his analysis of 1,334 patients, and as other authors have also done (2–4), it is the overwhelming acceptance and satisfaction with PCA that makes it distinct as an analgesic modality. Why is PCA so well accepted? Perhaps the work of Johnson et al. (7) and the issue of "control" supply us with an initial answer (16).

Hospitalization and subsequent surgery are anxiety-laden events for people, fraught with opportunities for losing control over the most basic human rights. The patient is forced into unfamiliar regimentation and loses mobility and privacy. Superimposed upon this is the possibility of new stress—severe postoperative pain.

The ability to immediately self-administer pain medication without the need to negotiate with physicians and nurses may afford patients a sense of control over their pain. Instead of being a passive recipient of perhaps painful intramuscular injections, the patient is now an active participant in his or her own care. Certainly, the role of psychologic factors, as well as the issue of control, need to be further explored in future research.

Although appealing, the hypothesis that "titration" of opioid use occurs in accordance with the endogenous opioid content of the CSF is probably overly simplistic, given the complex interactions of numerous neurotransmitters at the level of the spinal cord or more rostrally. Indeed, recent work suggests the relationship proposed by Tamsen may not apply for postoperative pain relief in obstetric patients (20). However, such novel investigations should not be abandoned. Future research with PCA should address the role of opioid receptor subtypes, various neurotransmitters, and hormones (e.g., progesterone) upon analgesic requirements with opioid and nonopioid analgesics (e.g., ketorolac).

Do we really understand how a particular individual uses PCA? In short, the answer is: not really. We have developed a hierarchy of response from pharmacokinetic to pharmacodynamic to psychologic considerations. Certainly, future research with PCA must address this most basic of all questions.

REFERENCES

1. Ferrante FM, Orav EJ, Rocco AG, Gallo J. A statistical model for pain in patient-controlled analgesia and conventional intramuscular opioid analgesia and conventional intramuscular opioid regimens. *Anesth Analg* 1988;67:457–461.
2. Rayburn WF, Geranis BJ, Ramadei CA, Woods RE, Patil KD. Patient-controlled analgesia for post-cesarean pain. *Obstet Gynecol* 1988;72:136–139.
3. Eisenach JC, Grice SC, Dewan DM. Patient-controlled analgesia following cesarean section: a comparison with epidural and intramuscular narcotics. *Anesthesiology* 1988;68:444–448.
4. Harrison DM, Sinatra R, Morgese L, Chung JH. Epidural narcotic and patient-controlled analgesia for post-cesarean section pain relief. *Anesthesiology* 1988;68:454–457.
5. Welchew EA. On-demand analgesia. A double-blind comparison of on-demand intravenous fentanyl with regular intramuscular morphine. *Anaesthesia* 1983;38:19–25.
6. Magnani B, Johnson LR, Ferrante FM. Modifiers of patient-controlled analgesia efficacy. II. Chronic pain. *Pain* 1989;19:23–29.
7. Johnson LR, Magnani B, Chan V, Ferrante FM. Modifiers of patient-controlled analgesia efficacy. I. Locus of control. *Pain* 1989;39:17–22.
8. Ausin KL, Stapleton JV, Mather LE. Multiple intramuscular injections: a major source of variability of analgesic response to meperidine. *Pain* 1980;8:47–62.
9. White PF. Patient-controlled analgesia: a new approach to the management of postoperative pain. *Semin Anesth* 1985;4:255–266.
10. Austin KL, Stapleton JV, Mather LE. Relationship between blood meperidine concentrations and analgesic response: a preliminary report. *Anesthesiology* 1980;53:460–466.
11. Tamsen A, Hartvig P, Fagerlund C, Dahlstrom B. Patient-controlled analgesic therapy, Part II: Individual analgesic demand and analgesic plasma concentrations of pethidine in postoperative pain. *Clin Pharmacokinet* 1982;7:164–175.
12. Tamsen A, Bondesson U, Dahlstrom B, Hartvig P. Patient-controlled analgesic therapy, Part III: Pharmacokinetics and analgesic plasma concentrations of ketobemidone. *Clin Pharmacokinet* 1982;7:252–265.
13. Dahlström B, Tamsen A, Paalzow L, Hartvig P. Patient-controlled analgesic therapy, part IV:

Pharmacokinetics and analgesic plasma concentration of morphine. *Clin Pharmacokinet* 1982;7: 266–279.
14. Tamsen A, Sakurada T, Wahlström A, Terenius L, Hartvig P. Postoperative demand for analgesics in relation to individual levels of endorphins and substance P in cerebrospinal fluid. *Pain* 1982;13: 171–183.
15. Tamsen A. Patient characteristics influencing pain relief. In: Harmer M, Rosen M, Vickers MD, eds. *Patient-controlled analgesia*. Oxford: Blackwell Scientific Publications, 1985;30–37.
16. Egan KJ. What does it mean to a patient to be "in control"? In: Ferrante FM, Ostheimer GW, Covino BG, eds. *Patient-controlled analgesia*. Boston: Blackwell Scientific Publications, 1990;17–26.
17. Rotter JB. Generalized expectancies for internal versus external control of reinforcement. *Psychol Monagr* 1966;80:1–28.
18. Rotter JB. Some problems and misconceptions related to the construct of internal versus external control of reinforcement. *J Consult Clin Psychol* 1975;43:56–67.
19. Wallston KA, Wallston BS, DeVillis R. Development of the multidimensional health locus of control (MHLC) scales. *Health Educ Monogr* 1978;6:160–170.
20. Eisenach JC, Dobson CE II, Inturissi CE, Hood DD. Do spinal enkephalins mediate analgesia in pregnancy? (abstract). *Anesth Analg* 1989;68:S78.
21. Ferrante FM. Patient characteristics influencing effective us of patient-controlled analgesia. In: Ferrante FM, Ostheimer GW, Covino BG, eds. Patient-controlled analgesia. Boston: Blackwell Scientific Publications, 1990;51–60.

DISCUSSION (Chapters 22 and 23)

Dr. Stephen Cooper: In our studies, we find patients who are particularly sensitive to the instructions we give them. Couldn't the manner by which patients are told to use PCA influence them?

Dr. Harlan Hill: In our PCA studies, we use a standard set of instructions covering operation and safety features of the equipment and encourage the patients to request morphine as often as they want in order to be as comfortable as possible. I suspect that PCA would be less successful without such instructions.

Dr. Charles Berde: I think the different authors have illustrated the extent to which the findings in a PCA study depend very much on the characteristics of the study population. For example, our study of PCA in children having orthopedic surgery used a control group that received bolus morphine in a fairly generous way, and showed that this control group and the experimental group used equivalent amounts of morphine. The PCA groups had better analgesia, however, and the side effect incidences were the same. Conversely, a colleague of mine studied children having thoracotomies at an institution that was historically less liberal about administering opioid postoperatively. In this population, the children getting PCA self-administered more opioid than the control group and had better analgesia.

Finally, I would like to make an additional point about the effect of age on these studies. In children ages 7 to 19 using PCA in an orthopedic situation, the younger patients used less drug, even when drug intake was normalized per kilogram.

Dr. C. R. Chapman: Although group means are presented in studies of PCA, there is actually enormous variation in the pattern of drug use from day to day. There are many reasons for this. Part of it is that patients engage in a trial and error process. Although we tell them about comfort, we don't train them in a strategy that is effective for self-control of pain, largely because we don't know what that should be. Another factor concerns changes in the patient's environment. If there is a spouse in the room telling the patient to stop taking the drug, or if there are health care professionals or family members in the room demanding the patient's time, or if the patient gets tired and nods off, then the pattern of self-administration changes. These variabilities all creep into the data set. Behavior has many determinants and we need to identify what those are.

Dr. Henry McQuay: Patients using PCA do not press the button until they reduce pain to zero. In all the groups we have looked at, this remains a solid finding. Even the nociceptive cancer pain patients do not get down to a pain score of zero using the machine. We do not yet have an explanation for this phenomenon.

Dr. Harlan Hill: I think we have to be extremely careful about what "level pressing" means in human beings, especially in the pain context. By itself, the amount of analgesic used or the rate of self-administration means very little. The real question is whether patients gain incremental pain relief from self-administration of the drug.

Dr. Michael Cousins: Many studies look at new method X, which may be well tuned, such as PCA, versus a highly disorganized old method Y, such as routine intramuscular administration, in which drug is very sparingly given. To compare modalities, we must develop strategies that allow us to optimize the two treatments we are comparing. A second issue concerns the question of the primary and secondary response variables. Does it really matter that there is a 10% difference in the TOTPARs or SPIDs or whatever? We may need to look at other things, such as patient satisfaction scales. One of the members of my department, for example, found that rather small changes in VAS scores for obstetrical pain will result in very big changes in patient satisfaction. Unless that happens, I don't think it matters if there is a small difference in the pain score profile.

Dr. Russell Portenoy: I think that there is an important distinction between the use of PCA as a dependent measure in analgesic studies designed to address other issues and the use of PCA as the independent variable in studies that assess the value of PCA compared to other kinds of treatments. In the latter type of study, when one compares PCA with other types of treatment, we do not know which variables are important to evaluate. Descriptive studies are needed in which trained interviewers simply ask patients who are using PCA why they selected the dosing pattern they did.

Advances in Pain Research and Therapy, Vol. 18,
edited by M. Max, R. Portenoy, and E. Laska,
Raven Press, Ltd., New York © 1991.

24

Pharmacokinetic Considerations in Analgesic Study Design

Charles E. Inturrisi

*Department of Pharmacology, Cornell University Medical College, New York,
New York 10021; and Pain Research Program, Memorial Sloan-Kettering
Cancer Center, New York, New York 10021*

The intensity of the therapeutic and toxic effects of most drugs is a function of drug concentrations at receptor or other sites of action. Pharmacokinetics provides a quantitative description of the time course of drug disposition in the body. Drug disposition includes the rates and extent of absorption, distribution, biotransformation, and elimination. The quantitative relationship between drug dose and concentration can be described by an equation (i.e., a pharmacokinetic model) that is shown schematically in Figure 1.

The major impetus to pharmacokinetic studies has been the demonstration of significant interindividual variation in the kinetic processes of drug disposition that determine the concentration of drug available at the site(s) of action after a given dose. Furthermore, pharmacokinetic studies have revealed that the dose-concentration relationship can also be significantly affected by the age of the patient, genetic constitution, disease, and concomitant drug therapy (1). Pharmacokinetic analysis can provide information that can be used to allow a more rational choice of drug dose, route, and frequency of administration; such information can be useful in adjusting dosage to compensate for changes in drug disposition that can result from alterations in the clinical status of the patient. For many drugs, pharmacokinetic studies have provided guidelines for individualizing doses to provide a desired range (i.e., therapeutic range) of drug concentrations (1,2). The practical clinical utility of the pharmacokinetic approach depends, of course, on the extent to which the pharmacokinetic model (Fig. 1) yields concentrations that are capable of producing the desired intensity of therapeutic effect. Therefore, implicit in pharmacokinetic studies aimed at optimizing drug dosage is a consideration of pharmacodynamics. Pharmacodynamics defines the relationship between drug concentrations and the intensity of the therapeutic and/or toxic pharmacological effects. This drug concentration-effect relationship can also be described by an equation (a pharmacodynamic model) shown sche-

(a) **PK MODEL**

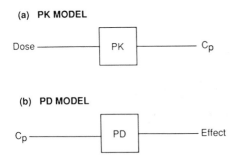

(b) **PD MODEL**

FIG. 1. A schematic representation of (a) the dose-drug concentration (C_p) relationship by use of a pharmacokinetic (PK) model and (b) the drug concentration (C_p)-effect relationship by use of a pharmacodynamic (PD) model.

matically in Fig. 1. Note that the common feature shared by both models is drug concentration. How these concentrations are obtained and analyzed is discussed below.

During the past several years approaches have been developed that allow integration of pharmacokinetic and pharmacodynamic data (PK-PD modeling). The United States Food and Drug Administration is strongly encouraging the routine incorporation of PK-PD modeling in the whole of drug development (3,4). Although the advantages of this approach for defining therapeutic concentrations are obvious, it may be of particular utility for analgesic drug development where patient factors, such as opioid tolerance and the intensity of the pain stimulus, can result in large interindividual variation, and approaches are required to define individual PK-PD relationships.

This chapter presents information and approaches that are of value in the design of studies whose objectives are to obtain essential pharmacokinetic data and define the relationships between the pharmacokinetics and pharmacodynamics of analgesics. While acknowledging the considerations that form the basis for the "classical" pharmacokinetic drug plan (5) used to develop the biopharmaceutical portion of a new drug application (NDA), the major emphasis of this chapter is on the collection and analysis of the pharmacokinetic and pharmacodynamic data that define the clinical pharmacology of the analgesic.

This chapter discusses study designs that are common to most pharmacokinetic studies as well as design issues that are of particular relevance to analgesics. Most of the examples are taken from studies of opioid analgesics, although the same or very similar approaches can be used with nonopioid analgesics. The discussion is not intended to develop the theoretical framework for the choice of particular pharmacokinetic or pharmacodynamic models, although appropriate references are provided. For each approach I present there are acceptable alternate ways of generating and analyzing the data and it is recommended that wherever possible multiple approaches be utilized.

PRELIMINARY INFORMATION

Initial (Phase I) clinical studies of new drugs are usually carried out in healthy volunteers and are intended to evaluate limiting side effects. These studies are commonly called "tolerance" studies, a potentially confusing term that is best avoided when discussing analgesic studies. A secondary objective of these initial studies is to obtain preliminary human pharmacokinetic data. These studies may include single and multiple doses as well as a mass balance study that attempts to account for the fate of the entire dose using a radiolabeled drug. The latter studies provide information about the human metabolic profile of the drug and, together with prior disposition studies in animals, may identify potentially active metabolites.

The analytical methods employed in pharmacokinetic studies must be both selective in excluding metabolites that interfere with the quantitation of the study drug and sensitive in their ability to measure the drug after test or therapeutic doses. The sensitivity of the method will often determine the required size of the biofluid sample (see below) and the ability to adequately characterize the biofluid concentration-time profile. This, in turn, may profoundly affect estimates of pharmacokinetic parameters such as half-life. Analytical methods should include an internal standard to compensate for variation in losses during the sample preparation procedure. A standard curve should define the linear range of the detector response used to quantitate the study drug, and samples should be diluted if necessary so that their response falls within the linear range of the standard curve. Information on whether other commonly used drugs (e.g., other analgesics) or their known metabolites interfere with the assay of patient samples should be provided. In addition, it is useful to test any new method by screening samples from patients who have received drugs (e.g., analgesics) other than the compound of interest; this helps to ensure that unknown or poorly characterized metabolites of drugs commonly used by a study population (e.g., cancer patients) do not interfere with the assay.

In general, analytical methods that employ a combination of solvent extraction followed by a separation method, such as gas-liquid chromatography or high performance liquid chromatography coupled to sensitive detectors, are preferred over radioimmunoassay (RIA) procedures. The accuracy of the latter procedure may be reduced by antisera that may cross-react with metabolites (6). Unfortunately, for some of the more potent opioids, e.g., fentanyl and buprenorphine, RIAs have provided the requisite sensitivity not yet available from other methods (7). Regardless of the analytical method selected, each assay should indicate the lower limit of sensitivity for a given biofluid volume as well as the inter- and intraassay coefficient of variation.

The development of appropriate analytical methods must be given a very high priority in drug development. Analytical methods have been used to measure simultaneously opioids and their active metabolites (8–13) and to separate and quantitate the optical isomers of ibuprofen (14). Analytical methods useful with the nonsteroidal antiinflammatory drugs (NSAIDs) are found in the citations reviewed by Verbeeck et al. (15). Since the identity of active metabolites may not always be known during the initial human studies, the process of analytical methods development must be viewed as an ongoing one, adapting to new information and requirements as development progresses throughout clinical studies.

SUBJECTS AND SAMPLE COLLECTION

The issues that should be considered when choosing an appropriate population for pharmacokinetic studies have been reviewed by Brazzell and Colburn (16). Since concurrent collection of pharmacokinetic and pharmacodynamic data, (i.e., PK-PD studies) are to be a critical part of the design, studies in patients with pain are essential. Initially, however, studies may be conducted in normal volunteers since this approach enhances the convenience of the study and minimizes the influence of other drugs on the assessment of safety and on the collection of pharmacokinetic data.

Reports of pharmacokinetic studies should include information on the clinical characteristics of the subjects (17). Such information includes age, sex, weight, and, as appropriate, disease, diagnosis, current analgesic dosage, and clinical laboratory values relating to renal and hepatic function. Information on pain intensity, site, and character should be included in PK-PD studies (18).

The objective of the study, the route of administration, and the drug itself may influence the type of biofluid sample or samples that are collected. Studies designed to estimate standard pharmacokinetic parameters and bioavailability usually collect blood samples and recover plasma for analysis. If the drug is unstable in blood, it may be necessary to collect, aliquot, and freeze the blood sample at the patient's bedside (11).

Historically, plasma has been used because it is easier to manipulate after freezing and thawing and provides a sample with less interference from endogenous substances (6). However, with a combination of solvent extraction and an appropriate chromatographic procedure blood, plasma, or serum can be used, although this needs to be verified for each new method. Collection of plasma samples permits analysis both by RIAs, which usually require plasma or serum, as well as by use of chromatographic procedures.

A physiologically based pharmacokinetic parameter, such as clearance (see below), is derived from consideration of the blood concentrations of a drug entering and leaving an organ (19). Thus, drug concentrations in blood are the least equivocal sample, if not the most convenient. For many drugs, plasma concentrations are proportional to blood concentrations, and estimation of the whole blood/plasma concentration ratio on a representative sample from each subject allows conversion of plasma drug concentrations to blood drug concentrations where this may be required (4,20). In sum, blood, plasma, or serum samples may be used for systemic pharmacokinetic studies. However, once selected, the type of biofluid should remain the same for each subsequent study. With the advent of newer modes of opioid administration (i.e., epidural and intrathecal) the collection of CSF is required to provide a more complete pharmacokinetic profile (21). Synovial fluid is sometimes collected in pharmacokinetic studies of NSAIDs (14,15).

The majority of pharmacokinetic studies sample venous blood, usually from the arm. Recently, Chiou (22,23) has reviewed pharmacokinetic studies of drugs that exhibit differences in the plasma or blood concentration-time profiles when arterial sampling is compared with venous sampling. This sample site dependence can influence estimates of pharmacokinetic parameters and may lead to complications when attempting to interpret relationships between peripheral venous blood drug concentration and pharmacodynamic effects (PK-PD relationships). Although not yet demonstrated for analgesics, this sample-site dependence is most apparent when the elimination half-life ($t\frac{1}{2}$) is less than 2 to 4 hrs and measurements are made after IV bolus injection when arteriovenous differences are maximal (23). Although a drug may exhibit marked arteriovenous concentration differences after a single dose, at steady state there should be no difference in arterial and venous drug concentrations (22,23). Thus, it would appear prudent to use either only arterial or only venous sampling for pharmacokinetic studies and to compare estimates of pharmacokinetic parameters obtained after a single dose with those determined under steady-state conditions (see below).

The sampling schedule is dictated by the objective of the study. If the objective is to accurately characterize the concentration-time profile by use of a pharmacokinetic model, then sampling frequency is adjusted to the expected rate of change of concentration, as anticipated from preliminary studies. In simple terms, the sampling schedule after an IV bolus is designed to capture the rapid initial phase and slow "postdistribution" phases. After other routes of administration (e.g., oral), sampling is adjusted as necessary to characterize the peak blood concentration (C_{max}) and the peak time (T_{max}). Generally, the sampling schedule should be twice as long as the mean half-life of the drug. This goal may be difficult to achieve when the drug has a very long half-life (i.e., >24 hrs) or when assay sensitivity becomes limiting. To illustrate approaches to these difficulties, Plummer et al. (13) have compared sampling schedules for methadone pharmacokinetic studies and Endrenyi (24) has proposed an optimal sampling method wherein the number of time points sampled depends on the number of parameters to be estimated.

Collection of total voided urine provides valuable additional information including the quantitative contribution of this route, the urinary metabolite pattern, and an estimate of renal drug clearance (Cl_R) as a fraction of the total blood clearance (Cl_B) (Table 1). As with blood samples, the duration of urine collection after a single dose is based on estimates of the half-life of the drug. The pH of urine should be noted since the urinary excretion of some drugs (e.g., opioids) may vary as a function of urinary pH (12,20). The subject's renal status should also be measured since alteration in renal function may profoundly affect the pharmacokinetics and pharmacodynamics of analgesics (25).

When pharmacokinetic and pharmacodynamic data are concurrently collected, the design of a biofluid sample schedule must include consideration of the time-

TABLE 1. *Methadone pharmacokinetic parameter estimates in chronic pain patients after a single intravenous dose[a]*

Parameter	Mean	±1 SD
$t_{\frac{1}{2}}\pi$ (min)	1.2	0.6
$t_{\frac{1}{2}}\alpha$ (min)	29.6	10.6
$t_{\frac{1}{2}}\beta$ (hr)	27.3	12.0
V_c (liters)	10.6	5.3
V_{area} (liters)	237.0	7.0
Cl_B (ml/min)	142.1	72.2
Cl_R (ml/min)	6.6	4.6
ER	0.09	0.05

[a] Data are mean values from eight patients. $t_{\frac{1}{2}}\pi$, $t_{\frac{1}{2}}\alpha$, dispositional (distribution) half-lives; $t_{\frac{1}{2}}\beta$, terminal elimination half-life; V_c, apparent volume of distribution of the central compartment; V_{area}, apparent volume of distribution during the postdistribution phase; Cl_B, blood clearance; Cl_R, renal clearance; ER, hepatic extraction ratio.
Modified from ref. 20, with permission.

effect curve of the drug and be adjusted accordingly. For example, after a single dose, the analgesic effects of methadone occur during the first 4 to 6 hrs, and predominantly during the early distribution phase (20); the pharmacodynamic measurements should therefore focus on this early time period, whereas more extended sampling is required for pharmacokinetic characterization.

PK-PD studies in patients with pain often present practical considerations that impose limits on the frequency and sometimes on the duration of pharmacokinetic sampling as well as on the duration of pharmacodynamic measures. For example, the total volume of blood per 24-hr period that can be collected from a patient may be limited by hospital regulations. Within these limitations, however, it is usually possible to obtain adequate pharmacodynamic data by collecting the data more frequently than blood samples. Although the relative frequency of PD-only sampling to simultaneous PK and PD sampling may vary, we have limited those times that PD data are collected alone to 15% or less of the total sampling times. This important issue requires a systematic evaluation.

Clearly, patients with persistent pain cannot abstain from analgesics during the extended sampling schedules required to characterize long half-life analgesics. Our approach is to provide an opioid analgesic on request by the patient. The remedication analgesic cannot be the study drug or a drug that interferes with the analytical method. Once the patient is remedicated during a study, no additional pharmacodynamic data are collected but blood sampling is continued. In the case of methadone, it has been possible to compare the pharmacokinetic data from a number of subject groups including normals and patients without pain where remedication was not an issue to data from pain patients, and to demonstrate that remedication does not confound the pharmacokinetic parameter estimates (20). However, whenever alterations in the "general" format such as those indicated above are introduced, the data analysis should be conducted with and without the "new" points to evaluate their contribution to final estimates.

The opioids are bound to both the alpha-glycoprotein and albumin fractions of plasma. Disease states can alter albumin, generally decreasing the concentration, whereas inflammation, infection, or malignancy can increase alpha-glycoprotein levels (6,26). Abramson (26) has shown that the unbound (free fraction) of methadone, which is highly bound to alpha-glycoprotein, varies fourfold in plasma samples from cancer patients. Thus, the plasma protein binding of methadone may be a source of interindividual variation in methadone disposition. The clinical significance of this observation, however, remains to be determined. For drugs with relatively high plasma protein binding (e.g., >50%) a predose plasma sample should be collected from each subject for *in vitro* analysis of drug binding. This information can be used to estimate whether a measure of drug clearance (hepatic clearance) is restricted to the free, circulating drug or is nonrestricted (6,19,20). This sample also provides an indication of whether a particular patient's disease state has dramatically altered drug binding. Excellent reviews of the theoretical and clinical aspects of drug binding are available (6,27).

ESTIMATING STANDARD PHARMACOKINETIC PARAMETERS

Pharmacokinetic studies should be designed to assess intra- and interindividual variation as well as the linearity of pharmacokinetic (concentration-time) profiles, and to generate reliable pharmacokinetic parameters in the dose range of pharmacodynamic interest. These pharmacokinetic studies can identify the pharmacokinetic equation (Fig. 1) to be used in subsequent PK-PD modeling.

The pharmacokinetic profile obtained after an IV bolus provides the best estimate of "intrinsic" pharmacokinetic parameters (i.e., not subject to errors associated with input functions such as absorption). The pharmacokinetic parameters are obtained from the pharmacokinetic profiles by use of both model-dependent and (relatively) model-independent data analysis. Model-independent approaches refer to parameter estimates that do not require, for their computation, assumptions about a model equation (e.g., Fig. 1) that relates drug input to drug disposition.

It is beyond the scope of this review to present the theoretical development and assumptions that underlie the selection of pharmacokinetic models and the estimation of pharmacokinetic parameters. This information is described in several texts and articles (see 1,2,5,6). Rather than describe every pharmacokinetic parameter that can be estimated by these approaches, the following discussion will focus on those parameters I have found most useful in describing the pharmacokinetics of analgesics.

Since the disposition of most drugs [a notable exception being the elimination of aspirin (28)] is by first-order processes in which the rate of elimination is proportional to the amount present at that time, the simplest and most useful data analysis involves fitting the plasma (or blood) concentration–time data to an exponential equation, such as the following:

$$C_p = Ae^{-\alpha t} + Be^{-\beta t} \qquad [1]$$

where Cp is the drug concentration in the central (plasma) compartment, α and β are the fast and slow disposition rate constants, respectively, and A and B are the corresponding zero-time intercepts (1,2).

Iterative weighted nonlinear least-squares regression computer programs (e.g., 10,18) are used to fit the plasma concentration-time data to the exponential equation. Many pharmacokinetic models have been developed (1,2), the most common being models described by two or three exponentials. Exponential equations have been used to describe the IV bolus pharmacokinetics of morphine (29), methadone (8,13,20), meperidine (9), fentanyl (7,30), alfentanil (7,30,31), and heroin (11).

Another useful approach to pharmacokinetic analysis involves the application of clearance concepts. This approach is based on the efficiency of any organ in removing drug irreversibly from the perfusing blood (19). The rate of drug removal from the body can be described by the total body (or systemic) clearance (Cl)

$$Cl = \frac{D_{IV}}{AUC} \qquad [2]$$

where D_{IV} is the intravenous dose and AUC is the area under the plasma or blood concentration-time curve. Clearance estimates are also obtained from the model-dependent analysis. Comparison of model-independent and model-dependent estimates for this parameter provides some insight into the appropriateness of the model selected to generate the model-dependent estimate of clearance. The clearance parameter together with the volume of distribution parameters (see below) are important because they assist in the determination of the frequency and size of doses.

Figure 2 shows an example of the plasma concentration-time profile following the IV administration of methadone to a patient with chronic pain (12,20) and the theoretical curves generated from the computer-estimated pharmacokinetic parameters. The pharmacokinetic parameters obtained from the model-dependent and model-independent approaches (Table 1) describe methadone as a drug with rapid and extensive distribution phases ($t_{1/2\pi}$ and $t_{1/2\alpha}$) followed by a slow elimination phase ($t\frac{1}{2}\beta$). The mean apparent volume of distribution of the central compartment (V_c) of 10.6 liters was equal to 15% of average body weight, whereas

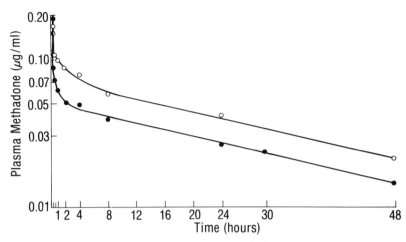

FIG. 2. Plasma concentration-time profiles of methadone after a single intravenous dose of 20 mg (●) or 30 mg (○) of methadone hydrochloride (HCl) administered to the same patient 1 week apart. *Points* denote observed concentration; the *solid line* is a theoretical line obtained by fitting the data with a triexponential equation. (From ref. 12, with permission.)

the apparent volume of distribution during the postdistribution phase (V_{area}) of 237 liters was equal to approximately 3.5 times average body weight.

It is important to recognize that a volume of distribution does not, per se, represent a physiological volume (e.g., blood volume). Rather, it is a constant that allows conversion between the dose (amount of drug) and the concentration in the sampled biofluid compartment (i.e., dose/volume = concentration). Thus a volume of distribution can be used to calculate the dose (loading dose) necessary to "fill" a volume of the body and rapidly produce a desired blood concentration.

The blood clearance or Cl_B (Table 1) can be used to calculate the hepatic extraction ratio (ER), a measure of the efficiency of the hepatic clearance of drug (20). In our example, methadone was found to have an average ER value of 0.09, which indicates that less than 10% of the available methadone is cleared from the blood as it passed through the liver. Thus, methadone can be classified as a low-extraction (hepatic) drug. In contrast, morphine has an ER of 0.70 and is an example of a high-extraction drug. The implications of these characteristics of methadone are discussed elsewhere (20).

Replication of parameter estimates provides a measure of the precision of these estimates. We found that whereas the interindividual variation in methadone's terminal elimination half-life and blood clearance were four- and fivefold, respectively, that these parameters vary, on the average, less than 30% in patients who participated in a second study (12,20).

Bioavailability studies, which may include studies in both normals and patients, can be conducted throughout the development process. The intent of these studies is to evaluate the systemic availability of new drug or new (or modified) dosage forms, and compare this to a reference, which most appropriately is an intravenous dose. When two formulations are compared by the same route of administration, the term "bioequivalence" is used to describe the intent of the study. A variation of the standard bioavailability study evaluates the effect of food, which can increase or decrease the absorption of orally administered drugs (5). The bioavailability of opioid analgesics has been compared after oral (29), intramuscular (29), and epidural (29,32) administration. Shepard (33) has compared the bioequivalence of immediate- and controlled-release oral dosage forms of morphine.

Figure 3 shows plasma concentration-time profiles for oral methadone and intravenous deuterium-labeled methadone after simultaneous administration of methadone in the naturally occurring and stable isotope forms to a opioid-dependent patient undergoing detoxification (8). Bioavailability is quantitatively characterized (Table 2) in terms of the extent or fraction of drug absorbed (F) when drug is administered by the test route (e.g., F-oral) and the time of peak concentration (T_{max}). The biofluid drug concentration at peak time (C_{max}) is also noted. The absorption rate may also be described by the $t\frac{1}{2}$ ka (absorption half-life), a model-dependent parameter, which assumes a first-order absorption process (not shown in Table 2). Whereas T_{max} and C_{max} are empirically observed

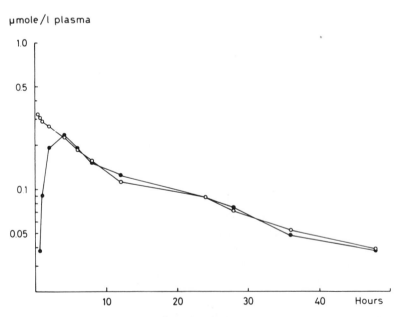

FIG. 3. Plasma concentration-time profiles of methadone (● — ●) and deuterium-labeled methadone (○ — ○) after the simultaneous oral (methadone hydrochloride, 20 mg) and intravenous (deuterium-labeled methadone hydrochloride, 20 mg) administration to an opioid-dependent patient undergoing detoxification. (From ref. 8, with permission.)

TABLE 2. *Methadone bioavailability parameters obtained after simultaneous administration of 20 mg of methadone orally and 20 mg of deuterium-labeled methadone intravenously in eight opioid dependent subjects*

Parameter	Mean	±1 SD
T_{max} (hr)	3	1.40
C_{max} (μmole/liter)	0.27	0.16
AUC po (μmole/liter $\times$ hr)	7.48	4.40
AUC IV (μmole/liter $\times$ hr)	9.61	5.23
F-oral	0.79	0.21

T_{max}, time to peak (maximum) plasma concentration after oral dosing; C_{max}, peak (maximum) plasma concentration; AUC po, area under the plasma concentration-time curve after oral dosing; AUC IV, area under the plasma concentration-time curve after intravenous dosing; F-oral, fraction of the methadone dose that is bioavailable after oral (po) administration.
From ref. 8, with permission.

values, F is estimated from the AUCs calculated by the trapezoidal rule (1,2) as follows:

$$F = \frac{(D_{IV})(AUC_r)}{(D_r)(AUC_{IV})} \quad [3]$$

where D_{IV} is as above for equation [2] and r is the test route of administration.

Multiple-dose studies are designed to identify changes in the pharmacokinetic profile with repeated dosing. The primary objective is to determine if the drug concentrations increase in a linear and predictable manner as the dose is repeated and/or increased over time. Other information obtained from these studies may include the extent of drug accumulation, the length of time required to attain steady state, the degree of interdose fluctuation in drug concentrations at steady state, and the relative rate of accumulation of parent and metabolites (1,2,5).

Multiple-dose studies may also employ more limited biofluid sampling to evaluate steady-state pharmacokinetics. Figure 4 illustrates the correlations observed by Sawe (34) between the total daily dose of morphine and mean steady-state plasma morphine and the metabolite concentrations obtained from a pre-dose sample. These results suggest that the concentration of morphine and metabolites are linearly related to the daily dose over the range tested. Additional information can be obtained from this type of study if within-subject time-dependent changes are compared.

When more extensive sampling is employed, multiple estimates of pharmacokinetic parameters can be made in the same patient. For example, similar clearance estimates were obtained during different periods of a continuous infusion of heroin (a drug with a very short elimination half-life), where each successive period was characterized by a higher infusion rate that resulted in increasing apparent steady-state blood levels (11). This observation indicated

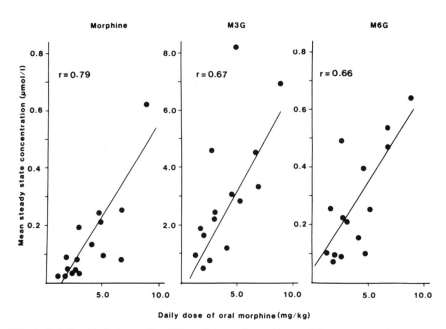

FIG. 4. Relationship between the daily oral dose of morphine and the mean steady-state concentrations of morphine and its metabolites, morphine-3-glucuronide (M3G) and morphine-6-glucuronide (M6G). Data are from cancer patients who have received chronic dosing with morphine. (From ref. 34, with permission.)

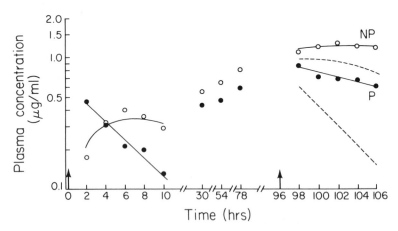

FIG. 5. Plasma concentration-time profiles of propoxyphene (●) and norpropoxyphene (○) observed during and following 13 consecutive 130 mg oral doses of propoxyphene HCl. The *arrows* indicate the time of administration of dose 1 (0 hr) and dose 13 (96 hrs). The values of 30, 54, and 78 hrs are plasma concentrations determined at 6 hrs after the 4th, 7th, and 10th dose, respectively. The *solid lines* represent the theoretical line obtained by independently fitting the dose 1 and dose 13 data with equations that describe the concentration-time profiles of propoxyphene (P) and norpropoxyphene (NP) in plasma during and following consecutive doses of propoxyphene (8), and the *dashed lines* represent the dose 13 plasma concentrations expected using dose 1 parameter estimates. (From ref. 10, with permission.)

that, at least for the range tested, heroin's kinetics remain linear (11). In contrast, a different result was observed in a study of the accumulation of propoxyphene and its active metabolite, norpropoxyphene (10). Figure 5 shows that the pharmacokinetics of propoxyphene (P) and norpropoxyphene (NP) change during repetitive-dose administration and that these changes result in a more extensive accumulation of P and NP than would be predicted from the single (first dose) profiles. The dash lines in Figure 5 represent the values predicted from the PK parameters obtained from analysis of the first dose, and the solid lines and the circles are the actual observed values (after the 13th dose). Compared to the first dose values the clearance of P and NP after the 13th dose are decreased 50%, the AUCs for P and NP are doubled, and the elimination $t_{1/2s}$ for P and NP are increased 4 to 6 times. Thus, the kinetics of P and NP do not appear to remain linear during repetitive dosing. Multiple-dose studies of analgesics are receiving much greater attention (see Chapter 5), and it is hoped that PK-PD studies will become an integral part of this effort.

STUDIES IN SPECIAL RISK POPULATIONS

The disposition of an opioid analgesic may be altered by disease. Renal failure results in the accumulation of active and potentially toxic metabolites of meperidine, propoxyphene, and morphine, whereas cirrhosis decreases the clearance of meperidine, propoxyphene, and pentazocine (25). The clearance of morphine is decreased in individuals over the age of 50 (25), and perhaps also as a result of pharmacodynamic changes, older patients demonstrate greater sensitivity to therapeutic doses of morphine, fentanyl, and alfentanil (25,30). All of the above observations were made after the drugs had been marketed. However, future drug development studies should include some assessments in special risk populations including the elderly and patients with renal dysfunction or hepatic disease. The objective of these studies is to determine if dose adjustments are required in these patients owing to measurable pharmacokinetic and/or pharmacodynamic differences. Recognizing that it may be difficult to enter a sufficient number of patients in this type of study, some suggestions have been made with respect to inclusion criteria for pharmacokinetic studies based on specific disease markers (5).

POPULATION PHARMACOKINETICS

The previous discussion has focused on the design of studies aimed at collecting data for analysis by what can be described as "classical" pharmacokinetic methods. An alternate approach uses knowledge of average pharmacokinetic parameters and their variation within the population to design dosing regimens. This approach, population pharmacokinetics, employs designs that use a limited number of measurements from many individuals and statistical models that can then be used to "individualize" a patient's pharmacokinetics or pharmacodynamics (5,35,36). This aspect of population pharmacokinetics may have particular utility in anesthesiology when the methodologies for simultaneously measuring plasma drug concentrations and degree of drug effect during anesthesia become available (6).

COLLECTION OF PHARMACODYNAMIC DATA

The concurrent collection of pharmacokinetic and pharmacodynamic data can provide a knowledge base that is useful for establishing the optimal dose range and choosing dosing regimens for chronic administration. Furthermore, these data are essential to understand the relationship between biofluid concentration-time profiles and analgesic time-effect curves. At present, whereas two formulations of a particular analgesic may be assumed to provide equivalent analgesia if they produce concurrent curves of active drug in the blood, controlled clinical trials are necessary to demonstrate the clinical relevance of any significant difference observed in the concentration-time profiles produced by different formulation of an analgesia unless PK-PD data (see below) are available to provide an estimate of the consequences, if any, of this variation.

Thus, pharmacodynamic measures should be included in pharmacokinetic studies whenever possible. Likewise, sample collection for pharmacokinetic (PK) determinations should be included in "classical" pharmacodynamic (PD) studies whenever possible. For example, in a relative potency analgesic assay patients may elect to participate only in the analgesic assay (PD study) or, alternatively, in a study designed to collect both PK and PD data. The effect data obtained then can be analyzed with and without the PK and PD subgroup data to determine whether biofluid sample collection significantly altered the outcome of the analgesic assay. Even limited PK sampling (e.g., one or a few biofluid samples) collected with PD data obtained in analgesic studies may allow some insight into sources of variation in analgesic responses when responders are compared with dropouts, sustained responders, or those with unexpected toxic effects.

As is discussed elsewhere (see Chapter 4), a methodology has developed for the clinical evaluation of analgesic drugs that involves the use of categorical (descriptor) and visual analogue (VAS) scales (37,38). Although the ordinal values of the categorical scales may not be linearly related, they have generally been treated as equally spaced ordinal data by investigators in the field (38). Regression of ordinal and VAS measures of changes in pain and pain relief after the administration of analgesics demonstrates extremely high correlations (38). In general, VAS scales have been found to be reliable indices, acceptable to the patients and more sensitive to changes than categorical scales (38). Both categorical and VAS scales have been empirically validated in studies estimating relative analgesic potency (37,38). Wallenstein (38) has shown that the pain descriptors that have a power function relationship to the intensity of the stimulus in experimental pain bear a similar relationship to the VAS scales used in the assessment of clinical pain where the intensity of the stimulus cannot be directly measured.

ANALYSIS OF CONCURRENTLY COLLECTED PK-PD DATA

Pharmacodynamic Models

The objective of studies in which pharmacokinetic and pharmacodynamic data are concurrently collected is to determine what relationships exist between a change in drug concentrations and a change in effect. In quantitative terms, this relationship can be described by an equation, i.e., a PD model (Fig. 1), that relates biofluid drug concentration to effect. A number of PD models have been described (39–42) and it is useful to test PK-PD data sets with more than one of these models. Figure 6 shows a representation of the concentration-effect relationship that is predicted for a receptor-mediated effect such as opioid analgesia. It is a sigmoid curve that defines the plasma opioid concentration-effect relationship from 0 (no effect) to 1.0 (the maximum effect). This type of concentration-effect relationship is described by a PD model which Holford and Sheiner (41) have called the Sigmoid Emax model. The model equation is:

$$FR = \frac{(C_e)^\gamma}{(C_{ss}50)^\gamma + (C_e)^\gamma} \qquad [4]$$

where FR is the fraction of maximum effect, C_e is the concentration of drug at the effect site, $C_{ss}50$ is the steady-state concentration of drug at half maximum effect and a measure of individual sensitivity to the drug, and γ is a slope factor that determines the steepness of the concentration-effect curve.

Both FR and C_e can be considered to be experimentally measurable quantities. FR is the observed effect, (e.g., pain relief, VAS) transformed to a scale that extends from 0 to 1.0, and C_e can be obtained from the pharmacokinetic model

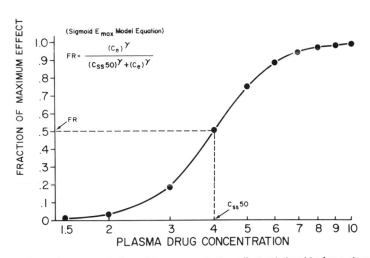

FIG. 6. A schematic representation of the concentration-effect relationship for a drug with a sigmoid concentration-effect curve.

that describes the concentration-time relationship (see below). Equation [4] also contains two constants or pharmacodynamic parameters, γ and $C_{ss}50$. These parameters are estimated from analysis of the experimental data by an iterative technique in the same manner as described above for the pharmacokinetic parameters. Thus, if γ and $C_{ss}50$ could be estimated from each patient's data set, a complete plasma concentration-effect curve could be generated using equation [4]. These curves could be used to determine the plasma drug concentrations above which the majority of patients respond and those concentrations above which the majority develop limiting side effects (i.e., a therapeutic range). The onset and duration of effect can be described in terms of the time required to reach and leave the therapeutic range (42). The acquisition of this type of data for clinical populations is certainly one of the goals of PK-PD modeling of analgesics.

Figure 7 shows a plot of plasma methadone concentrations and mean analgesic effect in six cancer patients using a pain relief (PR) categorical (CAT) scale and a pain intensity difference (PID) visual analogue scale following an intravenous dose of methadone. For methadone, higher plasma drug concentrations are associated with a greater intensity of analgesia and a concentration-effect relationship appears to exist over this range of plasma methadone. From Fig. 7 it might be possible to estimate the desired constants ($C_{ss}50$ and γ) without the need for a more rigorous analysis, i.e., the use of a PK-PD model equation. The limitations to this approach have been discussed elsewhere (20,40,41,43,44). One of the advantages of using a PK-PD model is that the model allows prediction of the entire concentration-effect relationship (Fig. 6) from the more limited data, i.e., data that do not encompass the entire range of effect from 0 to 1.0 (Fig. 7) usually obtained in individual patients. An additional consideration in analgesic studies

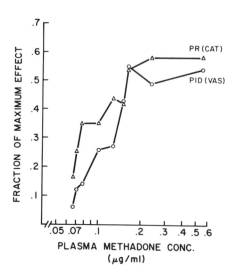

FIG. 7. The relationship between mean plasma methadone concentration and mean fractional analgesic effect, measured using pain relief (PR) CAT scales (△) and pain intensity difference (PID) VAS (○) following an intravenous dose of methadone to six cancer patients. (From ref. 43, with permission.)

is that the presence of endogenous analgesics and/or prior exogenously administered analgesics may influence initial pain intensity and the concentration-effect relationships obtained (18). Colburn and Gibson (45) have described PD models that include consideration of baseline responses. These approaches require more extensive measurements of baseline responses than are available from typical PK-PD study design and therefore must be considered during the design of the study.

Pharmacokinetic-Pharmacodynamic Models

The objective of PK-PD modeling is to link the dose-concentration relationship described by a PK model to the concentration-effect relationship obtained by use of a PD model. This may be accomplished directly by equating the concentration predicted by a PK model (Fig. 1) to the drug concentration at the effect site (C_e in equation [4]). This direct approach requires that there is rapid equilibration between drug in the biofluid "compartment" being sampled (e.g., plasma) and the effect site concentration (e.g., CNS opioid receptors). This approach can be used to describe the PK-PD relationship for methadone in cancer patients receiving an intravenous infusion (18). However, a more common observation is that there is a lag between the time course of effect and plasma drug concentration, giving rise to a hysteresis loop in the concentration-effect plot (40–43). Figure 8 shows a plot of plasma morphine concentration-effect data for a cancer patient during and following an intravenous infusion of morphine. Note that when the infusion is discontinued and plasma morphine concentrations decrease, the intensity of the analgesic effect lags behind the change in plasma drug concentration. This time-dependent lag of effect behind a change in plasma drug concentration is called hysteresis and has been reported for many drugs (41,42).

Plots of effect as a function of plasma drug concentration are useful for the

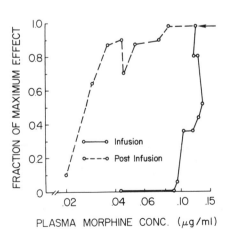

FIG. 8. A plasma concentration-effect plot for pain relief (VAS) data from a cancer patient who received a continuous intravenous infusion (20 mg/hr) of morphine sulfate. The *solid line* indicates data obtained during the infusion, the *arrow* indicates the point at which the infusion was discontinued, and the *broken line* indicates data collected during the post-infusion phase. Note the counterclockwise hysteresis (lag loop) for pain relief produced by morphine.

recognition of time-dependent changes between plasma drug concentration and effect. Data obtained from continuous IV infusions are particularly useful for hysteresis plots since this method insures increasing and decreasing plasma drug concentrations in the effect range. Figure 9 shows simulated hysteresis plots using a PK-PD model with an effect compartment for data obtained during and following an intravenous infusion. The plot in the center, labeled "Symmetrical," shows no evidence of hysteresis. This would occur if neither an equilibrium delay nor the development of tolerance occurred during the infusion so that the concentration-effect relationship during the infusion was identical to that seen during the postinfusion washout. This type of plot is seen with methadone infusions (18). The "Tolerance" plot shows a clockwise loop indicating that higher plasma drug concentrations are required to produce a given level of effect later in the study, e.g., during the postinfusion phase. This type of plot could, in theory, be obtained from a rapid change in receptor sensitivity or number during the study or from the accumulation of an antagonistic metabolite, although this mechanism is unlikely in the case of opioids. The plot labeled "Lag" shows a counterclockwise loop characteristic of an equilibrium delay between plasma drug concentration and effect-site concentration. Alternately, this type of loop would occur if an active metabolite is rapidly formed and the ratio of active metabolite to parent increases with time.

The practical consequence of the demonstration of hysteresis using a concentration-effect plot is that the measured plasma drug concentration (C_p) must be

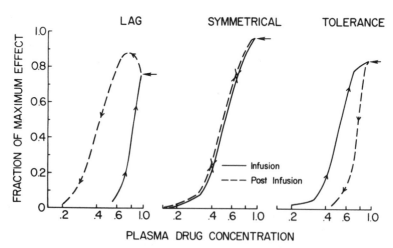

FIG. 9. Concentration-effect curves illustrating the presence and absence of hysteresis. These curves were simulated using an infusion PK-PD model (18) and the following parameter and constant values: $\alpha = 6.0$ hr^{-1}, $\beta = 0.06$ hr^{-1}, $k_{21} = 1.86$ hr^{-1}, $V_c = 4.8$ liters, infusion rate = 2.78 mg/hr, duration of infusion 6 hrs. For the Lag plot (counterclockwise hysteresis), $K_{e0} = 0.4$, $C_{ss}50 = 0.5$, and $\gamma = 5.0$. For the Symmetrical plot (no hysteresis), $k_{e0} = 100$, $C_{ss}50 = 0.5$, and $\gamma = 5.0$. For the Tolerance plot (clockwise hysteresis), $k_{e0} = 4.0$, $\gamma = 5.0$, and $C_{ss}50$ is changed from 0.5 to 1.0 beginning at 4 hrs into the infusion.

adjusted to reflect the temporal difference between a change in plasma drug concentration and a change in effect before it can be used in the PD model. This "adjustment" is accomplished by using the time course of the effect itself to define the rate of drug movement into a distinct "effect compartment" of negligible volume. The theoretical aspects of effect compartment models are discussed elsewhere (39–46). Figure 10 shows a representation of a PK-PD model with an effect compartment. The plasma drug concentrations are modeled by whatever PK model is appropriate to characterize the plasma drug concentration-time profile. The hypothetical effect compartment (E) is modeled as an additional exponential function. The rate constant for drug removal from the effect compartment is designated k_{e0} (Fig. 10) and will precisely characterize the temporal aspects of equilibration between C_p and effect; k_{e0} is a model parameter determined by nonlinear regression that will characterize the degree of hysteresis (39,40,42). Thus, by use of the observed C_p values and the estimates of k_{e0} obtained from the model (Fig. 10), the effect-site concentrations (C_e) are predicted and C_e values are used by the PD model to estimate the desired pharmacodynamic parameters, $C_{ss}50$ and γ (Fig. 10).

An example of this approach is given in Fig. 11, which shows the simultaneous fit of the plasma morphine concentration-time profile and analgesic effect data (pain relief, VAS) to a PK-PD model with an effect compartment (43). Table 3 lists the mean pharmacodynamic parameters estimated from the curve-fitting procedure. Good agreement was found between parameters obtained by use of categorical and visual analogue measures of analgesia. The k_{e0} parameter can be converted to a half-life value (Table 3) to provide a more direct illustration of the hysteresis lag. Thus, when plasma morphine concentrations are altered, the half-life for the analgesic effect to come into equilibrium with this change averages 15 to 20 min. The intrinsic sensitivity to morphine's analgesic effects in this group of patients (43) is given by the $C_{ss}50$ values which averaged 0.052 and 0.063 $\mu g/ml$ (Table 3). These values can be compared with $C_{ss}50$ values obtained in the same manner for other opioids (18). Estimating these pharmacodynamic parameters provides a quantitative method for determining whether patient variables such as age, sex, disease, or organ dysfunction alter drug effects by affecting kinetics, dynamics, or both (e.g., see 30).

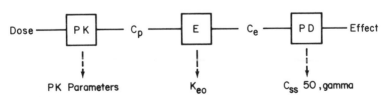

FIG. 10. A schematic representation of a PK-PD model with an effect compartment. The PK and PD models are linked by an effect compartment (E). The model yields both PK parameters and the PD parameters k_{e0}, $C_{ss}50$, and gamma.

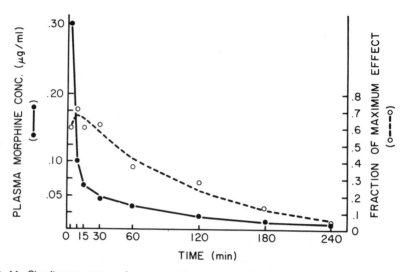

FIG. 11. Simultaneous mean plasma morphine concentration-time data (●) and mean fractional analgesic effect data measured as pain relief (VAS) (○) following intravenous administration of morphine to six burn patients. (From ref. 43, with permission.)

Figure 12 shows an example of a simulated plasma morphine concentration-effect curve generated from the pharmacodynamic parameters (Table 3) obtained from the fit of the pain relief (VAS) data for morphine shown in Fig. 11 by a PK-PD model (43). The γ value (slope function) of 1.4 (Table 3) predicts that the intensity of the analgesic effect of morphine will change from a value of 0.1 (10% of maximum) to 0.9 (90% of maximum) in response to a 25-fold increase in plasma morphine concentration (Fig. 12). Much steeper concentration-effect relationships have been reported for the effects of other opioids (18,20,30). These

TABLE 3. *Mean pharmacodynamic (PD) parameter estimates by simultaneous curve-fitting plasma morphine concentrations and measures of analgesia following intravenous administration of morphine to six burn patients*

PD parameters	Pain relief CAT	Pain relief VAS
k_{e0} (min^{-1})	0.034	0.046
$t\frac{1}{2} k_{e0}$ (min)	20.4	15.1
$C_{ss}50$ (μg/ml)	0.052	0.063
gamma	1.3	1.4

k_{e0}, elimination rate constant from the hypothetical effect compartment; $t\frac{1}{2} k_{e0}$, half-life for equilibration between plasma morphine concentration and analgesia ($t\frac{1}{2} k_{e0}$ = .693/k_{e0}); $C_{ss}50$ steady-state concentration of morphine when the effect is 50% of maximum; gamma, power factor which determines the slope of the concentration-effect curve; CAT, categorical scale; VAS, visual analogue scale.
Modified from ref. 43, with permission.

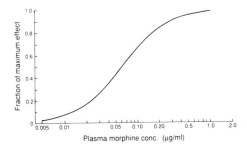

FIG. 12. A simulated plasma morphine concentration-effect curve for intravenous morphine in burn patients. The curve was generated by use of the sigmoid Emax equation (see equation [4]) and the pharmacodynamic constants given in Table 3.

results with morphine need to be extended to include other patient populations, but it is clear that information about intrinsic sensitivity ($C_{ss}50$) and the steepness of the concentration-effect curve (γ) can provide important new quantitative insights into the concentration-effect relationship and ultimately into the development of analgesic dosing regimens. When pharmacodynamic measures include desirable and undesirable effects, (e.g., analgesia and sedation) each of these effects can be analyzed and the pharmacodynamic parameters and concentration-effect curves compared within and between patients, thereby providing a more complete quantitative pharmacological profile (18).

The preceding discussion has focused on the use of parametric PK-PD models, since this approach has been used successfully with analgesic data. An alternate approach that may be of value utilizes a nonparametric method in which no *a priori* judgment is made about the form of the PK and or PD models and the value of K_{e0} is evaluated until the area within the hysteresis loop is minimized (collapsed) (44,47).

SUMMARY

Although the data analysis of simultaneously collected pharmacokinetic and pharmacodynamic data is in its infancy, it is clear that this approach provides a unique insight that, in addition to providing the most complete quantitative description of the clinical pharmacology of an analgesic, may also serve to streamline the drug development process. For example, PK-PD modeling permits predictions of concentration-effect relationships that extend beyond the observed data, allowing some extrapolation of the therapeutic dose range. PK-PD modeling can provide an efficient method for defining the relative contribution of parent and metabolites, or each stereoisomer, to the therapeutic and/or undesirable effects of an analgesic. This approach also has the potential to provide methods for quantitating the development of tolerance to the analgesic and other effects of opioids. Finally, I would emphasize that whereas the utility of any particular pharmacokinetic or pharmacodynamic analytical method discussed in this chapter needs to be validated by rigorous application to each analgesic and modified as required, the concept that analgesic study design must include concurrent collection and analysis of pharmacokinetic and pharmacodynamic data is not a hope for the future, but a necessity for the present.

ACKNOWLEDGMENTS

My research activities are supported in part by National Cancer Institute grant CA-32897 and National Institutes on Drug Abuse grants DA-01457 and DA-05130. Many colleagues have contributed to the clinical pharmacokinetic and pharmacodynamic studies conducted by the Analgesic Studies Section and the Pain Research Program of the Memorial Sloan-Kettering Cancer Center (MSKCC) and some of these studies are used as illustrations in this chapter. I wish to thank Dr. R. Houde and Dr. K. Foley of MSKCC and Dr. W. Colburn of Harris Laboratories for their continuing collaboration and strong support of these studies. I thank Dr. U. Meresaar of Mölndals Hospital, Sweden for generously providing additional data that is presented in Table 2, and Dr. R. Portenoy of MSKCC for helpful comments during the preparation of the manuscript.

REFERENCES

1. Greenblatt DJ, Shader RI. *Pharmacokinetics in clinical practice.* Philadelphia: WB Saunders, 1985.
2. Gibaldi M, Perrier D. *Pharmacokinetics,* 2nd ed. New York: Academic Press, 1981.
3. Peck CC, Collins JM. First time in man studies: a regulatory perspective—art and science of phase I trials. *J Clin Pharmacol* 1990;30:218–222.
4. Peck CC. The randomized concentration-controlled clinical trial (CCT): an information-rich alternative to the randomized placebo-controlled clinical trial. *Clin Pharmacol Ther* 1990;47: 148.
5. Colburn WA, Olson SC. Classic and population pharmacokinetics. In: Welling PG, Tse G, eds. *Pharmacokinetics, regulatory, industrial: academic perspectives.* New York: Marcel Dekker, 1988;337–384.
6. Mather LE, Stanski DR. Drug disposition: basic pharmacokinetics. In: Benedetti C, Chapman CR, Giron G, eds. *Advances in pain research and therapy,* vol 14. New York: Raven Press, 1990;143–170.
7. Hill HF, Chapman CR. Tailored infusion of opioids. In: Benedetti C, Chapman CR, Giron G, eds. *Advances in pain research and therapy,* vol 14. New York: Raven Press, 1990;203–215.
8. Meresaar U, Nilsson M-I, Holmstrand J, et al. Single dose pharmacokinetics and bioavailability of methadone in man studied with a stable isotope method. *Eur J Clin Pharmacol* 1981;20:473–478.
9. Pond SM, Tong T, Benowitz NL, Jacob P, Rigod J. Presystemic metabolism of meperidine to normeperidine in normal and cirrhotic subjects. *Clin Pharmacol Ther* 1981;30:183–188.
10. Inturrisi CE, Colburn WA, Verebey K, Dayton HE, Woody GE, O'Brien CP. Propoxyphene and norpropoxyphene kinetics after single and repeated doses of propoxyphene. *Clin Pharmacol Ther* 1982;31:157–167.
11. Inturrisi CE. Pharmacokinetics of oral, intravenous, and continuous infusions of heroin. In: Foley KM, Inturrisi CE, eds. *Advances in pain research and therapy,* vol 8. New York: Raven Press, 1986;117–127.
12. Inturrisi CE, Colburn WA. Pharmacokinetics of methadone. In: Foley KM, Inturrisi CE, eds. *Advances in pain research and therapy,* vol 8. New York: Raven Press, 1986;191–199.
13. Plummer, JL, Gourlay GK, Cherry DA, Cousins MJ. Estimation of methadone clearance: application in the management of cancer pain. *Pain* 1988;33:313–322.
14. Day RO, Williams KM, Graham GG, et al. Stereoselective disposition of ibuprofen enantiomers in synovial fluid. *Clin Pharmacol Ther* 1988;43:480–487.

15. Verbeeck RK, Blackburn JL, Loewen GR. Clinical pharmacokinetics of non-steroidal anti-in-flammatory drugs. *Clin Pharmacokinet* 1983;8:297–331.
16. Brazzell RK, Colburn WA. Controversy I: Patients or healthy volunteers for pharmacokinetic studies? *J Clin Pharmacol* 1986;26:242–247.
17. Sheiner LB, Benet LZ, Pagliaro LA. A standard approach to compiling clinical pharmacokinetic data. *J Pharmacokinet Biopharm* 1981;9:59–127.
18. Inturrisi CE, Portenoy RK, Max MB, Colburn WA, Foley KM. Pharmacokinetic-pharmaco-dynamic (PK-PD) relationships of methadone infusions in patients with cancer pain. *Clin Pharmacol Ther* 1990;47:565–577.
19. Wilkinson GR, Shand DG. A physiological approach to hepatic drug clearance. *Clin Pharmacol Ther* 1975;18:377–390.
20. Inturrisi CE, Colburn WA, Kaiko RF, Houde RW, Foley KM. Pharmacokinetics and pharma-codynamics of methadone in patients with chronic pain. *Clin Pharmacol Ther* 1987;41:392–401.
21. Max MB, Inturrisi CE, Kaiko RF, Grabinski PY, Li CH, Foley KM. Epidural and intrathecal opiates: cerebrospinal fluid and plasma profiles in patients with chronic cancer pain. *Clin Pharmacol Ther* 1985;38:631–641.
22. Chiou WL. The phenomenon and rationale of marked dependence of drug concentration on blood sampling site. Implications in pharmacokinetics, pharmacodynamics, toxicology and ther-apeutics (Part I). *Clin Pharmacokinet* 1989;17:175–199.
23. Chiou WL. The phenomenon and rationale of marked dependence of drug concentration on blood sampling site. Implications in pharmacokinetics, pharmacodynamics, toxicology and ther-apeutics (Part II). *Clin Pharmacokinet* 1989:17;275–290.
24. Endrenyi L. Design of experiments for estimating enzyme and pharmacokinetic parameters. In: Endrenyi L. ed. *Kinetic data analysis.* New York: Plenum Press, 1981;271–284.
25. Inturrisi CE. Effects of other drugs and pathologic states on opioid disposition and response. In: Benedetti C, Chapman CR, Giron G, eds. *Advances in pain research and therapy,* vol 14. New York: Raven Press, 1990;171–180.
26. Abramson FP. Methadone plasma protein binding: alterations in cancer and displacement from alpha-acid glycoprotein. *Clin Pharmacol Ther* 1989;32:652–658.
27. MacKichan JJ. Protein binding drug displacement interactions. Fact or fiction? *Clin Pharmacokinet* 1989;16:65–73.
28. Levy G. Pharmacokinetics of salicylate elimination in man. *J Pharm Sci* 1965;54:959–967.
29. Dahlstrom B, Hedner T, Mellstrand T, Nordberg G, Rawal N, Sjostrand U. Plasma and cere-brospinal fluid kinetics of morphine. In: Foley KM and Inturrisi CE, eds. *Advances in pain research and therapy,* vol 8. New York: Raven Press, 1986;37–44.
30. Scott JC, Stanski DR. Decreased fentanyl and alfentanil dose requirements with age. A simul-taneous pharmacokinetic and pharmacodynamic evaluation. *J Pharmacol Exp Ther* 1987;240:159–166.
31. Stanski DR Jr, Hug CC. Alfentanil—a kinetically predictable narcotic analgesic. *Anesthesiology* 1982;57:435–438.
32. Glynn CJ, Mather LE, Cousins MJ, Graham JR, Wilson PR. Peridural meperidine in humans: analgetic response, pharmacokinetics, and transmission into CSF. *Anesthesiology* 1981;55:520–526.
33. Shepard KV. Review of a controlled-release morphine preparation. In: Foley KM, Bonica JJ, Ventafridda V, eds. *Advances in pain research and therapy,* vol 16. New York: Raven Press, 1990;191–202.
34. Sawe J. Morphine and its 3- and 6-glucuronides in plasma and urine during chronic oral ad-ministration in cancer patients. In: Foley KM, Inturrisi CE, eds. *Advances in pain research and therapy,* vol 8. New York: Raven Press, 1986;45–55.
35. Whiting B, Kelman AW, Grevel J. Population pharmacokinetics. Theory and clinical application. *Clin Pharmacokinet* 1986;11:387–401.
36. Maitre PO, Ausems ME, Vozeh S, Stanski DR. Evaluating the accuracy of using population pharmacokinetic data to predict plasma concentrations of alfentanil. *Anesthesiology* 1988;68:59–67.
37. Houde RW, Wallenstein SL, Beaver WT. Clinical measurement of pain. In: deStevens G, ed. *Analgetics.* New York: Raven Press, 1965;75–127.
38. Wallenstein SL. Scaling clinical pain and pain relief. In: Bromm B, ed. *Pain measurement in man. Neurophysiological correlates of pain.* New York: Elsevier Science Publishers BV, 1984;389–396.

39. Sheiner LB, Stanski DR, Vozeh S, Miller RD, Ham J. Simultaneous modeling of pharmacokinetics and pharmacodynamics: application to d-tubocurarine. *Clin Pharmacol Ther* 1979;25:358–371.
40. Colburn WA. Simultaneous pharmacokinetic and pharmacodynamic modeling. *J Pharmacokinet Biopharm* 1981;9:367–388.
41. Holford NHG, Sheiner LB. Understanding the dose-effect relationship: clinical application of pharmacokinetic-pharmacodynamic models. *Clin Pharmacokinet* 1981;6:429–453.
42. Tucker GT. Pharmacokinetic and pharmacodynamic models. In: Benedetti C, Chapman CR, Giron G, eds. *Advances in pain research and therapy,* vol 14. New York: Raven Press, 1990;181–201.
43. Inturrisi CE, Colburn WA. Application of pharmacokinetic-pharmacodynamic modeling to analgesia. In: Foley KM, Inturrisi CE, eds. *Advances in pain research and therapy,* vol 8. New York: Raven Press, 1986;441–452.
44. Sheiner LB. Clinical pharmacology and the choice between theory and empiricism. *Clin Pharmacol Ther* 1989;46:605–615.
45. Colburn WA, Gibson DM. Endogenous agonists and pharmacokinetic-pharmacodynamic modeling of baseline effects in pharmacokinetics and pharmacodynamics. In: Kroboth PD, Smith RB, Juhl RP, eds. *Pharmacokinetics and pharmacodynamics, vol 2: current problems, potential solutions.* Cincinnati: Harvey Whitney Books, 1988;167–184.
46. Colburn WA. Combined pharmacokinetic/pharmacodynamic (PK/PD) modeling. *J Clin Pharmacol* 1988;28:769–771.
47. Unadkat JD, Bartha F, Sheiner LB. Simultaneous modeling of pharmacokinetics and pharmacodynamics with nonparametric kinetic and dynamic models. *Clin Pharmacol Ther* 1986;40:86–93.

DISCUSSION

Dr. Laurence Mather: The objectives of pharmacokinetic analysis are twofold: to provide a description of the drug circulating in the blood and to provide a model to represent the interaction of the drug and the organism. The requirement for representative sampling applies to both. Traditional pharmacokinetic studies rely by convenience on sampling from a vein in the arm. However, if the drug is being removed anywhere or being added to the system, there are many regions in which the blood concentrations of drugs differ. In fact, the idea that venous blood correctly represents all drug blood concentrations is physiological nonsense. Arterial and venous gradients are important. Arterial drug concentrations represent those being supplied to the tissues. Venous concentrations reflect the rate and extent of drug equilibration in the tissues. Venous samples have very little to do with brain concentrations of the drug, except under steady-state conditions.

A second point relates to the choice of model. How does one decide upon a pharmacokinetic model? There are several kinds, including those based on simple empirical equations, multicompartment pool models, physiological models, and empirical descriptive models. Depending on the purpose of the exercise, one may choose a better or worse model to represent the data. The majority of investigators rely upon compartment models because of their simplicity. However, the interpretation of such data is extremely dangerous without experience. In many cases, simple empirical models, such as looking at the time of maximum concentration and the concentration itself, may be perfectly adequate. What we really want to know, of course, are the concentrations in the organs that have effect; that is, we need a physiological model. Unfortunately, the difficulty obtaining data for construction of such a model prohibits its widespread use and we make do with second best.

Given the extent of pharmacokinetic and pharmacodynamic variability, it is not surprising to discover that there is a mismatch between standardized dosing regimens and actual dose requirements after surgery. In short, when it comes to narcotic analgesics, I believe that the simple approach of close patient observation during dose titration is far more important than trying to decide in advance what the pharmacokinetic parameters are and then dosing on some predetermined dosing schedule that cannot account for the unknown characteristics of an individual patient.

Dr. Charles Inturrisi: I think the issue of blood concentration-effect relationships is, at this point, largely an empirical one; that is, if you can develop a relationship and that relationship has some predictive value, then I think you ought to use it. I think that it is clear for some analgesics that there is a very simple relationship between drug concentration in venous blood and effects (1). In other situations, or for other analgesics, it may be much more complicated and require the aid of models (2). More complicated approaches to handling the data are being developed, and these approaches may be able to address placebo effects and other baseline factors more directly (3).

Dr. Robert Kaiko: I would like to raise an issue. Has sufficient thought been given to appropriate controls and ways to minimize bias in these pharmacokinetic-pharmacodynamic studies? Some studies use placebo and others do not, but perhaps a placebo is not necessary. However, there does seem to be an inherent order effect in these studies. One is infusing a drug and, of course, with plasma levels rising, therapeutic effects go up, and when the infusion is turned off, they both go down. These changes do not necessarily imply a causal relationship. Moreover, these studies do not really randomize patients or sample, if you will, at random within each patient.

REFERENCES

1. Inturrisi CE, Portenoy RK, Max MB, Colburn WA, Foley KM. Pharmacokinetic-pharmacodynamic (PK-PD) relationships of methadone infusions in patients with cancer pain. *Clin Pharmacol Ther* 1990;47:565–577.
2. Inturrisi CE, Colburn WA. Application of pharmacokinetic-pharmacodynamic modeling to analgesia. In: Foley KM, Inturrisi CE, eds. *Advances in pain research and therapy,* vol 8. New York: Raven Press, 1986;439–450.
3. Colburn WA, Gibson DM. Endogenous agonists and pharmacokinetic/pharmacodynamic modeling of baseline effects in pharmacokinetics and pharmacodynamics. In: Kroboth PD, Smith RB, Juhl RP, eds. *Pharmacokinetics and pharmacodynamics, vol 2: current problems, potential solutions.* Cincinnati: Harvey Whitney Books, 1988;167–184.

Advances in Pain Research and Therapy, Vol. 18,
edited by M. Max, R. Portenoy, and E. Laska,
Raven Press, Ltd., New York © 1991.

Commentary

Pharmacokinetic/Pharmacodynamic Models in Analgesic Study Design

Raja Velagapudi,* John G. Harter,**
Ralf Brueckner,† and Carl C. Peck††

*Division of Biopharmaceutics, **Pilot Drug Evaluation Staff, †Division of
Experimental Therapeutics, Walter Reed Army Institute of Research,
Washington, DC 20307, ††Center for Drug Evaluation and Research,
Food and Drug Administration, Rockville, Maryland 20857*

The kinetic/dynamic approach described by Inturrisi in Chapter 24 to characterize opioid analgesics is generally applicable to other analgesic drugs. For both ketorolac, a parenteral, nonsteroidal antiinflammatory agent, and dezocine, a mixed agonist-antagonist that were both recently approved by the Food and Drug Administration (FDA) for use in minor or postoperative pain, this type of analysis had a very striking effect on speeding the approval process. The labels for these new analgesics look considerably different than traditional drug labels, because the sponsoring companies had sufficient information in their new drug applications to enable the FDA to undertake a state-of-the-art kinetic/dynamic analysis that resulted in useful parameters. Moreover, in the case of ketorolac, the FDA approved the drug at a dosing regimen that had never been studied. This was possible because the company had sufficiently characterized the kinetics and dynamics among the possible dosing regimens. Hence, the FDA felt comfortable in taking a calculated risk in approving a drug for marketing with a regimen that was near the studied doses, with a commitment from the company to confirm, in the postmarketing phase, the efficacy and toxicity of the new regimen.

An important message here is if a drug company has done its homework on pharmacokinetics/pharmacodynamics, it may be able to compress the drug development and regulatory review time. A pharmacokinetic/pharmacodynamic analysis is not burdensome and enhances drug development. It should, if properly applied, compress the drug development time rather than expand it, and perhaps more importantly, enable the development of more optimal dosing regimens at the time of first marketing.

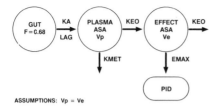

ASSUMPTIONS: Vp = Ve

FIG. 1. Combined PK/PD model for aspirin.

To exemplify the power of the kinetic/dynamic approach we briefly describe here our recent work on aspirin analgesia (1). We analyzed averaged data from a double-blind study in which subject groups were given either effervescent aspirin or placebo in parallel fashion. The groups consisted of 28 healthy patients who entered the study with moderate to severe pain following surgical removal of third molar(s) under local anesthesia. A single 1,000 mg dose of an effervescent aspirin formulation (buffered solution) was ingested with a standard meal. Blood samples were collected at 0, 10, 20, 30, 40, 60, 90, and 120 min, and pain assessments were made at 0, 15, 30, 60, 120, 180, and 240 min following the dose. The pain intensity was evaluated on a scale of 0 to 3 (0 = none, 1 = slight, 2 = moderate, and 3 = severe). The pain intensity difference (PID) was measured as the difference in the average pain intensity scores of the aspirin and placebo groups subtracted from their respective baseline. Plasma concentrations of aspirin (ASA) and salicylic acid (SA) were determined using a high performance liquid chromatography (HPLC) procedure.

A nonparametric analysis (2) of ASA versus PID revealed collapsible, counterclockwise hysteresis. The half-life of the equilibration rate constant ($t_{\frac{1}{2}}$ K_{e0}) for the hypothetical effect compartment was 20 min. However, the SA versus PID did not yield any definitive collapsible model. Initially, a parametric model

TABLE 1. *Final estimated model parameters*

Description	Parameter estimates
Lag (hr)	0.11
KA $t_{\frac{1}{2}}$ (hr)	0.08
VI (L)	22.48
KMET $t_{\frac{1}{2}}$ (hr)	0.36
K_{E0} $t_{\frac{1}{2}}$ (hr)	0.33
Emax (PID Units)	2.58
C50 (mcg/ml)	5.31
Hill's N	1.34

KA $t_{\frac{1}{2}}$, absorption half-life; KMET $t_{\frac{1}{2}}$, aspirin disposition half-life; K_{E0} $t_{\frac{1}{2}}$, effect compartment equilibrium half-life; Emax, maximum effect; C50, concentration in effect compartment required to reach half maximal effect; Hill's N, Hill's coefficient.

was developed, in which a linear one-compartment pharmacokinetic model was linked to a pharmacodynamic model wherein both ASA and SA contribute to the total PID through their respective sigmoid Emax models. Analysis, however, indicated that there was no contribution of SA to the total PID estimations. The part of the model that utilizes the ASA data alone was determined to be adequate to predict the total effect. Therefore, the model was reduced (Fig. 1) to accommodate ASA data alone.

The final parameters obtained are shown in Table 1. The results indicated that the maximum pain intensity difference that could be obtained was 2.6 PID units (out of a possible 3) over the placebo. The Hill's coefficient or the sigmoidicity factor (N) was 1.35, which indicated that the actual underlying pharmacodynamic model approximates an Emax model. This model reasonably predicted analgesic intensity as well as time to peak analgesic effect (Fig. 2), which occurred 20 to 30 min after time to peak ASA (30 min). This model was also helpful in providing insights as to why there was detectable analgesic effect at a time when plasma ASA was below detection limits. For example, pharmacological effects that persist after disappearance of the parent drug in plasma may be owing to delayed biochemical or subcellular events, actions of active metabolites, etc. It indicated that SA at these concentrations may not yield significant analgesic

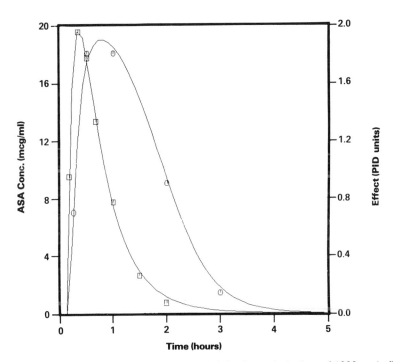

FIG. 2. Plasma concentration (□), PID (○) of aspirin following a single dose of 1000 mg buffered solution. The *solid line* is the computer-fitted line.

effect. This kind of pharmacokinetic/pharmacodynamic modeling is useful for better understanding of efficacy data, especially when the shapes of the plasma concentration curves are altered using different dosage forms during clinical trials. Hence, as in the ketorolac example cited above, it is easy to envision that the consequences of alternative various dosage forms, routes of administration, or dosage regimens can be predicted once the pharmacokinetic/pharmacodynamic profile of an analgesic drug has been mapped. This may be especially useful early in drug development as a guide to selection of dosage regimens for Phase II evaluation that are most likely to demonstrate effectiveness at the lowest effective doses. Finally, the approach may also provide some insights as to whether metabolite(s) are contributing to the total effect, as in the present example.

REFERENCES

1. Velagapudi R, Brueckner R, Harter JG, Peck CC, Viswanathan CT, Sunshine A, Laska EM, Mason WD, Byrd WG. Pharmacokinetics and pharmacodynamics of aspirin analgesia (abstract). *Clin Pharmacol Ther* 1990;47:179.
2. Verotta R, Sheiner LB. Simultaneous modeling of pharmacokinetics and pharmacodynamics: an improved algorithm. *Comput Appl Biosci* 1987;3:345–349.

Advances in Pain Research and Therapy, Vol. 18,
edited by M. Max, R. Portenoy, and E. Laska,
Raven Press, Ltd., New York © 1991.

Commentary

Pharmacokinetic Considerations in Analgesic Study Design

Laurence E. Mather

*Department of Anaesthesia and Intensive Care, School of Medicine, Flinders University
of South Australia, Bedford Park, SA 5042, Australia*

To many prescribers and/or administrators of drugs, pharmacokinetics provides
about as much useful information about a drug as its melting point or its ultraviolet spectrum, i.e., information recorded at some stage of a drug's development
by a backroom scientist that can safely be ignored in clinical practice. After all,
dosage regimens of most drugs can be constructed empirically and these, particularly when it comes to analgesic agents, may or may not correspond to "the
pharmacokinetics"—it doesn't particularly matter. An unenlightened view?
Maybe, but certainly not an unpopular view. A more enlightened view about
pharmacokinetic considerations in analgesic study design will develop only if
the purposes of "the pharmacokinetics" are clearly defined and the potential
pitfalls are fully appreciated.

PHARMACOKINETIC CONSIDERATIONS

A suitable starting point is to consider some of the definitions of pharmacokinetics. Many definitions have been presented over the past 30 to 40 years,
during which pharmacokinetics has grown into a self-contained subdiscipline of
pharmacy and pharmacology. John Wagner, who was extremely influential in
the establishment of pharmacokinetics theory and practice during the 1960s and
1970s, has discussed at length the origins of pharmacokinetics (1–3). He points
out that the definition of pharmacokinetics by Professor F. H. Dost who, in
1955, coined the word, was ". . . the science of the quantitative analysis between
drug and organism." This is an appealing definition as it brings together all of
the key elements involved in drug treatment. Wagner does not entirely approve
of the commonly used World Health Organization (WHO) definition ". . . the
study of the absorption, distribution, metabolism, and elimination of drugs . . ."
which has been taught in undergraduate pharmacology lectures for several de-

cades. Instead he prefers a definition based on ". . . the quantitation of the time-course of drug and/or metabolite in biological fluids and of pharmacological response and of the construction of models to represent such data" (2). Undoubtedly, contemporary pharmacokinetics does contain all of the elements described above. It is always quantitative and always involves a time course (i.e., kinetics) but it should be remembered that models constructed to represent such data need only to be sufficient for the purpose of better using or explaining the data from which they were generated. They are only representations of the system (i.e., the interaction between drug and organism). Problems come when pharmacokineticists lose sight of the purpose of the exercise and sacrifice the reality of the experiment that created the data for the myths of the model, so that the model, once created, is believed at the expense of the data. After all, the principle of using a model is to represent reality; the modeler is obliged to compare the models to reality and to revise it in the light of discrepancies, not discard data to make the data fit the models. The problems become compounded when journal editors, reviewers, and regulatory authorities require their use, regardless of their fidelity, and thereby perpetuate the myths.

PHARMACOKINETIC PROPERTIES

By any definition, the pharmacokinetic properties of a drug relate drug and/ or metabolite concentrations in biological fluids and/or tissues to drug dose and time. The fundamental pharmacokinetic properties of any drug are the *rate and extent of dilution* in the body and the *rates and route(s) of elimination* from the body. Mathematical formulae for the calculation of these parameters are generally unambiguous and are given in many standard sources (2,4). Other fundamental properties such as clearance, half-life, and mean transit time can be educed from these (3,5). If the drug has to be introduced into the body by some process involving absorption, then the *rate and extent* of the absorption process(es) become of interest also. However, the fundamental pharmacokinetic properties can only be determined if there is no preceding absorption process so that the drug has immediate access to the appropriate biological reference fluid. Since the latter is usually the blood, drugs are typically administered intravascularly. The absorption properties can be determined with certainty only when the fundamental pharmacokinetic properties are known. Hence "fundamental pharmacokinetic properties" calculated after intramuscular or other routes of administration that are presumed not to involve some kind of first-pass drug clearance are almost invariably in error because the extent of absorption within the observed time frame is unknown. Better experimental designs involve either sequential, or preferably, concurrent (with stable isotopically differentiated forms of the drug) doses, with appropriate numerical deconvolution techniques to determine the absorption pharmacokinetics (6,7).

In all cases, it is assumed that the dose of drug is known accurately and the time course of concentrations in the appropriate biological reference fluid can be determined with sufficient sensitivity by representative sampling of this fluid. The fluids most relevantly used in analgesic studies are blood (plasma or serum), sometimes cerebrospinal fluid, occasionally saliva, and, rarely, urine. Each has its uses in particular experimental designs and its associated pitfalls. Dr. Inturrisi has presented a survey of these considerations (see Chapter 24). This commentary is intended to supplement Dr. Inturrisi's chapter by discussing additional pharmacokinetic considerations that impinge upon the design and interpretation of analgesic drug clinical trials.

Let us consider a simplistic study, say blood drug concentrations after an oral dose of an analgesic medication. What might be suitable pharmacokinetic objectives of such an analysis? First, descriptive data might be sought to reduce a concentration-time data set to a few summary variables. Such values could then be used *to compare* different experiments, e.g., between different drugs, formulations, recipients of drugs, etc. Descriptive data can be useful, to characterize the maximum concentration in blood (C_{max}) and the time at which it occurred (T_{max}), or perhaps the rate of change of blood drug concentrations after T_{max}. The former might be useful *to predict* C_{max} and T_{max} from a different dose, the latter for when another dose might be necessary. Second, drug concentrations may be used to generate a pharmacokinetic model. The use of a dose-C_{max} relationship to predict the outcome of different doses implies a model (involving linearity?). More complicated models are not possible without knowledge of the rate and extent of drug absorption because it is not possible to determine the actual dose available to the reference fluid (and not just "administered"). Third, drug concentrations may have a relationship to pain relief. Estimating the C_{max} and T_{max} might also be useful in estimating the magnitude of effect and of the time of its occurrence, if there was additional knowledge of this relationship (8). These issues highlight a range of legitimate pharmacokinetic objectives: (a) for evaluating pharmaceutical dosage forms and methods of drug administration, (b) for understanding individual differences in the handling of drugs in the body, and (c) for resolving (at least partially) differences observed in the effects of drugs. They necessarily lead to considerations of anatomical-physiological and statistical veracity in pharmacokinetics that are often neglected.

SYSTEMIC PHARMACOKINETICS

The first consideration is the use of an appropriate biological reference fluid. For most pharmacokinetic studies, "blood" is the chosen reference fluid, implying that *systemic pharmacokinetics,* i.e., the relationships between drug dose, systemic blood concentrations, and time, are being studied. For convenience without undue invasion (at least in human subjects), the concentrations of the test drug and/or metabolite are measured in blood (or plasma or serum) usually drawn from a vein in the arm.

Several points are pertinent to this approach:

1. Whether blood, serum, or plasma is used as the reference fluid needs to be specified accurately by investigators; often it isn't. The choice of the fluid often depends on analytical considerations, but it should depend, principally, on the use to which the data will be put. If the purpose is comparative, then plasma concentrations will usually suffice. If the purpose is absolute, e.g., calculation of physiological mass balance, blood concentrations are usually required. If the drug equilibrates quickly and distributes uniformly between blood cells and plasma, then blood and plasma are equivalent in usefulness. There is a common practice of measuring drug concentrations in plasma and then converting them to "blood concentrations" by dividing by "the blood/plasma concentration ratio" previously determined *in vitro*. This practice may be erroneous if the ratio is concentration dependent, is acid-base sensitive, or is subject to other experimental variables *in vivo* that are not completely accounted for *in vitro*. Blood concentrations are best measured, not calculated (9).

2. It is implied in most pharmacokinetic models or calculations that the blood was drawn from a well-mixed pool. This is, of course, anatomical and physiological nonsense. Blood is not a well-mixed pool: if drug is being added to or removed from the body, there is no well-mixed pool! There are affluent-effluent gradients of virtually all solutes in the body (10). If, as is shown in Figure 1, the

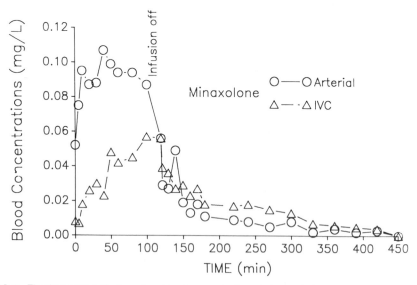

FIG. 1. The time course of minaxolone blood concentrations during and after infusion of minaxolone citrate (an aminosteroid anesthetic agent) at 0.36 mg/min for 124 min in a sheep. The differences in arterial and inferior vena caval (IVC) (draining the hindquarters, distal to hepatic and renal veins) blood concentrations would lead to entirely different conclusions about pharmacokinetics and blood concentration-response relationships for this drug.

pharmacokinetics of the steroidal anesthetic agent, minaxolone, were to be determined from the time course of arterial or inferior vena caval blood concentrations, then entirely different conclusions would be reached (11). This example has been chosen to exaggerate the point, but the point is clear: measuring in the effluent of any region shows the influence of the region on the concentrations of the solute. Thus, drug concentrations in blood sampled from a vein of the arm will show the influence of the rate of equilibration of the solute with the tissues being drained. Although a minor point in the conduct of most pharmacokinetic studies, it is assumed that arterial concentrations are the same at all points. This is not strictly true, as short and long circuits may need to be considered. Although it seems almost ludicrous to have to comment upon it, some investigators still choose blood sampling sites downstream of the drug administration sites, thereby unintentionally sampling drug-enriched blood. Others still use the same catheter for both administering drug and sampling blood. Despite flushing, a residue even of micrograms may contaminate samples drawn for high sensitivity analysis!

3. Factors influencing tissue blood flow or the distribution of tissue blood flow (e.g., skin/muscle) have the potential to influence the measured pharmacokinetics. If such changes are time dependent, then the pharmacokinetics may appear to show time-dependent effects. A frequently encountered example would be in studying drugs during neural blockade. For example, during epidural anesthesia, upper body vasoconstriction occurs as the compensatory response to lower body vasodilatation. Thus the time course of venous blood drug concentrations will be influenced by the time course of the neural blockade and the pharmacokinetics of the drugs will differ markedly whether arterial or venous blood concentrations are measured (12).

REGIONAL PHARMACOKINETICS

Few drugs act by being in the blood. For most drugs the blood is only a means of transport to sites of action, distribution, and clearance. Therefore, the kinetics of drug uptake and elution in regions of drug response is of importance to understanding drug effects and side effects, although uptake into nonresponsive regions is also important because of its influence in modulating drug concentrations in responsive regions. Much misunderstanding and mystique in pharmacokinetics and pharmacodynamics can be traced to the confusion generated by the failure of investigators to think in terms of regional pharmacokinetics. The expectations that drug concentrations sampled in a vessel of the arm will correlate (in some way, eventually) with drug effects has spawned a cult of pharmacokinetic-pharmacodynamic modeling intent on "abolishing the hysteresis" in "blood concentration-effect" data. This is not to decry this work, which has been developed to offset the limitations of less than ideal experimental designs, but it is to point out that there is no need to expect that drug concentrations in, say, the cephalic vein would relate to events in discrete areas of, say, the myocardium or the brain that produce the observed pharmacological effects.

Regional pharmacokinetics involves the relationship between the concentrations of a drug in affluent and effluent blood and in individual regions and tissues of the body. A *region* may be regarded as any anatomical area of the body contained between specified afferent and efferent blood vessels. A region, therefore, may be a single organ, such as the myocardium as defined by the coronary arteries and the coronary sinus, or group of organs, such as the hepatosplanchnic system as defined by the aorta and the hepatic veins. Using such anatomical reference points and applying the law of conservation of matter to each regional drug (± metabolite) concentration gradient and blood flow, the rates of drug distribution (or the net drug flux) may be determined and, when normalized for the affluent concentration, allow calculation of regional clearance. The time integral of the net flux gives the extent of drug distribution into each region (i.e., the regional net drug mass, or content, which, if divided by the organ mass, gives the regional drug concentration). From the total body and the measured regional fluxes and clearances of a drug and metabolites, its total fate in the body may be accounted for by mass balance (13). A particular benefit of this methodology is that the effects of physiological or pathological perturbations on global and regional drug mass balance can be assessed.

Several pertinent examples of regional mass balance from the author's laboratory can illustrate this principle.

1. Much recent attention has been directed toward the pulmonary first-pass extraction of drugs, and rightly so because the lungs, apart from vascular endothelium, are the first region encountered by a drug admitted to the venous blood. There is considerable evidence that the lungs act to impede the transit of most drugs, including opioid analgesics. For these agents, the lung "uptake" (rather ill-defined pharmacokinetically) or first-pass extraction increases in magnitude with the lipophilicity of the drugs, e.g., approximately 80% extraction of fentanyl, approximately 50% of meperidine, and approximately 20% of morphine (14–18). The first-pass extraction is assessed by comparison of drug concentrations entering (in pulmonary arterial blood) and leaving (in arterial blood) the lungs in relation to those of an intravascular marker substance (typically indocyanine green dye) administered simultaneously. This effect takes on an important role when drugs are admitted rapidly into the blood, causing arterial concentrations to be attenuated (19), thereby moderating their effects on vital organ systems. There has been a tendency by some to identify "pulmonary uptake" with metabolic clearance in the lungs. However, this view has not been substantiated. In almost every case in which it has been tested (in sheep) (10,20,21), no extraction under "steady-state" conditions has been found for either opioid analgesics or local anesthetics (22–25). Unless there is elimination, drug lost to the lungs is regained as the initial concentration gradient from blood to tissue is dissipated. Most reports contain only the first pass (positive) extraction, i.e., usually over

only the first minute or so after IV bolus administration, and imply that this is clearance. They do not indicate the extended time course showing negative extraction or release back into the blood. This is not to say that drugs are not cleared by the lungs. They may be, but apart from volatile or gaseous substances, there are relatively few examples in which the lungs have been proven to act as a major site of drug clearance during drug treatment. The lungs, like the kidneys and many other tissues, are well perfused, contain a rich supply of drug metabolizing enzymes capable of drug metabolism, and are readily shown to metabolize drugs *in vitro,* but, *in vivo,* the higher concentrations of the enzymes in the liver contribute usually the major proportion of drug metabolism (26–28).

2. During the past 6 years, much has been written about the effects of renal dysfunction on morphine elimination. Early claims that morphine elimination was impaired in patients with renal dysfunction (thereby suggesting an appreciable amount of renal clearance and/or metabolism of morphine) were repudiated on the basis of nonspecific morphine radioimmunoassays unintentionally also measuring morphine metabolites (29,30). However, many of the repudiating claims were made on the basis of systemic pharmacokinetics derived from drug concentrations in arm or mixed venous blood and (systemic) pharmacokinetic compartment models (31–33). Although these conclusions may be correct, unequivocal conclusions are not possible based only on systemic pharmacokinetics derived from arm or mixed venous blood sampling because the balance between sites and rates of clearance may be altered without there being a net change in the systemic pharmacokinetics. In fact, the author's studies in the chronically cannulated sheep preparation (20,21) have shown that morphine is both cleared by the kidneys and excreted into urine (34). Renal clearance determined directly by the product of the renal extraction ratio and the renal blood flow indicates that about 35% of the total body clearance is renal; however, only about 13% of the dose is excreted into urine (34). This difference indicates that the sheep kidney both excretes and metabolizes morphine, but this could not have been determined from conventional studies of renal clearance and systemic pharmacokinetics.

3. Although the liver and kidneys, and sometimes the lungs and the gut, are the putative principal regions of drug clearance, other regions that may also be involved cannot be detected or quantitated unless appropriate regional pharmacokinetic studies are performed. Other studies in the chronically cannulated sheep preparation (20,21) have shown that meperidine is extracted by the liver and kidneys but not by the lungs or gut (23). However, the discrepancy between the total body and the summed visceral clearances indicated that sundry nonvisceral regions also must be involved to a major extent. The only remaining regions with sufficient blood flow to account for the magnitude of the discrepancy in clearance were nonvisceral (i.e., regions not usually recognized as important in drug clearance). In a subsequent study (35), cannulation of the venous drainage of the sheep hindquarters showed that mean steady state meperidine extraction ratio was 0.4 and the corresponding clearances were approximately 0.8 l/min

(20% of total body clearance). Similar extraction ratios would occur in regions of similar anatomical composition such as forequarters and chest wall, with clearances in proportion to the regional blood flows. In this case, an appreciable portion of the total body clearance was unexpectedly accounted for by nonvisceral clearance. Whether significant nonvisceral clearance of drugs occurs in other species remains for systematic studies.

4. The pharmacokinetics of propofol were studied in the same sheep preparation (36). Propofol anesthesia is of brief duration, consistent with its very high total body clearance, which was confirmed in these studies, and has been suggested to be owing to extrahepatic clearance (37). A mean total body clearance of propofol of 3.15 L/min was found, consistent with a mean hepatic extraction ratio of 0.87 and mean hepatic clearance of 1.12 L/min. The difference between total and hepatic clearances principally consisted of pulmonary clearance, but its extent was variable. However, propofol in humans has been observed to have a long terminal plasma half-life and this has been ascribed to its washout from a very large apparent volume of distribution (37). In the sheep experiments, it was observed that there was propofol "production" by the kidney (i.e., a negative renal extraction ratio was found). This was interpreted as arising from a propofol metabolite formed elsewhere being further metabolized back to propofol in the kidney and thereby producing renovascular recycling (analogous to enterohepatic recycling). This therefore suggests an alternative explanation for the balance between the high total body clearance and long plasma half-life found in patients (38). For other drugs and other species, unexpected results such as these are perhaps going unnoticed or being dismissed as artifact.

5. The completion of distribution equilibrium in individual regions may take appreciably more time than is predicted from the old pharmacokineticists' rule of "five times the distribution half-life" of the drug. In studies of the equilibration of a number of drugs in the hindquarters of sheep (e.g., Fig. 1), it was observed that blood/tissue equilibration during intravenous infusion may take so long to occur that it can masquerade as clearance if determined by conventional pharmacokinetic calculations (11,39).

6. Another relevant physiological consideration in pharmacokinetics is that of *stationarity,* i.e., the constancy in time of "the system" being studied. Violation of this assumption most commonly occurs in the perioperative period—a popular time for analgesic drug trials—and presents another example of physiological infidelity. A frequently encountered study design involves the intraoperative study of analgesic agents administered as part of, or shortly after, induction of anesthesia, with the continuation of blood sampling for drug analysis through the perioperative course. In some studies, the evaluation of the drug may even be given preoperatively (Fig. 2), perhaps as premedication (40). The resultant serial blood concentration-time data are then analyzed and an "appropriate" pharmacokinetic model is applied to all of the data as if the pharmacokinetics were the same throughout the studied period. Various components of the perioperative period (anaesthesia, surgery, ventilation, alterations in acid-base bal-

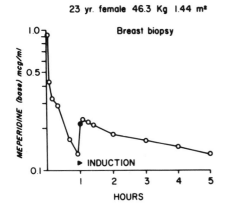

23 yr. female 46.3 Kg 1.44 m²

FIG. 2. Plasma concentrations of meperidine from the vein of the arm of a surgical patient. Meperidine HCl (50 mg) was administered intravenously as premedication, anesthesia was induced as shown, and the meperidine concentrations were measured into the postoperative period (data from ref. 40). The *closed circle* indicates the first concentration measured after induction of anesthesia. A difference in pharmacokinetics caused by anesthesia has been documented with virtually all anesthetic agents in current use (see ref. 41).

ance, alterations in fluid balance, etc.) may each markedly influence pharmacokinetics. It is clear that the results of such a time-averaged pharmacokinetic analysis may bear no relationship to the "true pharmacokinetics" of any individual period (Fig. 3); the dominant influence may be the effect of, say, anesthesia on drug distribution and/or clearance (41). For example, in a recent study on the effects of propofol anesthesia on meperidine disposition using steady-state methodology, arterial blood meperidine concentrations increased by approximately 100% and recovered to baseline values approximately 3 hrs after anes-

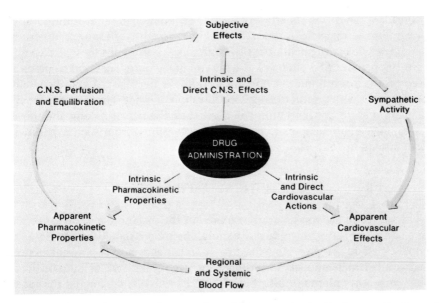

FIG. 3. A depiction of interaction between the variables associated with pharmacokinetics and pharmacodynamics in intact subjects. Intrinsic pharmacokinetic parameters are sought but the measured or apparent pharmacokinetics are the result of the influences as shown.

thesia; the mean values of hepatic meperidine clearance decreased to 79% of baseline values in parallel to decreased hepatic blood flow; the respective mean values of renal meperidine clearance decreased to 69% of baseline; and the respective mean values of hindquarter pethidine clearance decreased to 49% of baseline (35). By considering all of the perioperative drug concentration-time data as a continuum, a pharmacokinetic model can be produced, but the value of such a model is dubious as it combines the pharmacokinetic properties of the drug with the physiological perturbations of the perioperative period. Under strictly controlled conditions, it may be possible to reproduce a dose-drug blood concentration relationship but this is not the "true pharmacokinetics." If it is not the true pharmacokinetics and the point of the exercise is not the study of perioperative variables on the pharmacokinetics, why bother? It is emphasized that pharmacokinetic model formed by sampling only blood can be used only to predict systemic blood concentrations. However, sampling regional blood and or tissue drug concentrations allows pharmacokinetic modeling which preserves anatomical and physiological veracity and insight that cannot be gained by studying systemic pharmacokinetics alone. Unfortunately, the difficulty of performing such experiments makes them inaccessible for most researchers and most drugs.

ANATOMICAL INFIDELITY

Anatomical infidelity in analgesic drug trials is not infrequently encountered in consideration of CSF pharmacokinetics, say after epidural or intrathecal administration of analgesic agents. An investigator might, for example, determine the time course of drug in lumbar CSF and calculate from this the CSF clearance and the apparent CSF volume of distribution of the drug. These calculations are based on the assumption that the sampled fluid is well mixed and is therefore homogeneous with respect to drug concentration. It is not! This is totally invalid; it is plain that the concentration will depend on the rate of mixing and the site of sampling. Pharmacokinetic parameters determined from such experiments are of limited use at best.

STATISTICAL INFIDELITY

The choice of the model used to represent the disposition of the drug is an issue related to statistical veracity. Plainly, the model should be chosen as the simplest method of representing the data. A decade ago, most pharmacokineticists used compartment models to estimate the extent and rate of dilution in the body (apparent volume of distribution and its rate of change) and the rate of elimination (clearance and rate constants). Now it is recognized that it is difficult to determine which of a variety of generally similar compartment models most validly represents the data. Hence, there is a trend for pharmacokineticists to express results in terms of simple equation parameters that allow interpolation of drug concentrations at times other than those measured and/or allow the determination of dilution and rate of elimination without reference to a particular structural model. This helps to overcome the difficulty arising from the imposition of a particular structural model onto the data. However, it does not help to increase the confidence in pharmacokinetic parameters that have to be calculated from the data obtained from the less than perfect experimental designs that usually have to be used in practice.

Several problems remain. How does one report the half-life of a drug that cannot be determined accurately because the slope of the blood concentration-time curve cannot be sampled frequently enough or for long enough for any of a variety of valid reasons? How does one report the total body clearance or the half-life of a drug that cannot be determined accurately because the sensitivity of the assay is insufficient to follow its blood concentrations for long enough to enter the "terminal phase"? How does one report the pharmacokinetic parameters of a drug that differ between bolus and infusion administration? For example, it is well known that the terminal half-life of some drugs, e.g., fentanyl, gets longer over the years because the ability to detect the slow washout from some tissues increases with improved analytical methodology or with the doses that are used (42). Different experimental designs, viz., bolus versus infusion, may maximize one or the other element of perfusion limitations (bolus) or diffusion limitations (infusion) in determining the extent of blood/tissue equilibration during washin and washout and, thereby, the pharmacokinetic parameters. Thus, the pharmacokinetic considerations of the choice of a model will get back to the purpose of creating the model and the quality of the data used in its construction.

ANALYTICAL INFIDELITY

Lastly, but very significantly, it has been assumed in the foregoing commentary that the drug under consideration can be measured faithfully over its time course and that inadvertent interference from metabolites or other substances does not occur. If this assumption is not correct, the rest is a worthless exercise. If, however, the activity of the drug is partly or wholly resident in a metabolite of the drug, then it is plain that the pharmacokinetics of the metabolite—its rates and regions of synthesis, its regional distribution, and its elimination—need to be documented also. The recent vast literature on the 3- and 6-glucuronides of morphine provide a timely example of the complexities of understanding the effects of the oldest analgesic agent.

The recent attention given to enantioselectivity in pharmacokinetics and pharmacodynamics is timely (43–45). It points to one common way in which the assumption of analytical fidelity in pharmacokinetics is violated. Many drugs used in clinical practice (including some opioids, e.g., methadone and most cyclooxygenase inhibitor antalgics) exist as enantiomeric pairs of stereoisomers with most, sometimes all, of the pharmacological activity residing in one of the enantiomers. The fundamental pharmacokinetics of the enantiomers usually differ and inversion of one enantiomer (to the other) may occur as a metabolic reaction. Most drug assays are not enantioselective, thus the measured time courses of the drugs consist of the sum of the enantiomers, which, if the pharmacokinetics differ, will be a time-dependent mixture. To date, most of pharmacokinetic literature on racemic drugs has been presented as if only one compound was involved. Ignorance of pharmacokinetic enantioselectivity can lead to misinterpretation of data, especially when blood drug concentration–pharmacologic response data and comparisons of species or patients are involved. In fairness, the principal reason for this has been the lack of suitable methods for enantioselective analysis of these agents. However, pharmacokinetic treatment of data that ignores this issue in interpretation or subsequent modeling exercises can only be seen as erroneous.

CONCLUSIONS

The conclusions reached by the writer after both successes and failures in this area indicate that pharmacokinetics do, indeed, need to be documented as fundamental information about a drug. Such information does provide a basis for *understanding* the time course of drug action, the influence of pathology on the time course, and many of the individual or unexpected differences in response to drugs. However, in documenting such information, it is important for all involved to keep an open mind as to (a) the limitations of most pharmacokinetic experiments that can reasonably be performed and of pharmacokinetic models used, so that there is no overinterpretation, (b) the physiological and biochemical capability of the various body regions to perform pharmacokinetic functions, (c) the rate at which regional distribution equilibration of drug occurs and of the potential pitfalls in assuming that perfusion rather than diffusion limitations apply, and (d) the compatibility of pharmacokinetic data (particularly of analgesics) derived from anesthetized and unanesthetized subjects. If these caveats are recognized, the pharmacokinetic data may be useful for the comparative and predictive purposes for which they were intended. Whether they can be safely ignored in clinical practice is a different issue.

The writer has personal sympathy with the position that, however interesting, pharmacokinetics should not dictate clinical practice over clinical observation. Opioid analgesics, by and large, are safe enough for the treatment of acute pain that they can be administered "until the patient stops hurting or stops breathing, whichever comes first," *but only if the patient is under such close observation that the dose can be adjusted exactly when needed.* This, unfortunately, is the exception rather than the rule. Pharmacokinetic studies of opioid absorption have been invaluable in pointing to reasons for the inefficient treatment of pain and have suggested improved methods of using the same agents. In the case of cyclooxygenase inhibitor antalgics, it should be remembered that they, too, can have serious side effects.

The recent tragedy of deaths of elderly patients following the use of benoxaprofen (46,47) is notable as evidence of the use of pharmacokinetics, regrettably *in hindsight,* to rationalize unexpected drug effects (48). Potentially fatal cholestatic jaundice and renal papillary necrosis were unexpected side effects of benoxaprofen. Benoxaprofen was known from early pharmacokinetic studies in healthy volunteer subjects to have a long half-life (30 to 35 hrs) (49) and this was used to advantage in once daily dosage regimens. Despite knowledge of the impairment of benoxaprofen clearance in patients with renal dysfunction (50), dosage modification for patients with age-related decreased renal function leading to a longer half-life, with or without concomitant alterations in benoxaprofen plasma binding (46) leading to greater accumulation of active drug, was not generally used. Thus, accumulation of active benoxaprofen may have contributed to its toxicity in the elderly patients (48).

For the present, pharmacokinetics provides a methodology to investigate drugs more intensively and, through rational design of dosage regimens, of using them more effectively. This methodology cannot be safely ignored in the design of analgesic drug trials but does, itself, require innovative thought and experiments.

ACKNOWLEDGMENTS

The support of the National Health and Medical Research Council of Australia is acknowledged.

REFERENCES

1. Wagner JG. Pharmacokinetics. *Annu Rev Pharmacol* 1968;8:67–94.
2. Wagner JG. *Fundamentals of clinical pharmacokinetics.* Hamilton, Illinois: Drug Intelligence Publications, 1975.
3. Wagner JG. History of pharmacokinetics. *Pharmacol Ther* 1981;12:537–562.
4. Tozer TN. Concepts basic to pharmacokinetics. *Pharmacol Ther* 1981;12:109–131.
5. Nakashima E, Benet LZ. General treatment of mean residence time, clearance, and volume parameters in linear mammillary models with elimination from any compartment. *J Pharmacokinet Biopharm* 1988;16:475–492.
6. Burm AGL, Van Kleef JW, Vermulem NPE, Olthof G, Breimer DD, Spierdijk J. Pharmacokinetics of lidocaine and bupivacaine following subarachnoid administration in surgical patients: simultaneous investigation of absorption and disposition kinetics using stable isotopes. *Anesthesiology* 1988;69:584–592.
7. Tucker GT. The determination of in vivo absorption rate. *Acta Pharm Tech* 1983;29:159–164.
8. Holford NHG, Sheiner LB. Kinetics of pharmacological response. *Pharmacol Ther* 1982;16:143–166.
9. Morgan D, Thiel WJ, La Rosa C, Mather LE. The blood/plasma concentration ratio of pethidine. *J Pharm Pharmacol* 1986;38:557–558.
10. Mather LE, Runciman WB. The physiological basis of pharmacokinetics: concepts and tools. In: Stoeckel HO, ed. *Quantitation, modelling and control in anaesthesia.* Stuttgart: Georg Thieme Verlag, 1985;12–40.

11. Upton RN, Mather LE, Runciman WB, Nancarrow C, Carapetis RJ. The uptake and elution of chlormethiazole, meperidine and minaxolone in the hindquarters of the sheep: implications for clearance calculations. *J Pharm Sci* (in press).
12. Tucker GT, Mather LE. Physicochemical properties, absorption and disposition of local anesthetics: pharmacokinetics. In: Cousins MJ, Bridenbaugh PO, eds. *Neural blockade in clinical anesthesia and management of pain,* 2nd ed. Philadelphia: JB Lippincott, 1988;47–110.
13. Upton RN, Mather LE, Runciman WB, Nancarrow C, Carapetis RJ. The use of mass balance principles to describe regional drug distribution and elimination. *J Pharmacokinet Biopharm* 1988;16:13–29.
14. Persson MP, Hartvig P, Wiklund L, Paalzow L. Pulmonary disposition of pethidine in postoperative patients. *Br J Clin Pharmacol* 1988;25:235–241.
15. Persson MP, Wiklund L, Hartvig P, Paalzow L. Potential pulmonary uptake and clearance of morphine in postoperative patients. *Eur J Clin Pharmacol* 1986;30:567–574.
16. Roerig DL, Kotrly KJ, Vucins EJ, Ahlf SB, Dawson CA, Kampine JP. First pass uptake of fentanyl, meperidine and morphine in the human lung. *Anesthesiology* 1987;67:466–472.
17. Roerig DL, Kotrly KJ, Ahlf SB, Dawson CA, Kampine JP. Effect of propranolol on the first pass uptake of fentanyl in the human and rat lung. *Anesthesiology* 1989;71:62–68.
18. Taeger K, Weninger E, Schmelzer F, Adt M, Franke M, Peter K. Pulmonary kinetics of fentanyl and alfentanil in surgical patients. *Br J Anaesth* 1988;61:425–434.
19. Bokesch PM, Casaneda AR, Ziemer G, Wilson JM. The influence of a right-to-left cardiac shunt on lidocaine pharmacokinetics. *Anesthesiology* 1987;67:739–744.
20. Runciman WB, Ilsley AH, Mather LE, Carapetis R, Rao M. A sheep preparation for studying the interaction of regional blood flow and drug disposition. I: Physiological profile. *Br J Anaesth* 1984;56:1015–1028.
21. Runciman WB, Mather LE, Ilsley AH, Carapetis R, McLean CF. A sheep preparation for studying the interaction of regional blood flow and drug disposition. II: Experimental applications. *Br J Anaesth* 1984;56:1117–1129.
22. Mather LE, Runciman WB, Carapetis RJ, Ilsley AH, Upton RN. Hepatic and renal clearances of lidocaine in conscious and anaesthetised sheep. *Anesth Analg* 1986;65:943–949.
23. Mather LE, Runciman WB, Ilsley AH, Carapetis RJ, Upton RN. A sheep preparation for studying interactions between blood flow and drug disposition. V: Pethidine disposition. *Br J Anaesth* 1986;58:888–896.
24. Nancarrow C, Mather LE, Runciman WB, Upton RN, Plummer JL. The influence of acidosis on the distribution of lidocaine and bupivacaine into the myocardium and brain of the sheep. *Anesth Analg* 1987;66:925–935.
25. Rutten AJ, Mather LE, Nancarrow C, Sloan PA, McLean CF. Cardiovascular effects and regional clearances of ropivacaine in sheep. *Anesth Analg* 1990;70:577–582.
26. Rawlins MD. Extrahepatic drug metabolism. In: Wilkinson GR, Rawlins MD, eds. *Drug metabolism and disposition.* Lancaster (U.K.): MTP Press, 1985;21–33.
27. Wahlström A, Winblad B, Bixo M, Rane A. Human brain metabolism of morphine and naloxone. *Pain* 1988;35:121–127.
28. Yue Q, Odar-Cederlöf I, Svensson JO, Säwe J. Glucuronidation of morphine in human kidney microsomes. *Pharmacol Toxicol* 1988;63:337–341.
29. Moore RA, Sear JW, Baldwin D, Allen M, Hunniset A, Bullingham R, McQuay H. Morphine kinetics during and after renal transplantation. *Clin Pharmacol Ther* 1984;35:641–645.
30. Sear JW, Hand CW, Moore RA, McQuay HJ. Studies on morphine disposition: influence of renal failure on the kinetics of morphine and its metabolites. *Br J Anaesth* 1989;62:28–32.
31. Aitkenhead AR, Vater M, Achola K, Cooper CMS, Smith G. Pharmacokinetics of single-dose i.v. morphine in normal volunteers and patients with end-stage renal failure. *Br J Anaesth* 1984;56:813–818.
32. Säwe J, Odar-Cederlöf I. Kinetics of morphine in patients with renal failure. *Eur J Clin Pharmacol* 1987;2:377–382.
33. Säwe J. High dose morphine and methadone in cancer patients. Clinical pharmacokinetic considerations of oral treatment. *Clin Pharmacokinet* 1986;11:87–106.
34. Sloan PA, Mather LE, McLean CF, Rutten AJ, Nation RL, Milne W, Runciman WB, Somogyi AA. The physiological disposition of morphine in sheep. *Pain* 1990;Suppl 5:S170.
35. Mather LE, Selby DG, Runciman WB. The effects of propofol and of thiopentone anaesthesia on the regional kinetics of pethidine in the sheep. *Br J Anaesth* 1990;65:365–372.

36. Mather LE, Selby DG, Runciman WB, McLean CF. Propofol: assay and regional mass balance in the sheep. *Xenobiotica* 1989;19:1337–1347.
37. Langley MS, Heel RC. Propofol: a review of its pharmacodynamic and pharmacokinetic properties and use as an intravenous anaesthetic. *Drugs* 1988;35:334–372.
38. Campbell GA, Morgan DJ, Kumar K, Cranskshaw DP. Extended blood collection period required to define distribution and elimination kinetics of propofol. *Br J Clin Pharmacol* 1988;26:187–190.
39. Upton RN, Runciman WB, Mather LE, McLean CF, Ilsley AH. The uptake and elution of lignocaine and procainamide in the hindquarters of the sheep described using mass balance principles. *J Pharmacokinet Biopharm* 1988;16:31–40.
40. Mather LE, Tucker GT, Pflug AE, Lindop MJ, Wilkerson C. Meperidine kinetics in man: intravenous injection in surgical patients and volunteers. *Clin Pharmacol Ther* 1975;17:21–30.
41. Runciman WB, Mather LE. Effects of anaesthesia and drug disposition. In: Feldman SA, Scurr CF, Paton W, eds. *Mechanisms of Action of Drugs in Anaesthetic Practice.* London: Edward Arnold, 1987;87–122.
42. Varvel JR, Shafer SL, Hwang SS, Coen PA, Stanski DR. Absorption characteristics of transdermally administered fentanyl. *Anesthesiology* 1989;70:928–934.
43. Ariëns EJ, Wuis WE, Veringa EJ. Stereoselectivity of bioactive xenobiotics. A pre-Pasteur attitude in medicinal chemistry, pharmacokinetics and clinical pharmacology. *Biochem Pharmacol* 1988;37:9–18.
44. Caldwell J, Hutt AJ, Fournel-Gigleux S. The metabolic chiral inversion and the dispositional enantioselectivity of the 2-arylpropionic acids and their biological consequences. *Biochem Pharmacol* 1988;37:105–114.
45. Tucker GT, Lennard MS. Enantiomer specific pharmacokinetics. *Pharmacol Ther* 1990;45:309–329.
46. Editorial: Benoxaprofen. *Br Med J* 1982;285(6340):459–460.
47. Brooks PM, Birkett D. Release of new drugs. The lessons of benoxaprofen. *Med J Aust* 1983;(i):251–252.
48. Upton RA, Williams RL, Kelly J, Jones RM. Naproxen kinetics in the elderly. *Br J Clin Pharmacol* 1984;18:207–214.
49. Smith GA, Goulbourn RA, Burt RAP, Chatfield H. Preliminary studies of absorption and excretion of benoxaprofen in man. *Br J Clin Pharmacol* 1977;4:585–590.
50. Aronoff GR, Ozawa T, DeSante KA, Nash F, Ridolfo AS. Benoxaprofen kinetics in renal impairment. *Clin Pharmacol Ther* 1982;32:190–194.

Advances in Pain Research and Therapy, Vol. 18,
edited by M. Max, R. Portenoy, and E. Laska,
Raven Press, Ltd., New York © 1991.

25

Evaluating Endogenous Mediators of Pain and Analgesia in Clinical Studies

Kenneth M. Hargreaves* and Raymond A. Dionne**

*Department of Restorative Sciences, University of Minnesota School of Dentistry,
Minneapolis, Minnesota 55455; **Clinical Pharmacology Unit, Neurobiology
and Anesthesiology Branch, National Institute of Dental Research,
National Institutes of Health, Bethesda, Maryland 20892*

New analgesic drugs are generally developed from one of three research strategies. These strategies include drug development based on insight into mechanisms of pain (e.g., recognizing the importance of cyclooxygenase in inflammation), synthesis of congeners of a successful prototype drug (e.g., derivatives of propionic acid) or neurotransmitter, or the application of a preexisting drug to a new disease state (e.g., use of amitriptyline for diabetic neuropathy).

This chapter focuses on the first research approach, evaluating physiologic mechanisms of pain and inflammation by measuring mediators of pain and analgesia. Demonstration that "mediator X" is important in a clinical pain model provides a strong rationale for the development of drugs which alter either its synthesis, its release, or its receptor. This research approach consists of:

1. Characterizing the time-response profile of the mediator following a stimulus to determine its participation in the physiologic response to the stimulus.
2. Evaluating whether pharmacologic agents that block the mediator's actions alter the physiologic response in a predictable fashion and whether agents that stimulate mediator release have the opposite effect.
3. Characterizing regulatory mechanisms controlling the release or production of the mediator by administration of prototype and novel pharmacological agents.

For example, our research on β-endorphin (β-END) release in the oral surgery model has demonstrated that (a) immunoreactive β-END is released into blood during surgical stress and postoperative pain; (b) low doses of dexamethasone suppress β-END levels and increase postoperative pain, whereas corticotropin-releasing hormone (CRH) stimulates β-END levels and decreases postoperative pain; and (c) that naloxone, ibuprofen, diazepam, methylprednisolone, and epinephrine all modulate stress-induced release of β-END. These clinical studies and parallel animal studies have characterized the response of an endogenous opioid peptide to stress and pain, and have led to the hypothesis that opioids act at peripheral sites of inflammation (1). This illustrates that clinical studies incorporating biochemical measures as dependent variables contribute knowledge of the physiologic responses to pain, inflammation, and stress that can lead to improved analgesic therapy.

EVALUATING CHEMICAL MEDIATORS OF PAIN AND INFLAMMATION

A common response to tissue damage is development of the signs of inflammation: pain, edema, hyperthermia, erythema, and loss of function. Inflammation occurs in clinical conditions such as arthritis and burns, as well as after surgery. Even minor surgical procedures, such as oral surgery, evoke postoperative inflammation (Fig. 1). Controlled clinical studies using this surgical model indicate that patients generally report moderate to severe levels of pain by 3 to 5 hrs after surgery (2) and that edema reaches peak levels by 48 to 72 hrs after

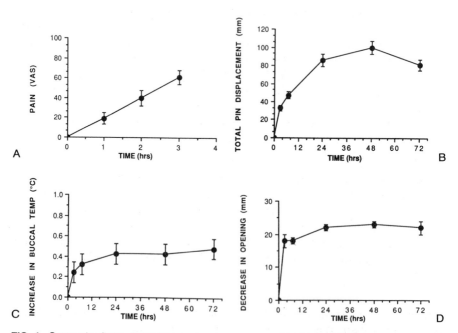

FIG. 1. Composite figure illustrating oral surgery as a model of inflammation. Four of the five classic signs of inflammation, pain (**A**), edema (**B**), hyperthermia (**C**), and loss of function (**D**), were assessed in 24 patients undergoing the surgical extraction of impacted third molars. The process of inflammation occurs in dental procedures involving tissue damage (usually less than one hr), whereas inflammatory signs continue for greater than 72 hrs. (Modified from ref. 3, with permission.)

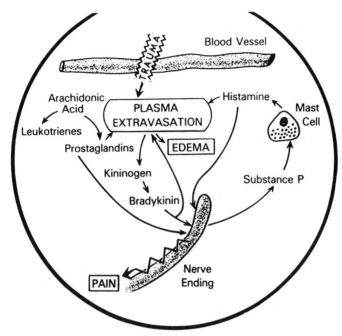

FIG. 2. Pain with inflammation. Trauma activates a cascade resulting in the synthesis or release of prostaglandins, bradykinin, substance P, and histamine (as well as other mediators not shown). The interrelationships of these inflammatory mediators form a positive feedback loop allowing inflammation to persist far beyond cessation of the dental procedure. (Modified from ref. 8, with permission.)

surgery (3,4). To a great extent, the effectiveness of oral surgery as a clinical model for evaluating analgesics (5–8) resides in the predictable development of postoperative inflammation.

The development of inflammation is a consequence of the release and interaction of literally dozens of putative inflammatory mediators and neuroendocrine substances (Fig. 2). For the interested reader, detailed reviews are available on tissue mediators of pain and inflammation (9–11) and the neurophysiology of pain perception (12,13). The following section reviews results and design issues of clinical trials evaluating pharmacologic modulation of inflammatory mediators in a variety of conditions.

Bradykinin

Bradykinin is a putative inflammatory mediator with a wide spectrum of proinflammatory actions. This peptide activates nociceptive afferent nerves, increases vascular permeability, promotes vasodilation, and induces positive chemotaxis of leukocytes (9,14–17). Several animal studies have demonstrated that agents that block either bradykinin synthesis (18) or receptors (19–21) produce analgesic/antiinflammatory effects. Collectively, these studies provide impetus for clinical research evaluating bradykinin levels and their modulation in inflammatory diseases.

Bradykinin is liberated by the enzymatic cleavage of its precursor, kininogen, by the enzyme kallikrein (Fig. 2). The precursors and enzymes for the plasma kinin system, prekallikrein and kininogen, circulate in the vascular compartment. Since kallikrein is activated as part of the intrinsic clotting cascade, bradykinin can be locally released whenever there is damage to blood vessels. The synthetic capability of the bradykinin system is immense; plasma levels of bradykinin can increase nearly 10,000-fold under appropriate *in vitro* conditions (22).

Elevated blood levels of immunoreactive bradykinin have been observed in a clinical model of acute inflammation. Using oral surgery patients, circulating levels of immunoreactive bradykinin increased fourfold from preoperative to intraoperative samples (Fig. 3) and remained elevated in the postoperative period (18). The kinin system can be activated during blood collection, requiring the use of a collection procedure that immediately inactivates and precipitates both the enzymes and the precursors of the bradykinin system, leaving only the kinin peptides in the supernatant. Although this collection method permits measurement of circulating levels of bradykinin, until recently levels of bradykinin in the biologically relevant compartment, the inflamed tissue, remained unknown.

Previous attempts to measure tissue levels of mediators generally used methods such as the push-pull catheter, in which saline was pumped into the tissue and then collected. Although this approach has been used in both humans (23,24) and animals (22,25,26), there are several limitations. First, inflamed tissue contains substantial enzymatic activity (27). Peptidase activity may lead to low levels of measured peptide, via peptide degradation, or may even lead to high levels of measured peptide, either by continued *in vitro* synthesis (e.g., bradykinin production owing to kallikrein cleavage of kininogen) or by interference with radioimmunoassays through tracer degradation (28). Second, the precursor (e.g., kininogen) is collected in the perfusate where it may interfere with subsequent

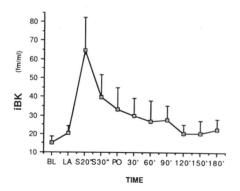

FIG. 3. The effects of oral surgery on blood levels of immunoreactive bradykinin (iBK) in 19 patients. *, $p < 0.05$; **, $p < 0.01$. (From ref. 18, with permission.)

assays (i.e., cross-reactivity of the antiserum with the precursor). Third, it is impossible to determine actual tissue levels of mediators since the saline dilutes their concentration by an unknown factor. And fourth, the process of inflammation is altered by pumping saline into the tissue, leading both to dilution of mediators and to activation of some peptidases.

A new method that avoids these limitations is microdialysis (Fig. 4). By implanting a probe having a semipermeable membrane (molecular weight cutoffs can range from 3,000 to 20,000 daltons), it is possible to collect a dialysate that contains only the inflammatory mediators (most of which have a molecular weight less than 1,500 daltons). The advantages of the microdialysis method are (a) immediate exclusion of peptidases and precursors, (b) quantitation of tissue levels of the mediators (based on *in vitro* calibration studies), and (c) minimal disruption of the inflamed tissue. Preliminary studies using this method appear promising; tissue levels of immunoreactive bradykinin increase progressively after surgical extraction of an impacted third molar, peaking near 15,000 fm/ml (29). This is approximately 200-fold greater than peak plasma levels of immunoreactive bradykinin (Fig. 3). The peak in tissue levels of immunoreactive bradykinin precedes peak levels of pain and the two are significantly correlated. In a second double-blind microdialysis study in oral surgery patients, pretreatment with methylprednisolone (125 mg IV, 2 hrs preoperation) reduced tissue levels of bradykinin by 66% as compared to placebo-treated patients (29). Thus, this technique appears useful for measuring tissue levels of mediators of pain/inflammation and their modulation by drugs.

Several clinical studies have also measured components of the kinin system during chronic inflammation. Using rheumatoid arthritis (RA) as an example of chronic inflammation, circulating levels of prekallikrein (30) and kininogen (31) are elevated as compared to levels observed in control patients. Changes in the activity of these bradykinin precursors probably contributes to elevated levels of immunoreactive bradykinin observed in patients with RA (Fig. 5); as compared

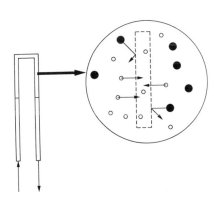

FIG. 4. Schematic depiction of the principle of microdialysis for measuring local tissue levels of substances such as inflammatory mediators. The U-shaped microdialysis probe, which is placed under the mucosa at the extraction site, has a semipermeable membrane (*stippled* portion of the tubing) that permits substances smaller than the molecular weight cutoff (*open circles in insert*) to cross the membrane; substances larger than the molecular weight cutoff (*filled circles in insert*) cannot cross the membrane. The application of this collection method to measuring inflammatory mediators relies on the uniform small molecular weight (generally less than 1,500) of mediators whereas their degradative enzymes are generally much larger (i.e., >30,000).

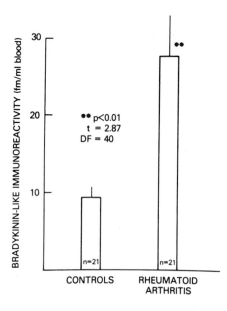

FIG. 5. Comparison of blood levels of immunoreactive bradykinin in patients with rheumatoid arthritis and age- and sex-matched controls. (From ref. 18, with permission.)

to age- and sex-matched controls, RA patients have two- to threefold greater levels of immunoreactive bradykinin (18). In addition, samples of synovial fluid have been demonstrated to have elevated levels of kallikrein-like activity (32), decreased levels of kininogen (33), and increased levels of kinins (34).

The effect of aspirin-like drugs on the kinin system has been evaluated in clinical trials. In arthritis patients, plasma levels of kininogen are reduced by 35% within 30 min of administration of indomethacin (50 mg po), with the maximal reduction of kininogen coinciding with maximal blood levels of indomethacin (35). Similar findings have been reported after one week of aspirin treatment (975 mg qid po) to RA patients (31). In addition, administration of diclofenac reduced urinary kallikrein activity by about 50% after 15 days of treatment (36). These studies suggest that aspirin-like drugs may have multiple effects on modulating inflammatory mediators. These actions of aspirin-like drugs may still be related to their inhibition of cyclooxygenase, possibly owing to prostaglandins acting in this case not as inflammatory mediators but as inhibitor modulators of endocrine secretory activity (37).

Eicosanoids and Prostaglandins

Products of arachidonic acid metabolism also have strong support as inflammatory mediators. Eicosanoids, the family name for this class of mediators, are end products of arachidonic acid metabolism and are synthesized as needed. Under conditions of tissue damage, phospholipase A_2 and other enzymes liberate arachidonic acid from phospholipids embedded in cell membranes (Fig. 2). At this point, enzymatic oxidative metabolism can proceed along two divergent pathways to produce several active compounds. The first pathway uses the enzyme cylcooxygenase and the second pathway uses the lipoxygenase enzymes. The action of cyclooxygenase upon arachidonic acid leads to the synthesis of prostaglandins, thromboxanes, and prostacyclin. The second pathway of arachidonic acid metabolism is catalyzed by the enzyme lipoxygenase and results in the formation of the leukotrienes. Results from animal models of inflammation suggest that prostaglandin E_2 and prostacyclin are probably synthesized in local tissues, whereas leukotriene B_4 (LTB_4) and thromboxanes are probably derived from polymorphonuclear leukocytes (38).

Products of arachidonic acid are released in clinical conditions of inflammation or tissue injury. Prostaglandins of the E and F series are elevated in inflamed tissue collected from patients having rheumatoid arthritis (39,40), osteoarthritis (41), ultraviolet radiation (42), allergic reactions (24), menorrhagia (43), dysmenorrhea (44), periodontitis (45), and ulcerative colitis (46). LTB_4 levels are elevated in tissue samples collected from patients having gout (47), rheumatoid arthritis (47–49), spondylarthritis (48), psoriasis (50), and ulcerative colitis (46).

The effects of prototype drugs on peripheral and systemic levels of eicosanoids have been evaluated in several of these clinical models of inflammation. An equilibrium dialysis sampling method (similar in concept to Fig. 4) has been used in patients with ulcerative colitis. The results indicate that prednisolone (1.5 mg/kg/day po $\times$ 3 days) significantly reduced tissue levels of PGE_2, $PGF_{2\alpha}$ and LTB_4, whereas administration of indomethacin (150 mg/day po) reduced levels of PGE_2 and $PGF_{2\alpha}$ with no significant change in levels of LTB_4 (46). Another dialysis study revealed that topically administered prednisolone (25 mg) was sufficient to reduce tissue levels of PGE_2 and LTB_4 in colitis patients (51). In patients suffering from menorrhagia, oral administration of mefenamic acid (250 mg q6h $\times$ 3–5 days) significantly reduced endometrial prostaglandin levels as compared to placebo-treated patients (43). Other studies have demonstrated that nonsteroidal antiinflammatory drugs (NSAIDs) significantly reduce synovial levels of PGE_2 (52), blood levels of thromboxane A_2 (53), gingival crevicular concentrations of prostaglandins (54), and urinary levels of prostaglandins (55).

Several therapeutic implications arise from these types of studies. First, elevated tissue levels of eicosanoids may provide a quantitative, biochemical index of disease severity (51,54) useful for identifying susceptible subgroups of patients or for predicting flare-ups of the disease. Second, demonstration of elevated tissue levels of mediators suggests that topical administration of drugs into the inflamed tissue can produce a highly effective and locally restricted reduction of eicosanoid synthesis, providing an efficacious treatment with minimal systemic side effects (51). And third, tissue measurement studies provide mechanistic information on both disease etiology and drug activity. For example, the demonstration that both flurbiprofen and indomethacin produce equivalent *in vivo* reduction of eicosanoids in periodontal disease but that flurbiprofen is more effective in halting disease activity (i.e., bone loss), has led to the suggestion that flurbiprofen has an additional mechanism of action beyond inhibition of cyclooxygenase (45).

Other Inflammatory Mediators

Additional substances have been implicated as biochemical indices of inflammation including histamine, serotonin, platelet activating factor (PAF), cytokines, substance P, calcitonin gene-related peptide, vasoactive intestingal peptide (VIP), α-1-acid-glycoprotein, and still-unidentified factors (56,57). Although space precludes consideration of these substances, the interested reader is referred to several excellent reviews (9–11,58).

Although relatively few clinical trials have evaluated these substances, there are theoretical implications for their evaluation in controlled analgesic trials. For example, animal studies have repeatedly demonstrated that opiates suppress the release of substance P from both central (59,60) and peripheral sites (61–63). Accordingly, substance P levels may provide a useful biochemical marker for evaluating time-, dose-, or drug-related changes in patients following administration of opioids. Biochemical markers may complement subjective markers of efficacy, e.g., pain relief, or may replace them in conditions where the patient is unable to respond, e.g., general anesthesia. In addition, the finding that elevated levels of peptides occur in some clinical settings, e.g., VIP release after allergen challenge (64), suggests that peripheral administration of neuropeptide receptor antagonists may have clinical efficacy in selected diseases.

EVALUATING CHEMICAL MARKERS OF STRESS OR ANALGESIA

A number of neuroendocrine substances are released under conditions of stress or pain. Collectively, these factors play a key role in initiating and coordinating behavioral, cardiovascular, metabolic, and immunologic responses to a provoking stimulus. This section reviews clinical studies evaluating circulating markers for stress or pain modulation; space limitations restrict the review to a prototype endocrine response, activation of the pituitary-adrenal axis, and to a prototype neural response, stimulation of the sympathoadrenal axis. The interested reader is referred to several recent reviews for more detailed information on markers of stress (65–67) and endogenous analgesic systems (12,68).

Pituitary-Adrenal Axis

A major endocrine response to a variety of stressors is activation of the pituitary-adrenal axis, which originates with hypothalamic secretion of corticotropin-releasing factor (CRF). In turn, CRF stimulates the pituitary corticotroph cell to cosecrete adrenocorticotropin (ACTH), beta-lipotropin (β-LPH) and beta-endorphin (β-END). Although the physiologic properties of ACTH are recognized (i.e., adrenocortical steroidogenesis), the contributions of β-END and β-LPH, if any, to the adaptive response to stress are not known. However, results from several clinical studies suggest that pituitary β-END may modify the perception of pain. For example, blood levels of immunoreactive β-END (iβ-END) are inversely related to pain report in patients after oral surgery (69), laparotomy (70), dressing changes after major burns (71), and painful electrical shocks (72). Additional studies have demonstrated that stimulation of β-END secretion by administration of CRF to oral surgery patients is associated with decreased postoperative pain (73), whereas blockade of β-END secretion with low doses of dexamethasone results in increased levels of postoperative pain (74). Studies conducted in rats indicate that at least a portion of CRF-induced analgesia is owing to release of β-END (75), although other mechanisms may also operate (76). A potential target site for the analgesic activity of circulating opioid peptides is opiate receptors located in peripherally inflamed tissue (1,77). This finding may have clinical implications for the development of peripherally selective opioid analgesic drugs. These results indicate that activation of the pituitary-adrenal axis alters metabolic, immunologic, and nociceptive responses to stressors (78).

The oral surgery model is also useful for evaluating the pharmacologic modulation of pituitary β-END as circulating levels of β-END increase during the stress of oral surgery and acute postoperative pain (Fig. 6). Results from these studies indicate that CRF (73), ibuprofen (37), and naloxone (Fig. 6; 79) all increase iβ-END levels, whereas dexamethasone (74), methylprednisolone (37), diazepam (79), fentanyl (79), and epinephrine (80) all suppress the stress-induced increase in iβ-END levels.

Sympathoadrenomedullary Axis

A second major category of stress responses consists of neurally derived substances. The primary example of this category is the sympathoadrenomedullary system. Numerous studies indicate that stressors evoke increased circulating levels of epinephrine (EPI) from adrenomedullary secretion and norepinephrine (NE), primarily from sympathetic nerve terminal overflow (81). Plasma levels of these catecholamines can increase several-fold in response to acute stressors such as oral surgery [EPI: one- to threefold; NE: no change (80,82,83)], acute postoperative pain [EPI: zero- to onefold; NE: one- to twofold (79,82,83)], cardiopulmonary bypass [EPI: fivefold; NE: two- to threefold (84)], exercise [EPI: sixfold; NE: eightfold (85)], and cardiac arrest [EPI: 300-fold; NE: 32-fold (86)]. As suggested by their differential response to these stressors, the adrenomedullary and sympathoneural components can be regulated separately (80,81). Catecholamine release may also be regionally selective as stimulation of adrenomedullary outflow produces increases in systemic plasma levels of epinephrine,

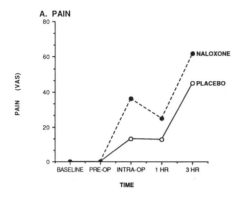

FIG. 6. The pain associated with oral surgery (A) is sufficient to increase circulating levels of immunoreactive beta-endorphin (B) and activate an endogenous opioid analgesic system. Twelve patients per group were injected IV with either placebo or naloxone (10 mg) and underwent the extraction of impacted third molars with 2% lidocaine and 1:100,000 epinephrine. (Modified from ref. 79, with permission.)

whereas sympathoneural release of norepinephrine (81,87) would be limited to a more restrictive locus. The physiologic consequence of increased catecholamine levels is increased cardiac output, skeletal muscle blood flow, sodium retention, inhibition of gut motility, cutaneous vasoconstriction (pallor), increased glucose availability, bronchiolar dilatation, and behavioral activation (81).

Several controlled clinical trials have evaluated the effects of various drugs on levels of circulating catecholamines. In the oral surgery model, both diazepam (79,82,83) and naloxone (79) suppress stress-induced release of norepinephrine, whereas CRF has no effect (73). Studies conducted in other clinical models (see ref. 88 for review) indicate that the stress-induced release of catecholamines is suppressed by muscle relaxants (89), enflurane (90), and large doses of fentanyl (75 μg/kg; 91).

Endogenous Pain Suppression System

Research over the last 20 years has documented the existence of endogenous pain suppression systems; one such system is the endogenous opioid peptides

(EOPs). The EOPs are a family of peptides that possess many of the properties of exogenous opioids and include β-endorphin, enkephalin, and dynorphin. Studies indicate that endogenous pain suppression systems can be activated by pain or stress. By using an opiate receptor antagonist, the relative activation of the EOPs can be determined. Although naloxone does not alter the perception of pain when injected into humans under basal conditions (92), it significantly increases the perception of pain when administered under conditions of stress. As seen in Fig. 6, naloxone-induced hyperalgesia is observed during oral surgery; pretreatment with the opiate antagonist results in significantly greater intraoperative pain as compared to placebo-treated patients (79). Moreover, naloxone increases pain experienced in the acute postoperative period after oral surgery (93,94). These findings indicate that the endogenous analgesic system can be activated in patients undergoing stressful clinical procedures or experiencing acute postoperative pain. In addition, the finding that naloxone more than doubles the amount of intraoperative pain as compared to placebo-treated patients (Fig. 6), provides an estimate of the magnitude of pain relief that accompanies activation of this endogenous pain suppression system.

DESIGN ISSUES FOR MEASURING CHEMICAL MEDIATORS

The measurement and functional evaluation of chemical mediators of pain and inflammation requires careful attention to a large number of variables that can confound the experimental design with resultant loss of sensitivity. Factors contributing to the variance of a study include the choice of clinical model, sampling methods/intervals, patient inclusion/exclusion criteria, the use of concurrent medications, variations in the clinical condition or procedure, and the sensitivity, validity, and reproducibility of the biochemical assay. Additionally, the influence of baseline variation between subjects often requires use of statistical techniques that account for this variability, such as analysis of covariance, data transformations, or nonparametric comparisons. This section briefly reviews strategies for controlling these factors in order to provide optimal conditions for evaluating the role of chemical mediators of pain and inflammation.

Choice of Clinical Model

The surgical removal of impacted third molars (oral surgery) is a suitable stressor for assessing acute neuroendocrine change. The oral surgery model utilizes healthy patients who receive minimal concurrent medications for the procedure and who experience a spectrum of stressful stimuli ranging from anticipatory anxiety preoperatively, acute surgical stress and pain intraoperatively, and moderate-to-severe pain for several hours postoperatively. Given the uncertainty of pharmacologic interactions that modulate neurohumoral release in man, the ability to limit the number and dose of agents favors use of the oral surgery model over other surgical models requiring general anesthesia, where a number of possible confounding agents are given. Conversely, the relatively minor degree of surgical trauma during oral surgery might provide an insufficient stimulus for activation of neurohumoral responses to major stressors, such as hemorrhagic shock or laparotomy. Patients should be selected or stratified to form homogeneous groups on the basis of age, difficulty of the surgical procedure, level of consciousness during the procedure, sex, and concurrent medications. Chronic responses are more readily studied in rheumatoid arthritis and other forms of chronic pain. Other factors that should be considered in selecting the clinical model include alterations in endocrine states (i.e., postpartum women undergoing episiotomy) and the effects of concurrent systemic disease on levels and release of the chemical mediator of interest.

Criteria for Patient Selection

Subtle but potentially significant variation can exist within the patient population eligible for inclusion in a clinical model. The intensity of surgical stimuli, in oral surgery patients for example, can vary widely, ranging from simple extractions to multiple full bony impactions requiring the elevation of mucoperiosteal flaps, bone removal, sectioning of teeth, possible trauma to the mandibular neurovascular bundle, occasional perforation of the maxillary sinus, and the placement of sutures. The surgical stress and resultant pain and inflammation from this latter situation represents a significant stimulus for neuroendocrine responses not comparable to the responses of patients with simple extractions. Comparability between groups can be prospectively sought by establishing inclusion criteria based on indices of anticipated surgical difficulty and the number of teeth to be extracted. The degree to which the treatment groups are homogeneous can be subsequently improved by additional prospective criteria for the actual degree of surgical trauma that occurred, the dose of concurrent medications used, the duration of the surgical procedure, minimum and maximum times for the onset of postoperative pain, and the occurrence of complications such as postoperative infections and hemorrhage.

The more specific these criteria can be made, the more homogeneous the patient sample will become, but this occurs at the expense of fewer potential subjects and increased time to complete the study. This is illustrated by a clinical trial evaluating the effects of low doses of the glucocorticoid dexamethasone on plasma beta-endorphin levels and postoperative pain (74). Subjects for this study were selected over the course of a year from a large patient pool. Of the 75 patients who underwent oral surgery, 23 were excluded at the time of surgery (under double-blind conditions) based on prospective criteria specifying the time to the loss of anesthesia and onset of pain, the degree of surgical trauma, and the dose of local anesthetic. The results of the study, however, demonstrated a significant difference between the experimental treatment and placebo using only 12 subjects per group. Similar sensitivity as a result of careful patient selection has been demonstrated for small sample sizes following hormonal and other types of pharmacologic manipulations (3,73).

Concurrent Medications

The choice of clinical model can largely dictate the number, type, and doses of drugs administered, in addition to the pharmacologic manipulation of interest. Required medications can range from single drug entities, such as local anesthetics, to combinations of general anesthetics, opioids, benzodiazepines, barbiturates, catecholamines (as vasoconstrictors with local anesthetics), and corticosteroids. As described above, the administration of an opioid, a benzodiazepine, catecholamines, an NSAID, or a glucocorticoid have all been demonstrated to alter the release of immunoreactive pituitary beta-endorphin; accordingly, these drugs could interfere with a study of a physiologic neuroendocrine response to stress or pain. Conversely, therapeutic administration of medications that alter patient apprehension and acute pain influences the perceived level of stress thereby providing insight into behavioral states regulating neuroendocrine responses.

Sample Collection and Measurement

Selection of time points for sampling should relate to the response of the biological process under study. In oral surgery studies evaluating the effects of drugs on endocrine markers of stress, patients experience different stressors over time ranging from preoperative apprehension, to intraoperative surgical stress, to postoperative pain. Anxiolytic drugs, such as diazepam, are generally more effective in suppressing stress hormones at time points when the major stimulus is anxiety, whereas analgesic drugs may be more effective when the major stimulus is pain. Although this issue is complicated by multiple sites of drug action [i.e., some drugs may have direct effects at the endocrine gland (37), in addition to their effects on stress (67)], it is evident that the choice of sampling times has a major influence on experimental outcome.

The stability of the measured substance and potential interfering factors also influence sample collection technique. The complexity of the sample collection protocol can range from minimal to quite involved. For example, the stability of cortisol permits blood samples to be simply collected and stored on ice; in contrast, the lability of bradykinin requires replicate blood samples to be collected using custom-made vacutainers containing ethanol and 100 mM 1,10-orthophenanthrolene to separate kinins from their precursors and to inactivate proteases (18). The assay sensitivity, specificity of the measurement technique, and the relative concentration of the substance of interest also must be considered in designing the sampling procedure. For example, cortisol and catecholamines can be easily measured with sample volumes less than 0.5 ml, whereas peptides such as beta-endorphin often require 5 to 6 ml of plasma. The larger the blood sample needed and the number of replicates required to overcome assay variability may limit the number of samples that can be collected per patient in the study.

Once the samples have been collected and are being stored under stable conditions, the frequency of assaying the clinical samples may introduce variability into the data. The desire to obtain results, coupled with concern over sample stability, compels many investigators to conduct several assays over the course of a clinical study. However, this must be tempered by consideration that the interassay variability of most radioimmunoassays is approximately twice the intraassay variability (95). All factors being equal, maximal statistical power is achieved by conducting the fewest possible assays over the course of the study. A compromise is to analyze the samples from clinical studies in two assays, to provide minimal additional sources of variability while generating interim data to evaluate whether the study design appears to be appropriate.

A second factor in assaying samples is the potential for a skewed distribution in the measured values. Both stress hormones and markers of inflammation have the potential for a positive (right-shifted) kurtosis in samples collected during stress/inflammation as compared to baseline samples. The skewness and kurtosis of the data can be calculated using available computer software (e.g., BMDP P2D; University of California Press, 1983). If the data is nonnormally distributed, it may require transformation (96,97) or analysis by nonparametric methods.

Use of Developmental Studies to Optimize Experimental Design

The measurement and evaluation of chemical mediators of pain and inflammation in clinical models is based on a relatively new and evolving body of literature. The measurement of plasma beta-endorphin has only become reliable within the past 5 to 10 years, and its role in pain and analgesia is undecided. In contrast, the evaluation of a new analgesic in man is based on experimental designs that have become standardized to the point that scientific innovation is not acceptable, owing to regulatory and industrial reluctance to deviate from traditional methods. As a consequence of the uncertainty in measurement, and variability in factors that influence the biological response under study, each series of experiments should be tailored on the basis of pilot studies that characterize the independent and dependent variables important to the study outcome.

The influence of factors reviewed above such as the duration of local anesthesia, the appropriate time and volume of biological fluid to sample, and the effects of adjunctive medications can be assessed in developmental studies in which the variables of interest are examined. This is illustrated by the dexamethasone study (74), in which the correct local anesthetic to provide a relatively uniform loss of local anesthesia required a preliminary study to assess the drug selected, the concentration of the solution to be used, and the total volume that would permit the oral surgical procedure but without prolonged anesthesia. Based on these considerations, the drug subsequently selected (mepivacaine) was used for the surgical procedure without a vasoconstrictor, but required that the solutions be prepared by the pharmacy at a concentration not commercially available (2%), and limited to 9 ml of total injected volume. A study was then conducted to determine the time to loss of mandibular paresthesia that resulted in exclusion criteria based on early or late anesthesia offset. An additional study was used to select a low dose of dexamethasone (0.1 mg) which suppressed pituitary beta-endorphin release without exerting a separate pharmacological effect to suppress inflammation. Thus, the use of serial developmental studies can permit the investigator to design a clinical experiment by examining each of the variables important to the biological process being studied under controlled conditions and then conducting a tightly controlled main study having a greater probability of a successful outcome.

CORRELATING CHEMICAL MARKERS
WITH EFFICACY MEASURES

A major objective of measuring chemical markers of inflammation or analgesia is to correlate their levels with other dependent measures of efficacy such as pain or edema. However, this is not a simple task, as indicated by studies using prototype analgesic drugs. For example, peak blood levels of morphine occur 20 min after IM injection, but at the time of peak pain relief (1 hr), blood levels of morphine have decreased to 50% of peak levels (98). Similar results are seen for ibuprofen, where peak blood levels occur at 1 to 2 hrs after oral administration whereas peak pain relief occurs at 2 to 3 hrs; the correlation coefficient between the two measures decreases from $r = 0.54$ at 1 hr to $r = 0.08$ at 3 hrs (99). In addition, we have observed that administration of CRF stimulates the pituitary-adrenal axis in postoperative patients, but that peak levels of iβ-END and cortisol precede peak pain relief by at least 1 hr (73).

These studies indicate that comparison between biochemical and physiological or subjective measures can be complicated by several factors, which collectively produce a temporal dissociation between peak measured levels in blood and other dependent measures. Prominent among these factors are diffusion/redistribution (i.e., collecting in a sampling site distinct from the target site), a delay between receptor occupancy and physiologic effect, and bioassay sensitivity. The correlation is generally good when the above three factors have minimal effects. For example, peak plasma levels of epinephrine correlate well with maximal cardiovascular activation and the two are altered similarly by drugs such as diazepam (80,82). However, the apparent correlation can be quite poor when one or more of these factors predominates. For example, the time for glucocorticoids to produce an observable effect appears to be owing to both protein synthesis and to the sensitivity of the bioassay, which is readily apparent if both are evaluated simultaneously. Other types of comparisons, such as evaluating the area under the time-response curve for several levels of an intervention (i.e., doses of a drug), may prove more useful in correlating measured levels of a substance with changes in other dependent variables.

CONCLUSIONS

Clinical analgesic trials incorporating biochemical measurement of endogenous substances can provide information about physiologic mechanisms of pain and analgesia as well as the mechanisms of prototype and novel drugs. This type of study, bringing the test tube to the clinic, may prove useful in developing and evaluating analgesic drugs.

REFERENCES

1. Joris J, Dubner R, Hargreaves KM. Opiate analgesia at peripheral sites: a target for opioids released during stress and inflammation? *Anesth Analg* 1987;66:1277–1281.
2. Cooper SA, Precheur H, Rauch D, Rosenheck A, Ladov M, Engel J. Evaluation of oxycodone and acetaminophen in treatment of postoperative pain. *J Oral Surg* 1980;50:496–501.
3. Troullos E, Hargreaves KM, Butler D, Dionne R. Comparison of two non-steroidal anti-inflammatory drugs, flurbiprofen and iburpofen, to methylprednisolone for suppression of post-operative pain and edema. *J Oral Surg* 1989;48:945–952.
4. Miles M, Desjardins P, Pawel H. The facial plethysmometer; a new instrument to measure facial swelling volumetrically. *J Oral Maxillofac Surg* 1985;43:346–450.
5. Cooper S, Beaver W. A model to evaluate mild analgesics in oral surgery outpatients. *Clin Pharmacol Ther* 1976;20:241–250.
6. Cooper SA. New peripherally acting oral analgesic agents. *Annu Rev Pharmacol Toxicol* 1983;23: 617–647.
7. Dionne R. Suppression of dental pain by the preoperative administration of flurbiprofen. *Am J Med* 1986;80:41–49.
8. Hargreaves KM, Troullos E, Dionne R. Pharmacologic rationale for the treatment of acute pain. *Dent Clin North Am* 1987;31:675–694.
9. Dawson W, Willoughby D. Inflammation—mechanisms and mediators. In: Lombardino J, ed. *Non-steroidal antiinflammatory drugs,* New York: Wiley, 1985;1–76.
10. Willoughby D. Inflammation. *Br Med Bull* 1987;43:247.
11. Gallin J, Goldstein I, Snyderman R. *Inflammation: basic principles and clinical correlates.* New York: Raven Press, 1988.
12. Dubner R, Bennett G. Spinal and trigeminal mechanisms of nociception. *Annu Rev Neurosci* 1983;6:381–418.
13. Willis, W. *The pain system.* Basel: S. Karger, 1985.
14. Basran G, Morley J, Paul W, Turner-Warwick M. Evidence in man of synergistic interaction between putative mediators of acute inflammation and asthma. *Lancet* 1982;1:935–937.
15. Mense S. Sensitization of group IV muscle receptors to bradykinin by 5-hydroxtyrptamine and prostaglandin E_2. *Brain Res* 1981;225:95–105.
16. Lim R, Miller D, Guzman F, et al. Pain and analgesia evaluated by the intraperitoneal bradykinin-evoked pain method in man. *Clin Pharmacol Ther* 1967;8:521–542.
17. Coffman J. The effect of aspirin in pain and hand blood flow responses to intra-arterial injection of bradykinin. *Clin Pharmacol Ther* 1966;7:26–37.
18. Hargreaves KM, Troullos E, Dionne R, et al. Bradykinin is increased during acute and chronic inflammation: therapeutic implications. *Clin Pharmacol Ther* 1988;44:613–621.

19. Steranka L, Dehass C, Vavrek R, et al. Antinociceptive effects of bradykinin antagonists. *Eur J Pharmacol* 1987;136:261–262.
20. Steranka L, Manning D, Dehass C, et al. Bradykinin as a pain mediator: receptors are localized to sensory neurons and antagonists have analgesic actions. *Proc Natl Acad Sci USA* 1988;85: 3245–3249.
21. Costello A, Hargreaves KM. Suppression of carrageenan-induced hyperalgesia, edema and hyperthermia by a bradykinin antagonist. *Eur J Pharmacol* 1989;171:259–263.
22. Hargreaves KM, Costello A, Joris J. The role of bradykinin in the development of hyperalgesia, edema and hyperthermia induced by carrageenan. (Submitted) 1989.
23. Chapman LF, Ramos A, Godell H, Wolff H. Neurohumoral features of afferent fibers in man. *Arch Neurol* 1961;4:617–650.
24. Greaves M, Sondergaard J, McDonald-Gibson W. Recovery of prostaglandins in human cutaneous inflammation. *Br Med J* 1971;2:258–260.
25. Imai Y, Saito K, Maeda S, et al. Inhibition of the release of bradykinin-like substances into the perfusate of rat hindpaw by neurotropin. *Jpn J Pharmacol* 1984;36:104–106.
26. Limaos E, Borges D, Souza-Pinto J, et al. Acute terpentine inflammation and kinin release in rat paw thermic edema. *Br J Exp Pathol* 1981;62:591–594.
27. Kumakura S, Tsurufuji S, Kurooka S, Sunhara N. Role of bradykinin generating and degrading systems in the vascular permeability response induced with kaolin in rats. *J Pharmacol Exp Ther* 1987;243:1067–1073.
28. DiAugustine L, Lazarus G, Jahnke G, et al. Corticotropin/beta-endorphin immunoreactivity in rat mast cells: peptide or protease? *Life Sci* 1980;27:2663–2668.
29. Hargreaves KM, Costello AN. Glucocorticoids suppress release of immunoreactive bradykinin from inflamed tissue as evaluated by microdialysis probes. *Clin Pharmacol Therap* 1990;48:168–178.
30. Teppo A, Pakkanen R, Maury C. Plasma total prekallikrein-kallikrein activity in rheumatoid arthritis with and without amyloidosis. *Acta Med Scand* 1985;217:397–402.
31. Sharma J, Zeitlin I, Brooks P, et al. The action of aspirin on plasma kininogen and other plasma proteins in rheumatoid patients: relationship to disease activity. *Clin Exp Pharmacol Physiol* 1980;7:347–354.
32. Sharma J, Zeitlin I, Deodhar S, et al. Detection of kallikrein-like activity in inflamed synovial tissue. *Arch Int Pharmacodyn* 1983;262:279–286.
33. Sawai K, Niwa S, Katori M. The significant reduction of high molecular weight-kininogen in synovial fluid of patients with active rheumatoid arthritis. *Adv Exp Med Biol* 1978;120B:195–202.
34. Eisen V. Plasma kinins in synovial exudates. *Br J Exp Pathol* 1970;51:322–327.
35. Sharma J, Zeitlin I, Brooks P, Dick W. A novel relationship between plasma kininogen and rheumatoid arthritis. *Agents Actions* 1976;6:148–153.
36. Gross W, Kroh J, Krebs A, Zoller H. Diclofenac sodium: blood concentration of the slow release form and influence on the metabolism of kallikrein. *Arzneimittelforschung* 1984;34:1327–1329.
37. Dionne R, Troullos E, Hargreaves KM. Ibuprofen elevates immunoreactive β-endorphin levels during surgical stress. (Submitted for the 1990 meeting of the American Society of Clinical Pharmacology.)
38. Higgs G. The role of eicosanoids in inflammation. *Prog Lipid Res* 1986;25:555–561.
39. Trang L, Granstrom E, Lovgren O, et al. Levels of prostaglandins $F_{2\alpha}$, and E_2 and thromboxane B_2 in joint fluid in rheumatoid arthritis. *Scand J Rheumatol* 1977;6:151–154.
40. Henderson B, Pettipher E, Higgs G. Mediators of rheumatoid arthritis. *Br Med Bull* 1987;43: 415–428.
41. Bombardieri S, Carrani P, Ciabattoni G, et al. The synovial prostaglandin system in chronic inflammatory arthritis: differential effect of steroidal and non-steroidal anti-inflammatory drugs. *Br J Pharmacol* 1981;73:893–901.
42. Graeves M, Sondergaard J. Pharmacological agents released in ultraviolet inflammation studied by continuous skin perfusion. *J Invest Dermatol* 1970;54:365–368.
43. Tsang B, Domingo M, Spence J, et al. Endometreal prostaglandins and menorrhagia: influence of a prostaglandin synthetase inhibitor in vivo. *Can J Physiol Pharmacol* 1987;65:2081–2084.
44. Chan W, Hill J. Determination of menstrual prostaglandin levels in non-dysmonorrheac and dysmenorrheac subjects. *Prostaglandins* 1978;15:365–370.
45. Williams R, Offenbacher S, Jeffcoat M, et al. Indomethacin or flurbiprofen treatment of peri-

odontitis in beagles: effect on crevicular fluid arachidonic acid metabolites compared with effect on alveolar bone loss. *J Periodont Res* 1988;23:134–138.

46. Lauritsen K, Laursen L, Bukhave K, et al. In vivo effects of orally administered prednisolone on prostaglandin and leucotriene production in ulcerative colitis. *Gut* 1987;28:1095–1099.

47. Rae S, Davidson E, Smith M. Leukotriene B_4, an inflammatory mediator in gout. *Lancet* 1982;2: 1122–1124.

48. Klickstein L, Shapligh C, Goetzl E. Lipoxygenation of arachidonic acid as a source of polymorphonuclear leukocyte chemotactic factors in synovial fluid and tissue in rheumatoid arthritis and spondylarthritis. *J Clin Invest* 1980;66:1166–1170.

50. Brain S, Camp R, Dowd D, et al. Psoriasis and leukotriene B_4. *Lancet* 1982;2:762–763.

51. Lauritsen K, Laursen L, Bukhave K, et al. Effects of topical 5-aminosalicylic adic and prednisolone on prostaglandin E_2 and leukotriene B_4 levels determined by equilibrium in vivo dialysis of rectum in relapsing ulcerative colitis. *Gastroenterology* 1986;91:837–844.

52. Higgs G, Vane J, Hart F, et al. Effects of anti-inflammatory drugs on prostaglandins in rheumatoid arthritis. In: Robinson H, Vane J, eds. *Prostaglandin synthetase inhibitors.* New York: Raven Press, 1974;165–173.

53. Heavey D, Barrow S, Hickling N, et al. Aspirin causes short-lived inhibition of bradykinin-stimulated prostacyclin production in man. *Nature* 1985;318:186–188.

54. Offenbacher S, Odle B, Gray R, et al. Crevicular fluid prostaglandin E levels as a measure of the periodontal disease status of adult and juvenile periodontis patients. *J Periodont Res* 1984;19: 1–13.

55. Levine R, Petokas S, Nandi J, et al. Effect of non-steroidal anti-inflammatory drugs on gastrointestinal injury and prostanoid generation in healthy volunteers. *Dig Dis Sci* 1988;33:660–666.

56. Hargreaves K, Costello A, Joris J. Release from inflamed tissue of a substance with properties similar to corticotropin releasing factor. *Neuroendocrinology* 1989;49:476–482.

57. Carr D, Ballantyne J, Osgood P, Kemp J, Szyfelbein S. Pituitary-adrenal stress response in the absence of brain-pituitary connections. *Anesth Analg* 1989;69:197–201.

58. Hargreaves KM, Dubner R. Mechanisms of pain and analgesia. In: Dionne R, Phero J, eds. *Management of pain and anxiety in dentistry.* New York: Elsevier Press, (in press) 1990; chapter 2.

59. Jessell T, Iversen L. Opiate analgesics inhibit substance P release from rat trigeminal nucleus. *Nature* 1977;268:549–551.

60. Yaksh T, Jessell T, Gamse R, et al. Intrathecal morphine inhibits substance P release from mammalian spinal cord in vivo. *Nature* 1980;286:155–157.

61. Brodin E, Gazelius B, Panopoulos P, et al. Morphine inhibits substance P release from peripheral nerve endings. *Acta Physiol Scand* 1983;117:567–570.

62. Yonehara N, Iami Y, Inoki R. Effects of opioids on the heat stimulus-evoked substance P release and thermal edema in the rat hind paw. *Eur J Pharmacol* 1988;151:381–387.

63. Yaksh T. Substance P release from knee joint afferent terminals: modulation by opioids. *Brain Res* 1988;458:319–327.

64. Tonnesen P, Hindberg I, Schaffalitzky O, et al. Effect of nasal allergen challenge on serotonin, Substance P, and VIP in plasma and nasal secretions. *Allergy* 1988;43:310–317.

65. Carr D, Carr J. Role of brain opiates in pain relief. In: Stoll B, Parbhoo S, eds. *Bone metastasis: monitoring and treatment.* New York, Raven Press, 1983;375–393.

66. Carr D, Murphy M. Operation, anesthesia and the endorphin system. *Int Anesthesiol Clin* 1988;27: 199–205.

67. Hargreaves KM. Neuroendocrine markers of stress. *Anesth Prog* 1990;37:99–105.

68. Basbaum A, Fields H. Endogenous pain control systems: brainstem spinal pathways and endorphin circuitry. *Annu Rev Neurosci* 1984;7:309–338.

69. Hargreaves K, Dionne R, Mueller G. Plasma beta endorphin-like immunoreactivity, pain and anxiety following administration of placebo in oral surgery patients. *J Dent Res* 1983;62:1170–1173.

70. Pickar D, Cohen M, Dubois M. The relationship of plasma cortisol and beta endorphin immunoreactivity to surgical stress and post-operative analgesic requirement. *Gen Hosp Psychiatry* 1983;5:93–98.

71. Szyfelbein S, Osgood P, Carr D. The assessment of pain and plasma beta-endorphin immunoreactivity in burned children. *Pain* 85;22:173–182.

72. Facchinetti F, Sandrini G, Petralgia F, et al. Concomitant increase in nociceptive flexion reflex threshold and plasma opioids following transcutaneous nerve stimulation. *Pain* 1984;19:295–303.

73. Hargreaves KM, Mueller G, Dubner R, Goldstein D, Dionne R. Corticotropin releasing factor (CRF) produces analgesia in humans and rats. *Brain Res* 1987;422:154–157.
74. Hargreaves K, Schmidt E, Mueller G, Dionne R. Dexamethasone alters plasma levels of beta-endorphin and post-operative pain. *Clin Pharmacol Ther* 1987;42:601–607.
75. Hargreaves KM, Flores C, Dionne R, Mueller G. The role of pituitary β-endorphin in mediating corticotropin releasing factor (CRF)-induced antinociception. *Am J Physiol* 1990;258:E235–E242.
76. Hargreaves KM, Dubner R, Costello A. Corticotropin releasing factor (CRF) has a peripheral site of action for antinociception. *Eur J Pharmacol* 1989;170:275–279.
77. Stein C, Millan M, Shippenberg T, et al. Peripheral effects of fentanyl upon nociception in inflamed tissue of the rat. *Neurosci Lett* 1988;4:225–228.
78. Munck A, Guyre P, Holbrook N. Physiological functions of glucocorticoids in stress and their relation to pharmacological actions. *Endocr Rev* 1984;5:25–44.
79. Hargreaves KM, Dionne R, Goldstein D, et al. Naloxone, fentanyl and diazepam modify plasma beta-endorphin levels during surgery. *Clin Pharmacol Ther* 1986;40:165–171.
80. Troullos E, Hargreaves K, Goldstein D, Stull R, Dionne R. Epinephrine suppresses stress-induced increases in plasma immunoreactive beta-endorphin in humans. *J Clin Endocrinol Metab* 1989;69:546–561.
81. Goldstein D. Stress-induced activation of the sympathetic nervous system. *Baillieres Clin Endocrinol Metab* 1987;1:253–278.
82. Dionne R, Goldstein D, Wirdzek P: Effects of diazepam premedication and epinephrine-containing local anesthetic on cardiovascular and plasma catecholamine responses to oral surgery. *Anesth Analg* 1984;63:640–646.
83. Goldstein D, Dionne R, Sweet J, Gracely R, Brewer B, Gregg R, Keiser H. Circulatory, plasma catecholamine, cortisol, lipid, and psychological responses to a real-life stress (third molar extraction): effects of diazepam sedation and of inclusion of epinephrine with the local anesthetic. *Psychosom Med* 1982;44:259–272.
84. Moore R, McQuay H. Neuroendocrinology of the post-operative state. In: Smith G, Covino B, eds. *Acute pain.* London: Buttersworth, 1985;133–154.
85. Halter J, Stratton J, Pfeifer M. Plasma catecholamines and hemodynamic responses to stress states in man. *Acta Physiol Scand* 1984;572(suppl):31–38.
86. Wortsman J, Frank S, Cryer P. Adrenomedullary response to maximal stress in humans. *Am J Med* 1984;77:779–784.
87. Havel P, Veith R, Dunning B, Taborsky G. Pancreatic noradrenergic nerves are activated by neuroglucopenia but not by hypotension or hypoxia in the dog. *J Clin Invest* 1988;82:1538–1545.
88. Finn R, Moss J. Effect of anesthetics on endocrine function. *Anesthesiol Clin North Am* 1987;5:411–442.
89. Derbyshire D, Chmiewski A, Fell D, et al. Plasma catecholamine responses to tubal intubation. *Br J Anaesth* 1983;55:855–860.
90. Hamberger B, Jarnberg P. Plasma catecholamines after surgical stress: differences between neurolept and enflurane anaesthesia. *Acta Anaesthesiol Scand* 1983;27:307–310.
91. Lappas D, Fahmy N, Slater E, et al. Catecholamines, renin and cardiovascular responses to fentanyl-diazepam anaesthesia. *Anesthesiology* 1980;53:S14.
92. Grevart P, Goldstein A. Endorphins: naloxone fails to alter experimental pain or mood in humans. *Science* 1978;199:1093–1095.
93. Gracely R, Dubner R, Wolskee P, Deeter W. Placebo and naloxone can alter post-surgical pain by separate mechanisms. *Nature* 1983;306:264–265.
94. Levine J, Gordon N, Fields H. The mechanism of placebo analgesia. *Lancet* 1978;2:654–657.
95. Chard T. *An introduction to radioimmunoassay and related techniques.* Amsterdam: North Holland Pub. Co., 1978.
96. Box G, Cox D. An analysis of transformations. *J R Stat Soc* 1964;26B:211–252.
97. Hancock A, Bush E, Stanisic D, et al. Data normalization before statistical analysis: keeping the horse before the cart. *Trends Pi* 1988;9(abstract):29–32.
98. Grabinski P, Kaiko R, Rogers A, Houde R. Plasma levels and analgesia following deltoid and gluteal injections of morphine and methadone. *J Clin Pharmacol* 1983;23:48–55.
99. Laska E, Sunshine A, Marrero I, Olson N, Siegel C, McCormick N. The correlation between blood levels of ibuprofen and clinical analgesic response. *Clin Pharmacol Ther* 1986;40:1–7.

DISCUSSION

Dr. Dwight Moulin: Dr. Hargreaves presents data showing that dexamethasone inhibited endogenous opioid analgesia in oral surgery patients by suppressing their release of pituitary β-endorphin. Dexamethasone itself can be a powerful analgesic; we frequently use it to treat intractable cancer pain because it has such dramatic pain-relieving effects. Why didn't the analgesic effects of dexamethasone overwhelm the effects of endorphin suppression? Also, does postoperative naloxone cause an increase in pain?

Dr. Hargreaves: In three studies in the dental impaction model, neither methylprednisolone nor dexamethasone produced profound analgesic effects, even at high doses, although they did inhibit many other signs of inflammation. In the dexamethasone study described in the preceding chapter, the dose, 0.1 mg, was deliberately chosen to be well below the classic antiinflammatory dose of dexamethasone, in the range of 10 mg. We were trying to selectively inhibit pituitary-adrenal responses without having concurrent antiinflammatory effects.

Regarding naloxone, Gracely at the National Institute for Dental Research and Levine and Fields from the University of California at San Francisco have shown that administration of 10 mg naloxone following third molar extraction causes an increase in pain. We extended that finding in a double-blind trial where we administered naloxone just prior to third molar extraction, to see whether that stress is capable of releasing opioid peptides. We found that naloxone increased intraoperative pain two- or threefold, even though all patients also had local anesthetic.

Dr. Laurence Mather: I greatly admire the work presented by Drs. Hargreaves and Dionne, but would like to add one piece of caution regarding the interpretation of blood concentrations of hormones. In addition to synthesis and release, one must pay attention to clearance, because it is the balance among those three processes that determines the measured concentrations. Simply measuring concentrations without other information such as regional blood flow may be a misleading index of production and release.

Dr. Kathleen Foley: We have given β-endorphin to patients, and have found that even high systemic levels do not produce significant analgesia. We assumed that this was because this opioid doesn't cross the blood-brain barrier, although Herz and others have also shown peripheral effects. Do you think the β-endorphin effect you saw was a central or peripheral effect?

Dr. Hargreaves: I don't know. The peripheral effect, I'd like to add, has only been detected in inflamed tissues. When we inject opioid into a normal paw of a rat, we don't see any effect on behavioral responses to noxious stimuli. It isn't yet clear whether the peripheral opioid effect is mediated through leukocytes or is a direct effect on the peripheral nerve.

Advances in Pain Research and Therapy, Vol. 18,
edited by M. Max, R. Portenoy, and E. Laska,
Raven Press, Ltd., New York © 1991.

Commentary

Caveats in the Evaluation of Stress Hormone Responses in Analgesic Trials

Daniel B. Carr

Analgesic Peptide Research Unit, Massachusetts General Hospital and Shriners Burns Institute, Boston, Massachusetts 02114; and Departments of Anesthesiology and Medicine (Endocrinology), Harvard Medical School, Boston, Massachusetts 02114

The scholarly survey provided by Drs. Hargreaves and Dionne touches upon many important aspects of drug design and evaluation. Of the many topics in their review that might be commented upon, one in particular stands out as quite relevant to analgesic trials. Measurements of circulating hormones are widely used to supplement other indices of analgesic efficacy, to the point that inhibition of a "stress hormone" response is now equated with successful analgesia in advertisements for new clinical analgesics. Yet rarely does one see any discussion of shortcomings of this approach, or appreciation that a new drug's ability to inhibit hormonal responses may not impact upon clinical outcome. The purpose of this discussion, therefore, is to offer the reader several caveats regarding the use of hormone levels as markers of stress or analgesia.

WHAT IS A STRESS HORMONE?

Experimental studies of glandular changes provoked by environmental challenges well antedate the coinage of the terms "stress" or "homeostasis." Selye in his 1949 treatise (1) cited numerous 19th century investigations of what would now be termed stress physiology, a topic that has thus been under continuous study for over a century. At present, the concept of a stress hormone has well permeated the collective medical consciousness, yet it remains quite vague. A standard modern endocrinology reference defines hormone as "a substance that is secreted by one cell and travels through the circulation, where it exerts actions on other cells" (2). Compounding this broadness is the wide range of circumstances, not all of which are clearly noxious, within which hormonal responses have been evaluated: physical exercise (3), sauna, and even weightlessness (4). If a hormone level changes during pain or trauma, it need not be interpreted as a sign that the body is experiencing pain, but might equally as well reflect anxiety (5), immune activation (6), or overzealous fluid replenishment (7). Thus, I would submit that the concept of "stress hormone" has become less and less meaningful as more and more hormones have been characterized and their levels have been demonstrated to change in response to a broader and broader variety of stimuli.

When we read that endothelin levels rise during operation (8), or atrial natriuretic peptide levels increase during fluid challenge (9), do we consider that we have learned something about "stress hormone" regulation? Would it be advantageous to administer a drug solely to inhibit such responses? Although my answers to these questions are no, they are not too far from a common justification for administering opioids perioperatively—namely, that pituitary-adrenal activation is blunted by doing so, signifying a reduction in perioperative stress and improved clinical outcome (10). Insofar as one may justifiably use a term as broad as "stress hormone," one is safest in restricting its use to plasma markers of pituitary-adrenal or sympathomedullary activation, time-honored responses to threats to the integrity of the organism. In specific circumstances where the literature supports doing so, other hormones may be grouped under this heading, e.g., plasma melatonin during exercise (11), but not during psychological stress.

OPIOIDS AND THE STRESS RESPONSE: CAVEATS

During the 1970s and 1980s, numerous clinical investigators have employed the pituitary-adrenal response to operation as a benchmark of stress against which the presumptive antistress effects of opioids have been titrated (12–26). Because intraoperative opioid analgesics are now given daily with such studies in mind, it is worthwhile to examine this practice by posing two questions. First, if a stress hormone response is diminished by opioid administration, is this the result of improved analgesia? Second, if a stress hormone response is unaffected by administration of an opioid analgesic, should we have given a higher dose? Several lines of evidence argue that the answer to both questions is no.

Because commonly measured stress hormones of the pituitary-adrenal group include adrenocorticotropin (ACTH), beta-endorphin, and cortisol, one must recall that opioids exert short-loop negative feedback control of a classical endocrine nature (27). That is, the stress-induced release of corticotropin-releasing hormone (CRH) is under inhibitory opioid control (28); naloxone administration during stress interrupts this feedback loop and augments pituitary beta-endorphin secretion (29). To observe a lowering of plasma ACTH, beta-endorphin, or cortisol levels after opioid administration is therefore a physiological conundrum. It is no more a proof of analgesia than might be a lowering of luteinizing hormone levels after estrogen administration or a fall in parathyroid hormone levels as serum calcium rises. Given that many clinical pains are resistant to opioids (30), one can readily imagine a situation in which opioid administration might be ineffectual as an analgesic, yet promptly lower plasma measures of pituitary-adrenal activity.

As to the significance of a persistent stress response in the face of opioid analgesic administration, it is clear that cells of the immune system contain and may secrete neuropeptides including ACTH and opioids (31). Other white cell products such as interleukin-1 possess significant CRH-like activity (32), raising the possibility that circulating immune mediators resulting from peripheral inflammation may reach the pituitary via the systemic circulation and thereby trigger a "stress response" that has no relation to nociception or even cognition. Hargreaves and colleagues' (33) preliminary characterization of a peripherally derived corticotropin-releasing substance strengthens this view, as does our recent finding of a pituitary-adrenal stress response in rats bearing pituitary-to-kidney autotransplants (6). These findings, together with others detailed in recent reviews of bidirectional neuroimmune interactions, make a compelling case that secretion of neurohormones may reflect immune activation as well as painful stimuli (34–36). These immune-derived neuropeptide responses may not necessarily reflect levels of pain, and hence it may not always be possible to draw conclusions concerning the relative painfulness or stress of different circumstances by comparing the magnitudes of the respective stress hormone responses (37). Intriguingly, the hypothesis that tissue injury factors may trigger a stress response appears to have been prophesied by Selye himself in an early letter to *Nature* (38). He wrote that "the 'general adaptation syndrome' . . . might be compared to other general defence reactions such as inflammation or formation of immune bodies" and speculated that "an essential part in the initiation of the syndrome is the liberation of histamine or some similar substance which may be released from the tissues either mechanically in surgical injury or by other means in other cases."

In light of the above we may further ask whether one typically observes suppression of pituitary-adrenal responses during successful opioid analgesia. Kehlet (39), in studies of hormone responses during postoperative analgesia by different techniques, has shown that analgesic doses of epidural morphine do not prevent a plasma cortisol rise. It is possible that cerebrospinal fluid levels of opioid, tachykinin, or other neurotransmitters may be influenced by analgesic interventions, but these are not reflected in concentrations in the systemic circulation from which blood is normally sampled for analysis. Indeed, the compartmental nature of stress responses is well recognized: depending upon the particular circumstance examined, central and peripheral beta-endorphin levels may rise in concert (29) or be entirely dissociated (40,41). Just as the regulation of opioid secretion may be highly compartmentalized, the mode of action of opioid analgesia may be qualitatively different at different sites. The recent demonstration that opioids can produce analgesia by acting directly upon the inflammatory process in the periphery (42) undermines still further our tendency to view opioid analgesia as a process limited to the central nervous system and tightly coupled to the secretion of hormones from the pituitary or adrenal into the circulation.

OPIOIDS AND STRESS RESPONSES: PARADOXES

Pituitary-adrenal activation is certainly not the only hormonal measure of stress, even if one restricts attention to anterior pituitary products. Rises in growth hormone or prolactin, or falls in gonadotropins are likewise interpreted as responses to stress (2,3,5). Yet opioid administration to unstressed subjects is well recognized to stimulate growth hormone and prolactin secretion, as well as to lower gonadotropin levels (27,43–45). Thus if one were to restrict attention to other indices of hormonal stress responses besides pituitary-adrenal activation, one might deduce that exogenous opioid administration causes stress rather than reducing it. Supporting this paradoxical view (that opioid analgesics provoke stress) are reports that giving morphine to unstressed subjects produces hormonal (46) and cardiovascular (47) signs of a sympathoadrenal response. Moreover, if morphine or other narcotics happen to provoke nausea, then the emetic response by itself may trigger a robust outpouring of hormones such as vasopressin (2), whose magnitude far exceeds that found during physiological stress (48). In aggregate, then, the physiological effects of opioids are quite context dependent, with numerous reports of hormone inhibition during stress balanced by findings of hormone stimulation in the basal state. The implication for analgesic trials is that even as seemingly objective a measure as an analgesic's capacity to alter a hormone level might be affected by many aspects of the clinical context of the subjects studied.

Assuming one were able to solve the problem of heterogeneous basal levels of stress, other problematic effects of opioids upon hormone levels would remain. Opioids constitute a diverse series of compounds: their structures may differ widely, and they may have selective affinity for one or another opioid receptor type or subtype (49). Whether an opioid stimulates or suppresses pituitary hormone secretion, and the precise profile of hormones affected, depend upon its receptor selectivity (50–55). Certain opioids (e.g., butorphanol or nalbuphine) act as agonists at one opioid receptor and antagonists at another type of opioid receptor; the hormonal response to their administration is a mixture of mu opioid receptor antagonism and kappa opioid receptor occupancy (56). Thus, with respect to mu opioid receptor-mediated hormone secretion or respiratory depression, administering the opioid analgesic nalbuphine will in part produce responses resembling those seen after naloxone (57).

CONCLUSIONS

This commentary has addressed the common practice of using "stress hormone" levels to gauge the analgesic benefit of intra- and perioperative opioids.

A common finding in many clinical studies during the 1970s (12–16) and 1980s (17–26), opioid suppression of pituitary-adrenal responses is now a marketing point in the 1990s. Pitfalls in this approach include its narrow focus upon the adrenal cortex and medulla, its disregard for compartmentalization of stress hormone responses, and its ignoring peripheral sources of these hormones or their releasing factors. Even if no questions existed regarding the techniques of hormone assay, there would still remain caveats in the interpretation of the findings. Lowered cortisol is a confirmation that feedback is intact but may mean little as regards pain. Peripheral opioid effects are ignored in a model that sees all their effects resulting from actions within the central nervous system. Opioid actions upon pituitary hormones are complex and at times paradoxical, the direction of the effects dependent upon the particular hormone scrutinized and whether it is studied in basal or stressed subjects. Side effects such as nausea can trigger striking hormonal responses that may dwarf those owing to the clinical stress itself. Finally, analgesia or stress hormone suppression may occur independently.

Given the neuroanatomy of the inputs to the hypothalamus that culminate in pituitary hormone secretion (58,59), it has previously been tempting to view measurements of pituitary stress hormone responses as a sort of limbic visual analogue scale. Indeed, if considered cautiously along with other measures of analgesic efficacy (e.g., pain scales, disability or quality-of-life indices, length of hospital stay, measures of hyperalgesia), they may in particular contexts remain worthwhile adjuncts in clinical trials of novel analgesics. Nonetheless, in light of the above arguments it is no longer appropriate to regard hormone measurements uncritically as objective outcome measures of analgesic therapy.

REFERENCES

1. Selye H. *Stress.* Montreal: Acta, 1949.
2. Felig P, Baxter JD, Broadus AE, Frohman LA, eds. *Endocrinology and metabolism,* 2nd ed. New York: McGraw-Hill, 1987.
3. Carr DB, Bullen BA, Skrinar GS, Arnold MA, Rosenblatt M, Beitins IZ, Martin JB, McArthur JW. Physical conditioning facilitates the exercise-induced secretion of beta-endorphin and beta-lipotropin in women. *N Engl J Med* 1981;305:560–563.
4. Tigranian RA, Kalita NF, Macho L, Kvetnansky R, Vigas M. Changes of some pituitary hormones in cosmonauts after space flights of different duration. In: Usdin E, Kvetnansky R, Axelrod J, eds. *Stress: the role of catecholamines and other hormones.* New York: Gordon and Breach, 1984;1003–1010.
5. Carr DB, Sheehan DV, Surman OS, Greenblatt DJ, Heninger GR, Jones KJ, Spiro T, Levine PH, Watkins WD. Neuroendocrine correlates of lactate-induced panic and their response to chronic alprazolam therapy. *Am J Psychiatry* 1986;143:483–494.
6. Carr DB, Ballantyne JC, Osgood PF, Kemp JW, Szyfelbein SK. Pituitary-adrenal stress response in the absence of brain-pituitary connections. *Anesth Analg* 1989;69:197–201.
7. Carr DB, Athanasiadis CG, Skourtis T, Fishman SM, Fahmy NR, Lappas DG. Quantitative relationships between plasma beta-endorphin immunoactivity and hemodynamic performance in preoperative cardiac surgical patients. *Anesth Analg* 1989;68:77–82.
8. Hirata Y, Itoh K-I, Ando K, Endo M, Marumo F. Plasma endothelin levels during surgery. *N Engl J Med* 1989;321:1686.

9. Raine AEG, Erne P, Burgisser E, Muller FB, Bolli P, Burkart F, Buhler FR. Atrial natriuretic peptide and atrial pressure in patients with congestive heart failure. *N Engl J Med* 1986;315: 533–537.
10. Carr DB, Murphy MR. Operation, anesthesia and the endorphin system. In: Napolitano LM, Chernow B, eds. *Stress responses during anesthesia (International Anesthesia Clinics,* vol 26). Boston: Little, Brown, 1988;199–205.
11. Carr DB, Reppert SM, Bullen BA, Skrinar GS, Beitins IZ, Arnold MA, Rosenblatt M, Martin JB, McArthur JW. Plasma melatonin increases during exercise in women. *J Clin Endocrinol Metab* 1981;53:224–225.
12. George JM, Reier CE, Lanese RR, Rower JM. Morphine anesthesia blocks cortisol and growth hormone response to surgical stress in humans. *J Clin Endocrinol Metab* 1974;38:736–741.
13. Newsome HH, Rose JC. The response of human adrenocorticotropic hormone and growth hormone to surgical stress. *J Clin Endocrinol* 1971;33:481–487.
14. Brandt MR, Korshin J, Hansen AP, et al. Influence of morphine anaesthesia on the endocrine-metabolic response to open-heart surgery. *Acta Anaesthesiol Scand* 1978;22:400–412.
15. Hall GM, Young C, Holdcroft A, Alaghband-Zadeh J. Substrate mobilisation during surgery: a comparison between halothane and fentanyl anesthesia. *Anaesthesia* 1978;33:924–930.
16. Stanley TH, Philbin DM, Coggins CH, et al. Fentanyl-oxygen anesthesia for coronary artery surgery: cardiovascular and antidiuretic hormone responses. *Can Anaesth Soc J* 1979;26:168–172.
17. Stanley TH, Berman L, Green O, Robertson D. Plasma catecholamine and cortisol responses to fentanyl-oxygen anesthesia for coronary-artery operations. *Anesthesiology* 1980;53:250–253.
18. Haxholdt O, Kehlet H, Dyrburg V. Effect of fentanyl on the cortisol and hyperglycaemic response to abdominal surgery. *Acta Anaesthesiol Scand* 1981;25:434–436.
19. Cooper GM, Paterson JL, Ward ID, Hall GM. Fentanyl and the metabolic response to gastric surgery. *Anaesthesia* 1981;36:667–671.
20. Walsh ES, Paterson JL, O'Riordan JBA, Hall GM. Effect of high-dose fentanyl anaesthesia on the metabolic and endocrine response to cardiac surgery. *Br J Anaesth* 1981;53:1155–1165.
21. Sebel PS, Bovill JG, Schellekens APN, Hawker CD. Hormonal responses to high-dose fentanyl anaesthesia. *Br J Anaesth* 1981;53:941–948.
22. Zurick AM, Urzua J, Yared J-P, Estafanous FG. Comparison of hemodynamic and hormonal effects of large single-dose fentanyl anesthesia and halothane/nitrous oxide anesthesia for coronary artery surgery. *Anesth Analg* 1982;61:521–526.
23. Campbell BC, Parikh RK, Naismith A, et al. Comparison of fentanyl and halothane supplementation to general anaesthesia on the stress response of upper abdominal surgery. *Br J Anaesth* 1984;56:257–261.
24. Hynynen M, Lehtinen AM, Salmenpera M, et al. Continuous infusion of fentanyl or alfentanil for coronary artery surgery: effects on plasma cortisol concentration, beta-endorphin immunoreactivity and arginine vasopressin. *Br J Anaesth* 1986;58:1260–1266.
25. Dubois M, Pickar D, Cohen MR, et al. Effects of fentanyl on the response of plasma beta-endorphin immunoreactivity to surgery. *Anesthesiology* 1982;57:468–472.
26. Cork RC, Hameroff SR, Weiss JL. Effects of halothane and fentanyl anesthesia on plasma beta-endorphin immunoreactivity during cardiac surgery. *Anesth Analg* 1985;64:677–680.
27. Carr DB, Rosenblatt M. Endorphins in the normal and abnormal pituitary. In: Black PMcL, Zervas N, Ridgway EC, Martin JB, eds. *Secretory tumors of the pituitary gland (Progress in endocrine research and therapy,* vol 1). New York: Raven Press, 1984;245–261.
28. Plotsky PM. Opioid inhibition of immunoreactive corticotropin-releasing factor into the hypophysial-portal circulation of rats. *Regul Pept* 1986;16:235–242.
29. Carr DB, Bergland RM, Hamilton A, Blume H, Kasting NW, Arnold MA, Martin JB, Rosenblatt M. Endotoxin-stimulated opioid peptide secretion: two secretory pools and feedback control in vivo. *Science* 1982;217:845–848.
30. Payne RM. Pain in peripheral neuropathy. In: Foley KM, Payne RM, eds. *Current therapy of pain.* Philadelphia: Decker, 1989;235–244.
31. Smith EM, Blalock JE. Human lymphocyte production of corticotropin and endorphin-like substances: association with leukocyte interferon. *Proc Natl Acad Sci USA* 1981;78:7530–7534.
32. Woloski BMNRJ, Smith EM, Meyer WJ, et al. Corticotropin-releasing activity of monokines. *Science* 1985;230:1035–1037.
33. Hargreaves KM, Costello AH, Joris JL. Release from inflamed tissue of a substance with properties similar to corticotropin-releasing factor. *Neuroendocrinology* 1989;49:476–482.

34. Blalock JE, Smith EM. A complete regulatory loop between the immune and neuroendocrine systems. *Fed Proc* 1985;44:108-111.
35. Dougherty PM, Dafny N. Neuroimmune intercommunication, central opioids, and the immune response to bacterial endotoxin. *J Neurosci Res* 1988;19:140-148.
36. Di Marzo V, Tippins JR, Morris HR. Neuropeptides and inflammatory mediators: bidirectional regulatory mechanisms. *Trends Pharm Sci* 1989;10:91-92.
37. Hamilton AJ, Carr DB, LaRovere JM, Black PMcL. Endotoxic shock elicits greater endorphin secretion than hemorrhage. *Circ Shock* 1986;19:47-54.
38. Selye H. A syndrome produced by diverse nocuous agents. *Nature* 1936;138:32.
39. Kehlet H. Modification of responses to surgery by neural blockade: clinical implications. In: Cousins MJ, Bridenbaugh PO, eds. *Neural blockade in clinical anesthesia and management of pain,* 2nd ed. Philadelphia: Lippincott, 1988;145-188.
40. Arnold MA, Carr D, Togasaki DM, Pian M, Martin JB. Caffeine stimulates beta-endorphin release in blood but not cerebrospinal fluid. *Life Sci* 1982;31:1017-1024.
41. Steinbrook R, Carr DB, Datta S, Naulty JS, Lee C, Fisher J. Dissociation of plasma and cerebrospinal fluid immunoactive beta-endorphin during pregnancy and parturition. *Anesth Analg* 1982;61:893-897.
42. Joris J, Dubner R, Hargreaves KM. Opioid analgesia at peripheral sites. *Anesth Analg* 1987;66: 1277-1281.
43. Morley JE. The endocrinology of the opiates and opioid peptides. *Metabolism* 1981;30:195-209.
44. Barraclough CA, Sawyer CH. Inhibition of the release of pituitary ovulatory hormone in the rat by morphine. *Endocrinology* 1955;57:329-337.
45. Zimmermann E, George R, eds. *Narcotics and the hypothalamus (Kroc Foundation Symposia, number 2).* New York: Raven, 1974.
46. Van Loon GR, Appel NM, Ho D. Beta-endorphin-induced stimulation of central sympathetic outflow: beta-endorphin increases plasma concentrations of epinephrine, norepinephrine, and dopamine in rats. *Endocrinology* 1981;109:46-53.
47. Vatner SF, Marsh JD, Swain JA. Effects of morphine on coronary and left ventricular dynamics in conscious dogs. *J Clin Invest* 1975;55:207-217.
48. Kasting NW, Carr DB, Martin JB, Blume H, Bergland RM. Changes in CSF and plasma vasopressin in the febrile sheep. *Can J Physiol Pharmacol* 1983;61:427-431.
49. Carr DB. Opioids. In: Firestone LL, ed. *Molecular basis of anesthetic drug action in anesthesia (International Anesthesia Clinics,* vol 26). Boston: Little, Brown, 1988;273-287.
50. Spiegel K, Kourides IA, Pasternak GW. Prolactin and growth hormone release by morphine in the rat: different receptor mechanisms. *Science* 1982;217:745-747.
51. Pfeiffer A, Pfeiffer DG. Differential involvement of central opiate receptor subtypes in prolactin and gonadotropin release. *Endocrinology* 1983;112(suppl):189.
52. Koenig JI, Mayfield MA, McCann SM, Krulich L. Differential role of the opioid mu and delta receptors in the activation of prolactin and growth hormone (GH) secretion by morphine in the male rat. *Life Sci* 1984;34:1829-1837.
53. Pechnick R, George R, Poland RE. Identification of multiple opiate receptors through neuroendocrine responses. I. Effects of agonists. *J Pharm Exp Ther* 1985;232:163-169.
54. Pechnick RN, George R, Poland RE. The effects of the acute administration of buprenorphine hydrochloride on the release of anterior pituitary hormones in the rat: evidence for the involvement of multiple receptors. *Life Sci* 1985;37:1861-1868.
55. Iyengar S, Kim HS, Wood PL. Effects of kappa opiate agonists on neurochemical and neuroendocrine indices: evidence for kappa receptor subtypes. *Life Sci* 1986;39:637-644.
56. Eisenberg RM. Plasma corticosterone changes in response to central or peripheral administration of kappa and sigma opiate agonists. *J Pharmacol Exp Ther* 1985;233:863-869.
57. Zsigmond EK, Durrani Z, Barabas E, et al. Endocrine and hemodynamic effects of antagonism of fentanyl-induced respiratory depression by nalbuphine. *Anesth Analg* 1987;66:421-426.
58. Ganong WF, Dallman MF, Roberts JL, eds. The hypothalamic-pituitary-adrenal axis revisited. *Ann NY Acad Sci* 1987;512:218-236.
59. Joseph SA, Pilcher WH, Knigge KM. Anatomy of the corticotropin-releasing factor and opiomelanocortin systems of the brain. *Fed Proc* 1985;44:100-107.

Advances in Pain Research and Therapy, Vol. 18,
edited by M. Max, R. Portenoy, and E. Laska,
Raven Press, Ltd., New York © 1991.

26

The Nurse-Observer

Observation Methods and Training

James A. Forbes

*Department of Psychiatry, Johns Hopkins University School of Medicine,
Baltimore, Maryland 21205*

Analgesic studies are usually executed by a research nurse referred to as a "nurse-observer" or "analgesic study nurse." Few publications address the duties or training of this individual (1,2). This chapter outlines the role of the nurse-observer in postoperative analgesic studies (3–6) my associates and I have completed; discussions with other investigators suggest these procedures are representative. I refer to the nurse-observer as female since all of our study nurses have been women; however, there are male nurse-observers.

INPATIENT ANALGESIC STUDIES

In the typical study, the nurse-observer controls the day-to-day activity of the clinical trial. It is the nurse-observer who selects patients, instructs patients concerning the study purposes and procedures, obtains written informed consent, administers the study medication, periodically interviews the patients in order to assess pain and its relief, remedicates the patients if necessary, follows the patients until adverse effects are resolved, completes appropriate study and institutional records, and keeps the research team and institutional staff informed. These activities are conducted according to a study protocol approved by the local institutional review board (IRB) and are under the supervision of the study's principal investigator.

The nurse-observer begins by reviewing the operating room schedule for the next working day. She will circle the name of any potential study patient, considering only those patients who are scheduled for a surgical procedure compatible with the inclusion/exclusion criteria of the study protocol, and whose attending physician is cooperating with the analgesic evaluation program.

Record Review

The hospital records for a potential patient should be thoroughly reviewed. Patients must meet the inclusion/exclusion criteria specified in the study protocol. In general, patients are excluded from studies if they are pregnant or lactating; have any history of hypersensitivity or serious adverse reaction to any agent similar to the study medications; have any clinically significant condition that would affect the absorption, metabolism, or excretion of the study medications; or require concomitant medication that might confound quantitating analgesia. Long-term users of analgesics or tranquilizers are also excluded. We also routinely exclude patients having a history of drug or alcohol dependence and patients who are known to have developed a tolerance to any medications similar to the study medications.

The nurse-observer cannot always accept the hospital records as gospel; she must question the patient directly if there is any reason to suspect an entry in the patient's official record. For example, it is not unusual to find a patient's hospital record flagged to indicate an allergy to aspirin or codeine when in fact the patient has experienced a dose-related adverse effect, e.g., nausea or dizziness to codeine, or dyspepsia and tinnitus following treatment with aspirin. A patient may deny alcohol or drug addiction on admission, then confess when symptoms suggestive of withdrawal appear postoperatively. Experience at several hospitals indicates it is impractical and unwise to attempt to correct the patient's hospital records in order for the patient to participate in a research study. As a matter of courtesy to the patient and hospital staff, we routinely note apparent discrepancies in official records in hopes that appropriate corrections will be made at a later date. For example, a patient whose chart is mislabeled "allergic to codeine" may be denied necessary and appropriate treatment.

In our initial studies, our nurse-observers contacted potential patients prior to surgery. This procedure was not satisfactory; some patients were anxious concerning the impending surgery and could not concentrate on the nurse-observer's presentation. In addition, we obtained written informed consent from patients who, for one reason or another, did not participate in the study after surgery. We decided to recruit patients postoperatively. This procedure was questioned by the local IRB since patients were being asked to participate in the study when they had pain. Some members of the IRB thought patients might feel under pressure to enter the study; these fears were dispelled when it was clear to the IRB that patients were offered a choice of routine analgesic or the study medication.

If the nurse-observer, after reviewing the patient's records, considers the patient eligible for the study she flags the patient's chart and medication record. The flag indicates the patient might participate in a pain study and requests the nurse-observer be notified before any analgesic medication is administered.

Our nurse-observer starts early in the morning before patients have awakened for breakfast. Experience indicates that patients often awaken and request analgesic medication when the ward nurses change shift. The nurse-observer tries to flag the charts of all potential patients before analgesic medication is requested or routinely administered. It is best to give the study medication as the first analgesic of the day. Since most patients will have slept during the night, the washout period following the last analgesic will be maximized. Otherwise, if routine analgesic is administered prior to the study medication, it might be 3 to 6 hrs before the patient needs additional medication for pain. The nurse-observer may be faced with the decision of not entering the patient in the study or potentially staying at the hospital late in the day if the patient participates in a 6- or 8-hr study and has relief for the entire period. Our nurse-observers are on duty only during the day shift and we prefer the patient to be evaluated by one nurse.

After flagging charts for potential patients, the nurse-observer locates the attending nurse in order to determine the patient's current status, whether the patient is alert and capable of fluent communication, and whether there are any contraindications that might preclude the patient's participation in the study. A special effort is made to thank the staff nurses for their assistance. It is impossible to conduct an analgesic study without the complete cooperation of ward personnel. If time permits, our nurse-observers will help ward nurses with routine tasks.

Patient Interview

After reviewing all charts and interviewing appropriate attending staff, the nurse-observer waits to be notified that one of her patients has requested medication for pain. Experience has taught us to respond promptly to messages from the attending nurse. If potential patients have to request pain medication a second time, the attending nurse will probably medicate the patient instead of continuing to wait for the nurse-observer.

Purpose and Procedures of the Study

Although the nurse-observer has a considerable amount of information about the patient before their first meeting, the initial interview is a complex social situation. The nurse-observer must establish rapport with the patient quickly, decide if the patient is acceptable, and if all is satisfactory, completely brief the patient and obtain written informed consent in 5 to 10 min. Our nurse-observers have found it best to be concise and businesslike.

Initially, our approach was to have the nurse-observer explain who she was and discuss the nature of the study as soon as she entered the patient's room. We have revised our procedures in order to address the patient's complaint first and discuss the study second.

The nurse-observer begins her first meeting with the patient by saying, "How are you doing?" This very general question gives the patient an opportunity to express any symptoms; usually the patient will indicate that he has pain and medication has been requested. The nurse-observer will then ask the following questions and record the appropriate data:

> Do you have pain now? Where is the pain located? Can you describe the pain; for example, is it dull, pulling, sharp, etc? Would you describe your pain as mild (slight, a little), moderate (a medium amount), or severe (a lot)? Do you need to take medication to relieve the pain?

If a visual analogue scale (VAS) is being used, the nurse-observer will ask the patient to mark the VAS line indicating the severity of their pain. Appropriate information is recorded on a worksheet. If the patient has moderate or severe pain, indicates the need for medication, and is acceptable, the nurse-observer introduces herself and outlines the purpose and procedures of the study. *It must be made clear at this time that participation in the study is voluntary and routine medication can be administered immediately instead of discussing the study further.* If the patient is unacceptable the nurse-observer or attending nurse will medicate the patient with a routine analgesic.

This initial interview is very demanding and calls for clinical judgment on the part of the nurse-observer. She must decide if the patient has clinically significant pain and whether the patient will be cooperative. There are many reasons for rejecting patients, e.g., a patient's pain may be too severe for the study medications. The nurse-observer always makes the final decision concerning the acceptability of a patient, if protocol criteria are met and approval has been granted by the attending physician.

As indicated, acceptable patients are given a choice of taking the analgesic ordered by their physician or being informed about the study by the nurse-observer. Patients interested in participating are thoroughly briefed concerning all aspects of the study for legal, ethical, and scientific reasons. The patient must understand what drugs are being studied, and the potential analgesic response to each, in order to prevent having a biased anticipatory set favoring a particular response. For example, if one were evaluating 1,000 mg diflunisal, 650 mg aspirin, and placebo, and diflunisal was discussed longer and more enthusiastically than the aspirin standard it might leave the patient with the impression that their dose of study medication would be the long-acting diflunisal.

In the previous example, the nurse-observer would emphasize, "You will get only *one* of the three treatments: diflunisal, aspirin, or placebo. I do not know and you will not know which medication you will get. You could have complete relief for 8 hrs, no relief at all, or a medium amount of relief for a few hours." Patient responses indicate that they do not expect a specific result from the medication following these instructions; instead, they are open to any treatment outcome. In this case, patients would also understand their chance of receiving placebo would be 1 out of 3.

Written Informed Consent

It is not easy to obtain written informed consent and fulfill the true intent of this requirement. Unfortunately, consent forms have become lengthy, often legalistic documents that are difficult for the average patient to understand. The study consent form is a matter for the principal investigator and the IRB to resolve; however, pharmaceutical company sponsors often attempt to dictate the format and content of consent forms. In some cases, the sponsor adds terminology to limit its liability to study patients. IRBs, on the other hand, seem to have gone in the direction of portraying every study as very high risk. It is difficult to give a balanced presentation of a study in a consent form approvable by both the company sponsor and the IRB.

It is mandatory that the nurse-observer describe the adverse effects that have occurred with the study medications and important for her to discuss the relative incidence of these effects in order for the patient to truly understand the potential risks. We have had some problems over this issue since IRBs object to the nurse-observer saying anything that might seem to diminish the patient's concern about entering the study. For example, when evaluating a new nonsteroidal antiinflammatory drug (NSAID) that had undergone extensive clinical evaluation and had a very low incidence of adverse effects, the nurse-observer could not say, "Patients have had fewer adverse effects with this drug than with a routine dose of aspirin," despite data supporting this conclusion.

Although a witness is required for informed consent, it is often difficult, or impossible, to have a staff member present during the entire briefing. Frequently the nurse-observer will explain the study in detail, have the patient read the consent form, and then call the attending nurse. At that time the nurse-observer might say, in the presence of the attending nurse, "I have completely explained the study to Mr. Smith, he has read the consent form, I have answered his questions, and he is willing to volunteer to participate in the study. Is that correct Mr. Smith?" If the patient affirms his willingness to enter the study, the patient will date and sign the consent form in the presence of the staff nurse, then the staff nurse and nurse-observer will date and sign the consent form.

Baseline and Interval Evaluations

When the patient is found to be acceptable and has signed the consent form, the nurse-observer will administer the study medication recording the time and baseline pain severity on a study worksheet. She places a copy of the signed consent form in the patient's records and notes the administration of the study medication in the patient's chart, usually in the nursing notes and medication record. The flags on the patient's chart and medication record will be changed to indicate that the patient *is participating* in the "pain study" and should not be medicated without notifying the nurse-observer.

Interval evaluations of the patient should be consistent in content and format; the nurse-observer asks the same questions in the same manner at each interview. She always offers all alternative descriptors for pain, relief, and acceptability. The patient's position and/or activity should be relatively the same at each interview, and each interview should be conducted within 5 min of the scheduled time, awakening the patient if necessary. The nurse-observer must question the patient concerning any adverse effect observed or reported in order to determine the adverse effect's nature, onset, duration, and level of severity. If she has any questions concerning the patient's behavior or vocal responses she requests a clarification or explanation.

The nurse-observer must make every effort to be objective in interacting with the patient, emphasizing that the patient give an honest appraisal of the medication whether it is good or bad. In general the nurse-observer will avoid agreeing with or approving of the patient's responses, since this may inadvertently reinforce the patient and bias his or her response. Interaction with the patient should be limited to behavior, questions, and responses that are related to the patient's pain, relief, or emergent symptoms. The nurse-observer should not become involved with the patient while the patient is on the study since this may influence the patient's response. For example, if the patient likes the nurse-observer, the patient may be reluctant to say the medication is not working. The placebo effect may be enhanced if the nurse-observer is too friendly and assuring. Despite these cautions, the patient must not have the feeling of being rushed during interviews and must feel confident that his pain will be treated if relief from the study medication is inadequate.

The nurse-observer will ask the following questions and record the appropriate data at each interval evaluation.

General

"How are you doing?" This gives the patient a chance to express his symptoms and describe any changes since the last interview.

Pain

"Do you have pain now?" If the patient has pain, ask "Would you describe your pain as mild, moderate, or severe?" Then ask, "Where is the pain located?" This helps assure that the patient is talking about the same pain described at baseline. "Can you describe the pain, for example, is it dull, pulling, sharp, etc.?"

Relief

"How much relief from the starting pain is the study medication giving you now: none, a little (slight), some (a moderate amount), a lot, or complete relief?"

50% Relief

"Remember the pain you had when you took the study medication? Is that pain at least half gone: yes or no?"

Acceptability

The patient's overall evaluation or acceptability of the study medication will be determined by asking, "Taking into consideration: how much relief you have had, if any; how quickly the medication worked; how long the medication worked; and any other effects you experienced, would you rate this medication as being poor, fair, good, very good, or excellent?"

Adverse Effects

The nurse-observer should note *any* effects she observes and *any* effects reported by the patient. She will attempt to determine the time of onset, the duration, and the severity of any potential adverse effects. In the event of a clinically significant adverse effect, the first objective is to treat the patient as needed; the nurse-observer will notify the attending nurse, principal investigator, attending physician, and local IRB in a timely manner. Any clinically significant, serious, or unanticipated adverse effect will be reported to the sponsor as soon as practical by telephone and subsequently in a formal written report signed by the investigator and nurse-observer. Decisions concerning the relationship of the adverse effects to the study medication are made jointly by the nurse-observer and the investigator.

Remediation

If the patient completes the study, the nurse-observer or the attending nurse will remedicate the patient with the routine, ordered analgesic if additional medication is needed. The nurse-observer should administer routine, ordered analgesic if after 2 hrs, or the agreed-upon waiting period, the patient *requests* medication for pain and (a) the patient *stays* at baseline pain and is experiencing no relief; (b) the patient's pain *returns* to baseline level and he is experiencing no relief; (c) the patient's pain *increases* and he is experiencing no relief; or (d) in the opinion of the nurse-observer it is in the best interest of the patient to remedicate him at that time.

Entry and Exit Notes

The nurse-observer must record certain information in the hospital records describing the patient's participation in the study; usually this is recorded in the nursing notes. For example, the nurse-observer might record the following: "Ms. Smith reported moderate postoperative pain at 10:15 AM and became Patient 106 in Vicodin Study 8922. Two tablets of study medication were administered po at 10:20 AM". Adverse effects occurring anytime during the study period should be recorded in the nursing notes. The nurse-observer should note the nature of the adverse effect, time of onset, severity, termination time, and whether the effect required treatment, e.g., "Ms. Smith reported moderate dizziness at 12:05 PM ending at 6:30 PM; no treatment required." In addition, a copy of the signed consent form must be inserted in the patient's record.

After the patient has completed the study, the nurse-observer should indicate when the patient was last evaluated, the patient's general condition with respect to pain at that time, and indicate whether the patient's response to the study medication was satisfactory. Many patients will require remediation with a routine analgesic before the end of the study evaluation period. The nurse-observer should evaluate the patient after the administration of the backup analgesic in order to assure that the patient is getting satisfactory relief; response to the routine analgesic should also be recorded in the nursing notes.

Early Termination From Study

Evaluation of the patient may be terminated by the nurse-observer prior to completion of the scheduled interviews, if (a) the patient refuses to be interviewed; (b) it is necessary to administer a medication that conflicts with the study; or (c) the nurse-observer thinks it is in the best interest of the patient to end his participation in the study.

OUTPATIENT ANALGESIC STUDIES

In the typical oral surgery outpatient study the nurse-observer selects patients, instructs them concerning the study procedures, issues study medication and materials, debriefs patients at a postoperative follow-up visit, and follows the patient until any adverse effects or postoperative complications are resolved. She controls the day-to-day activity of the clinical trial and is completing what Sidman (7) would call an "exact replication" of the experiment completed on the previous patients; each patient receives the same instructions, study materials, etc. Therefore, differences in outcome, i.e., analgesic efficacy, are, it is hoped, owing to drug effect as opposed to other factors, such as variations in instructions given by the nurse-observer.

The following discussion outlines the role of the nurse-observer in our oral surgery outpatient analgesic trials (8–10, see Chapter 15). These procedures should be applicable to other outpatient populations, such as those with pain related to orthopedic surgery, dysmenorrhea, podiatric surgery, etc.

Study Procedures

Potential subjects are interviewed preoperatively by the nurse-observer. The purposes and the procedures of the study are explained to participants in detail after the presurgical consult and on the day of surgery. Patients must give written informed consent. The participation of minors requires the written informed consent of a parent or legal guardian, in addition to that of the minor.

On the day of surgery, after a briefing on the study procedures, each patient receives a packet of materials containing: a Patient Self-Rating Record-1 (PSRR-1) to be used to evaluate the study medication; the study medication; a common kitchen timer; a supply of a standard analgesic (e.g., codeine phosphate 30 mg with acetaminophen 325 mg) to be used as a backup if additional pain relief is needed after taking the study medication; and a Patient Self-Rating Record-2 (PSRR-2) to be used as a diary for the backup analgesic or to evaluate doses subsequent to dose 1 in repeat-dose studies. Patients are instructed to take the study medication when (a) their pain is steady, as opposed to transient; (b) the pain is moderate or severe in intensity; and (c) they feel they must take an analgesic to relieve the pain. They record the time and intensity of their baseline pain when they medicate. Then they are required to complete the following statements at periodic intervals (e.g., hourly) for the duration of the study period or until remedication is necessary: my pain at this time is: none (0), slight (1), moderate (2), severe (3); my relief from starting pain is: none (0), a little (1), some (2), a lot (3), complete (4); my starting pain is at least $\frac{1}{2}$ gone: no (0), yes (1). A visual analogue scale for pain intensity, relief, or some other measure, e.g., anxiety, may also be employed.

At the end of the evaluation period, e.g., hour 8 in an 8-hr study, or at the time the patient takes backup analgesic, the patient makes an overall evaluation of the study medication as poor (0), fair (1), good (2), very good (3), or excellent (4), taking into consideration the onset, level, and duration of relief as well as any other effects experienced. Adverse effects are noted on the self-rating record. Patients are asked to give the study medication at least 2 hrs to manifest an effect before taking the first dose of the backup medication, not to remedicate as long as they are having any relief, not to remedicate if their pain is less than moderate, and to complete the next scheduled evaluation of the study medication before remedicating.

The nurse-observer instructs the patient as to study procedures, but unlike the inpatient study, she is not present to assure patient compliance. In a sense, the nurse-observer is training the patient to be an investigator or researcher. Instructions must be complete and she must have some way of determining whether the patient understood; this requires clinical experience with patients. Written instructions attached to the PSRRs and medication serve only to remind the patient of the nurse-observer's briefing; they cannot be depended upon to control the patient's behavior after he has left the office. We think lengthy written instructions often confuse the patient.

Postoperative Follow-up

The nurse-observer will make a telephone call to each of her patients the evening of surgery in order to determine their medical status, e.g., bleeding, and ask if there are any questions concerning the study. The telephone follow-up is usually very brief and cannot substitute for thorough instructions at the preoperative briefing.

When patients return to the oral surgeon's office 5 to 7 days after surgery for suture removal the nurse-observer will conduct a study debriefing with the patient by reviewing both PSRRs and counting returned medication. She will try to clarify any discrepancies in the patient's report forms. If patients have a postoperative complication, or need additional analgesic, they are terminated from the study, given appropriate treatment, and followed by the nurse-observer until all problems are resolved.

The postoperative debriefing is a critical part of the study. It is, in most instances, the nurse-observer's last opportunity to ask the patient questions concerning responses on the PSRRs. It is very easy to overlook missing data and/or inconsistencies. We have found it very useful to have the nurse-observer review the patient's study behavior chronologically starting with the completion of surgery. For example, she might say to a patient, "You completed your surgery at 2:30 PM last Tuesday. You took both tablets of study medication at 5:15 PM for moderate pain. At 6:20 PM your pain was moderate, you had a little relief, but your starting pain was not half gone. At 7:15 PM . . .", etc. Following this procedure, the nurse-observer will probably note missing evaluations, illegible entries, instances where the patient has multiple-rated (e.g., selected more than one descriptor), entries that lack internal consistency (e.g., both pain and relief increase simultaneously), and other discrepancies. While participating in the review of the PSRRs the patient might observe an error and bring it to the attention of the nurse-observer. Inconsistent responses are questioned; however, there is no pressure on the patient to change the response. Ultimately, the investigator will review the PSRRs and determine whether the patient's efficacy ratings are valid; this decision is made before the blind is broken. A reason must be given for invalidating a patient's efficacy data (e.g., evaluations were too far off schedule, the patient did not take all of the study medication, etc.). Table 3 in Chapter 15 summarizes the reasons for invalidating efficacy data in more than 20 oral surgery outpatient studies.

Entry and Exit Notes

As in the inpatient study, the nurse-observer must record certain information in the office records describing the patient's participation in the study. Usually she notes the date and time, the study designator, patient's assigned number, description of the study medication issued, description of the backup medication issued, and any other pertinent information. A copy of the signed consent and study case report forms (CRFs) are maintained in the oral surgeon's office. Information recorded in the office records (e.g., health history) must be consistent with the entries on the CRFs. Study patients may have been seen in the office previously over a period of years; data (e.g., weight, current medications, telephone number, etc.) must be updated when the patient is screened for the study.

TRAINING

All of our nurse-observers have been Registered Nurses (RN), which has had several advantages. Their training is more comprehensive than that of other nursing personnel, e.g. a Licensed Practical Nurse. One must be an RN in order to administer narcotics and parenteral medications at some institutions. The nurse-observer, as an RN, is able to deal with hospital nursing personnel on an equal footing. It is not necessary for the nurse-observer to have had any previous experience in research; however, it is helpful for the nurse to have had some experience with the patient population being evaluated.

Observation of An Experienced Nurse-Observer

Initially, a new nurse-observer is scheduled to observe a working, experienced nurse-observer for several days. She sees all phases of her new job and is exposed to the mechanics of the situation. The trainee sees the nurse-observer schedule patients, conduct briefings, fill out CRFs, conduct postoperative debriefings, make entries in the patient's chart, secure study medications, and interact with non-study staff members.

Reading Assignments

The nurse-observer must have a working knowledge of numerous subjects related to analgesics and their evaluation. Our nurse-observers have found it useful to read *Analgesic Drugs* by Parkhouse, Pleuvry, and Rees (2). It gives an overview of pain mechanisms, the pharmacology of analgesics, and has a brief section on controlled clinical trials of analgesics including the "use of trained observers."

Reprints by Beaver (11–13), our group, and other investigators are read and discussed. We want the nurse-observers to understand concepts such as the placebo effect, assay sensitivity, upside assay sensitivity, plateau effect of NSAIDs, the lack of plateau effect with narcotics, additivity of narcotic and nonnarcotic analgesics, study designs (parallel and crossover), the effect of error variance on discrimination, relative potency studies, relative potency of narcotics by various routes of administration, and interpretation of time-effect curves. The nurse-observer takes a written test after discussing these concepts.

Although some investigators have a new nurse-observer conduct a pilot study for training purposes (see commentary p. 630), we do not find this necessary.

Our nurse-observers start with a sponsored study. The nurse-observer and I review the study protocol, CRFs, worksheets for inpatient studies, Patient Self-Rating Records 1 and 2 (PSRR-1 and -2) for outpatient studies, consent form, IRB submission, investigational brochure, and any applicable reprints. The nurse-observer is issued a current *Physicians' Desk Reference* (PDR) (14), *Physicians' Desk Reference For Nonprescription Drugs* (15), a copy of *The Merck Manual* (16), and a medical dictionary. These she can use to reference standard analgesics and concomitant medications employed in the study.

After reading, reviewing, and discussing the aforementioned information I prepare what our nurse-observers call a "spiel" or "presentation." This an outline of the nurse-observer's presentation to the patient; it starts with the nurse-observer introducing herself and includes all information pertinent to the patient's participation in the study.

Nurse-observers conducting an outpatient study are issued a sample packet containing a PSRR-1 with dummy medication attached, a PSRR-2, dummy backup medication, a felt-tipped pen, and a common kitchen timer. Using these materials she practices reading the presentation and showing the appropriate forms to any willing helper. She repeatedly briefs another experienced nurse-observer. After experienced nurse-observers approve of the trainee's performance the trainee gives the presentation to my assistant, and finally gives the presentation to me as if I were a potential patient. She may have to "brief" me for the study several times before being approved to work with patients.

Next she starts the study under the supervision of an experienced nurse-observer. When the supervisor thinks it appropriate, the new nurse-observer works alone for one week, requesting assistance if necessary. The new nurse is then periodically monitored by someone from my staff.

Our study protocols are signed by each member of the research team; this indicates each member has reviewed the protocol and all associated documents, and intends to conduct the study as outlined. Patients sign PSRR-1 and PSRR-2. Only the nurse-observer and I, acting as principal investigator, sign the CRFs in addition to the PSRRs. Our signatures indicate we have reviewed the CRFs and attest to their accuracy to the best of our knowledge. I discuss any discrepancies with the nurse-observer and there is a resolution before CRFs are signed and released to the study sponsor. These discussions also serve as a potential teaching device; they are an opportunity to remind the nurse-observer of the standardized procedures.

Corrections on CRFs or PSRRs are made by drawing a line through the incorrect entry, entering the correct data nearby, then initialing and dating the transaction.

Monitoring the Performance of the Nurse-Observer

In some respects, the nurse-observer's first study is the easiest for the investigator. Most new nurse-observers are very concerned about performing well and adhere to their instructions religiously. They do not want to have a study with poor assay sensitivity, e.g., a "big placebo effect." The new nurse-observer is alert and conscientious. That attitude sometimes changes after the nurse-observer has completed one or more successful analgesic trials.

Parkhouse (1) comments on this phenomenon:

> There is a large element of human interest, but this tends to be offset by the need for a measure of detachment and avoidance of personal involvement with the patient. With time there comes a staleness and here the "within-observer" variation is likely to arise.

This seems to be an increasing problem over time; the rigid standardization becomes more flexible and variation creeps into the study results. Parkhouse uses the term "staleness" to describe this phenomenon; boredom and overconfidence may play a role. The nurse-observer may fail to adhere to inclusion/exclusion criteria, reduce the time to brief a patient, miss a postoperative debriefing, or miss discrepancies on the PSRRs. There seems to be an attitude that "everything will work out." Although most analgesic models are reasonably robust, they are not bulletproof.

The investigator must establish some system for monitoring the activities of the nurse-observer and the quality of the data in order to ensure compliance with standardized procedures. This is best done by periodically observing the nurse-observer briefing and debriefing patients, using the reviews of CRFs and PSRRs as a teaching device, holding routine training and discussion sessions with all staff nurse-observers, and having the nurse-observers monitor each other.

In the past we have used interim analyses of study data to monitor the system of measurement. Unfortunately, in studies done by the pharmaceutical industry, there is almost a complete ban on using interim analyses and the result may very well be a decrease in the quality of research trials (see pp. 88–89).

Part of our monitoring program includes annual meetings for our nurse-observers. These 3- to 5-day sessions involve lectures and open discussions concerning all aspects of an analgesic trial. Studies completed by our nurse-observers are presented and discussed. Usually a comprehensive examination is given. Nurses are encouraged to discuss problems and solutions in conducting clinical studies.

Finally, the nurse-observer must be considered a full member of the research team and must be involved in decisions concerning the conduct of the study. In addition, the nurse-observer should be a coauthor on any manuscript published from her work.

CONCLUSIONS

The nurse-observer, or analgesic study nurse, is the central figure in an analgesic study. She provides the day-to-day standardization for the system of measurement. Appropriate selection, training, and monitoring of the nurse-observer increases the probability of being able to repeatedly conduct sensitive analgesic assays.

ACKNOWLEDGMENTS

I am indebted to current members of my research team (Irene A. Edquist, Katherine F. Jones, Carolyn J. Kehm, Janet A. Saltzer-Bates, Christina Adolfsson, Eva Nyqvist), previous nurse-observers (Billie A. Barkaszi, Geraldine A. Butterworth, Bette M. Chachich, Virginia M. Foor, Charlene D. Grodin, Ethel M. Moore, Barbara A. Newman, Martha S. Reuss, Christine C. Yorio), and to Alice Lawrence Forbes for her assistance in training and monitoring our staff nurses and in preparation of this manuscript.

REFERENCES

1. Parkhouse J. Subjective assessment of analgesics. *Anaesthesia* 1967;22:37–42.
2. Parkhouse J, Pleuvry BJ, Rees JMH. *Analgesic drugs.* London: Blackwell Scientific Publications, 1979.
3. Forbes JA, Kolodny AL, Beaver WT, Shackleford RW, Scarlett VR. A 12-hour evaluation of the analgesic efficacy of diflunisal, acetaminophen, an acetaminophen-codeine combination, and placebo in postoperative pain. *Pharmacotherapy* 1983;(3:Pt 2):47S–54S.
4. Forbes JA, Kolodny AL, Chachich BM, Beaver WT. Nalbuphine, acetaminophen, and their combination in postoperative pain. *Clin Pharmacol Ther* 1984;35:843–851.
5. Forbes JA, Kolodny AL. An evaluation of a hydrocodone-acetaminophen combination, a codeine-acetaminophen combination, and placebo in postoperative pain. 1990 (submitted).
6. Bostrom A, Forbes JA, Sevelius H, Bynum L, Beaver WT. A repeat dose evaluation of naproxen sodium and a naproxen sodium-codeine combination in postoperative pain. *Clin Pharmacol Ther* 1987;41:228.
7. Sidman M. *Tactics of scientific research.* New York: Basic Books, 1960.
8. Forbes JA, Butterworth GA, Burchfield WH, Yorio CC, Selinger LR, Rosenmertz SK, Beaver WT. Evaluation of flurbiprofen, acetaminophen, an acetaminophen-codeine combination, and placebo in postoperative oral surgery pain. *Pharmacotherapy* 1989;9:322–330.
9. Forbes JA, Butterworth GA, Burchfield WH, Beaver WT. An evaluation of ketorolac, aspirin, and an acetaminophen-codeine combination in postoperative oral surgery pain. *Pharmacotherapy* 1990;10.
10. Forbes JA, Kehm CJ, Grodin CD, Beaver WT. An evaluation of ketorolac, ibuprofen, acetaminophen, and an acetaminophen-codeine combination in postoperative oral surgery pain. *Pharmacotherapy* 1990;10.
11. Beaver WT. Measurement of analgesic efficacy in man. In: Bonica JJ, Lindblom U, Iggo A, eds. *Advances in pain research and therapy,* vol 5. New York: Raven Press, 1983;411–434.
12. Beaver WT. Maximizing the benefits of weaker analgesics. In: *Refresher courses on pain management.* Seattle: International Association for the Study of Pain, 1987;1–25.
13. Beaver WT. Nonsteroidal antiinflammatory analgesics and their combinations with opioids. In: Aronoff GM, ed. *Evaluation and treatment of chronic pain,* 2nd ed. Baltimore: Urban & Schwarzenberg, (in press).
14. *Physicians' desk reference,* 44th ed. Oradell, NJ: Medical Economics Company, 1990.
15. *Physicians' desk reference for nonprescription drugs,* 10th ed. Oradell, NJ: Medical Economics Company, 1989.
16. Berkow R, ed. *The Merck manual of diagnosis and therapy,* 15th ed. Rahway, NJ: Merck & Co., 1987.

Advances in Pain Research and Therapy, Vol. 18,
edited by M. Max, R. Portenoy, and E. Laska,
Raven Press, Ltd., New York © 1991.

Commentary

The Nurse-Observer and the Conduct of Clinical Trials

Ada G. Rogers

*Pain Service, Department of Neurology, Memorial Sloan-Kettering
Cancer Center, New York, New York 10021*

James Forbes has meticulously documented the importance of the study nurse observer as a member of the research team, and has described the observation and training methods employed in his group. Some groups have employed non-nursing personnel and physician assistants as observers. The advantage of employing nurses rather than nonnursing personnel is that nurses have the experience at the bedside, can legally administer analgesics, and have the necessary medical knowledge to scrutinize medical charts and assess the capability of the patient to communicate (1).

INPATIENT ANALGESIC STUDIES

Forbes states that contact between the nurse-observers and investigator may be unusual. This is probably true when you have group of experienced nurse-observers with one acting as the coordinator or supervisor; however, when you have only one nurse-observer, contact with the investigator is necessary and essential. The nurse-observer needs someone with whom to discuss the day's events and resolve problems. It takes a nurse-observer several months before she feels comfortable conducting the studies. A feeling of isolation may be very discouraging even for an experienced nurse-observer. The investigator or his designee should meet with the nurse-observer as often as she feels is necessary. At Memorial Sloan-Kettering Cancer Center, the clinical coordinator meets with nurse-observers at the end of each day for a daily report. The clinical coordinator has access to the investigator at all times. This promotes continuity and a feeling of being an important part of the research team.

Record Review

Over the past 38 years, we have conducted analgesic studies in cancer patients with chronic or postoperative pain. For the most part, patients selected to participate in postoperative analgesic studies have not been tolerant to narcotics and tend to respond as other patients who have undergone surgery (2). In chronic pain, patients fall into two groups: those who are not tolerant to narcotics and those who are. Even postoperative patients may have received narcotics perioperatively or immediately postoperatively, e.g., in the recovery room; therefore, in these situations there are relatively few narcotic-naive patients. In the cancer population, patients are selected based on the type of pain, class of drugs, route of administration, and dosage of the analgesics to be studied. The narcotic-tolerant patients would not be suitable for a postoperative study of an agonist-antagonist or a nonnarcotic analgesic. A patient who is receiving chemotherapy may not be selected to participate in an analgesic study. The emotional impact of a cancer diagnosis may indeed affect the study results but this may be reduced by using a crossover design where the patient serves as his own control.

Patient Interview

The choice of whether to interview patients for study before or after surgery depends on the hospital institutional review board (IRB) and in some instance the sponsor and the FDA. Forbes points out that they were unsuccessful in obtaining patients for study before surgery. We prefer interviewing patients preoperatively. Our nurse-observer may often come in on Sunday to screen and interview patients scheduled for surgery on Monday. Although our patients are probably more anxious about their surgeries, they also are concerned about adequate pain control after surgery. The advantage of seeing them before surgery gives us the opportunity to assess the patient's ability to communicate without anesthesia or analgesia on board, to explain the study fully while they are not in pain, and to obtain informed consent in a patient who is alert. Our interview may take at least 15 min to explain the purpose of the study and acquaint patients with the questions to be asked, the type of drugs to be studied, and any possible adverse effects. At times, we may leave the consent with the patient and return later to answer any questions about the study. We have found that even the day after surgery, some patients are too sleepy or confused to obtain an informed consent. We also have found that patients will not participate in a study if they are satisfied with their present analgesic. The best time may depend on the type of patient, surgery performed, and the general setting.

When we obtain consent, consents and IRB protocols are inserted in the patient's chart and a note written on the progress sheet indicating that the patient has consented to participate in a postoperative analgesic study starting the first day after surgery. During the study, notes are written on the progress sheet rather than in the nurse's notes. The chart, patient's door, and medication cardex are flagged. On the first postoperative day, our nurse-observers start their first round between 8 and 9 AM seeing every patient that has signed a consent and checking their charts for the outcome of the surgery, their stay in the recovery room, and the analgesics received in the last 24 hrs. They will medicate the patient with a test drug if 3 hrs have elapsed since their last analgesic and the patient reports at least a moderate amount of pain. If the patient does not require medication at that time, the patients will be seen every hour thereafter until the patient has sufficient pain to medicate with the test preparation.

The patient's appearance or behavior (watching television, putting curlers in her hair) is not used to determine the patient's suitability to enter the study. We have been trained to accept the patient's verbal reports of pain. We will delay starting the study if the patient appears to be too sleepy, confused, disoriented, or does not report moderate or severe pain on moving or coughing. Each patient is assessed for any activity that the patient states makes the pain worse. Pain may increase when patients cough, move, turn from side to side, sit up in bed, elevate, or move extremities. These activities should be assessed before the administration of a test medication. It is simple to ask what makes the pain worse. If coughing makes the pain worse then the instruction to the patient is "Tell me how much pain you have while you are coughing—no pain, slight pain, moderate pain, or severe pain." Same for relief. The same position and activity should be done at each subsequent observation; however, there may be times when the position may not be exactly the same, e.g., patient may be in bed for the first few observations and then may be in a chair. The difference is not really that great. The patient could be moved or coughed while in the chair. The patient should always be requestioned if the nurse-observer feels that the patient's answers are inconsistent or that the patient does not seem to understand the questions or the assessment tool being used, e.g., the patient reports "no pain" but reports the relief as a lot rather than complete. Patients should be requestioned for pain intensity and pain relief. In using visual analogue scales, make sure the patient realizes which end of the scale is the least possible pain and which end is the worst possible pain (3). This sometimes is confusing for the patient and may cause inconsistent reports. The scale can easily be explained without leading the patient. At no time should the patient be told that the middle of the 100-mm line represents moderate pain.

Some ward activities may interfere with the study observations. This can be overcome by a full explanation to the ward personnel and by coordinating the patient's activities with the study observations, e.g., asking the patient's nurse when she plans to get her out of bed, etc. The same with the physical therapist and x-ray technician. The nurse observer has a leeway of 10 min to complete her observation when some of these activities may have to be done.

Since we need a 6-hr period to interview the patient after the test medication is administered, patients will not receive the test medication after 11 AM unless the nurse-observer decides to work later that day if necessary. During some of our pharmacokinetic studies the nurse observer may be required to work as long as 12 hrs on a 1- or 2-day study. I agree with Forbes that the nurse-observer makes the final decision to accept the patient for study.

OUTPATIENT STUDIES

Our outpatient studies most often involve patients with chronic pain. Patients are selected primarily from patients seen on in-hospital pain consults who have been discharged or those who are attending our pain clinic. The studies may involve the assessment of analgesic response, pharmacokinetics, or both.

Patients may come into the clinic and stay for a period of 8 hrs for a short-term study. Other studies may take 3 to 30 days to complete. In these long-term studies, the nurse-observer will call the patient at home every day, including weekends, to assess analgesia and adverse effects. When necessary, the nurse-observer will make a home visit to draw bloods and assess the patient. When a protocol dictates obtaining a series of blood samples for several days, a "high tech" home care agency may be employed. These studies require an nurse-observer with sufficient experience to coordinate all of the technical aspects of such studies. Patients who participate in long-term outpatient studies need continuous instructions and assessment to prevent misunderstanding and errors. Since many cancer patients are candidates for complications from their disease, the nurse-observer must be aware of any physical or mental changes in the patients on a daily basis, which are then reported to the investigator.

TRAINING AND MONITORING THE NURSE-OBSERVER

Methods used for training and monitoring the nurse-observer are similar to those outlined by Forbes. We do not conduct a pilot study and our nurse-observers also start with a sponsored study. There is no doubt that some nurse-observers may become less diligent and start "cutting corners." On the other hand, there are those who become more proficient the longer they conduct studies. What makes the difference? I agree with Parkhouse, quoted by Forbes, "that the best way to keep the nurse-observer interested and efficient is to insure that the observer is a true member of the team, with a 'stake' in the project and its aims and to encourage discussion of the results and the design of future trials." Dr. Houde has always asked for my opinion on any study that he was considering before he made the commitment to do the study. For example, when we were considering an intramuscular study where two separate injections were to be administered at the same time he asked me if this was feasible and would this be accepted by the patient (4). In turn, I have asked our nurse-observers their opinion on similar situations. Although the nurse-observer's principal responsibility is the selection of study patients and the collection of study data, she can assist the investigator in planning studies, in suggesting possible study designs, in the analysis of the data, and in being the liaison between the investigator and the hospital personnel. She should be included in the preliminary discussions with sponsors and review all protocols being proposed. When studies are completed, the nurse-observer should assist in the writing of the reports or manuscripts and, at times, present these papers at meetings. The daily contact and close monitoring of the nurse-observers and patients on study will help to recognize some discrepancies, problems, or change of attitude or mood in the nurse-observers. My nurse-observers were always encouraged to discuss any problem with me or Dr. Houde and for the most part, they did. A poor assay sensitivity may not be the nurse-observer's fault. Study design, patient population, and drug efficacy may be the culprits. There is nothing more discouraging to a nurse-observer than to be told prematurely that she is to blame for a poor assay.

SELECTION OF THE NURSE-OBSERVER

We have had 32 nurse-observers and one medical student in 38 years conducting studies on a full-time basis. Their median length of employment has been $1\frac{1}{2}$ years, ranging from 1 month to 38 years. Not all nurses make excellent study observers. Experience has taught me to consider certain factors in the selection of the nurse-observer. The following suggestions may be helpful when interviewing for the position.

1. Qualifications. We prefer the nurse-observer to have at least two years recent bedside experience with the type of patient to be studied, e.g., cancer, surgical, or pediatric. A nurse that has been away from the bedside too long may not be familiar with recent advances in medicine. For pharmacokinetic studies, blood drawing experience is important. Advanced degrees may not be necessary. Some of the best nurse-observers have graduated from a diploma school of nursing. Having a master's degree does not insure better understanding or execution of the studies.

2. I always explain to the applicant the advantages and disadvantages of the position. She needs to know what her responsibilities will be. It is essential to determine how she feels about giving investigational drugs blindly, how she might feel when a patient does not want to participate in a study, and whether she is secure enough not to take personally a patient's refusal to participate. How would she feel when a patient does not get relief on a test medication or has adverse effects? An important part of the job is screening for potential candidates, which is time-consuming and tedious. Many nurses become discouraged when they cannot find patients for study. This is part of the job that may cause a great deal of stress and the new applicant must be aware of this.

REFERENCES

1. Houde RW, Wallenstein SL, Rogers A. Clinical pharmacology of analgesics: 1. A method of assaying analgesic effect. *Clin Pharmacol Ther* 1960;1:163–174.
2. Wallenstein SL, Rogers AG, Kaiko RF, Heidrich G III, Houde RW. Relative analgesic potency of oral zomepirac and intramuscular morphine in cancer patients with postoperative pain. *J Clin Pharmacol* 1980;20:250–258.
3. Fishman B, Pasternak S, Wallenstein SL, Houde R, Holland JC, Foley KM. The Memorial Pain Assessment Card: a valid instrument for the evaluation of cancer pain. *Cancer* 1987;60:1151–1158.
4. Beaver WT, Wallenstein SL, Houde RW, Rogers AG. A comparison of the analgesic effects of pentazocine and morphine in patients with cancer. *Clin Pharmacol Ther* 1966;7:740–751.

Advances in Pain Research and Therapy, Vol. 18,
edited by M. Max, R. Portenoy, and E. Laska,
Raven Press, Ltd., New York © 1991.

Commentary

The Nurse-Observer

Additional Issues

Nancy Z. Olson

Abraham Sunshine, M.D., P.C.
New York, New York 10021

The purpose of this commentary is to address some issues discussed by Forbes
in which our experience differs and where alternate viewpoints are available. It
must be pointed out that there are many ways to conduct good clinical trials.
Each of us, through our years of experience, has developed a methodology that
has worked well for our respective situations.

SCREENING PROCEDURES FOR INPATIENTS

The degree of involvement of the principal investigator, co-investigator, or
the patient's attending physician varies from institution to institution. Although
Forbes states that the nurse-observer often does not have day-to-day contact
with the investigator, we would emphasize that the nurse-observer's expertise
must include knowing when to contact the principal investigator or co-investigator if she has a concern about a particular study issue or patient. It is particularly
important in the inpatient surgical setting that the nurse-observer have access
to a study physician if the need arises (e.g., serious adverse reaction, patient
complaint, etc.).

The screening procedure is determined by the policy and requirements of the
specific institution as well as one's experience. Surgical inpatients can be screened
either prior to or after surgery. The nurse-observer reviews the operation schedule
for the next day to identify those patients with surgical procedures eligible for
the study. We recommend using a "Screening Worksheet" on which to log all
possible study patients identified from the operation schedule. This worksheet
allows one to follow the patient until the patient is either placed on the study or
is clearly determined not to be suitable for the study. The worksheet provides
the patient's name, the floor and room number, the patient's attending physician,
the patient's surgical procedure, and space for comments by the nurse-observer.
The nurse-observer makes routine daily rounds (approximately every hour) to

meet and identify the appropriate surgical patients as they come to the floor from the recovery room. We find that having the nurse-observer make routine rounds results in a patient-nurse relationship that helps the nurse-observer in making a judgment as to the suitability and cooperativeness of a patient for a given study. It also allows the nurse-observer the opportunity to identify potential study patients to the floor staff.

When the nurse-observer determines that a patient is eligible for a particular study, the patient's chart is flagged indicating the patient is being considered for a research study and that the nurse-observer should be notified immediately if the patient complains of pain that requires an analgesic. Providing the nurse-observer with a beeper has proven to be an effective way to decrease the number of patients lost to study as a result of the nurse-observer not being readily available to medicate the patient in pain.

In providing informed consent to the patient, again one must comply both with the requirements of the specific institution as well as the pertinent FDA regulations. Although informed consent can be obtained either pre- or postsurgery, our experience is that obtaining informed consent after surgery works best for us. When this was done prior to surgery we found that we were obtaining consent from many patients who actually never went on study, e.g., patients developed postoperative complications and were placed in the ICU; patients never developed postoperative pain; patients were discharged soon after surgery, etc. However, the preoperative period can be utilized to familiarize patients with the research program and the nurse-observer.

In terms of patient screening and enrollment, one should try not to set rigid limits with respect to the time of day when a patient can enter a study. This varies with the institution. In one institution patients are enrolled between 7:00 and 8:00 AM; the nurse-observer begins her shift at 6:00 AM. In a second institution the majority of patients are enrolled between 10:00 AM and noon because in this institution the night shift staff medicates patients at about 6:00 AM and a 4-hr washout period is required by most protocols. Our experience has been that a nurse-observer will stay for the duration of the study even if it means working unusually long days.

As we all know, there are days when there are no patients suitable for study enrollment. On such days, one can consider allowing the nurse-observer the flexibility of leaving earlier to make up for those days when she stayed later to complete the study observations. This flexibility allows one to maximize patient enrollment based on the availability of patients and not be restricted by a nurse-observer's fixed work schedule. The nurse-observer is a vital member of our research team and to make the project a success, both the number of patients enrolled in a study and the quality of the assessments made must be optimized. The careful and concerned activities of the nurse-observer determine the assay sensitivity of the study; if the nurse-observer adheres to standardized procedures, the study will distinguish between standard and placebo and between graded doses of analgesic. If the nurse-observer is uninterested and inconsistent, the study will probably have poor assay sensitivity.

OUTPATIENT ORAL SURGERY MODEL

A modification to the outpatient self-rating model described by Forbes has been implemented by us and used successfully in many studies (1–4) including pharmacokinetic/pharmacodynamic studies to correlate drug blood levels with analgesic effect (5–7). The modification is that patients are medicated in a dental clinic rather than being sent home with the study medication to self-medicate when they develop pain. Patients are scheduled for extraction of their impacted third molars and are given a briefing of the study. For patients agreeing to participate in the study, the written consent form is given to them on their initial visit; the consent is taken home for review and discussed with the parents in the case of a minor. Patients return the following week with the signed consent form and have the surgery performed. Following surgery patients remain in the clinic area. If the study requires frequent blood samples, an indwelling catheter unit may be placed in the patients' forearm; a baseline blood sample is drawn and all subsequent blood samples may be drawn from the catheter unit eliminating the need for additional "sticks."

When a patient develops pain of moderate or severe intensity and requests an analgesic, he is medicated by the study nurse. The patient remains in the clinic for a specified fixed time following which he goes home and continues the remaining observations. This procedure allows the research nurse to have a period of up to 4 hrs to brief the patient on the self-assessment procedures. For the shorter-duration studies (i.e., 4 hrs) the entire study can be completed in the clinic and the assessments can be done either by the nurse-observer or using a patient self-rating form. For studies longer than 4 hrs, the first 4 hrs of the study are completed in the clinic, and the subsequent observations (i.e., 12, 24 hrs, etc.) are completed at home by the patient following the exact procedures used in the clinic during the first 4 hrs. The patient returns one week later for removal of the sutures and for debriefing. At debriefing the nurse-observer reviews the patient's diary and checks it for completeness and consistency.

Some special features of this model are:

1. It allows one the opportunity to conduct pharmacokinetic-pharmacodynamic studies that could not otherwise be done if the patient was sent home immediately after surgery.
2. The nurse-observer medicates the patient, assuring us that the patient is actually taking the study medication, and for a pain level specified by the protocol.
3. It provides a period of up to 4 hrs in which to brief patients and observe them as they carry out the self-assessments.

4. It enables us to minimize the number of patients who are dropped as a result of protocol violations often reported with other outpatient studies.

TRAINING OF THE NURSE-OBSERVER

The need for the proper training of a nurse-observer cannot be overstated. Our training procedures are similiar to those described by Forbes. However, once we feel that the nurse-in-training has acquired an understanding of the research procedures and methodology we place her on a pilot training study. The pilot studies are conducted as randomized, double-blind studies using patient informed consent and following a protocol approved by the institutional review board. For oral studies, the pilot study is a double-blind comparison of placebo versus graded doses of an oral standard. The parenteral pilot study is a double-blind comparison of a low- versus high-dose injectable standard analgesic. A nurse may be on a pilot training study for 3 to 6 months before acquiring the proven ability to differentiate treatments. Data are analyzed periodically. When the data confirm that the nurse can statistically distinguish the active treatments from placebo, or preferably distinguish the graded doses of the active treatments, the nurse can be transferred to an actual study depending on the specific needs of the study.

We feel that the time used to run a pilot training study is a worthwhile investment as it provides an accurate and reliable measure of the nurse's ability to conduct a study with good assay sensitivity.

REFERENCES

1. Sunshine A, Marrero I, Olson NZ, Laska EM, McCormick N. Oral analgesic efficacy of suprofen compared to aspirin, aspirin plus codeine and placebo in patients with postoperative dental pain. *Pharmacology* 1983;27(Suppl 1):31–40.
2. Sunshine A, Marrero I, Olson N, McCormick N, Laska EM. Comparative study of flurbiprofen, zomepirac sodium, acetaminophen plus codeine, and acetaminophen for the relief of postsurgical dental pain. *Am J Med* 1986;80(Suppl 3A):50–54.
3. Olson N, Sunshine A, Marrero I, Ramos I, Laska EM. Piroxicam, aspirin and placebo in dental pain (abstract). *Clin Pharmacol Ther* 1987;41(2):162.
4. Sunshine A, Marrero I, Olson NZ, Tirado S, Kaiko R, Grandy R, Siegel C. Analgesic efficacy of choline magnesium trisalicylate (Trilisate) alone and in combination with codeine contin for the treatment of postsurgical dental pain. Presented at the 80th Annual Scientific Meeting of the American Pain Society, October 26–29, 1989, Phoenix, Arizona (Abstract No. 100).
5. Laska EM, Sunshine A, Marrero I, Olson NZ, Siegel C, McCormick N. The correlation between blood levels of ibuprofen and clinical analgesic response. *Clin Pharmacol Ther* 1986;40:1–7.
6. Sunshine A, Marrero I, Wagner D, Freshwater L, Olson NZ, Siegel C, Laska EM. Correlation of aspirin blood levels and analgesic response (abstract). *Clin Pharmacol Ther* 1988;43(2):141.
7. Velagapudi R, Brueckner R, Harter JG, Peck CC, Viswanathan CT, Sunshine A, Laska EM, Mason WD, Byrd WG. Pharmacokinetics (PK) and pharmacodynamic (PD) of aspirin analgesia (abstract). *Clin Pharmacol Ther* 1990;47(2):179.

Advances in Pain Research and Therapy, Vol. 18,
edited by M. Max, R. Portenoy, and E. Laska,
Raven Press, Ltd., New York © 1991.

27

Analgesic Trials to Clinical Practice

When and How Does It Happen?

Charles S. Cleeland

*Pain Research Group, Department of Neurology, WHO Collaborating
Center for Symptom Evaluation in Cancer Care,
University of Wisconsin, Madison, Wisconsin 53706*

Once a clinical trial produces a finding that would be of major benefit to pain patients, how does this finding influence the practice of caring for patients in pain? In an ideal world, the finding would be immediately translated into every encounter between a health care professional and a patient who could benefit from the finding. In reality, we know that seldom happens. Although some patients, especially those of the researchers conducting the trial, may benefit immediately, the majority of patients will not receive the benefits for some time, if ever. Many factors contribute to an inertia that must be overcome before practice habits will be modified by clinical trials data. Yet practice does change, and at least some scientific findings dictate this change. Which findings are selected, and how does it happen that they are implemented?

This chapter examines some of the dynamics of practice change in response to new information, with an emphasis on new information about analgesics. We look at some of the attributes of findings from analgesic trials in terms of their potential for adoption. We examine the literature on what is known about diffusion of research findings in general, as well as active attempts by various groups to have these findings incorporated into patient-physician encounters. We look at how practice change can be evaluated. Finally, we offer some recommendations that might shorten the time between the emergence of knowledge about relieving pain and its implementation.

For the sake of this presentation, we make several assumptions: (a) the clinical trial to be considered (or a collection of clinical trials interpreted by a consensus group) identifies a "finding" that should provide more adequate pain management for a given group of patients; (b) the finding is impeccable, so that few recognized experts would argue that adoption of the finding would not be of benefit; and (c) the finding is at variance from the typical practice of many physicians who treat patients in pain, so that there is room for practice change to occur in the direction indicated by the finding.

Unfortunately, the last assumption is all too easy to grant. The undertreatment of pain in a variety of conditions has been well documented. Of patients with postoperative pain or with pain owing to cancer, more than half may receive inadequate analgesic treatment. The other assumptions can also often be met. The literature does provide guidelines, supported by clinical trials, that indicate appropriate choices for types and dosages of analgesics for various painful conditions. Such guidelines have been provided by the American Pain Society (1). At a global level, the World Health Organization's Guidelines for Cancer Pain Relief (2) is a prominent example of the consensus recommendations of a group of experts for cancer pain relief.

THE ATTRIBUTES OF A CLINICAL FINDING: EFFECTS ON ADOPTION

Obviously, not all clinical findings will be equal in impelling practice change. Certain attributes or dimensions of the finding will help define its power to change practice. Analgesic findings often assume positions on these dimensions that will determine whether or not they are adopted, or the rate of their adoption. Findings can be categorized in several ways, the first being the risk of not adopting them. For example, some findings indicate that a practice is at high risk for mortality or significant morbidity, and the risk is immediate. An example here is the identification of an agent found to be toxic. One can assume that response to this type of information, once received, is relatively rapidly adopted by most physicians who have access to the information. Rapid adoption of new technologies also occurs when some innovation is represented as having an effect on a life-threatening disease for which no current therapy is available (3).

Most other clinical trial findings are adopted at a more leisurely rate. For example, some findings indicate that risk is present, but that the risk is more remote in time. Findings concerning the benefits of specific preventative measures fall in this category. Finally, there are findings that do not appear to modify risk at all, but implementing them may increase the comfort of the patient. Findings of analgesic trials obviously fall in this category. No systematic study has been done on the rate of adoption of findings as a function of this risk dimension, but it is reasonable to assume that findings lower in implications for risk will receive lower priority for adoption.

A second attribute that operates to influence the rate of adoption is the complexity of the action required by the finding. Simple substitution of a more effective drug for one already being used marks the low end of this dimension. Midway along this dimension is a finding that suggests a specific course of action ("order mammogram") at specific intervals in time, requiring increasing monitoring of patient data. At the extreme end of this dimension are complex action plans involving multiple steps of assessment and the simultaneous use of multiple treatments. Findings of analgesic trials may vary greatly along this dimension. For example, a simple substitution of a more effective analgesic might be implemented relatively easily. At the other extreme, a finding that several medications need to be used simultaneously, or that nondrug therapies need to be included in the treatment plan probably will face a slower rate of adoption.

Complexity of adoption is closely related to a third dimension, the *economic implications* of the finding for the practice setting. Some findings may significantly increase the cost of care, but not be balanced by increased revenues. Examples are increases in nonprofessional contact time or increased density of surveillance. Some findings may even indicate eliminating procedures that have been economically beneficial for the practice, such as the elimination of surgeries shown to be ineffective. Here, economic factors could impede implementation. In some instances, however, adoption of a technique may add a new dimension that attracts more patients or revenues. Increasingly, consumer demand is becoming a significant factor influencing practice behavior. Examples from analgesic practice are also distributed along this economic dimension. Increased surveillance for pain may not be offset by new revenues. On the other hand, the introduction of sophisticated technology (such as implantable analgesic delivery systems) may dramatically increase practice revenue and attract new patients. Findings positively influencing practice revenues would be expected to be adopted more readily.

The literature on diffusion and adoption of innovations also indicates other attributes that may influence adoption rate (4). Some of these are obvious, such as the ease with which the finding can be communicated and understood by potential adopters. Some are less obvious, such as the compatibility of the innovation with the existing values, attitudes, and past experiences of the adopter. Many recommendations for analgesic practice will run counter to currently held attitudes. The most obvious example is the recommendation that opioids be used for the management of cancer pain, and that they be used in high enough does to control pain. This recommendation runs counter to long-established concerns about addicting patients to psychoactive drugs, concerns reinforced on a daily basis by multimedia campaigns against drug addiction. In this instance, these concerns are supported by similar concerns held by the general public, patients, and families (5). A more general barrier to the adoption of improved analgesic practice is the low priority that conventionally has been given to efforts for pain and symptom control. Excellence in pain and symptom management has rarely been adopted as the "mission" of practitioners.

Thus, the attributes of the finding, its implications for patient survival, its complexity, salience for potential users, and its economic implications will operate to determine the speed with which the finding is adopted, even before active attempts are made to change practice. Analgesic findings don't extend life, will often be complex to implement, and may add to practice burden without associated increases in revenue. These characteristics suggest that the adoption of analgesic findings will be slow, and those who wish to promote change will have to exert more ingenuity and effort to produce it.

A finding about appropriate pain management will be but a drop in a sea of information inundating the practicing health professional. Once a finding is accepted, the word has to get out. Some of the attributes of analgesic findings already discussed will also determine the attention they receive in the systems of communication that influence practice. For instance, analgesic findings will rarely appear in the most widely read medical journals or on popular physician-education television programs. Few analgesic findings become the subject of major news distribution following their publication.

Many findings that have altered practice have had the advocacy of major players in the health field. The most unimpeachable finding needs authority. As yet, there has been no surgeon general's report on pain and its management. There is no national institute on pain that can issue specific advisories for pain practice. Although the American Pain Society has begun to issue analgesic practice guidelines (6), no widely based disease-oriented groups (such as the American Cancer Society or the American Heart Association), have publicized the need to change pain management practice.

THE PROCESS OF ADOPTION

In a comprehensive and landmark study, Coleman et al. (7) examined patterns of physician adoption of a new antibiotic medication over an 18-month period following release of the drug. Several general principles were substantiated by this study. Sample physicians were easily categorized by their time of adoption of the new drug, from early to late. Early adopters were characterized by being specialists, frequent visitors to other medical centers and professional meetings, and readers of many journals. A major finding was the insufficiency of any single channel of influence in the adoption process, and that different channels contributed to various steps of the adoption process, from initial information about the drug to final introduction into practice. Rates of adoption were related to frequency of exposure to the various channels.

The relatively isolated practitioner was liable to be the slowest to adopt. The more "integrated" early adopter was linked by institutional ties and professional contacts. Even the frequency of social contacts with other physicians had a role. Professional networks demonstrated their effects very early in the process, with social networks demonstrating their importance later. Friendship networks were more influential in smaller towns. In its sociometric analysis, this study documented the importance of opinion leaders who were frequently contacted by other practitioners for advice and information.

The adoption or diffusion of a new practice by any group seems to have some consistency and be subject to similar influences, whether it be a practice change in medicine or the adoption of new agricultural techniques or new methods of manufacture. Rogers (4) has attempted one synthesis of this literature. He characterizes five definite stages in the adoption process. The first, "awareness" of a new finding or process, is often random in nature. The second, "interest," is that period of actively being receptive to new information about the process. In this stage, the degree to which information is highlighted in the mass media will be an influence. This, in turn, may focus attention on reports of the finding in the professional literature. The third stage, "evaluation," has been described as a "mental trial" stage. During this period, potential adopters actively seek technical information about how to implement the change and about its costs and liabilities. This stage is also characterized by the formation of an affective stance toward the innovation—"I think this will work. I like this." Personal information from other adopters is very important at this stage. Based on the outcome of this stage, the potential adopter will decide whether or not to institute a "trial." Moving from evaluation to trial appears to be the part of the adoption process that encounters the most resistance. Consistently across the history of innovations, the awareness-to-trial period is longer than the trial-to-adoption period. Social reinforcement for having undertaken the trial is often critical to the outcome of the trial stage, which can either be "adoption" or rejection ("discontinuance").

Certain personal characteristics seem to define how readily a person will adopt a new innovation. Early adopters tend to be younger, are more often members of a professional specialty group, have higher social and financial status and higher intelligence, and rely on larger numbers of information sources than do later adopters. Like antibiotics, analgesics are a staple of practice across a wide variety of practitioners. For instance, the severe pain of terminal cancer is liable to be managed by isolated physicians in many instances. Diffusion of information to specialty groups, those more likely to be most receptive to new information, is not sufficient to assure that a majority of patients will benefit.

Two factors seem to influence the rate of the awareness-to-trial stage. The first is the activity of various *change agents* who promote the new practice. In health care, the pharmaceutical detail person is an obvious example of such an agent. The advocacy of disease-oriented societies, such as the American Heart Association, also operates as a major factor in acceptance of new practice patterns. The second factor that can speed the adoption process is engaging potential adopters in a trial of the innovation. Active involvement in a trial can speed its adoption by months or years (4). Recognizing the importance of participation in trials, pharmaceutical companies will often provide free medications for a period of time. They may also involve physicians in simple protocols to acquaint them with products.

METHODS OF CHANGING PRACTICE: WHAT WORKS?

The evidence suggests that the mere presence of clinical trials findings in the literature will have little effect on practice (8–10). If change is to occur, an active attempt will have to be made to implement the change. The less impelling the change, the greater the effort that will be involved in the implementation. The attributes of an analgesic finding are such that successful implementation will require a significant effort.

Wide dissemination of consensus reports has been one method of presenting findings to practicing physicians. In one study of the effectiveness of such reports in modifying physician practice (11), changes following the 1984 Joint National Committee Consensus Report on High Blood Pressure were examined. Sixty-two percent of the physician sample was aware of the report one year after its release. Despite this awareness, and familiarity with its content, most indicated that there had been very little if any change in their practice behavior. In this instance, much of the information contained in the report had already been incorporated into practice.

Another consensus panel developed by the American Heart Association in 1977 recommended that patients with mitral valve prolapse (MVP) receive antibiotic prophylaxis prior to procedures with risk for bacterial endocarditis. One year after the report was published, only 37% of patients with MVP admitted to a university medical center had the prophylaxis recommended (12).

A Canadian study followed the release of a widely distributed and nationally endorsed consensus statement recommending decreases in the use of cesarean sections (13). Although most obstetricians were aware of the guidelines and agreed with them, and one-third of the hospitals and obstetricians reported modifying their practice as a result of the recommendations, data on actual practice demonstrated little change. The authors concluded that dissemination of research evidence in the form of practice guidelines "is unlikely to have much effect on inappropriate practices that are sustained by powerful nonscientific purposes."

ACTIVE ATTEMPTS TO MODIFY PRACTICE

If new information from clinical trials, even when endorsed by expert or consensus panels, has negligible impact, how can practice be modified? What do we know about active attempts to modify health care practice? It may be a fair conclusion that we know more about what doesn't work than what does. Two of the most commonly used methods of conveying findings—printed material and traditional continuing medical education—probably have much less effect on practice than is widely believed. In isolation, printed material, from package inserts to drug bulletins to articles, doesn't change practice or does so for only a limited time (14). For example, one study targeted the impact of a drug bulletin suggesting that aspirin or acetaminophen be substituted for propoxyphene for the treatment of mild pain because of the latter drug's high cost, limited efficacy, and potential toxicity. Propoxyphene use decreased by almost 50% in the first 2 weeks following the mailing, but thereafter returned to premailing levels (15).

Most states mandate participation in continuing medical education (CME) as a condition of licensure, as a way of upgrading medical performance and improving patient outcomes. A significant portion of this effort is to review new findings from clinical trials and introduce new methods of patient care. Although there is evidence that such programs improve physician knowledge, the evidence that actual practice performance changes is slim. Traditional CME, the weekend workshop, has little research support to back up its effectiveness. Lewis and Hassanein (16) found little evidence that such programs affect physician behavior. Because of the failure of many such programs, more aggressive and innovative approaches have been studied. For example, Sibley et al. (17) introduced a program of individualized educational packages for family physicians in Ontario. Outcome was studied by extensive chart review. Although the physicians demonstrated a significant increase in their knowledge of package information, there was little evidence of improvement in quality of care.

More positive benefits were described for a program of "academic detailing," a method specifically modeled after pharmaceutical sales strategies. Targeting the excessive use of several medications (including one analgesic, propoxyphene), Avorn and Soumerai (18) studied the effects of personal educational visits by doctoral-level pharmacists to doctors in their offices. This intervention had many aspects, including printed summaries of information prepared with the help of marketing consultants, as well as patient literature on the targeted changes, recognizing that consumer demand influences practice. The pharmacists made two visits to each physician in the face-to-face contact group. During these visits, the pharmacists presented the pharmacologic rationale for physicians altering their prescribing practice. This intervention successfully reduced the usage of three of the four targeted drugs, including propoxyphene, when the face-to-face group was compared with a control group as well as a group receiving the printed material only.

In contrast to other medical education programs, this program was multimodal as well as cost intensive. It also included an element known for decades to be effective by the pharmaceutical companies: information presented in the office setting on a one-to-one basis.

In one review of the literature (19), the most effective techniques for modifying physician practice were those that involved immediate feedback or prompting of physicians to take a specific action. Computers have been used to aid this process in several studies. Physicians increased use of tests required for medication monitoring when reminded to do so by a computer (20). Although a summary of performance (monthly feedback) was only marginally effective, immediate reminders to perform preventative care increased compliance (21). Simple checklists can be effective, at least during the duration of the study (22). In all of the above studies, although improvement was shown, this improvement was less than 50% of optimal practice. Even the effects of such prompting, however, may be fragile. Dombal et al. (23) studied the effect of a computer-aided diagnosis in patients with acute abdominal pain. Clinician diagnosis improved markedly during the trial, but continued monitoring indicated that performance reverted toward pretrial levels. Not all prompting programs work, even during the study period. A computer-based system was developed to detect and to provide feedback on the overutilization of laboratory tests (24). In addition to notifying physicians, a program of education was organized. The program was not effective in reducing overutilization.

In summary, computer-generated prompting for specific practice performance may work in some instances, and might be helpful for improving analgesic practice. But this improvement will probably affect only about half of the instances where practice change is indicated, and the computer prompting probably cannot be withdrawn without a return to baseline practice performance.

THE EFFECTS OF ESTABLISHING A PROTOCOL

Recently, there has been much interest in the effects of explicit *protocols* for improving specific health practices. Grimm et al. (25) have reported that use of a standardized protocol for the diagnosis and treatment of sore throat significantly altered the practice behavior of several groups of health professionals, despite physician opinion that protocols were most suitable for health professionals other than physicians. Acceptance of a protocol, with or without compliance prompted by a checklist, dramatically improved compliance with specified procedures in primary care (26). One study evaluated the relative influence of physician participation in research protocols on patterns of care in small cell lung cancer (27). In this study, physicians involved in clinical research provided a higher percentage of items indexed by the patterns of care review than did physicians not participating in protocols, even for their patients who were not included in protocols.

As yet, no studies report the establishment of an analgesic protocol as a method of improving pain management, but the studies just reviewed suggest that institutional or research protocols might be effective methods for practice change. Why might protocols work when more comprehensive educational programs have marginal effect? Following a protocol certainly requires less individualized decision making in the press of clinical work. By invoking institutional authority, a protocol "externalizes" the acceptance of the need to follow specific practice steps, yet preserves some of the practitioner's autonomy by his or her agreement to use the protocol. Following a protocol may also be more compatible with health practitioner culture than computer reminders or checklists, a positive attribute for the acceptance of an innovation (4).

Where an innovation is conceptually and technically quite new for the health professionals involved, a protocol may take on the characteristics of a demonstration project, such as the ones in cancer pain relief being conducted by the World Health Organization (28). Here, simple program implementation is complicated by additional variables, such as regulatory and supply barriers, professional inexperience with the classes of analgesics to be used, and lack of patient knowledge that pain is treatable. Such demonstration projects must assist with many more steps in the process than required by simple protocol acceptance.

Whether or not such demonstration projects work in changing practitioner practice and, perhaps, in diffusing practice to other institutions, is currently being evaluated.

EXTERNAL INCENTIVES

Agreeing to perform a protocol usually implies personal agreement with a standard. Increasingly, health practice is monitored by external agents, including professional standards review organizations, third-party payers, quality assurance policies, and state and federal bureaucracies. The results of malpractice actions have also become a driving force in the conduct of practice. The role of patients as consumers has become more prominent in dictating how patients will be treated. The impact of these forces on practice are only now being studied, although many of those frustrated with traditional medical education look to these influences to reduce the variability of adherence to optimal practice standards.

The role of cost-containment sanctions is probably limited in the promotion of optimal analgesic practice, although some patients may be spared ineffective procedures. At this date, malpractice law has yet to test the rights of a patient to adequate pain management. Quality assurance and consumer demand are probably much more promising for improvement of pain relief.

Quality assurance depends on indicators of performance that can easily be monitored. If quality assurance is to encompass pain relief, a major first step will be the introduction of pain measures into routine practice, coupled with the charting of the results as a routine practice (6). Once this is done, it is quite reasonable to establish an "incident" of poorly controlled pain that calls for review. An example might be to use the midpoint on an accepted pain rating scale as the point which defines poorly controlled pain.

Williamson (29) has argued that education for health practice change must be based on an evaluation encompassing both outcomes and process. Only when outcome data indicate deficiencies is process evaluation warranted and educational intervention mandated. He suggests starting with the most preventable or remediable health impairments as being of highest priority. His strategy begins with a standard of care that can be reasonably operationalized. An example of how this strategy might be implemented in the analgesic area is suggested by a study of Zelman and Cleeland (30). In this study, an index of pain management was derived from a combination of patient pain report and the World Health Organization's recommendations (2) for cancer pain management. The WHO's "stepladder" of analgesic prescription specifies aspirin-class analgesics for mild pain, codeine-class for moderate pain, and morphine-class for severe pain. The index ranges from 0 to 3, with 3 (a patient with severe pain receiving no analgesics) representing extreme mismanagement. Unfortunately, this index does not take into account whether or not the appropriate dose of the primary analgesic or other adjuvant drugs are being ordered. However, this simple index is able to differentiate patient pain management among different treatment settings. Patients from a cancer pain survey done in Wisconsin hospitals, clinics, and hospices were subjects for whom the index was computed. Using even this conservative index, 27% of patients in the sample were mismanaged. Both codeine and morphine-level analgesics were underutilized. Mismanagement, as estimated by the index, was significantly correlated with mood disturbance (depression, tension, and anger as measured by the Profile of Mood States) and with sleep disturbance in patients who had moderate to severe pain.

An alternative to the "incident" approach might be the use of such an index. Following Williamson's strategy, each institution would set a maximum acceptable level for the index. If outcome index data were above this level, process evaluation and education would be invoked. The outcome evaluation process would then be repeated to determine the extent of improvement.

CONSUMER DEMAND

Pharmaceutical companies are quite aware of the role of the patient as consumer in guiding health practice, as attested by their increasing promotion of prescription drugs in national media. Although not mentioning the product name (but featuring the name of the sponsoring company), the ads indicate that relief for a given condition is available and urge potential patients to see their physician.

In a recent study, physicians' attitudes and behavior concerning their approach to screening for and treating high cholesterol were measured in two communities, one of which had a very active public education program directed at the prevention of cardiovascular disease (31). This same city also had an active CME focus on the same topic. Although CME-related activities seemed to have little impact on the study city's physicians, the public education program was identified as a significant factor in modifying physician practice behavior. More of the study city's patients directly requested cholesterol screening and counseling, and fewer were reported to be noncompliant owing to poor understanding of the importance of therapy. In turn, physicians in the study city set lower limits for "normal" lipids, and initiated diet or drug therapy at lower levels as well. In this study, patients were informed of the results of clinical trials, and they then modified the practice of physicians.

The state cancer pain–initiative movement may serve as a similar force in modifying pain management practice. Started in Wisconsin, state initiatives are multiprofessional and organizational efforts that provide patient, public, and professional education and support for improved cancer pain relief (32). State cancer pain initiatives are now active in almost half the states. In Wisconsin and in several other states initiative activity has been accompanied by extensive media coverage concerning the undertreatment of cancer pain and the right of patients to adequate pain management. One focus of the initiatives has been to inform the public, the patients, and their families that poor management of cancer pain should not be tolerated and that patients and families should ask for appropriate care. The initiatives also advocate making pain management a priority in cancer care, educating health care practitioners in current pain management, and including pain management in quality assurance policies. Although it is much too early to evaluate the impact of state initiatives on analgesic practice, evidence beginning to accumulate in other areas of practice change indicates that consumer demand can be a very powerful force for practice change.

EVALUATION OF PRACTICE CHANGE METHODS

Interventions for analgesic practice change call for evaluation as much as for specific analgesic practices submitted to clinical trials. Several evaluation models exist that have been used to study the effectiveness of continuing medical education. Some of these models are intuitively and logically more attractive than others. Unfortunately, the most compelling of these designs are also the most complex and expensive to implement. Since practice change usually spreads most rapidly within a single practice setting, evaluation studies of this type might randomize institutions or practice settings into intervention and control sites. Some studies obtain outcome measures prior to and following the intervention, using treatment before the intervention as an historical control. With this latter type of study, changes in practice may be subject to variables (new information, new products) outside the control of the evaluation process.

The best evaluations of practice change will adhere to the standards applied to clinical trials in general. In addition to randomized assignment of the units of study (physicians, patients, or clinic sites), evaluators should ideally be blind as to the group from which the data comes. Subjective measures (measures of pain severity and quality, and subjective functional measures) should be brief, comprehensible to patients and staff, and should have demonstrated reliability and validity (33). Criteria for measures to be derived from record review should be unambiguous and high inter-rater reliability should be demonstrated. The question that the trial is designed to answer should be stated in such a way that the data will provide clear confirmation or disconfirmation of the question.

We are most likely to be convinced that a practice change intervention has made a difference if evidence for a change in *patient outcome* variables can be demonstrated. In evaluations of this sort, a set of criteria for better versus worse patient outcome needs to be developed in advance of the intervention trial. Examples of variables that might be used to evaluate these criteria include patient report of pain severity, some index of patient functioning, and an index of the severity of side effects. Depending on the focus of evaluation, other variables (such as patient understanding of therapy recommendations and compliance with recommended treatment) might assume importance. Some thought must be given to *when* these outcome data are collected. For example, the results of a visit for the treatment of pain might be best assessed after sufficient time has elapsed for the patient to have reasonably responded to the treatment. Satisfaction with care can also be examined. If outcome data are obtained by study personnel independent of the clinic and blind to the presence or absence of the intervention, the results are stronger (34). In some instances, specific patients with symptoms that are the target of the practice change being studied might be tracked for clinicians in both intervention and control groups (35).

A more common outcome measure (because of cost and ease of data collection) is the use of physician response to a *patient scenario* as a way of judging physician practice. A typical scenario will describe a patient with pain in some detail, then offer the physician the opportunity to respond with a treatment plan. Usually, the responses are multiple choice and not open-ended. Criteria for evaluation might include choice and dose of the most appropriate analgesic and adjuvant medications, side effect management, and what next step in analgesic management might be taken should the suggested treatment fail. The physician might also be asked to respond to a set of questions that probe specific reasons for the choice of treatment. Data of interest would be physician scenario responses prior to and after the practice intervention. A major reservation about scenario evaluation is whether the responses given by the clinician actually reflect practice behavior. Several studies, already reviewed in this chapter, have demonstrated that improvement in clinicians' knowledge is not always translated into practice.

If the targeted practice change is relatively simple, such as the frequency with which a given analgesic is prescribed, or the appropriate use of analgesic and adjuvant combinations, the evaluation can also be simplified. Computer-based *pharmacy records* are a very convenient data set comparing pre- and postintervention questions (36). Physicians can also be asked to make copies of their prescriptions for the study period, or evaluators can inspect prescriptions at the pharmacies used by the clinicians.

The most typical way of monitoring practice change, chart review, is also the most problematic. Whereas most medical charts are complete in their recording of major diagnostic and surgical procedures, they may be "silent" regarding treatment of lower priority medical issues, including prevention measures and, we might assume, measures taken for patient palliation (37). Studies based on chart review must identify criteria that can be unequivocally classified as being met or not met by study chart reviewers (e.g., pain assessment recorded, pain consult requested). Chart review–based evaluations are obviously facilitated in settings where the medical record is computerized.

SUMMARY AND RECOMMENDATIONS

The attributes of many analgesic practice findings are such that they will be slow to be adopted. Analgesic findings are often seen as low priority, complicated, and adding costs to practice without adding revenue. If they are to be of maximum benefit, they must be adopted by a wide range of practitioners, including those described as isolated, the slowest group to modify practice. Certain recommendations, such as the use of opioid analgesics for severe cancer pain, may not be compatible with the "antidrug" values that most practitioners hold, or with the past experience of the potential adopter with addicted patients. Analgesic findings that dictate a change in practice are not likely to make the evening news, or to be reported in the most broadly disseminated professional literature, retarding the awareness and interest stages of the adoption process. Analgesic findings have also traditionally lacked the advocacy of well-established and well-funded disease-oriented associations.

Regardless of their attributes, most clinical findings are not readily adopted without an active effort to promote them. The mere presentation of information in the literature, or even in traditional CME course format, will likely lead to minimal practice change. Computer prompting and feedback improve practice adequacy, but this improvement tends to degrade following withdrawal of the program. Cost-intensive programs involving personal contact with physicians in their office (supported with information presented in a multimodal format) do seem to work, but these interventions have only been studied with relatively simple recommendations ("discontinue drug X").

There are some approaches to changing practice that have demonstrated efficacy. Accepting a protocol improves practice and this improvement may spread to the care of patients not on the protocol. Increasing the health information of patients about specific health topics may also modify practice related to those topics. State cancer pain initiatives are already attempting to change the way patients regard cancer pain and its treatment.

An examination of the "dose-response" curve of practice change may suggest that changing analgesic practice is liable to require large doses at frequent intervals. Looking once again at the adoption process, specific interventions might speed up each stage.

Awareness and interest in the finding might be enhanced by strengthening the American Pain Society's review (1) and publication of consensus evaluations of pain therapy. Support of major disease-related societies, such as the American Cancer Society, would be extremely helpful. Specific recommendations for therapy from one of the NIH institutes would also be supportive. Publication of clinical trial findings in more general professional journals would appear to be essential. Promotion of findings in the public media would also be extremely helpful.

The evaluation stage might be accelerated by public and patient demand for more adequate care, and by professional advocacy and information at the local level of the practitioner's associates. It is at the evaluation stage that the values and experience of the potential adopter need to be addressed. Such steps as including pain as a quality assurance issue in local institutions (6) should facilitate evaluation as well as subsequent stages of adoption.

Trial and adoption of findings should be accelerated by the introduction of protocols for the management of pain. These protocols should be the products of consensus groups with impeccable credentials. They might be implemented locally, on the basis of quality assurance recommendations, or nationally through recommendations of major professional societies or clinical trials groups, such as those formed for studying treatments for major diseases, such as cancer or AIDS.

Optimizing pain management practice will require considerable effort, organization, and money, but might produce substantial benefit for patients in pain.

REFERENCES

1. American Pain Society. Principles of analgesic use in acute pain and chronic cancer pain, Skokie, IL: American Pain Society, 1989.
2. World Health Organization. *Cancer pain relief.* Geneva: WHO, 1986.
3. Warner KE. A "desperation-reaction" model of medical diffusion. *Health Serv Res* 1975; Winter: 369–383.
4. Rogers EM. *Diffusion of innovations.* New York: Free Press, 1962.
5. Cleeland CS. Effects of attitudes on cancer pain. In: Hill CS, Fields WS, eds. *Drug treatment of cancer pain in a drug-oriented society.* New York: Raven Press, 1989.
6. Max MB, Donovan M, Porteney RK, et al. American Pain Society standards for monitoring quality of analgesic treatment. In: Bond M, ed. *Proceedings of the Sixth World Congress on Pain.* Amsterdam: Elsevier, 1991, in press.
7. Coleman J, Katz E, Menzel H. *Medical innovation: a diffusion study.* Indianapolis: Bobbs-Merrill, 1966.
8. Chalmers TC. Impact of controlled trials on the practice of medicine. *Mt Sinai J Med (NY)* 1974;41:753–759.
9. Stross JK, Harlan WR. The dissemination of new medical information. *JAMA* 1979;241(24): 2622–2624.
10. Kessner DM. Diffusion of new medical information. *Am J Public Health* 1981;71:367–368.
11. Hill MN, Levine DM, Whelton PK. Awareness, use, and impact at the 1984 joint national committee consensus report on high blood pressure. *Am J Public Health* 1988;78(9):1190–1194.
12. Retchin SM, Fletcher RH, Buescher PC, Waugh RA, Battaglini SW. The application of official policy-prophylaxis recommendations for patients with mitral valve prolapse. *Med Care* 1985;23(10):1156–1162.
13. Lomas J, Anderson GM, Domnick-Pierre K, Vayda E, Enkin MW, Hannah WJ. Do practice guidelines guide practice? The effect of a consensus statement on the practice of physicians. *N Engl J Med* 1989;321:1306–1311.
14. Soumerai SB, Avorn J. Economic and policy analysis of university-based drug "detailing." *Med Care* 1986;24:313–331.
15. Berbatis CG, Maher MJ, Plumridge RJ, Stoelwinder JU, Zubrick SR. Impact of a drug bulletin on prescribing oral analgesics in a teaching hospital. *Am J Hosp Pharm* 1982;39:98–100.
16. Lewis CE, Hassanein RS. Continuing medical education–an epidemiological evaluation. *N Engl J Med* 1970;282:254.
17. Sibley JC, Sackett DL, Neufeld V, Gerrard B, Rudnick KV, Fraser W. A randomized trial of continuing medical education. *N Engl J Med* 1982;306(9):511–515.
18. Avorn J, Soumerai S. Improving drug-therapy decisions through educational outreach: a randomized controlled trial of academically based "detailing." *N Engl J Med* 1983;308(24):1457–1463.
19. Haynes RB, Davis DA, McKibbon A, Tugwell P. A critical appraisal of the efficacy of continuing medical education. *JAMA* 1984;251(1):61–64.
20. McDonald CJ. Use of a computer to detect and respond to clinical events: its effect on clinical behavior. *Ann Intern Med* 1976;84:162–167.

21. Tierney WM, Hui SL, McDonald CJ. Delayed feedback of physician performance versus immediate reminders to perform preventive care: effects on physician compliance. *Med Care* 1986;24(8):659–666.
22. Cohen DI, Littenberg B, Wetzel C, Neuhauser D. Improving physician compliance with preventive medicine guidelines. *Med Care* 1982;20(10):1040–1045.
23. Dombal FT, Leaper DJ, Horrocks JC, Staniland JR, McCann AP. Human and computer-aided diagnosis of abdominal pain: further report with emphasis on performance of clinicians. *Br Med J* 1974;1:376–380.
24. Eisenberg JM, Williams SV, Garner L, Viale R, Smits H. Computer-based audit to detect and correct overutilization of laboratory tests. *Med Care* 1977;15(11):915–921.
25. Grimm RH, Shimoni K, Harlan WR, Estes H. Evaluation of patient-care protocol use by various providers. *N Engl J Med* 1975;292(10):501–511.
26. Sullivan RJ, Estes HE, Stopford W, Lester AJ. Adherence to explicit strategies for common medical conditions. *Med Care* 1980;18(4):388–399.
27. Ford L, Feigl P, Diehr P, Yates J. Do protocol patient receive better care? Results of a pattern of care study in small cell lung cancer. Presented at the American Society of Clinical Oncology, 1987.
28. Cleeland CS. Demonstration projects for cancer pain relief. In: Foley KM, Bonica JJ, Ventafridda V, eds. *Second International Congress on Cancer Pain.* New York: Raven Press, 1989;465–474.
29. Williamson JW. Evaluating quality of patient care: a strategy relating outcome and process assessment. *JAMA* 1971;218(4):564–569.
30. Zelman D, Cleeland CS. A preliminary index of cancer pain management/mismanagement. Presented at the 1987 International Association for the Study of Pain, Hamburg, Germany.
31. Block L, Banspach SW, Gans K, Harris C, Lasater TM, Lefebvre C, Carleton RA. Impact of public education and continuing medical education on physician attitudes and behavior concerning cholesterol. *Am J Prev Med* 1988;4(5):255–260.
32. Dahl JL, Joranson DE. The Wisconsin Cancer Pain Initiative. In: Foley FM, Bonica JJ, Ventafridda V, eds. *Second International Congress on Cancer Pain.* New York: Raven Press, 1989;499–504
33. Cleeland, CS. Assessment of pain by subjective report. In: Chapman CR, Loeser J, eds. *Pain measurement.* New York: Raven Press, 1989;391–403.
34. Linn BS. Continuing medical education: impact on emergency room burn care. *JAMA* 1980;244(6):565–570.
35. Evans CE, Haynes RB, Birkett NJ, Gilbert JR, Taylor DW, Sackett DL, Johnston ME, Hewson SA. Does a mailed continuing education program improve physician performance? *JAMA* 1986;255:501–504.
36. Avorn J, Soumerai SB, Taylor W et al. Reduction of incorrect antibiotic dosing through a structured educational order form. *Arch Intern Med* 1988;148:1720–1724.
37. Feigl P, Glaefke G, Ford L, Diehr P, Chu J. Studying patterns of cancer care: how useful is the medical report? *Am J Public Health* 1988;78(5):526–533.

Advances in Pain Research and Therapy, Vol. 18,
edited by M. Max, R. Portenoy, and E. Laska,
Raven Press, Ltd., New York © 1991.

Commentary

Analgesic Trials to Change Clinical Practice

Marilee I. Donovan

Oregon Health Sciences University, Portland, Oregon 97201

I would like to expand on several points addressed in Dr. Cleeland's chapter and suggest some strategies for beginning to improve the clinical practice of analgesic therapy.

Dr. Cleeland identified risk as one of the factors affecting the adoption of a practice change. Practitioners are seldom acquainted with the risk of not treating pain: increased pain, longer hospitalization, decreased respiratory function, and mental changes (1–4). In fact, few even realize that such risks actually exist. But every practitioner, regardless of discipline, is well versed in the real and assumed risks associated with the various methods of treating pain. A recent report of the knowledge of 2,459 nurses who attended pain workshops across the United States reconfirmed a pervasive overestimate of the risk of addiction related to the use of opioids for pain relief; only 25% correctly estimated the risk to be <1% and more than 15% estimated the risk to be at least 50% (5). The overconcern for the risks of treating pain unbalanced by any concern for the risks of not treating pain may explain the observation that nurses and physicians report that their goal for patients in pain is less than total pain relief (6–8).

One cannot emphasize too strongly that education to improve knowledge and education to change behavior are totally different processes. When practices, like those involving pain management, are sustained by myth, misinformation, undue concern with treatment risks, and other nonscientific reinforcers, traditional rational educational strategies are of questionable value. An alternative is, a strategy termed "Contracts and Gaps" was developed to stimulate and evaluate behavior change. Learners were asked to identify the "gaps" between the reality of actual care given in their practice setting and the ideal being taught in the course. Then each learner selected one to three gaps based on patient need, agency need, personal abilities to change the involved practices, and resources available. The learner, with faculty consultation, developed a realistic plan for eliminating the gap and this plan was formalized in a contract between the learner, his/her employer, and the educational program. The contract explained what the learner planned to do, how it would be done, and the approximate time period in which it would be accomplished. After a reasonable period of time, a member of the faculty of the educational program visited the employing institution and evaluated the extent to which the contract was fulfilled. Eighty-one percent of the contracts were in the process of being implemented when the follow-up visit was made (9).

Industries that are known for quality and innovation strive to develop systems for continuous improvement rather than attempting to meet an arbitrarily established standard (10–12). Health care institutions have yet to accept this approach. The system itself is often a more important determinant of the outcome than the performance of the individuals within it. System-based impediments to effective pain treatment include the procedures established to meet the demands of regulatory agencies; peer censorship for using "too much" narcotic; failure of pharmacies to stock certain opioids; procedures for opioid distribution and record keeping; and poor systems of documentation and recall of information regarding pain, pain therapy, and pain relief. Holding the practitioner responsible for problems created by the system is counterproductive. Evaluation of the processes of pain relief and a commitment to the continuous improvement of these processes is an even greater challenge than the challenge of professional education.

Several strategies are appropriate to begin the process of changing practice related to the use of analgesics. First, additional research is warranted to fully understand undertreatment of pain in general, and specifically, the failure to change practices related to analgesic use. When a model of this process is developed, the variables that influence these practices can be systematically modified. Second, the systems related to providing pain relief need to be changed. Examples of this type of change include (a) the Wisconsin State Cancer Pain Initiative (13), a joint effort of federal, state, and private agencies and dedicated individuals that is apparently altering analgesic use in Wisconsin, and (b) model quality assurance standards for postoperative and cancer pain that are being developed by the American Pain Society (14) with the intention of improving the diagnosis and treatment of pain in these groups of hospitalized patients. In addition, consumers must be mobilized. Patients need to recognize the critical role they play in their own pain relief and appreciate that they have a right to pain relief and that pain relief without disastrous side effects is possible. The history of the consumer movement suggests that consumer activism could dramatically improve pain relief, even if little additional effort were directed to professional education or system restructuring. For example, when pregnant women began to demand prepared, awake childbirth, a revolution in obstetrics occurred.

Finally, improvement in clinical practice may be facilitated by collaboration with other agencies, including insurance companies, drug company representatives, and other national and international organizations that already exist to improve pain relief practices. For example, the wide dissemination of the International Association for the Study of Pain Task Force on Acute Pain report, which will be distributed soon, may be very useful in increasing awareness of the problem and educating practitioners about the availability of a solution.

REFERENCES

1. Yeager MP, Glass DD, Neff RK, Brinck-Johnsen T. Epidural anesthesia and analgesia in high risk surgical patients. *Anesthesiology* 1987;66:729–736.
2. Cleeland CS. The impact of pain on patients with cancer. *Cancer* 1984;54:2635–2641.
3. Melzack R. The tragedy of needless pain. *Sci Am* 1990;262(2);27–33.
4. Wall PD. The prevention of post-operative pain. *Pain* 1988;33:289–290.
5. McCaffery M, Ferrell B, O'Niel-Page E, Lester M, Ferrell B. Nurses' knowledge of opioid analgesics and psychological dependence. *Cancer Nusr* 1990;13(1):21–27.
6. Charap AD. The knowledge, attitudes and experience of medical personnel treating pain in the terminally ill. *Sinai J Med* 1978;45(4):561–580.
7. Marks RM, Sachar EJ. Undertreatment of medical inpatients with narcotic analgesics. *Ann Intern Med* 1973;78:172–181.
8. Watt-Watson J. Nurses' knowledge of pain issues: a survey. *J Pain Sympt Manag* 1987;2(4):207–211.
9. Donovan M, Wolpert P, Yasko J. Gaps and Contracts. *Nurs Outlook* 1981;29(8):467–471.
10. Deming WE. *Out of the crisis.* Cambridge, Massachusetts: MIT Press, 1982.
11. Peters T, Austin N. *A passion for excellence.* New York: Random House, 1985.
12. Walton M. *The Deming Management Method.* New York: Perigee Books, 1986.
13. Joranson DE, Dahl JL. Achieving balance in drug policy: the Wisconsin model. *Adv Pain Res Ther* 1989;11:197–204.
14. Max MB, Donovan M, Portenoy RK, et al. Standards for monitoring quality of analgesic treatment of acute pain and cancer pain. In: Bond M, ed. *Proceedings of the VI World Congress on Pain.* Amsterdam: Elsevier, 1991, in press.

Advances in Pain Research and Therapy, Vol. 18,
edited by M. Max, R. Portenoy, and E. Laska,
Raven Press, Ltd., New York © 1991.

28

The Food and Drug Administration's Regulation of Clinical Studies in the United States

Charles W. Prettyman

Regulatory Affairs, The Purdue Frederick Company, Norwalk, Connecticut 06856

The purpose of this chapter is to familiarize academic clinicians and researchers in medicine with the United States Government's role in regulating the conduct of clinical research investigations involving pharmaceuticals. It is intended as a general guide for the individual researcher interested in performing clinical trials but unfamiliar with the U.S. Government's oversight of clinical research.

HISTORY OF THE FOOD AND DRUG ADMINISTRATION DRUG REGULATION DEVELOPMENT

With the enactment of the 1938 Food, Drug, and Cosmetic Act (FD&C Act or "the act") (1) and the amendments to that act of 1962, Congress gave the Food and Drug Administration (FDA or "agency") authority over the research, development, and marketing of pharmaceutical products in the U.S. The law itself can be found in Chapter 5, Section 505(b), New Drugs, in the act, and FDA's regulations pertaining to the law can be found in the Code of Federal Regulations, Title 21, Part 312, titled "Investigational New Drug Applications" (2). This is the regulation with which we will be concerning ourselves in this chapter, which focuses on the regulation of clinical research with new drugs. Interested readers can also refer to Part 314 in the Code of Federal Regulations that pertains to the submission of New Drug Applications and the federal requirements for obtaining marketing approval for a new drug.

Hutt traces the evolution of the 1938 act following the elixir of sulfanilamide tragedy, which resulted from the use of a product manufactured by the Massengill Company that contained diethylene glycol as a solvent. Shortly after the marketing of this product, more than 100 people died of diethylene glycol poisoning.

The act was designed to assure the future safety of all products that would be distributed into the U.S. marketplace and stipulated that any new drug that would be investigated in humans must comply with investigational new drug (IND) regulations promulgated by the FDA. Before marketing such a drug, a new drug application (NDA) must have been submitted to the agency, and if the agency did not disapprove the NDA within 60 days, the drug would become legally available to the marketplace. In 1962 came the thalidomide tragedy, which originated in Germany and spread throughout several European countries, but fortunately bypassed the U.S. In response to this episode, Congress strengthened the 1938 law and regulations by requiring that an NDA used to support the marketing of a drug must contain proof of effectiveness as well as proof of safety. Under the 1962 amendments, the FDA must grant approval of the NDA, rather than simply allowing the NDA to become passively approved within a 60-day period. May et al. note that the 1962 amendments also required that the FDA be notified about preclinical studies and given detailed descriptions of investigations before clinical trials could commence. For the first time, informed consent of clinical trial subjects was required along with progress reports on all clinical investigations (3,4).

In response to the recent pressures directed at the federal government to find treatments and cures for cancer and acquired immunodeficiency syndrome (AIDS), the federal government has revised its IND regulations to allow for special types of INDs called "Treatment Use INDs" and "Compassionate Use INDs." One should refer to two recent *Federal Register* publications that deal with Treatment Use INDs (5) and life-threatening and severely debilitating illnesses (6). In this chapter, we focus on the typical IND submission to the agency by an independent investigator wishing to conduct clinical trials. The Treatment and Compassionate Use INDs will also be reviewed.

STRUCTURE OF THE FDA

Before we begin discussing the details of an IND submission and FDA's clinical trial regulatory philosophy, we will quickly review the structure of the FDA with particular attention to the Center for Drug Evaluation and Research (CDER). The commissioner of the FDA answers to the secretary for health and human services, and, as commissioner, is responsible for all regulated activities pertaining to foods, drugs, and cosmetics (Fig. 1). This chapter focuses on clinical pharmaceutical products, including prescription drug products and over-the-counter (OTC) drug products. The FDA's authority stems from the movement of a drug through interstate commerce. The regulatory body within the FDA with primary responsibility for regulating new drug research and marketing is the CDER, which in turn has a number of offices and divisions reporting to it with various responsibilities in this area (Fig. 2). The two primary offices reporting to the center with the responsibility to approve new drug applications for marketing and oversee investigational research are the Office of Drug Review I and the

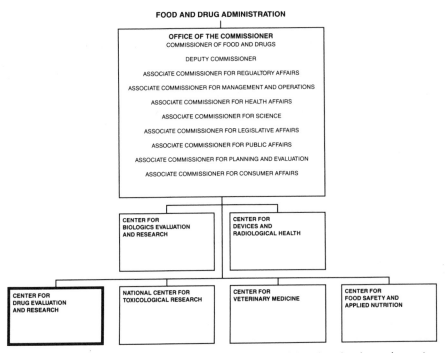

FIG. 1. Organizational chart of the U.S. Food and Drug Administration showing major centers with regulatory review responsibility.

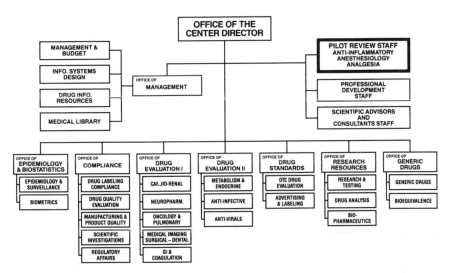

FIG. 2. Organizational chart of the FDA's Center for Drug Evaluation and Research showing office and division levels responsible for reviewing human pharmaceutical products, including the Pilot Review staff responsible for analgesic drug products.

Office of Drug Review II, both of which have a number of reviewing divisions each headed by a physician. These divisions, composed of medical officers, pharmacologists/toxicologists, chemists, and consumer safety officers (CSOs) and supported by statisticians and pharmacokineticists, review all IND and NDA applications received from various sponsors. Presently, there are nine review divisions within CDER, broken down primarily by the area of the drug's pharmaceutical activity, e.g., CNS active compounds or cardiovascular-type compounds. There is also a newly formed Pilot Review Division (Fig. 2). Currently, the responsibility for the review of analgesic drug products is vested in this unit, formally titled the Division of Anti-Inflammatory, Analgesic, and Anesthetic Pilot Review.

IND SUBMISSIONS

Definitions

At this point, a few definitions are in order. The term "IND" means an investigational new drug, and also means an investigational new drug application. IND is synonymous with "Notice of Claimed Investigational Exemption for a New Drug." An investigational new drug, in the opinion of FDA, is any new drug, antibiotic drug, or biological drug that is used in a clinical investigation. The term "investigator" means the person under whose immediate direction the drug is administered or dispensed to a subject. In the event that an investigation is conducted by a team of individuals, the principal investigator is the responsible head of that team, and other individuals involved in the trial are designated "subinvestigators." The term "sponsor" means a person who takes responsibility for and initiates a clinical investigation. The sponsor may be an individual, a pharmaceutical company, a government agency, an academic institution, or a private or public organization. The sponsor does not actually conduct the investigation unless the sponsor is considered a "sponsor-investigator." It is the sponsor who submits the IND to the FDA.

There are two basic types of INDs. A "commercial IND" is normally sponsored by a pharmaceutical company in support of an eventual NDA for marketing purposes. The other type of IND is an "independent investigator IND," usually submitted for research purposes only, or, in more recent times, for purposes of treating desperately ill people with unapproved drug products.

When an IND is Required

The question then arises as to when an IND is required for submission to the FDA. Institutional review boards (IRBs) and pharmaceutical companies often require proof of an IND on file with the FDA, or verification that an IND is not required, before permitting the conduct of a study or shipment of a drug. If, however, there is a doubt as to whether an IND should be filed or will be accepted by the agency, an investigator can call the FDA and determine whether or not the agency will require an IND. (One can contact the Office of Drug Review I at (301) 443-4330 or the Office of Drug Review II at (301) 443-2544, depending upon the nature of the drug and study.)

A clinical study of a lawfully marketed drug in the U.S. is *exempt* from IND requirements if:

1. The study is not intended to be submitted to the FDA in support of a new use or label change.
2. The study is not intended to support a change in advertising for the product.
3. The study does not involve a route of administration, dosage level, patient population, or other factor that increases the drug's risk or decreases the acceptability of risk with use.

These exemptions were intended to facilitate clinical research with already approved pharmaceutical products. However, even for a study exempt from IND requirements, IRB approval and patient informed consent must be obtained.

The revised IND regulations published in 1987(7) address studies that may be conducted without an IND. One must also not confuse the practice of medicine with drug research. Once a drug is approved by the FDA for marketing, a clinician is not bound to use the drug solely as indicated in the product labeling. However, the clinician must be willing to assume the responsibility for any extralabel use of a drug product. The FDA recognizes that good clinical practice and patient interests obligate the physician to use a marketed drug according to the best knowledge and judgment. Using a drug outside its labeled indications requires thorough information on the product and a solid scientific rationale for the use. Records should be kept reflecting use and side effects. The FDA recognizes that valid "new" uses of a marketed product are discovered and become accepted by the medical community before these uses become added formally to product labeling (8–10).

Phases of a Clinical Investigation

Clinical research is normally divided into three main phases that are somewhat arbitrary and sometimes not so distinct when progressing from one to the other. Phase I is the early clinical pharmacology phase that includes the initial introduction of an investigational drug in humans; studies are conducted in normal volunteer subjects and sometimes in patients. Phase I studies are designed to determine the metabolism and kinetics of the drug in humans and examine the side effects associated with increased doses of the drug. Preliminary information about efficacy can also be obtained. Normally, only single or an extremely limited number of doses are administered in Phase I studies, and the total number of patients usually involves anywhere from 20 to 100 patients. Phase I studies help permit the proper design of Phase II studies.

Phase II studies are controlled clinical studies conducted to evaluate the effectiveness of the drug for a particular indication or set of indications in patients with a disease or condition under study. Phase II studies also determine the common short-term side effects and risks associated with the drug and usually involve no more than several hundred subjects.

Phase III studies are expanded controlled and uncontrolled trials performed after preliminary evidence from Phase II studies shows effectiveness. These studies serve to collect additional information about effectiveness and safety that are needed for the overall evaluation of the benefit/risk ratio of the drug and involve anywhere from a few hundred to several thousand subjects. Phase I, II, and III studies, taken together, serve as the basis for product labeling. The FDA focuses its review on the safety of Phase I investigations and then includes consideration of the quality and scientific merit of the Phases II and III protocols.

Phase IV studies, also termed "postmarketing studies," may be requested by the FDA as a condition of a product's approval in order to answer specific toxicity or dosing questions. Alternately, they may be voluntarily conducted by a sponsor to add an indication, to expand a product's patient population, or to introduce a new dosage form. The FDA expects close monitoring during all phases of clinical investigation.

Preparation of an IND Submission

Once the investigator decides to submit an IND, he or she must follow the procedures briefly summarized below. Fye et al. (11) have prepared a thorough and well-structured review of the IND process. Much of the discussion in this chapter regarding IND content and procedure (this section and the section "Typical IND Submission") was patterned after this article.

Two government forms must accompany the submission of an IND. The first, form FDA 1571, serves as a two-page cover sheet identifying the sponsor of the IND, the name of the drug, the drug's indications or uses, what phase of clinical investigation will be conducted (i.e., Phase I, II, or III), and the required contents of the submission.

The second form that accompanies the IND submission, FDA 1572, provides pertinent information on the investigator of the clinical trial and any subinvestigators participating in the clinical trial. The back page of the form actually serves as a contract with the federal government by which the investigator commits to conducting the clinical trial under government regulations. The primary guiding principle used by the FDA when reviewing IND submissions is the assurance of the rights and safety of the subjects as specified on this form, as well as the adequacy of the proposed study in accomplishing its stated objective.

The IND application is submitted to the FDA as an original and two copies. Each subsequent submission to the IND is serially numbered using a single, three-digit serial number beginning with the number 000. The original IND submission is sent to a central mailing office at the FDA where a decision is made as to what review division will receive the IND and perform the review. The sponsor is notified of receipt of the IND by the appropriate review division and a 30-day waiting period begins.

The FDA will respond in writing, either confirming the initiation of the trial or detailing the reasons why the trial should not begin. Most of the written and telephone communications from the review division are performed by a CSO who acts as the liaison between the FDA and the IND sponsor. The IND is reviewed by a team normally consisting of a clinical or medical officer (generally a medical doctor), a chemist, and a pharmacologist, each of whom perform reviews of the relevant portions of the IND dealing with the clinical protocol and safety of human subjects, any pharmacology or toxicology derived from animal research in support of the proposed clinical trial, and the chemistry of the drug substance and the product to be used in the clinical investigation. These reviews are often supported by other teams within the FDA that address relevant statistical considerations, pharmacokinetics, and drug metabolism, and occasionally by outside consultants. Not infrequently, the commercial INDs for new chemical entities (NCEs) or major new uses, are discussed at advisory committee meetings that occur periodically at the FDA. Rarely do individual investigator INDs receive advisory committee review unless FDA considers the study to be controversial or outside of their area of expertise.

It should be noted that all of the information in an IND is considered confidential, except for material made previously available to the public, and is not released to the general public unless agreed to by the IND sponsor.

Once the sponsor has received approval to proceed with the clinical investigation, or if the sponsor did not receive word from FDA within 30 days of receiving the IND application that the trial could not proceed, the study may begin. Various reports are required to be submitted to the FDA on a periodic basis which inform the agency on the trial's progress and what has been learned to date. Any new protocols or alterations of the current protocols that affect patient safety or clinical outcome need to be submitted to the FDA for review, as do proposals to alter the composition of the drug product in any way.

ADVERSE DRUG REACTION (ADR) REPORTING

Of particular importance is the need to report any adverse events that occur during the conduct of the clinical trial to the agency. This involves the submission by telephone of 3-day safety reports (i.e., must be communicated to the review division within 3 days) for fatal or life-threatening events followed by a written description of the adverse event and by 10-day written reports to the agency for events that are both serious and unexpected. These reports must be submitted if the investigator believes that there is a reasonable possibility that the event may have been caused by the drug. The FDA considers a serious event to be one that meets one or more of the following conditions: fatal or life threatening, permanently disabling, requiring inpatient hospitalization, or involving congenital anomaly, cancer, or overdose. The FDA considers an unexpected event to be one that is not identified in nature, severity, or frequency in the investigator's brochure or the general investigational plan, or, for a marketed drug, does not appear in the product labeling (i.e., the package insert). In a multiinvestigator study the other investigators need to be notified of any 3-day or 10-day reports.

The FDA also requires that an annual report be submitted within 60 days of the anniversary date of the IND. This report summarizes the status of each ongoing study including the title of the study, the number of subjects, and their disposition. It must include a narrative or tabular summary showing the most frequent and most severe adverse experiences by body system for each study, a summary of all IND 3- and 10-day safety reports submitted during the year covered by the report, a list of all subjects who died or dropped out of the study with a description of the cause of death or reason for dropout, and a description of the general investigational plan for the coming year (See 21 CFR [Code of Federal Regulations] Sections 312.32 and 312.33).

SUBSTANTIAL EVIDENCE

The FDA requires that substantial evidence be submitted to support a new drug product approval or claim for a new indication. The term "substantial evidence" means that there must be adequate and well-controlled investigations to support the claims of effectiveness and safety.

The FDA has described the following characteristics of an adequate and well-controlled study (12,13):

1. There is a clear statement of the objective(s) of the investigation and a summary of the proposed or actual methods of analysis in the protocol for the study. If the protocol does not contain a description of the proposed analytical methods, the study report should describe how the methods used were selected.

2. The study uses a design that permits a valid comparison with a control to provide a quantitative assessment of drug effect. The protocol for the study and report of results should describe the design precisely (duration of treatment periods, whether treatments were parallel, sequential, or crossover, and whether the sample size was predetermined or based upon some interim analysis). Generally, FDA recognizes the following types of controls: (a) placebo concurrent control (usually randomized and blinded); (b) dose comparison concurrent control (at least two doses; usually randomized and blinded); (c) no treatment concurrent control (where objective measurements of efficacy are available and placebo effect is negligible; usually randomized); (d) active treatment concurrent

control (usually used when administration of placebo is not in the patient's interest; usually randomized and blinded; ability to detect differences between treatments needs assessing; why the drugs should be considered effective needs explaining); and (e) historical control (special circumstances, like diseases with high and predictable mortality or effect of drug, are self-evident). Placebo and/ or active treatment control are the two most frequently submitted to the agency in support of a study. To a lesser extent, dose comparison controls are used. It is important to realize that uncontrolled studies or even partially controlled studies are not acceptable to the agency as the sole basis for approval of claims of effectiveness. However, such studies are considered as supportive.

3. There is assurance that selected subjects have the disease or condition.

4. The method of patient assignment must minimize bias and assure comparability of treatment groups.

5. Efforts are made to minimize the required number of subjects, observers, and analysts.

6. Well-defined methods of assessment are used.

7. There is adequate analysis of results (See 21 CFR Section 314.26).

The FDA has also published a series of approximately 20 clinical guidelines (14) addressing clinical studies involving various types of pharmacological products, including "General Considerations for the Clinical Evaluation of Drugs" and "Guidelines for the Clinical Evaluation of Analgesic Drugs." These may be obtained at no charge from the Superintendent of Documents, U.S. Government Printing Office, Washington, D.C. 20402.

GOOD CLINICAL PRACTICE

In addition to the design and analysis of a clinical study, a sponsor and investigator must pay particular attention to good clinical practice (GCP) procedures (see ref. 15). GCP includes IRB approval, subject informed consent, proper record keeping, and reporting of adverse events. All clinical investigators need to understand the requirements stipulated in 21 CFR Parts 50 and 56.

TREATMENT USE, COMPASSIONATE USE, AND EMERGENCY USE INDS

In recent years, FDA has formalized or expanded upon already existing IND provisions for the treatment of seriously or desperately ill individuals using unmarketed drug products [(16) and 21 CFR Part 312, Sections 312.7, 312.34, and 312.35 (17)]. The two basic procedures are termed "Treatment Use IND" and "Compassionate Use IND," both of which differ from the typical IND studies that are designed to bring a new drug product to the market. The Treatment and Compassionate Use INDs are mechanisms by which a physician, under an

IND, can provide therapy to a desperately ill patient by using an unapproved new drug product.

Of the two mechanisms, only the Treatment Use IND is outlined at length in the regulations and in large part is owing to the need to provide any available treatment that shows promise of efficacy to AIDS patients, cancer patients, and others with serious or immediately life-threatening diseases for which no satisfactory alternative therapy exists.

Treatment Use INDs

The principles of Treatment Use IND date back to the late 1960s and early 1970s. At that time, a Compassionate or Humanitarian Use IND allowed patients to receive unapproved drugs for various illnesses. In 1987, FDA formalized regulations recognizing the Treatment Use IND under situations where there was sufficient evidence of safety and effectiveness of the drug and the potential benefits outweighed the risks.

The Treatment Use IND mechanism provides for accessibility to promising drugs prior to the completion of more formal studies necessary to obtain marketing approval. The Treatment Use IND regulations detail two procedures—one for immediately life-threatening diseases, and the other for serious diseases. Drugs for immediately life-threatening conditions are eligible for Treatment IND when there is reasonable evidence that the drug may be effective. This can occur as early as the initiation of Phase II trials. Drugs for serious conditions are held to somewhat more rigorous substantiation of safety and efficacy before their use will be allowed in a treatment program by the FDA. In this case, the sponsor must present sufficient evidence to support the drug's safe and effective use as proposed.

Although drugs for serious conditions may be available as early as Phase II, the FDA normally approves this type of treatment use during Phase III or upon the completion of the adequate and well-controlled trials. The FDA expanded on this effort by publishing an interim rule in 1988 (18) designed to speed up the investigational phases of new drug research for desperately ill patients, especially where no satisfactory alternative therapy exists, in order to obtain more prompt marketing approval. The key element in this provision is early consultation between sponsor and FDA to design trials and agree upon criteria for safety, efficacy, and minimal substantiation for marketing approval.

Compassionate Use INDs

The Compassionate Use IND is an umbrella phrase referring to a less formal regulatory process under which experimental unapproved drugs or uses of a marketed drug are made available to patients outside the traditional IND framework. The Compassionate Use IND or protocol is utilized on a more individual, less formal basis than the Treatment IND provisions. The drug may be a true experimental compound or a substance that has been studied or marketed abroad but lacks any U.S. experience.

Emergency Use INDs

There is one other mechanism worth mentioning by which experimental drugs can be made available on an individual basis, and it is referred to as the "Emergency IND." This procedure involves cases in an emergency situation that do not allow time for the regular submission of an IND (See 21 CFR Section 312.36). In this case, the FDA may authorize shipment of an experimental drug to a sponsor for a specified use in advance of submission of all the paperwork covering the IND. Emergency Use INDs are normally reserved for severe medical situations, typically when a patient is near death. In this situation, the physician explains the situation to the FDA by telephone. Usually, verbal FDA approval is obtained for the physician to use the drug. The physician will be assigned an IND number over the phone with permission to obtain a specified amount of drug. The sponsor must promptly submit a written IND submission for the situation. The September 1989 *U.S. Regulatory Reporter* provides an excellent overview of these special IND provisions (19).

These three types of IND special mechanisms may prove to be of particular utility in treating patients with novel agents for intractable pain. The investigator who contemplates using one of these procedures should call the Pilot Review Division and ask for the supervisory CSO to discuss the matter. It is worth noting that for all of these exceptions regarding Treatment Use, Compassionate Use, and Emergency Use INDs, the sponsor of the study must always provide FDA documentation demonstrating proof of informed consent, IRB approval, as well as the submission of the required government forms, FDA 1571 and 1572. Documentation must also be provided that describes the source of the drug, its purity, and other necessary chemical and physical characteristics. Any published or unpublished information supporting use of the drug will help expedite the FDA's review of these applications.

TYPICAL IND SUBMISSION

At this point, it is appropriate to review the typical IND submission to the FDA. As mentioned earlier, there are a variety of types of INDs and reasons for their submission: (a) the commercial IND, used by drug companies to begin the development of a new drug for eventual marketing approval in the U.S.; (b) the individual investigator IND, for research by an institution or an individual, often for already approved drugs; and (c) Treatment, Compassionate, and Emergency Use INDs normally used for the treatment of desperately ill patients for whom there is no available alternative therapy. What follows is a description of the usual process by which a sponsor files an IND with the FDA. In the case of the individual investigator IND, the sponsor often is also the investigator and usually refers the reviewer to a commercial IND, NDA, or drug master file (DMF) held by a commercial company, for information regarding the chemistry of the compound and preclinical or clinical work demonstrating the safety and effectiveness of the product. A drug sponsor submitting an IND must provide the agency with full details on the manufacturing controls of the new drug substance, the results of animal studies (short-term and long-term) that address the toxicity and metabolism of the drug substance, and the long-term effects of the drug including carcinogenicity and teratogenicity. All INDs require full details on the proposed protocol for use of the drug in the study situation, IRB approval, and patient informed consent. The FDA also requires the curriculum vitae (CV) of the principal investigator and a listing of all subinvestigators that participate in the study.

As stated earlier, the sponsor of any IND must submit two forms—FDA 1571, entitled "Investigational New Drug Application," and FDA 1572, entitled "Statement of Investigator." These forms may be obtained from: the FDA's Forms and Publications Distribution Center, AFC Warehouse (HFA-268), Consolidated Forms and Publications Distribution Center, 3222 Hubbard Road, Landover, Maryland 20785. In the case of a multicenter study, form FDA 1572 must be completed by each investigator at every study center. For an individual investigator performing his or her own study, an IND will normally require the assistance of the drug supplier or manufacturer. Once a manufacturer has agreed to supply a study drug, the sponsor-investigator needs a letter from the supplier granting the FDA permission to refer to their DMF, NDA, or their own IND already on file at the FDA, which generally satisfies the manufacturing data as well as the preclinical data requirement in Sections 12.7 through 12.10 of form FDA 1571. The FDA cannot legally refer to these data without the explicit authorization from the pharmaceutical company. Although form FDA 1571 is designed to serve as a cover sheet for the IND submission, it is advisable for a sponsor of an IND to submit a cover letter in addition, explaining the basis for wishing to submit this IND and conduct the study.

In addition to the cover letter and the two FDA forms, as well as any references of authorization from the manufacturer or supplier of the new drug substance, the sponsor must submit a detailed protocol describing the study, the patient population, and the exclusion and inclusion criteria, safety precautions that will be taken during the conduct of the study, and details of the planned statistical analysis.

As with all communications to the FDA regarding the IND, the IND application must be submitted in triplicate. (Registered or certified mail is suggested.) For studies involving products other than biological products, the *original* IND submission should be mailed to the Central Document Room, Center for Drugs Evaluation and Research, FDA, Park Building Room 214, 12420 Parklawn Drive, Rockville, Maryland, 20852. Upon receipt of the IND application, the FDA will assign an IND number to the application and issue a letter to the sponsor-investigator that provides identification of the submission and the person at

FDA with whom to communicate. In the case of analgesic drug products, the review division will be the new Pilot Review Division, designated HFD-007.

After an IND is submitted there is a mandatory 30-day waiting period during which time the sponsor must withhold initiation of the clinical trial(s) until FDA has either communicated by telephone or in writing that the study may proceed, or the 30 days have passed without FDA objection. The 30-day waiting period is defined as 30 days from the date the FDA receives the IND submission. If, during that 30-day period, the FDA reviewers find some serious deficiency in the proposed study, the sponsor will be notified by a (CSO) stating that the study has been placed on "clinical hold." Normally the sponsor will be notified verbally of the deficiencies followed by official written notification itemizing those deficiencies. The study may be initiated once these deficiencies have been corrected. Usually, the supplier of a drug will require proof of a filed IND with the FDA before the drug will be shipped to the sponsor or investigator. Normally, a copy of the FDA's letter acknowledging receipt of the IND submission is sufficient to satisfy this requirement.

IND Reporting Requirements

A sponsor of an IND has a number of responsibilities and reporting requirements once an IND becomes active. These involve any amendments (changes) to the original protocol, addition of any new investigators, IND safety reports, and annual reports. All IND submissions should be accompanied by a cover sheet and consecutively numbered (refer to Fig. 6, form FDA 1571). As stated earlier, the initial submission should be numbered serial no. 000. Any additional submissions should be numbered consecutively in the order in which they are submitted.

The types of submissions required during the course of an IND are:

1. Protocol amendments—new protocols, changes in protocol, new investigators.
2. Information amendments—new information on chemistry, pharmacology, toxicology, and clinical information.
3. IND safety reports—initial written and any follow-up reports (see above, Adverse Drug Reaction Reporting).
4. Responses to FDA requests for additional information.
5. Annual reports.
6. Response to a "clinical hold."
7. General correspondence.
8. Termination of the study.

Protocol amendments are required when there is any change in the *scope* or *direction* of the initial investigational plan submitted to the FDA by the investigator. This is especially important for any changes to the original protocol that affect the safety of the subjects or the benefit/risk considerations of the initial clinical plan. Examples of protocol changes requiring an IND amendment include an increase in drug dosage or duration of exposure, an increase in the number of study subjects, a significant change in study design, the addition of new test procedures, or the elimination of certain test procedures. New protocols or changes to existing protocols may not be initiated until the protocol amendment has been submitted to the FDA and approved by the IRB. The only exception to this requirement is a change made to eliminate an immediate hazard or risk to the patient. Such changes may be implemented immediately with subsequent notification to both the FDA and the IRB. Protocol amendments are also required whenever an investigator is added or replaced.

A form FDA 1572 must be completed by each investigator who will be assisting the sponsor at any collaborating institution. Normally, a CV will suffice for the required description of the education and experience of the investigator. Each investigator must also list the names of all subinvestigators. CVs for subinvestigators are not required to be filed with the FDA, but the sponsor and principal investigators should have them available.

The sponsor of an IND is required to promptly evaluate all information received from any source relevant to the safety of a drug. These requirements were previously detailed in the section Adverse Drug Reaction (ADR) Reporting. For each IND safety report submitted, the sponsor-investigator must identify all previous safety reports filed to this IND for similar experiences. The sponsor-investigator is also required to analyze the significance of this experience in light of the previous reports. The sponsor-investigator also has the obligation to inform all other investigators of any alarming or serious reactions submitted to the FDA.

The sponsor-investigator of an IND is also required to submit an annual progress report within 60 days of the anniversary date of the IND. The information in the annual report includes the following:

1. The status of the IND—that is, if it is still active or if it has been withdrawn or terminated.
2. All protocols and their current status, giving both the title and number of the protocol.
3. Plans for the upcoming year.
4. The progress of each completed or ongoing study, providing a brief description of the purpose and current status of the study.
5. The patient population, including the total number enrolled to date, the number of terminations or dropouts and the reasons for these; any interim analysis or final study results; a narrative or tabular listing of the most frequent and most severe adverse events for each of the protocols listed by body system; a summary of all IND safety reports submitted during the year; and a listing of any deaths and any study dropouts.

Conduct of a Clinical Investigation

It is extremely important for anyone contemplating being a sponsor or an investigator of an IND to familiarize themselves with the GCP regulations and the responsibilities and obligations of sponsors and investigators. In addition to

Part 312 of 21 CFR and general references such as Bert Spilker's Guide to Clinical Studies and Developing Protocols (20), one should familiarize themselves with the FDA notice "Clinical Investigations Proposed Rule—Obligations of Sponsors and Monitors" (21). Although never formalized into a regulation, these proposed rules still serve as the foundation for the FDA's GCP and the obligations and responsibilities of sponsors and investigators of an IND. By signing form FDA 1571, the sponsor or sponsor-investigator acknowledges the following obligations and responsibilities:

1. Selecting qualified investigators.
2. Obtaining commitments from investigators as described in form FDA 1572.
3. Monitoring investigator compliance with the protocol and commitments for data collection, drug accountability, protection of patient's rights, immediate reporting of serious adverse experiences, and obtaining IRB approval.
4. Discontinuing investigators who are not in compliance.
5. Keeping investigators informed of any new information concerning the drug, especially information with regard to safety.
6. Controlling accountability of study drug supplies.
7. Discontinuing the study if adequate data have been obtained or safety information indicates unreasonable and significant risk.
8. Conducting site visits preinvestigation, periodically during the investigation, and upon study completion. (The purpose of these site visits is to determine the adequacy of staff and facilities and to assure that investigators understand all obligations and adhere to the protocol, as well as comply with all FDA regulations, reporting requirements, and data capturing techniques.)
9. Data monitoring: the sponsor must promptly review all new data received from any investigator concerning the safety and effectiveness of the drug and periodically evaluate the accumulated data.
10. Satisfying the safety reporting requirements by immediately reviewing all information received from any source and reporting to FDA under the 3- or 10-day annual reporting requirements.
11. Reporting to FDA on an annual basis the progress of the study.

As an investigator, one acknowledges the following obligations by signing form FDA 1572:

1. Conducting and personally supervising the study in accordance with the protocol. Any changes require prior sponsor notification, except in the case of an emergency, in order to protect the safety of the subject.
2. Informing any subject or person used as a control that the study drug is being used for investigational purposes, and ensuring that all requirements pertaining to informed consent and IRB review and approval are met.
3. Reporting to the sponsor adverse experiences that occur in the course of the investigation that may be reasonably regarded as caused by the study drug. If such a reaction is alarming, the report must be made to the sponsor im-

mediately. Upon completion of the investigation, the sponsor must be provided with a final report of the study.

4. Reading and understanding the information provided in the investigator's brochure regarding the potential risks and side effects of the drug.

5. Maintaining adequate and accurate records. This includes accurate case histories and records of receipt and disposition of all study drugs during the study. These records are to be maintained for at least 2 years following completion of the study. Any unused drug supplies should be returned to the sponsor upon request.

6. Insuring that an appropriate IRB will be responsible for the initial and continuing review and approval of the clinical investigations; agreeing to promptly report to the IRB all changes in the research and any unanticipated problems that may arise, and agreeing not to make any changes in the research without IRB approval, except in the cases of immediate risk regarding the safety of the human subjects.

7. Complying with all of the requirements regarding the obligations of clinical investigators in the CFR, Part 312 (11).

FDA'S PILOT REVIEW DIVISION

Since this book is about the design of analgesic clinical trials, it is appropriate to conclude this chapter with some discussion of the recent experimental review division that has been established within CDER. This division is the Pilot Review Division, designated HFD-007. The division is responsible for the review and evaluation of all IND, NDA, and related information pertaining to analgesic drugs, nonsteroidal antiinflammatory drugs, anesthetic drugs, and the controlled substances.

There is also a good deal of interaction between the FDA reviewers and the sponsors with regard to study design, adequacy of data, and how the reviewers wish to have the data displayed in the IND or NDA reports. The division and sponsors may exchange data using electronic mail and personal computers. Although the Pilot Review Division readily accepts electronic data submissions, it is highly advisable for a sponsor contemplating the use of electronic communication with the FDA to speak with the division before committing to any particular equipment or format. Oftentimes, the sponsors and perhaps the investigators will visit the FDA and discuss the research issues with the FDA reviewers. Meetings with the division can be arranged by calling (301) 443-3741.

CONCLUSION

The best general advice one can give to a researcher interested in conducting clinical trials is to familiarize oneself with the rules and regulations pertaining to IND/NDA submissions (14,22,23). When in doubt, the sponsor-investigator should not hesitate to contact a CSO in the review division in order to obtain guidance regarding design and conduct of protocols and data submission. When an IND is required and submitted, Phase I studies are normally reviewed for safety reasons only, whereas Phase II and Phase III studies are reviewed for the adequacy and design of the proposed clinical investigations, to ensure that the study will indeed answer the questions proposed in the protocol.

As one can see from this brief overview, the FDA's regulation of clinical research is perhaps the most regulated activity overseen by the U.S. Government. By familiarizing oneself with these requirements and learning to work within the system, many investigators can avoid much of the delay and frustration associated with the government's regulation of clinical research.

REFERENCES

1. Federal Food, Drug, and Cosmetic Act of 1938, Chapter V, Section 505, New Drugs.
2. Investigational New Drug Application. *Code of Federal Regulations,* Title 21, Part 312.
3. Hutt PB. Investigations and reports respecting FDA regulations of new drugs (part I). *Clin Pharmacol Ther* 1983;33(4):537–538.
4. May MS, et al. New drug development during and after a period of regulatory change: clinical research activity of major United States pharmaceutical firms, 1958–1979. *Clin Pharmacol Ther* 1983;33(6):691–700.
5. Investigational new drug, antibiotic, and biological drug product regulations: treatment use. *Federal Register* May 22, 1987;52(99):19466–19477.
6. Investigational new drug, antibiotic, and biological drug product regulations: procedures for drugs intended to treat life-threatening and severely debilitating illnesses. *Federal Register* October 21, 1988;53(204):41516–41524.
7. New drug, antibiotic, and biologic drug product regulations, final rule. *Federal Register* March 19, 1987;52(53):(Docket No. 82N-0394).
8. Use of approved drugs for unlabeled indications. *FDA Drug Bulletin* April, 1982;12(1).
9. Use of drugs for unapproved indications: your legal responsibility. *FDA Drug Bulletin,* October, 1972.
10. Temple R. Legal implications of the package insert. *Prim Care* 1974;1(3):519–528.
11. Fye CL, et al. IND manual for sponsors/investigators. *Clin Res Pract Drug Reg Affairs* 1989;7(2):69–116.
12. New drug and antibiotic regulations; final rule. *Federal Register* February 22, 1985;50(36):7487–7488,7506–7507.
13. New drug application. *Code of Federal Regulations.* Title 21, Part 314.
14. Partial list of FDA guidelines for testing drugs:
    General considerations for the clinical evaluation of drugs; FDA 77-3-040; GPPO 017-012-00245-5.
    Guidelines for the clinical evaluation of analgesic drugs; FDA 80-3093; GPO 017-012-00283-8.
    Guidelines for the clinical evaluation of antiinflammatory drugs (adults and children); FDA 78-3054; GPO 017-012-00258-7.
15. Clinical investigations: obligations of sponsors and monitors, proposed rule. *Federal Register* September 27, 1977;42(187):49612–49630.
16. Investigational new drug, antibiotic, and biological drug product regulations: treatment use. *Federal Register* May 22, 1987;52(99):19466–19477.
17. Investigational new drug application. *Code of Federal Regulations,* Title 21, Part 312.
18. Investigational new drug, antibiotic, and biological drug product regulations: procedures for drugs intended to treat life-threatening and severely debilitating illnesses. *Federal Register.* October 21, 1988;53(204):41516–41524.

19. Treatment, compassionate use, and emergency INDs and parallel track: understanding it all. *U.S. Regulatory Reporter* September, 1989;6(3):3–6.
20. Spilker B. *Guide to clinical studies and developing protocols.* New York: Raven Press, 1984.
21. Clinical investigations: obligations of sponsors and monitors, proposed rule. *Federal Register* September 27, 1977;42(187):49612–49630.
22. Oates JA, Wood AJJ. The regulation of discovery and drug development, editorial. *N Engl J Med* 1989;320(5):311–312.
23. Kessler DA. The regulation of investigational drugs. *N Engl J Med* 1989;320(5):281–288.

Note: Copies of the *Federal Register* can be obtained from the U.S. Government Printing Office, Superintendent of Documents, Washington, D.C., 20402.

Advances in Pain Research and Therapy, Vol. 18,
edited by M. Max, R. Portenoy, and E. Laska,
Raven Press, Ltd., New York © 1991.

Commentary

Thoughts on the Relationship Between the Academic Investigator and the Drug Industry and the FDA in Developing Analgesic Drugs

William T. Beaver

*Departments of Pharmacology and Anesthesia, Georgetown University
School of Medicine, Washington, DC 20007*

It is particularly encouraging that this volume on the design of analgesic clinical trials represents the initiative primarily of the younger investigators in the field, because the central theme of my comments is the impact of some current trends in the administrative mechanisms of analgesic drug development on the role and even the viability of the academic investigator.

THE ACADEMIC INVESTIGATOR AND HIS VEXATIONS

Not all, but most academically oriented investigators who perform analgesic clinical trials are based in academic medical and dental centers, and there are many demands on their time and energies including teaching, patient care, institutional administration, lectures, other scholarly activities, and service for professional societies. They can devote only a portion of their time to analgesic research, and the creeping increase in institutional and external paperwork required to get a study under way puts further demands on what time is available.

At academic medical centers, the investigator is also confronted with a shrinking supply of suitable patients, inpatients in particular, as a result of recent rapid changes in medical practice: the massive increase in ambulatory surgery, diagnosis-related groups (DRGs) and the pressure to discharge patients as soon as possible, the routine use of patient-controlled analgesia (PCA) in the postoperative patient, and, in general, more clinical research chasing fewer patients. The situation is similar even for patients suffering from chronic cancer pain. At most major cancer centers, patients are admitted, receive multiple diagnostic and therapeutic modalities simultaneously, and are summarily discharged. Gone are the elegant, leisurely, complete-crossover studies that I did when apprenticed to Houde, Wallenstein, and Rogers at the Memorial Sloan-Kettering Cancer Center.

There are high fixed costs in doing this kind of research that are unrelated to the number of patients actually available for and completing the study. The investigator must recoup as much of his salary as possible including compensation for time and effort not directly related to carrying out a particular study. In addition, he or she must fund the entire salary of one or more highly trained nurse-observers, the costs of operating an office and a perennially increasing percentage for institutional overhead.

Considering these factors, it should come as no surprise that the academic investigator is usually not the most cost-effective source for analgesic clinical trials. He can rarely compete on a cost-per-patient basis with the proliferation of contract houses doing analgesic studies.

This brings us to the issue of potential sources of funding. There is a little federal government funding from the National Institutes of Health (NIH), National Cancer Institute (NCI), National Institute of Dental Research (NIDR), and National Institute of Drug Abuse (NIDA) grants and contracts. Whereas these fund a small but increasingly vital part of analgesic clinical research, by far most of the money comes from the drug industry; at one time, virtually all of the funding came directly or indirectly from the drug industry.

THE DRUG INDUSTRY

The drug industry is also, of course, where almost all of the new analgesics come from, with the exception of a few drugs of little commercial interest, such as heroin. Drug companies also provide most of the financial support for analgesic clinical trials. From my perspective, the relationship of the academic investigator to the drug industry has changed substantially over the last 10 to 15 years.

How were these studies formerly done? In the old days that Louis Lasagna discusses in Chapter 1, the drug company came to investigators with a drug. The company provided animal pharmacology and toxicology information, Phase I human safety data, and sometimes anecdotal reports of open-label, dose-ranging administration to a few patients. Occasionally, the data from the interim analysis of other investigators' controlled trials were also available. After reviewing this data and some discussion with the company about patient availability and what would constitute scientifically meaningful, feasible objectives, a consensus emerged as to appropriate control treatments and dose levels of the study medications. The company then provided these medications, often in bulk packages of dosage units, and someone in the study group or a hospital pharmacist was responsible for repackaging and coding them for the nurse-observer.

The design of the study and the analgesic scaling instruments were usually those the investigators had developed themselves and had used routinely in previous studies; periodically, the investigators modified or added new features to their study design. The investigators almost always did their own statistical analyses. Early on, if the study was to be done in the "usual way," there was often no formal written protocol. Subsequently, as detailed written protocols evolved, these were prepared or at least drafted by the investigators. A large number of excellent analgesic studies were performed this way, including the definitive studies on most opioids. Essentially all of the general methodologic features of modern controlled clinical trials were developed in this manner.

The mechanics of setting up studies and the division of labor between the drug company and the investigator have changed substantially in the interim, in some respects for the better. The company has assumed the chore of packaging and labeling study medications, and the extensive data monitoring, data processing, and statistical analysis resources provided by the company have certainly been helpful. On the other hand, certain changes have *not* been helpful, in particular, the tendency to exclude the investigator from participating in a meaningful way in the design of his own research. Up until a few years ago, I wrote the protocols for every study I ever did, and these protocols were relatively brief, eight to ten double-spaced typewritten pages at most. If necessary, the company could then append material related to administrative details and other necessary boilerplate.

Now, rather than being presented with a drug to study, the investigator is almost always presented with an excruciatingly detailed final protocol, and, although some drug companies are reasonably flexible in this regard, often there is great resistance to modifying this protocol. This is so in spite of the fact that the persons who wrote the protocol may never have been directly involved in the conduct of an analgesic study, whereas the investigator may have been designing and performing such studies for 15 or 20 years. There are many reasons for this anomalous state of affairs.

Over the years, the progressive increase in FDA regulation has spawned a massive counterbureaucracy in the drug industry. Every protocol change must be approved by multiple layers of this bureaucracy. I was told that in one company there are more than a dozen different persons and divisions that must sign off on a protocol, and, of course, if there is a change, they all must sign off on it again.

In addition, industry employees are really out on a limb if, after the study is submitted, the FDA does not like the way it was designed. If the employee exercises some initiative and modifies the protocol along the lines suggested by the investigator, and the FDA subsequently criticizes that study, that employee is potentially in trouble with his boss. To complicate matters, all sorts of rumors are constantly circulating through the industry as to the FDA's feelings at that moment concerning various fine points of analgesic study design. Sometimes these rumors are patently ridiculous, but they can cause concern nonetheless. So rather than sit down with the investigator and try to decide what study objectives and design features make good scientific sense, there is a tendency for the people in the drug company to try to guess what the people at the FDA want and design the protocol accordingly. A corollary to this approach is exclusive adherence to those study designs and data analyses that have recently found favor at the FDA to the exclusion of reasonable alternative approaches. None of this is conducive to innovation in the design of clinical trials.

This discussion would be incomplete without mention of the "holier than the FDA" approach to protocol design, which refers to the practice in some companies of inventing idiosyncratic policies that unnecessarily interfere with the conduct of analgesic trials. The investigator is often assured that an irksome requirement in the protocol represents an FDA requirement, when in fact it represents nothing more than the effort by someone in the company to adhere to an even higher standard of scientific purity than that required by the scientific community or the FDA. An example of this phenomenon is the evolution (and subsequent misapplication) of the concept of double-blinding in analgesic clinical trials.

Henry Beecher first applied the double-blind technique in his analgesic studies to minimize the bias potentially generated by the expectations of the patient and observer concerning the performance of a particular treatment. To achieve this goal, not everyone in the analgesic study team necessarily needs to be blind to the identity of the treatments; this decision rests on a consideration of which persons are interacting with patients or making judgments as to the acceptability of data. Subsequently, the scope of blinding has become more extensive to guard against unanticipated interactions among the study team and to discourage deliberate fraud, and this is probably a good idea to the degree that it does not impede the conduct of the study.

However, it is also a good idea for the investigator to examine the mean responses of patients to treatments (i.e., the analgesic time-effect curves) a few times during the course of the study to see whether some unanticipated problem is arising in the conduct of the study that should be sought out and corrected. A number of drug companies are resistant to this idea on the grounds that blinding will in some unexplained way be compromised, even though an individual numerical code is being used and the data in question have already been transmitted to the company. I have reviewed a number of studies in which this policy has resulted in a failed study and a substantial waste of time and money.

Recently, some companies don't even let their own people who are responsible for developing the drug see interim study results, presumably for fear of an ill-defined parapsychological interaction that might influence the investigator. There are costs associated with ignoring the biblical injunction concerning the blind leading the blind. Since the optimal design of subsequent studies depends on a knowledge of the results of previous studies, the above policies can prolong unnecessarily the drug development process and result in the exposure of patients to drugs in studies that will not be productive of useful results. Good science is simply not done this way.

THE FDA

Until quite recently, most analgesic investigators have had virtually no contact with the FDA other than in the context of a study audit. Other than that, the investigator and the FDA haven't really talked to each other. FDA medical reviewers are definitely not encouraged to phone the investigator and talk over a study under review, let alone discuss the investigator's general thoughts on a new analgesic. It is my impression that the FDA and the drug companies, being organized along comparable bureaucratic lines, would prefer to deal solely with each other, and neither wants the investigator intruding. The exception is the situation where things turn sour in this dialogue, in which case the drug company gets a token investigator or two to come to the FDA and plead the company's case.

The FDA has had a formidable impact on the analgesic investigator and his research, but for practical purposes, almost all of that impact has, in the past at least, been the indirect result of the FDA's interaction with the drug industry. Furthermore, as alluded to above, there is a real distinction between how people at the FDA perceive their message to the drug industry and how various companies perceive that message. More *direct* contact between the FDA and the academic investigator would certainly be helpful to both, and recent initiatives in that direction are encouraging.

THE FUTURE OF THE ACADEMIC INVESTIGATOR

My major concern is how much incentive this atmosphere provides for a new generation of academically oriented investigators. Will the prospect of just conducting analgesic clinical trials sponsored and designed by drug companies be of sufficient interest to capable young scientists to justify making a commitment to a career in analgesic clinical pharmacology?

Some companies are certainly more flexible than others in allowing investigators meaningful participation in the design of their own research, and some investigators are more adroit than others in bootlegging some innovative science into their studies or setting aside a portion of drug industry grants to do their own research. But it is my feeling that doing controlled analgesic trials for the drug industry is just not as much scientific fun as it once was. And fun, of course, is why people go into science. The kinds of people who can succeed as biomedical scientists have many career options and can choose among many fields of research.

My final question is whether we are going to be reduced to a kind of dual-track system for analgesic research, the beginnings of which are already evident. Namely, there will be a few academic clinical pharmacologists and others with a career interest in pain and its treatment doing intellectually exciting research, which is almost entirely funded by government grants, but doing very little work in collaboration with the drug industry. In order to generate the data necessary for the FDA approval of new drug applications (NDAs), there will be a second track consisting of clinicians with a primary commitment to other aspects of patient care with, at best, an ancillary interest in analgesic research and contract houses, and others who regard clinical trials solely as a profit-making business activity. The latter two groups will be turning the crank, no questions asked, to grind out industry protocols. I think that the academic investigator, the drug industry, the FDA, and the patient with pain would all be the losers should this dismal scenario come to pass.

DISCUSSION

Dr. Carl Peck: I would like to give a Center for Drugs (FDA) reaction to the thoughts expressed by Dr. Beaver. First of all, it seems to me that Bill Beaver is proof to the contrary of his thesis that an academic investigator can't undertake a creative career in analgesic research. He has undeniably overcome the obstacles he described.

Before I came to the agency in 1987, I was not an FDA watcher, and it is possible that, as Beaver claims, some combination of attitudes of industry and the FDA dampened the creative instincts of academic investigators. But we at the FDA Center for Drugs are now committed to promoting innovation. We recognize a problem in the INDs and NDAs that we presently see. There is often a surprising lack of innovation.

We are taking several steps to correct this. We have recently reconfigured the analgesics and drug abuse staff into a so-called pilot review staff, which is committed to developing innovative procedures for drug review. These include interaction with the drug industry and academic community early in the process of drug development, to encourage innovations in methodology.

In addition, we certainly do not have an ethic that discourages interaction with investigators. I note that companies often do not bring the investigators, and when they do, the investigators seem to be programmed to argue only one side of the question. This is unfortunate, because we are scientists and would like to have a balanced and candid discussion. We hope to work with the industry and academe to change that, because it should be a free-flowing, open, scientific environment.

Rather than being a barrier, I think, we are pushing the sponsors now for innovative designs. We are encouraging many sponsors in analgesics and other areas to "get modern," to quit looking at just dose and response, but consider how to get the right concentration of drug to the site of action, using modern concepts and techniques of pharmacokinetics and pharmacodynamics.

In summary, I would like to state that we are strongly in favor of innovation and promote involvement of academic investigators. We would like to work with you to eliminate any barriers to creative clinical research. For my part, if I were younger and starting out, I would be very excited about going into analgesiology. I think there is an enormous amount of new ground to break there. I am enthused about the kinetic and dynamic approach because I believe it offers an ability to more efficiently design studies and optimize dosing regimens, but there are many other areas for innovation as well.

Advances in Pain Research and Therapy, Vol. 18,
edited by M. Max, R. Portenoy, and E. Laska,
Raven Press, Ltd., New York © 1991.

29

Analytic Approaches
to Quantifying Pain Scores

Eugene M. Laska, Morris Meisner, and Carole Siegel

*Statistical Sciences and Epidemiology Division, Nathan S. Kline Institute for
Psychiatric Research, WHO Collaborating Center for Training and Research in Mental
Health Program Management, Orangeburg, New York 10962; and Department of
Psychiatry, New York University Medical Center, New York, New York 10016*

Despite the increasing use of visual analogue scales, statistical problems in clinical
trials frequently involve the analysis of data that are graded categorical response
variables. Usually an ad hoc *a priori* quantification is used to assign values to
these responses. For example, for pain intensity data collected in analgesic trials,
the usual equal-step approach is to set "no pain" equal to zero, "mild" equal to
one, "moderate" equal to two, and "severe" equal to three. Although this scheme
is widely utilized, few believe that the "true" magnitude of the differences between
pain intensity scores, were they knowable, are equal. Moreover, it is unlikely
that the pain intensity reported to be severe by a patient with uterine cramp is
as intense as that of a postoperative patient who uses the same adjective. In
short, the same words used to describe the pain intensity in different pain models
are likely to be quantitatively different. Many investigators are uncomfortable
with the arbitrariness of the numerical assignments to categories. Lasagna (1)
questioned whether the equal-step approach is legitimate, and he studied patient
perception of the relative importance of changes from one category to another.
He also attempted an approach using discriminant function analysis to find
"intervals in such a pain scale [that] serve most efficiently to separate active
from inactive drugs." He reported, "We have failed to come up with any weighting
of pain scores which serves to increase significantly the yield over that supplied
by the simplest (that is, the equal-step) approach. Houde and his colleagues at
Memorial Hospital in New York City have tried various manipulations of their
own data and have similarly failed to come up with a useful transformation" (1).

Absent an instrument to directly measure the numerical value of pain intensity
in a human being, we propose using, as a surrogate measure, the amount of a
standard analgesic necessary to change the verbal categorical response one unit.

It is likely that for different etiology, different doses of an analgesic may be required to obtain a comparable degree of relief for patients who report severe initial pain. If one can assume similar neural mechanisms of pain among several patient groups, the relative magnitude of the dosages needed to produce a comparable change can be used as a surrogate indicator of differences in the magnitude of a categorical pain intensity among types of pain.

To formalize these ideas, we present two mathematical models for quantifying categorical responses. In the first approach pain of only a single etiology is considered and the resulting scores maximize the least squares fit of the dose-response regression line. Numerical assignments based on this method result in estimates of the dose-response parameters that are at least as precise as those obtained using ordinary least-squares under the usual equal-step assumption. The optimal scores derived by this technique may then be used in other analyses, e.g., dose-related treatment contrasts or in a bioassay analysis to estimate the relative potency of two compounds.

In the second approach a quantal response model, i.e., one based on a binary response variable, allows the data to be used to estimate, for different pain etiologies, the numerical scores corresponding to verbal pain intensities.

We assume the following typical experimental situation. Two drugs, a test (T) and a standard (S), are to be studied and their relative potency (2) is to be estimated. A placebo may be studied as well. To accomplish this, at least one of the drugs and preferably both are to be studied at several dose levels. A patient receives a single dose of one or more of the treatments on a randomized, double-blind basis according to any one of the usual statistical designs: completely randomized parallel groups, Latin square, or partially balanced incomplete blocks. The patient is interviewed immediately preceding the administration of the study medication and again at various times thereafter so as to obtain subjective assessments of initial and postmedication pain intensity levels and relief. We note that the mathematical development given below does not require both a test and standard medication.

A REGRESSION MODEL OF DOSE RESPONSE

The linear log dose-response relationships usually postulated are expressed by

$$Y_S = \alpha_S + \beta \log x + \epsilon$$

and   [1]

$$Y_T = \alpha_T + \beta \log x + \epsilon$$

where Y_S and Y_T are numerical random variables, whose values are unknown, corresponding to the categories of responses of a patient receiving either the test T or standard S at the dose level x. Here ϵ represents random error in the model, and we assume that it has zero mean. Formally, equations [1] reflect the assumptions that the responses to dose x of medication S or T are random variables whose means lie on a straight line with respect to log dose. The line for S has an intercept α_S, the line for T has an intercept α_T and the two lines have a common slope, β.

Given the results of a clinical trial the standard regression problem is to determine estimates $\hat{\alpha}_S$, $\hat{\alpha}_T$, and $\hat{\beta}$ of the parameters α_S, α_T, and β in the model hypothesized in equation [1], so as to minimize the sum of the squares of the error given by

$$\sum_{i,\Delta} (y_{i\Delta} - (\alpha_\Delta + \beta \log x_i))^2. \qquad [2]$$

In the usual case $y_{i,\Delta}$ are the actual observed numerical values of the response of patient i who received dose x_i of a drug Δ, where Δ is either S or T. We denote by $\hat{y}_{i\Delta}$ the so-called predicted value of $y_{i\Delta}$ obtained by substituting x_i, the actual dose of drug Δ administered to patient i in the equation

$$\hat{y}_{i\Delta} = \hat{\alpha}_\Delta + \hat{\beta} \log x_i. \qquad [3]$$

The sum, over all observations, of the square of the difference between the predicting value of y, namely $\hat{y}_{i\Delta}$ and the observed value $y_{i\Delta}$ is referred to as the residual sum of squares or the unexplained variance. The least-squares procedure produces estimates $\hat{\alpha}_\Delta$, and $\hat{\beta}$, which minimize the unexplained variance.

The total variance of a set of data, independent of any hypothesized model is defined to be

$$\sum_{i,\Delta} (y_{i\Delta} - \bar{y})^2 \qquad [4]$$

where $\bar{y}$ is the grand mean. The algebraic relationship between the unexplained variance and the total variance is

$$\sum_{i,\Delta} (y_{i\Delta} - \bar{y})^2 = \sum_{i,\Delta} (y_{i\Delta} - \hat{y}_{i\Delta})^2 + \sum_{i,\Delta} (\hat{y}_{i\Delta} - \bar{y})^2. \qquad [5]$$

The last term on the right of equation [5] is referred to as the explained variance. Equation [5] states

Total variance = unexplained variance + explained variance.   [5A]

Since the total variance is a constant independent of the fit of the regression equation, the regression estimates of the variables α_S, α_T, and β that minimize the unexplained variance, equation [2], are the same estimates that maximize the explained variance. Therefore, the solution to the traditional least-squares problem also maximizes

$$R^2 = \frac{\text{explained variance}}{\text{total variance}}. \qquad [6]$$

The quantity R^2 is the square of the correlation between the observed $y_{i\Delta}$ and the predicted $\hat{y}_{i\Delta}$. Thus, R^2 may be interpreted as the fraction of total variance explained by the model given in equation [1].

We turn now to the problem we are considering, in which the numerical value of the observation $y_{iΔ}$ is unknown. Let Z_j be the unknown numerical value of the jth category of pain intensity. For a patient starting in pain category j, for example, and ending in category j', the response y representing the pain intensity difference (PID) is given by $Z_j - Z_{j'}$. The problem we consider is the simultaneous estimation of Z_j, $α_S$, $α_T$, and $β$ so as to maximize R^2, the fraction of the total variance explained by the regression. In a different context this problem was considered by Ipsen (3) and independently for clinical trials by Laska et al. (4,5). The mathematical details of the methods may be found in these references. The constants Z_j are shown to be the components of the eigenvector corresponding to the maximum eigenvalue of a certain matrix. The maximum eigenvalue is equal to the maximal value of R^2.

It is easy to see that the solution to the maximization problem is not unique for many values of the Z_j will maximize R^2. Suppose that a particular set of Z_j maximizes R^2. Then multiplying each of the Zs by a constant and/or adding a constant to each one leaves R^2 unchanged. Therefore, without loss of generality, the solution may be normalized so that the smallest value of Z_j is 0 and the largest value is 1. Under these constraints, the scores that minimize R^2 are unique.

It should be noted that in the above presentation no mathematical restriction has been made regarding the numerical ordering of the Z_j. Thus, although the verbal categories are ordered, that is, severe is greater than moderate, which in turn is greater than mild, this constraint was not built into the model. It is therefore possible that the estimated values of the Z_j for some sets of data will not be ordered, and it is possible that some of the values will not lie in the interval 0 to 1. For example, if the usual equispace scores contradict linearity, the resulting optimal scores will be consistent with linearity but would contradict the *a priori* pain order relationship. Lin and Tang (6) have developed algorithms that resolve this problem.

QUANTAL RESPONSE MODEL

As above, let z_{jt} represent pain intensity and let t be an indicator for pain etiology. In this model, values for z_{jt}, the jth pain intensity level for pain type t, are to be estimated. Any binary measure of effect can be used, but we shall illustrate the method by using complete relief (CR) or equivalently, zero pain intensity. The mathematical model assumes that the probability P that a patient obtains complete relief from x milligrams of a standard drug having pain of etiology t and initial pain severity z_{jt} is given by the expression

$$P(\text{complete relief} \,|\, t, z_{jt}, x) = 1 - F(λ_Δ z_{jt}^α x^{-β}).$$

Here $λ_Δ$, $α$, and $β$ are constant unknown parameters to be estimated from the data, $Δ = S$ or T, and F is the distribution of the random error. In some applications F may be assumed to be exponential or Weibull, both of which conveniently permit covariates to be added to the model.

The model is a special case of a general tolerance response variable W, of the form

$$W = -h(\lambda_\Delta, x, z) + \epsilon$$

where $h(\lambda_\Delta, x, z)$ is a function of λ_Δ, dose x, and severity z, and ϵ is the random error. Let Y be a quantal response variable indicating when $W > 0$. For example, W may represent pain intensity and Y is an indicator of complete relief. That is, Y takes the value 1 when $W > 0$ and zero otherwise. We obtain

$$P(Y = 1) = P(W > 0) = 1 - F(h[\lambda_\Delta, x, z]) \qquad [7]$$

where F is the probability distribution function of the random error, ϵ. The model described in this report corresponds to a multiplicative representation of h. Thus,

$$P = P(Y = 1) = 1 - F(\lambda_\Delta z^\alpha x^\beta). \qquad [8]$$

The parameters λ_Δ, α, and β are to be estimated from the data. The observations are (n_{ijt}, N_{ijt}) where n_{ijt} is the number of patients with CR among the N_{ijt} patients with severity level z_{jt} who received dose x_i.

In the classical situation, the method of maximum likelihood could be used to estimate the unknown values λ_Δ, α, and β based on the known observed numerical quantities z_{jt}, x_i, and N_{ijt}. Here, however, the observed values, which we shall call Z_{jt}, are verbally described pain categories, and their unknown numerical values z_{jt} are to be estimated as well. A different strategy is required. Let δ_{jt} be indicator variables running over the range of j and t. Thus, δ_{jt} takes the value 1 if the initial pain severity of the observation is z_{jt}, and the value zero otherwise. Introduce c_{jt} as the coefficient of the jth indicator variable.

The new maximum likelihood problem is to estimate the parameters λ_Δ, c_{jt}, and β by maximizing the likelihood which is proportional to

$$L(c_{jt}, \lambda_\Delta, \beta) = \Pi_{ij} F(\lambda_\Delta (\textstyle\sum c_{jt}\delta_{jt}) x_i^{-\beta})^{N_{ijt} - n_{ijt}} (1 - F(\lambda_\Delta (\textstyle\sum c_{jt}\delta_{jt}) x_i^{-\beta}))^{n_{ijt}} \qquad [9]$$

The estimates of c_{jt} are related to the estimates of z_{jt} through the equation $z_{jt}^\alpha = c_{jt}$.

Note that the maximum likelihood estimators are not unique, for if $\hat{c}_{jt}$ and $\hat{\lambda}_\Delta$ are maximum likelihood estimators and k is any nonzero constant, $\hat{c}_{jt}kd$ $\hat{\lambda}_\Delta/k$ are maximum likelihood estimators as well. Thus, the estimators of the severity constants are given, for any choice of k, by

$$\hat{z}_{jt} = {}_j k \qquad [10]$$

These equations do not lead to unique values of z_{jt}. However, all parameter estimators will be uniquely determined by arbitrarily choosing two values of z_{jt} perhaps equal to the values usually assigned to moderate and severe pain for some choice of t. Large sample properties of the estimators follow the standard theory for maximum likelihood estimation.

Suppose a unit dose of the drug suffices to produce CR for a patient with severity level $Z_{i't'}$. Then we define the "relative potency" ρ of severity level z_{it}

to $z_{i't'}$ to be the dose required by a patient with severity Z_{ij} to obtain CR. Under this model, for a fixed medication, i.e., $\Delta = S$ or T, ρ is easily shown to be given by

$$\rho(z_{it}, z_{i't'}) = (z_{it}/z_{i't'})^{-\alpha\beta}. \qquad [11]$$

It is easy to see that the relative potency estimator is not affected by the nonuniqueness of the estimates of the independence of the choices of the levels.

The relative potency ρ of S to T for any fixed severity level and etiology is given by

$$\rho(S, T) = (\lambda_S/\lambda_T)^\beta. \qquad [12]$$

Laska et al. (7) considered the question of the spacing between pain categories within and between pain types, and using the model described above concluded that the numerical values corresponding to pain intensity categories depend considerably on the pain model. They found that with respect to the ability of aspirin to completely relieve pain, the quantal model leads to estimates that suggest that severe initial pain intensity reported by surgical patients following cesarean section is numerically 1.4 times greater than severe initial pain intensity for episiotomy pain, which, in turn, is apparently 3.2 times greater than severe initial pain intensity for uterine cramping pain. This interestingly large range reflects the data well. As Fig. 1 shows, the 1,300-mg dose is insufficient to provide complete relief to even half of the patients with moderate or severe postepisiotomy or severe postsurgical pain. The model predicts that even 1,950-mg dose would not be large enough for half of the patients (ED_{50}) to obtain complete relief. In

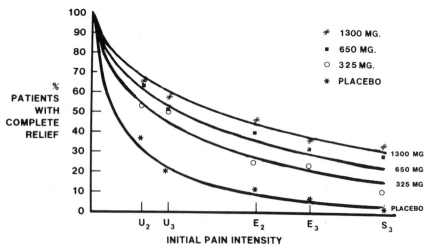

FIG. 1. Initial intensity—complete relief curves (8 studies) in response to three dose levels of aspirin. U_2, uterine moderate; U_3, uterine severe, etc. (From ref. 6, with permission.)

fact, no reasonable dose of aspirin would suffice. On the other hand, for severe uterine cramping pain, approximately 325 mg is the ED_{50}.

DISCUSSION

The quantal model postulates that severity levels for different pain etiologies are quantitatively different. Patients with more severe pain intensity are less likely to obtain complete relief for the same dose of a treatment than are patients with less severe pain; and this would be true for aspirin as well as for placebo and perhaps for any drug. If one accepts the hypothetical concept of an absolute amount of pain on some underlying universal scale, then it is clinically plausible that the intensity of postsurgical pain is more severe than the intensity of episiotomy pain, which, in turn is more severe than the intensity of uterine cramping pain. A patient's report of a level of pain intensity is made in the context of a clinical circumstance. The same word "severe" might be used in the maternity ward and after surgery, but if asked to compare the pain intensity of the two experiences, it seems likely that a patient would say that the latter was much greater than the former.

On the other hand, the quantal model does not rule out the possibility that there are different psychological profiles or mechanisms of action associated with pain of different etiology which may be different for different drugs. Two patients with equally severe pain, i.e., with identical "true" pain intensity levels but of different etiology, may be differentially susceptible to obtaining an analgesic effect from a particular drug or from all drugs. If this were true, an active drug such as aspirin as well as a placebo might provide different pain relief for patients with different etiology, whether or not the underlying initial pain intensities were identical. In the data presented above, both cesarean section pain and episiotomy involve incision of skin and muscle and early postoperative inflammation and might respond in similar fashion to aspirin, but uterine cramp might well have a somewhat different peripheral mechanism and sensitivity to prostaglandin inhibitors.

Although patients may give the same verbal description of their initial severity, the designer of a clinical trial that includes patients with pain of several types would be well advised to take into account the possibility that they may in reality have different levels of response for the same dose of a drug. Note that morphine 2 mg and morphine 16 mg would appear to be of equivalent efficacy in mild uterine cramp as well as in intractable pain. For the mild pain, everyone obtains complete relief, and for the severe pain no one is relieved. The clinician deciding on a dose of an analgesic should keep these differences in mind as well. Much additional research is required with standard and newer analgesics at a variety of dose levels and on patient populations with different kinds of pain. Such studies can provide a basis for more precise labeling information in package inserts. With such comparative information in hand, it is possible that more sensitive treatment and dose selections to match specific clinical needs of a patient can be made.

REFERENCES

1. Lasagna L. The clinical measurement of pain. *Ann NY Acad Sci* 1968;86:28–37.
2. Laska E, Gormley M, Sunshine A, Bellville JW, Kantor T, Forrest W, Siegel C, Meisner M. A bioassay program for analgesic clinical trials. *Clin Pharmacol Ther* 1967;8(5):658–669.
3. Ipsen J. Appropriate scores in bioassays using death-times and survivor symptoms. *Biometrics* 1955;11:465–480.
4. Laska E, Meisner M, Takeuchi K, Siegel C, Wanderling J. Quantifying pain scores: an analytic approach. *Proc Committee Drug Dependence* 1971;107–129.
5. Laska EM, Meisner M, Takeuchi K, Wanderling JA, Siegel C, Sunshine A. An analytic approach to quantifying pain scores. *Pharmacotherapy,* 1986;6(5):276–282.
6. Lin S and Tang D-I. A Unified Approach to Quantifying Ordered Response Categories. Technical Report. N. S. Kline Institute, 1990.
7. Laska EM, Sunshine A, Wanderling JA, Meisner MJ. Quantitative differences in aspirin analgesia in three models of clinical pain. *J Clin Pharmacol* 1982;22:531–542.

Advances in Pain Research and Therapy, Vol. 18,
edited by M. Max, R. Portenoy, and E. Laska,
Raven Press, Ltd., New York © 1991.

30

Statistical Methods in Univariate and Multivariate Bioassay

Eugene M. Laska and Morris Meisner

*Statistical Sciences and Epidemiology Division, Nathan S. Kline Institute for
Psychiatric Research, WHO Collaborating Center for Training and Research in Mental
Health Program Management, Orangeburg, New York 10962; and Department of
Psychiatry, New York University Medical Center, New York, New York 10016*

A bioassay experiment is designed to estimate the relative potency of a test analgesic (T) to a standard analgesic (S). The relative potency of T to S is defined as the dose of T that produces the same biological response as does a unit dose of S (1). Relative potency was developed under the assumption that a test compound is a dilution of the standard. However, the theory is often applied to two different compounds that have parallel dose-response curves over some range of doses. This case is known as a comparative assay.

A bioassay experiment may be either quantal or quantitative, direct or indirect. If the response measure is binary, the assay is said to be quantal (2). Otherwise, it is quantitative. In a direct assay the threshold dose required for a specifically defined response is determined for each experimental unit. Thus, the observed data are dose units and not response values. In an indirect assay the experimental unit receives one or more specified fixed doses of the preparation and the observed data may be either quantal (binary) or quantitative responses. Depending on the experimental design, several dose levels of T and S are given to the same or different experimental units.

In this chapter we discuss only indirect quantitative assays. We first review the elementary theory for the univariate case. Next, we summarize recent work that extends the theory to the multivariate situation. This theory enables the computations of a single estimate of relative potency based on many measures of outcome. For example, instead of obtaining different estimates of relative potency for summed pain intensity difference (SPID), total pain relief (TOTPAR), onset, etc., a single estimate based simultaneously on all of the response variables is obtained. The method also provides an approach for pooling results across experiments.

UNIVARIATE BIOASSAY

Estimating Relative Potency

The statistical analysis of a bioassay experiment requires a model that relates the average response to the dose of the preparations. If the average response is linearly related to the dose, and the line passes through the origin, the model is called a "slope-ratio assay." However, a more commonly used model is the "parallel line assay." In this assay, response is linearly related to the log dose, and the line need not pass through the origin. The mathematical setup of the parallel line assay is as follows. Let the dose of the standard (test abbreviations are in parentheses) preparation be denoted by z_S (z_T) and the log dose by $x_S = \log z_S$ ($x_T = \log z_T$). Let the response variable be denoted by Y_S for S and Y_T for T. The statistical model assumes that

$$Y_S = \alpha_S + \beta x_S + \epsilon_S$$
$$Y_T = \alpha_T + \beta x_T + \epsilon_T,$$

[1]

where ϵ_S (ϵ_T) is distributed normally with mean 0 and variance σ^2 for each value of x_S (x_T). In other words, $\alpha_S + \beta x_S$ is the average response owing to the dose x_S of S, and $\alpha_T + \beta x_T$ is the average response owing to the dose x_T of T. If T is a dilution of S, a dose, ρz_T, of the standard preparation will have an effect equal on the average to a dose, z_T, of the test preparation for every value of z_T in the range of doses for which the model holds. The relationships

$$z_S = \rho z_T$$

and

$$\alpha_S + \beta x_S = \alpha_T + \beta x_T$$

define the constant ρ, the relative potency of T to S. It follows that

$$\alpha_S + \beta \log \rho z_T = \alpha_T + \beta \log z_T$$

or

$$\log \rho = (\alpha_T - \alpha_S)/\beta.$$

[2]

This expression defines the log of the relative potency in terms of the parameters α_T, α_S, and β in equation [1]. The geometric interpretation of the quantity, log ρ, is given in Fig. 1.

To compute the point estimator of log ρ, the point estimators $\hat{\alpha}_S$, $\hat{\alpha}_T$, and $\hat{\beta}$ of the quantities α_S, α_T, and β are necessary. The latter three estimates are obtained by using ordinary least squares regression, and an estimate of log ρ is obtained by substituting the results into equation [2]. These regression estimators are computed in a manner similar to the computation of slopes and intercepts

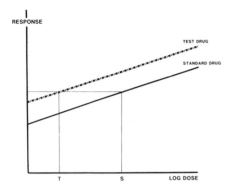

FIG. 1. Dose response for test and standard on a log dose scale. Log relative potency = S − T.

in the usual linear regression problem, but in this case, because of the assumption of parallelism, the slopes of the two lines are constrained to be equal.

A CONFIDENCE INTERVAL FOR RELATIVE POTENCY

Fieller's theorem (1,3,4) provides a method used to obtain a confidence interval for a ratio of parameters when the estimators of both the numerator and the denominator are normally distributed random variables. Its application to bioassay derives from equation [2], which expressed log relative potency as a ratio of the parameters $\alpha_T - \alpha_S$ to β from equation [1].

Let $\hat{\delta} = \hat{\alpha}_T - \hat{\alpha}_S$. From elementary regression theory it follows that $\hat{\delta}$ is a normal random variable with mean $\alpha_T - \alpha_S$, and $\hat{\beta}$ is a normal random variable with mean β. Then $E(\hat{\delta} - \mu\hat{\beta}) = 0$, where the notation E indicates expected value. In such a situation, Fieller's theorem asserts that

$$(\hat{\delta} - \mu\hat{\beta})^2 \le F_{1,\nu}(k_1\mu^2 - 2k_2\mu + k_3)s^2$$

defines a confidence region for $\mu = \log \rho$. Here s^2 is the point estimator of σ^2; k_1, k_2, and k_3 are constants that depend on the log doses and the number of test and standard observations; $\nu = N - 3$, where N is the total number of observations, and $F_{1,\nu}$ is the 95th percentile of an F distribution with 1 and ν degrees of freedom. The confidence interval is determined by the roots, A and B, of the quadratic equation

$$a\mu^2 + b\mu + c = 0,$$

where $a = \hat{\beta}^2 - F_{1,\nu}k_1$, $b = -2\hat{\delta}\hat{\beta} + 2k_2F_{1,\nu}$ and $c = \hat{\delta}^2 - F_{1,\nu}k_3$. If $a > 0$ then the confidence region is the interval [A, B]. But if $a < 0$ and $b^2 - 4ac > 0$, then the confidence region is the exterior of the interval [A, B], i.e., the set $\log \rho \le A$ and $\log \rho \ge B$. A third possibility is that the confidence region is the entire straight line. This uninformative consequence of Fieller's theorem occurs when $a < 0$ and $b^2 - 4ac < 0$. No other cases are possible (5).

TESTING THE VALIDITY OF ASSUMPTIONS

It is standard procedure to test the validity of the model of equation [1] via an analysis of variance (ANOVA) (1). In Table 1, the entry "Regression" tests the null hypothesis that the slope, β, is zero. This test is important for if β is zero, the concept of relative potency has no meaning because from equation [1] the relative potency parameter is undefined. The entry "Parallelism" is a test of the assumption that the dose response lines for test and standard are indeed parallel. The model of equation [1] assumes that the average response of Y_S depends linearly on the log dose, x_S. The true relationship between Y_S and x_S may be more complicated. They could be related by higher-order terms, such as a quadratic involving the square of x_S. "Linearity" is a test of the possibility that a linear model is an inadequate representation of the dose-response relationship. The entry "Preparations" examines whether the two treatments are being studied in the same range of effectiveness. It tests the null hypothesis that the weighted mean response of all doses of the standard equals that of all doses of the test used in the experiment. Even if the hypothesis is rejected, the assay may still be valid. The magnitude of the difference indicates how great an extrapolation in the effect range is involved.

Although the ANOVA is traditionally used to test validity, it is somewhat inconsistent with the analogous tests based on the model of equation [1]. Using likelihood-ratio theory all of the above-mentioned tests can be based on equation [1], thereby avoiding any possibility of inconsistencies. As an illustration, the estimator of σ^2 (required for instance by Fieller's theorem) resulting from the ANOVA model, is not the same as that resulting from the regression model of equation [1]. The dose-response relationship is ignored in the ANOVA model, but it is incorporated in the likelihood-ratio method (6).

TABLE 1. *Analysis of variance for parallel line assay based on a completely randomized (parallel groups) design*

Source of variation	Degrees of freedom[a]
Between doses	$K_S + K_T - 1$
Regression	1
Parallelism	1
Preparations	1
Linearity	$K_S + K_T - 4$
Within doses	$N_S + N_T - K_S - K_T$
Total	$N_S + N_T - 1$

[a] N_S (N_T) is the number of experimental units receiving the standard (test) preparation and K_S (K_T) is the number of different doses of the standard (test) preparation.

COMBINATION OF UNIVARIATE ASSAYS

The problem of combining bioassays (1,7–9) has received renewed attention in recent years. Suppose that several independent bioassay experiments designed to estimate the relative potency of the same test and standard analysis are performed. Each one produces a point and 95% confidence interval estimator of ρ. How can a single point and interval estimate of ρ be produced on the basis of all of the data? Clearly, such combined estimates will be more accurate than those produced by the individual experiments. By application of the method of maximum likelihood, a combined estimator can be obtained (7–9). We mention two features of the combined estimator: (a) the combined estimator of ρ depends not only on the individual estimates of ρ but on the sample sizes, experimental design, estimated residual error, and the statistics $\hat{\alpha}_T$, $\hat{\alpha}_S$, and $\hat{\beta}$ obtained in each of the experiments; and (b) the estimator of log ρ is obtained from the solution to a polynomial equation whose degree is greater than two. This latter situation does not occur if there is only one experiment where, for example, $\hat{\alpha}_T$ is obtained by solving a linear equation and the Fieller confidence interval is obtained by solving a quadratic equation. The new mathematical complication occurs because estimation of the common relative potency is a nonlinear problem.

As in the case of a single experiment, combining many bioassays involves first testing the validity assumptions in the individual studies. Even if a few studies fail to satisfy the validity tests, they need not be excluded from the analysis. Complications arise when the slope of the regression lines of one or two of the studies has a sign that is opposite to those of the other studies. The additional hypothesis requiring investigation is whether the drugs share a common relative potency across experiments. This hypothesis can also be tested by the likelihood-ratio approach. Mathematical complications arise here also because such a hypothesis is not linear. In particular, instead of minimizing a sum of squares as in straight-line regression theory, finding the likelihood-ratio test in this situation requires minimizing a function of the form

$$J(\mu) = \sum_{i=1}^{I} (\hat{\delta}_i - \mu\hat{\beta}_i)^2/(p_i\mu^2 + q_i\mu + r_i),$$

where p_i, q_i, and r_i are constants depending on the log doses in the ith experiment. I is the number of investigators and $\mu = \log \rho$. The value of μ that minimizes $J(\mu)$ is $\hat{\mu}$, the maximum-likelihood estimator of log relative potency. The solution can be found numerically. Another approach to finding the minimum is possible because $J(\mu)$ can be conveniently expressed as a ratio of two polynomials: $J(\mu) = P_1(\mu)/P_2(\mu)$. Standard techniques of differential calculus can then be used to obtain $\hat{\mu}$ as the root of a polynomial equation.

Finally, using likelihood-ratio methods, a Fieller-like confidence region, C for log ρ may be obtained. Likelihood-ratio theory requires the specification of two hypotheses, H_0 and H_1. In the above case, H_0 is the hypothesis that, across all experiments, the log relative potency is equal to a specified value, $\mu_0 = \log \rho_0$. C is the acceptance region of H_0, i.e., the set of all μ_0 for which H_0 is not rejected. An exact method and an asymptotic method, both of which use the same H_0, have been developed. They differ in the choice of H_1, the "alternative hypothesis." If H_1 is the hypothesis that all experiments share an unknown common relative potency, then asymptotic or large-sample distribution theory must be used. If H_1 is the general linear model of equation [1], a common relative potency across all experiments is not assumed, which results in the applicability of exact or small-sample distribution theory. The two approaches lead to different denominators in the likelihood ratio used to compute confidence regions. Nevertheless, the mathematical forms of the two confidence regions are very similar. Note that the word "region" rather than "interval" is used, for C may consist of one interval or many intervals. The possibility of many finite intervals in the confidence region does not occur when a confidence region for log ρ is computed for one bioassay. If C is the asymptotic confidence region, then $\hat{\mu}$, the combined estimator of log ρ, always belongs to C. The exact confidence region, however, may be empty. This situation, too, does not occur with a single bioassay experiment. However, when the exact confidence region C is not empty, $\hat{\mu}$ always belongs to it.

SINGLE AND COMBINED MULTIVARIATE BIOASSAYS

Several articles have discussed multivariate bioassay (6,10–13). Multivariate bioassay estimates a single relative potency when the observation of an experimental unit is not a single value but a vector of multiple responses, e.g., SPID, TOTPAR, PEAK, representing different, but possibly correlated, outcomes. As in a univariate assay, each of the responses of the two drugs S and T are assumed to follow a linear model. For the ith response variable, we assume the model

$$Y_{S,i} = \alpha_{S,i} + \beta_i \log z_S + \epsilon_{S,i} \qquad Y_{T,i} = \alpha_{T,i} + \beta_i \log z_T + \epsilon_{T,i} \qquad [3]$$

where, as before, z_T and z_S are the doses. For the ith response variable, equation [3] is identical to equation [1], the model in the univariate situation. Here, however, if there are, for example, three responses, the covariance between the error terms $\epsilon_{T,1}$, $\epsilon_{T,2}$, and $\epsilon_{T,3}$ play a major role. The vector $\epsilon_T = (\epsilon_{T,1}, \epsilon_{T,2}, \epsilon_{T,3})$ is assumed to be multivariately normally distributed with mean vector (0, 0, 0) and unknown variance-covariance matrix Σ. Note that, as in the univariate case, the standard and test formulations for each fixed i are assumed to have the same slope, β_i, although these slopes may be different for different response measures. If T is in fact a dilution or a new formulation of S, the relative potency should be the same, irrespective of the response measure used. The main goals of a multivariate bioassay are (a) to test the validity of the model of common slope for each variable; (b) to test the hypothesis that there is a common relative potency for each variable; (c) to estimate the scalar quantity, the common relative potency; and (d) to determine a confidence interval for the common relative potency.

If two or more independent bioassay experiments are performed on T and S, as in the univariate case, each experiment separately yields a relative potency. In addition to the above points, another goal of combining multivariate bioassays (13–15) is (e) to analyze the data of all the experiments simultaneously to obtain a single point and interval estimator of relative potency.

The mathematics of these problems are more difficult than those of corresponding problems that arise in the univariate situation. Goal (a) is easiest to reach because it can be formulated as a linear hypothesis with respect to a multivariate model, at the same time being somewhat more general than the multivariate model of equation [3]. The theory of tests of such linear hypotheses is well known. Thus, a test of (a) uses the F-test statistic. In short, (a) is treated as a special case of standard linear multivariate statistical theory. Hypothesis (b), on the other hand, does not arise univariately and is a nonstandard hypothesis testing situation because it is a nonlinear hypothesis. Asymptotic, i.e., large-sample, mathematical techniques are unavoidable. In the multivariate bioassay case, likelihood-ratio theory facilitates a large-sample test of the hypothesis of common relative potency. The same technique yields a maximum-likelihood estimator of the common relative potency and a corresponding 95% confidence interval. In a single multivariate bioassay experiment the methods that generate the tests and estimators described in (a)–(d) surprisingly turn out to require nothing more complicated than solving quadratic equations. However, analysis (e), combining several multivariate bioassays, involves solving higher-order polynomial equations, as in the situation that arises from combining several univariate bioassays. A maximum-likelihood solution to the problem of combining multivariate bioassays has just recently appeared. The mathematical detail of the statistical analyses of these experiments is given in references (13–15).

REFERENCES

1. Finney DJ. *Statistical method in biological assay.* New York: MacMillan, 1978.
2. Finney DJ. *Probit analysis. A statistical treatment of the sigmoid response curve.* Cambridge: Cambridge University Press, 1947.
3. Fieller EC. The biological standardization of insulin. *J R Stat Soc* 1940;137:1–53.
4. Fieller EC. A fundamental formula in the statistics of biological assay, and some applications. *Q J Pharm Pharmacol* 1940;17:117–123.
5. Buonaccorsi J. Letter to the editor. *Am Stat* 1979;33:162.
6. Laska E, Kushner HB, Meisner M. Reader reaction: multivariate bioassay. *Biometrics* 1985;41: 547–554.
7. Bennett BM. On combining estimates of relative potency in bioassay. *J Hyg* 1962;60:379–385.
8. Armitage P, Bennett BM, Finney DJ. Point and interval estimation in the combination of bioassay results. *J Hyg* 1976;76:147–162.

9. Williams DA. An exact confidence region for a relative potency estimated from combined bioassays. *Biometrics* 1978;34:659–661.
10. Rao CR. Estimation of relative potency from multiple response data. *Biometrics* 1954;10:208–220.
11. Volund A. Multivariate bioassay. *Biometrics* 1980;36:225–236.
12. Carter EM, Hubert JJ. Analysis of parallel line assays with multivariate responses. *Biometrics* 1985;41:703–710.
13. Srivastava MS. Multivariate bioassay, combination of bioassays and Fieller's theorem. *Biometrics* 1986;42:131–141.
14. Volund A. Combination of multivariate bioassay results. *Biometrics* 1982;36:225–236.
15. Meisner M, Kushner HB, Laska EM. Combining multivariate bioassays. *Biometrics* 1986;42:421–427.

Advances in Pain Research and Therapy, Vol. 18,
edited by M. Max, R. Portenoy, and E. Laska,
Raven Press, Ltd., New York © 1991.

Chapter 31

Onset and Duration

Measurement and Analysis

Eugene M. Laska,*,** Carole Siegel,*,**
and Abraham Sunshine,**

*The Nathan S. Kline Institute for Psychiatric Research, Orangeburg, New York 10962;
and **New York University Medical Center, New York, New York 10016

INTRODUCTION

The therapeutic effect of a treatment in a specific patient population may be
described in terms of (a) the magnitude of the effect over time; (b) the probability
of obtaining a clinically significant response, i.e., of achieving onset; (c) the probability distribution of time to onset; (d) the probability of cessation of the clinically
significant response; and (e) the probability distribution of the duration of effect.
Except for magnitude of effect over time, rarely is such information directly
obtained in clinical trials. The purpose of this chapter is to suggest that a simple
addition to standard protocols and the use of appropriate methods of statistical
analyses would provide much of this information.

The ideas we describe are general and relevant for many classes of drugs,
including, e.g., bronchodilators, antipsychotics, antidepressants, and analgesics.
In psychopharmacology, the time to onset for an antidepressant, measured in
weeks, is of critical importance because of the high risk of suicide. Also, antipsychotic agents are known to be differentially effective for different schizophrenic
patients so that to the clinician the probability of obtaining onset is important.
Obvious changes in the time-scale and in the clinically significant events that
define onset and duration will permit the principles and methods to be applied
in many other therapeutic classes. For ease of exposition, the concepts are presented in terms of analgesics.

In more than 30 years of analgesic research, clinical researchers have been
following essentially the same clinical trial paradigm for obtaining data from
patients and for analyzing and presenting the results to the medical community
(1). The experimental design is simple. A treatment is randomly assigned to a

---

This chapter reproduced with permission from *Clinical Pharmacology and Therapeutics,* Vol. 49,
No. 1, Mosby Year Book, 1991.

patient whose pain intensity is sufficient to require an analgesic. At subsequent fixed points in time, after baseline, usually at one-half hour, 1 hour, and hourly thereafter for 4 to 6 hours or even longer during the anticipated duration of effect, the patient is interviewed and asked about the current level of pain intensity and the amount of pain relief compared to initial baseline pain. These two measures of effect are usually scored on 4- or 5-point verbal categorical or continuous visual analogue scales.

If a patient drops out before a specified time, denoted by t, during the early stage of the clinical trial because of inadequate relief, a replacement patient is recruited. The rationale for this strategy is based on the belief that if the patient has not waited until t before receiving rescue medication, the drug has not been given an adequate opportunity to be effective (1). For studies of oral analgesics, t is often taken to be 1 hour, while for parenteral agents other times have been used. If a patient drops out after the specified time, the protocol of most studies simply calls for the value at the last actual assessment, usually reflecting no relief, to be imputed for each subsequent scheduled observation, as if the data had actually been observed. Despite compelling clinical arguments that seem to justify the last-observation-carried-forward approach, the analysis of this fictitious data can result in spurious and questionable statements of statistical significance, since, particularly toward the end of the trial, the analyses may be based on real data from only a small number of patients.

As discussed in Chapter 4, efficacy variables are usually derived from pain intensity and pain relief data. Pain Intensity Differences at time t (PID) are the differences between the pain intensity at baseline and at time t. The mean values of these variables are used to construct time-effect curves. Summary measures designed to characterize "total analgesia" over the course of the trial are formed on the basis of estimates of the area under the PID and the pain relief time-effect curves. These are given the acronyms SPID (Sum of the Pain Intensity Differences), and TOTPAR (Total Pain Relief).

Contrasts of mean PIDs, relief scores, the peak response, SPID, and TOTPAR are properly used to evaluate the difference in magnitude of effects among treatments. However, contrasts between the mean PIDs or relief scores have been used to characterize the onset and duration of a drug with considerable potential for error. For example, superiority of the mean effect level of one drug compared to another at the first observation is sometimes said to imply earlier onset, and superiority of mean effect level at the last observation has been said to indicate longer duration. In fact, all this shows is that the drug is more effective at these time points. Particularly because the data of patients who drop out before t are ignored and because for those who drop out after t the values used in the data analysis are imputed, such approaches are neither scientifically nor clinically adequate, and, worse, may be seriously misleading. The difficulty is illustrated by a hypothetical clinical trial comparing an active drug to placebo in which all placebo patients require rescue medication at t for lack of response. Comparisons of mean effect levels after t are therefore completely based on imputed values for placebo with a zero imputed mean effect and zero standard deviation. In such a case, the active drug will be erroneously reported to be statistically superior to placebo in mean effect long past its true duration.

Onset and duration are properties of a treatment that are measured in the time domain. It is almost axiomatic and seems obvious to say that it would be best to gather data about these variables directly in the time domain. Moreover, at the present time this information can only be obtained from the subjective viewpoint of the patient, i.e., in the same fashion as all other efficacy data about response to analgesic treatment are gathered. To accomplish this, we propose an experimental paradigm that augments the traditional fixed interview schedule and describe statistical models that can be used to analyze the data that are collected.

METHODS

Clinical Methods

At baseline, a participating patient is alerted to be sensitive to the time of onset and to the duration of pain relief. Although these times could be estimated retrospectively by the patient from memory (2), two stopwatches are provided to make the information more precise and to focus the patient's attention. They are started at baseline, and the patient is asked to stop one watch the moment a specifically defined, clinically significant amount of pain relief is first experienced. We shall call the time this occurs onset. Similarly, the patient is asked to stop the second watch when the clinically significant pain relief is no longer felt. We shall call this time point offset. Duration is defined as the length of the interval from onset to offset. For drugs of long duration, the offset could take place after the patient has left the clinic.[1]

Many possible clinical endpoints can be used to demark onset and offset. For example, onset could be measured as the time to just noticeable relief, meaningful relief, substantial relief, or complete relief. Offset could be measured as the time at which the patient feels that the pain has returned to the baseline level, is no longer noticeable, no longer meaningful, or that it is so severe that additional analgesic medication is needed. To be fully general, we shall denote the clinical endpoint corresponding to onset by E and to offset by $\bar{\text{E}}$.

For a patient in the trial who has onset at time t_o and offset at time t_d, the resulting data are the pair of numbers (t_o, t_d). However, for many patients t_o may

---

[1] With limited success, both PID and pain relief scores have been used to derive estimates of onset and duration (3). For example, onset time has been estimated as the time from baseline to the time that is midway between the timepoint of the first interview at which the patient reports a reduction of pain from the baseline and the timepoint of the preceding interview.

not be observable because E was not experienced during the course of the observation period. Some nonresponders may drop out of the clinical trial before the observation period is over, and some may hold out until the end. In either case, the time at which the observation of onset is censored[2] is recorded and denoted as t_o^+. Clearly, the true but unobservable value of t_o is greater than t_o^+. Similarly, t_d may not be observed because the patient may not have had onset; such an event is denoted by $(t_o^+, \text{\_\_})$. Or, the patient may have had onset but be lost to follow-up or may not have experienced $\bar{E}$ before the trial is over; such an event is denoted by (t_o, t_d^+). Thus, the possible outcomes for an individual patient in order of decreasing information are (t_o, t_d), (t_o, t_d^+) and $(t_o^+, \text{\_\_})$.

Statistical Methods

Depending on the underlying statistical assumptions that seem tenable, there are several methods that can be used to analyze and summarize onset and duration data. If there are no censored observations, an estimate of the probability of obtaining onset is the proportion of patients who obtained E before the observation period ends. For those who obtain onset, an estimate of the onset survival distribution, the probability of obtaining onset later than time t, may be derived from the histogram of the onset times of these patients. A univariate analysis of onset that estimates these two measures simultaneously is based on a mixture or cure model of the survival distribution H(t) of the observed random variables. Thus,

$$H(t) = P(\text{onset} > t) = 1 - p + pS(t).$$

Here p is the probability of having onset and S(t) is the conditional survival distribution representing the probability that onset occurs later than time t given that onset does ultimately occur. In the presence of censoring, Orazem,[3] Cupples et al,[4] and Laska and Meisner[4] have independently developed Kaplan-Meier-based nonparametric estimates of p and S(t). Gray and Tsiatis (5) have developed a rank test for testing equality of the probabilities p_i for two drugs (i = 1,2) under the assumption that the conditional survival distributions $S_i(t)$ are equal. Laska and Meisner[4] have developed a more widely applicable non-parametric likelihood ratio test for investigating whether the probabilities p_i are equal without the assumption of equality of the $S_i(t)$. Also, Orazem[3] has developed a rank procedure for testing if $S_1(t) = S_2(t)$ without the assumption of equality of the p_i.

Parametric procedures have also been proposed for cure models. Farewell (6)

---

[2] An observation is said to be censored if the patient does not complete the prescribed period of observation and is not evaluated with respect to the outcome of interest.

[3] Orazem J. Rank test to test equality of two survival distributions in a cure model. Ph.D. Thesis, Columbia University, New York, New York 1990.

[4] Laska EM, Meisner M. Nonparametric Testing and Estimation of the Survival Distributions for a Cure Model 1990. (submitted for publication).

has modeled p as a logistic distribution and S(t) as a Weibull distribution. Both components of the model permit the inclusion of covariates.

A similar statistical model may be used for offset or for duration as well. The cure model for duration is

$$P(\text{duration} > t) = (1 - r) + rU(t)$$

where r is the probability of $\bar{E}$, and U(t) is the conditional survival distribution describing the probability that duration is longer than t given that ultimately $\bar{E}$ will occur. The same univariate statistical methods described above for analyzing the onset cure model can be applied to duration data as well.

Laska, Lin, Meisner, and Siegel[5] have developed a parametric bivariate cure model treating onset and duration multivariately. Siegel et al. (7) applied the latter model to a clinical trial of meptazinol versus morphine in postoperative pain.

DISCUSSION

Describing the onset and duration of a drug in terms of four quantities, the probability p of the event E, the conditional survival distribution S(t) of time to onset given that the patient will have onset, the probability r of $\bar{E}$, and the conditional survival distribution U(t) of duration given that the patient had onset and that $\bar{E}$ will occur, appears to us to be clinically and logically compelling.

The design of a clinical trial in which onset and duration parameters are to be estimated needs to be carefully considered. For example, the choice of t determines a censoring point for onset and should be chosen late enough so that patients responding in the tail of the onset survival distribution are able to be observed. For the same reason, the length of the observation period for duration needs to be sufficiently long. Since effect levels need not be obtained in the late hours, the burden of a long follow-up post-medication may not be great. The choice of these time points can make a considerable difference in the precision with which the parameters can reasonably be estimated. Short follow-up time introduces the statistical problem of nonidentifiability, the inability to distinguish between a patient who will never achieve onset and one whose onset will occur late. Clearly, pharmacokinetic considerations will help make appropriate choices of these design parameters.

The onset and duration sample survival distributions can be reasonably summarized using a few percentile points, e.g., the twenty-fifth, the median, the seventy-fifth and perhaps the one-hundreth percentile as well. A summary of the onset properties of a drug might read as follows: "For patients whose pain is comparable to pain resulting from third molar extraction, it may be expected

---

[5] Laska EM, Lin S, Meisner M, Siegel C. A Bivariate Cure Model for Modeling Onset and Duration 1990. (submitted for publication).

that 80% will receive an effect from the drug. Of those who do have an effect, 25% will feel that they are obtaining meaningful relief by 10 minutes or less, half by 20 minutes or less, 75% by 60 minutes or less, and most all who obtain relief will have obtained it by 90 minutes." Such information can help the clinician decide whether the drug is appropriate for a particular patient. Also, if a medication is given and the patient feels no relief, it can help determine a reasonable point in time to administer additional medication. Similarly, a summary of the duration properties of a drug might read as follows: "For patients whose pain is comparable to pain resulting from third molar extraction and who obtain meaningful relief, it may be expected that 33% will require no further medication. Of those that do need an additional analgesic, 75% will require it after 5 hours, 50% after 6 hours and 25% after 8 hours."

It might be argued that the survival distribution of time to onset should include those patients for whom onset never occurs, in contrast to the approach suggested here. We believe that it would be confusing to include such patients as illustrated by the following example. Suppose in a 4-hour study, 51% of the patients on a treatment do not obtain onset, and 49% are completely relieved within 15 minutes; then, if all patients were included in the survival distribution, the estimated median time to onset would be greater than the length of the study. A more appropriate summary of the information is that the drug is effective in only about half of the patients, but in those for whom it does work, onset will occur with probability (near) one within the first 15 minutes.

Different clinical endpoints E used to define onset time, e.g., complete relief rather than meaningful relief, would also undoubtedly produce different probabilities of onset as well as different survival distributions of time to onset. Similar comments, of course, hold for duration. Further research that refines the clinical methodology is to be encouraged, but we believe it would be useful if investigators standardize on one definition of E and $\bar{E}$ so that comparable information across medications can be provided to the treating clinician.

Measurements of onset and duration may be different under different clinical conditions. These include factors such as the type and severity of the pain and psychological, physical, demographic, and medical characteristics of the individual patient. There are also, of course, factors related to the drug itself such as dose, route of administration and, for oral drugs, formulation parameters that influence absorption.

For onset and duration measures to be most clinically relevant, it will be necessary to develop a database of information on standard analgesics. The labelling of a new drug could provide the clinician with a comparative statement such as the following: "For patients with moderately severe postoperative pain, the percentage who may be expected to achieve onset with the new drug is 90%, which is somewhat higher than the 85% achieved with standard analgesic X. Also, for those who do respond, the median onset time was 40 minutes, which is considerably longer than the 25-minute median onset time of standard analgesic X. However, the median duration of effect was 8 hours compared to a median of about 4 hours for standard analgesic X. Finally, although 40% of patients on standard analgesic X do not need additional medication, 75% do not require it on the new drug."

A few clinical pharmacologists with whom these ideas have been discussed do not believe that the definitions described above properly characterize onset and duration. They argue that the time of onset of a medication coincides with the first point in time at which there is a statistically significant difference between the time-effect curve of the treatment and the time-effect curve of a placebo used as a control in the clinical trial. The idea behind this position is that many believe that every response to medication is composed of the sum of at least two parts. The first is the placebo response that would occur if the treatment contained no active ingredients. The second is the incremental contribution produced by the pharmacologically active component of the medication that brings the response above the placebo level. In this view, the patient's perception of a reduction in pain at a time that we have called onset may not, in fact, be due to the active component of the medication but may be due to the placebo component. Thus, until and unless there is a detectable difference between the effect level of the test treatment and placebo, only the effect of placebo is being observed. Onset then is the first instant in time at which the effect levels of the drug and placebo are different.

While the placebo comparison idea is understandable, it seems unlikely that such an instant of time could be reasonably detectable by any clinical study. Moreover, a placebo comparison definition does not take into account the fact that placebo itself is an effective treatment. A treatment is effective if within a reasonable period of time after its administration patients begin to feel some measure of benefit. To deny that individuals treated with placebo have onset leads to logical inconsistencies. For example, it forces the contradictory conclusion that patients whose pain is completely relieved by placebo did not have onset while patients whose pain was relieved by an active drug did have onset. Finally, the placebo-based definition confuses the issue of an appropriate definition of onset with the question of whether the onset of a test treatment and placebo are different. The definition of a clinical event whether relating to the magnitude of an effect or to onset or duration, must stand alone. Contrasts among treatments are necessarily answered in a randomized clinical trial that estimates the parameters and tests the null hypothesis of no difference in effect.

In a preliminary review of the pharmacodynamic data of two of our recent studies, it appeared that among nonresponders who had received strong, effective analgesics, a high percentage had inadequate blood levels indicating an inadequate dose, whereas among nonresponders who had received a weaker, less effective analgesic, many, apparently, had adequate blood levels indicating the limitation of the medication. Recent work (8,9) has begun to relate the patient specific onset time and the serum concentration curve. Many questions remain. We believe that an enlargement of such research will enhance our knowledge of the clinical pharmacology of analgesics.

ACKNOWLEDGMENT

Research in this grant was partially supported by NIMH Grant No. 42959 and a grant from Pfizer, Inc.

REFERENCES

1. Houde RW, Wallenstein SL, Rogers A. Clinical pharmacology of analgesics. *Clin Pharmacol Ther* 1960;1(2):163–174.
2. Laska EM, et al. A bioassay program for analgesic clinical trials. *Clin Pharmacol Ther* 1967;8(5): 658–699.
3. Laska EM, et al. Effect of caffeine on acetaminophen analgesia. *Clin Pharmacol Ther* 1983;33: 498–509.
4. Cupples LA, Terrin NC, Myers RH, D'agostino RB. Using survival methods to estimate age-at-onset distributions for genetic diseases with an application to Huntington Disease. *Gen Epidem* 1989;6:361–371.
5. Gray RJ, Tsiatis AA. A linear rank test for use when the main interest is in differences in cure rates. *Biometrics* 1989;45:899–1904.
6. Farewell VT. The use of mixture models for the analysis of survival data with long-term survivors. *Biometrics* 1982;38:1041–1046.
7. Siegel C, et al. Meptazinol and morphine in postoperative pain assessed with a new method for onset and duration. *J Clin Pharmacol* 1989;29(11):1017–1025.
8. Velagapudi R, et al. Pharmacokinetics (PK) and pharmacodynamics (PD) of aspirin analgesia. Abstract of paper presented at Ninety-First Annual Meeting of the American Society for Clinical Pharmacology & Therapeutics, March 21–23, 1990, Marriott Moscone Center, San Francisco, California. *Clin Pharmacol Ther* 1990;47:179.
9. Laska EM, et al. The correlation between blood levels of ibuprofen and clinical analgesic response. *Clin Pharmacol Ther* 1986;40(1):1–7.

Advances in Pain Research and Therapy, Vol. 18,
edited by M. Max, R. Portenoy, and E. Laska,
Raven Press, Ltd., New York © 1991.

32

Issues in Designing Trials of Nonpharmacological Treatments for Pain

C. Richard Chapman*,† and Gary W. Donaldson*

*Pain and Toxicity Program, Division of Clinical Research, Fred Hutchinson Cancer
Research Center, Seattle, Washington 98104; and †Department of Anesthesiology,
Department of Psychiatry and Behavioral Sciences, University of Washington
School of Medicine, Seattle, Washington 98195*

Nonpharmacological (NP) treatments for pain include such psychological interventions as relaxation, biofeedback and autogenics, operant conditioning, cognitive-behavioral therapy, and hypnosis. Some medical therapies are also nonpharmacological: for example, transcutaneous electrical nerve stimulation (TENS), acupuncture, and trigger-point injection or dry needling. Such treatments have become common methods for pain control, and the need for their rigorous evaluation is pressing. Despite this need, progress is slow because there are few precedents for how to conduct such studies and we lack strong theory to guide work in many NP areas.

This chapter explores the major issues that accompany research on such treatments. These issues fall into four categories: (a) goals of research on NP interventions; (b) setting therapeutic endpoints according to type of pain; (c) measurement of treatment effect; and (d) practical problems in experimental control. We also include a brief overview of methods for studying individual differences.

GOALS OF RESEARCH ON NP INTERVENTIONS

Studies of NP interventions typically address one of two goals: (a) determination of indications for a treatment, or (b) evaluation of the efficacy of a treatment. Determining the indications for a pain treatment necessarily precedes evaluating its efficacy, but investigators concerned with NP interventions are often tempted to skip or minimize this important first step. We emphasize here the importance of careful groundwork on indication for NP therapies.

Indications

Basic work on indications is the first step in evaluating an intervention for pain, even when there is anecdotal clinical evidence that the intervention helps patients. Before we can say how well a treatment "works," we must know which persons, which types of pain, and which specific pains or pathological states are candidates for the intervention. Indications begin with theory (scientific understanding of the nature of the problem and the therapeutic mechanism of the intervention), with clinical anecdotes (clinicians reporting therapeutic success), or in some cases with folklore.

TENS therapy emerged from gate control theory (1) and indications for treatment derive ultimately from our understanding of dorsal horn modulation of nociception. Currently some researchers link TENS to endogenous opioid modulation. Operant behavioral therapy for chronic pain followed from theory, once Fordyce defined pain as a behavior (2). Chemical hypophysectomy for cancer pain (3) eluded, and still eludes, explanation by theory but clinical reports of trial-and-error work have defined the indications for it (4).

Indications for acupuncture exist in folk medicine but are unsubstantiated by scientific knowledge. Some classic indications have proven false. When acupuncture first emerged in the United States, acupuncturists, including modern practitioners in China, made strong claims for its value in treating deafness, but research quickly ruled out hearing loss as an indication for this treatment. There were similar expansive claims for what acupuncture could do for various pain states, but the scientific community has yet to systematically address the issue of acupuncture indications (5).

Headache exemplifies the confusion on this topic. Acupuncture, according to its contemporary advocates and ancient records, can treat headaches, but headaches are subjectively defined events that occur intermittently and there are many types. Cluster headaches in males and premenstrual headaches in females may be wholly different phenomena. Today we distinguish migraine from tension headaches, allowing for "mixed" headaches, but these classifications differ from those used by the ancient Chinese, and there is no way to logically bridge the classifications used in the folk medicine with current medicine. Consequently, the assumption that we already know the indications for acupuncture therapy is tenuous.

The job of specifying indications is rarely a problem in pharmacological work on pain control. Pharmacological studies of therapeutic efficacy generally begin with well-specified indications defined by animal research and industry. However, investigators who deal with NP interventions rarely have the benefit of advanced theory and extensive preclinical work by a manufacturer. Often, they must define the indications for treatment from practitioners' claims, or even from guesswork.

The primary reason for conducting careful studies of indication is that we cannot proceed effectively with studies of efficacy until we define indications. We risk two types of errors: (a) falsely identifying an indication and subsequently undertaking needlessly elaborate studies of efficacy (e.g., acupuncture treats hearing loss); and (b) failing to identify an indication by being insufficiently precise about types of pain problems (e.g., "headache" covers many phenomena) and types of patients (age, sex, and psychologic status may be important). For the sake of example, suppose it is true that acupuncture at points on the ears reduces the intensity and frequency of cluster headaches. Suppose also that this treatment is ineffectual for tension headaches but it increases the frequency and intensity of migraine headaches. If an investigator were to conduct a study on headache patients without regard to type of headache, the mean scores for the mixed sample of patients might well reveal no effect and thus generate a false negative conclusion.

This example indicates that good clinical research must begin with rigorous attention to individual differences. Important differences among patients include sex, age, medical history, and genetic or other organismic predispositions. For the purposes of some studies, immediate stress level and neuroendocrine status, affective state, personality, intelligence, cultural heritage, immediate and long-term social surround, personal meaning of the pain, and resolve to get well can determine outcomes as well. There is much individual variation to explain in behavioral clinical data and some of it must be systematic. The same large variance that obscures treatment effect in studies with weak outcomes, looked at another way, represents opportunity. It is variance to be explained, and much of it may be related to differential treatment response. It is important to examine individual outcomes in early work with NP interventions, as is common practice in analysis of pharmacological data.

When individual differences are large in a data set, the mean represents any one subject poorly. Mean scores before and at repeated time points after treatment may display a pattern of response that reflects no individual's data. Or they may hide several patterns of treatment effects evident in subgroups of subjects. Investigators who venture boldly into large scale evaluations of NP interventions without careful individual subject work on indication risk sampling more than one population and failing to detect and account for the population differences.

We believe that many problems in research on NP interventions occur because researchers assume that they know the indications for therapies and seek to determine treatment efficacy expeditiously, without confirming their assumptions. Reviews of the literature on NP pain control (5–8) report rather modest effects. The results of many clinical trials have been disappointing and curiously at odds with the experience of clinicians who insist that nonpharmacologic interventions help patients (see, for example, the review of the acupuncture literature by Vincent and Chapman, 9).

In sum, work on indications for treatment defines the patients and pain problems that one can reasonably treat with a given NP intervention and protects future investigators from missing treatment effects because of important but undetected individual differences. Such work does not ascertain the magnitude or duration of treatment effect. These issues are part of the evaluation of efficacy.

Therapeutic Efficacy

When one conducts research for the purpose of hypothesis testing, it is only necessary to reject (or fail to reject) the null hypothesis. The criterion for statistical significance is set in advance. Whether the *P* value obtained barely exceeds or wildly exceeds one's criterion for significance makes no difference: scientific inference is the same. However, in studies of therapeutic efficacy, it is important to determine the magnitude of a treatment effect. It is quite possible for a skilled researcher to obtain statistically significant outcomes that are clinically trivial.

Clinicians generally want to know the size of a treatment effect and not just whether it "worked." We can ascertain this broadly from examining the amount of variability in the data set that the treatment explains, typically with multiple regression techniques. The square of the multiple regression coefficient, R^2, represents explained variance due to an intervention when treatments are entered as predictors. Recently, techniques for measuring effect size have emerged and a classification scheme for effect exists (10).

Meta-analyses use such techniques to examine the efficacy of a treatment across multiple studies. Reviewers of nonpharmacologic interventions have generally measured effect size as treatment-control differences in within-group standard deviation units. Miller and Berman (11) found that effect sizes of cognitive-behavioral therapy studies ranged between .21 and .83, which correspond to Cohen's (10) "small" and "large" effect magnitudes, respectively. Mullen et al. (12) found a mean effect size of .20 for psychoeducational interventions to reduce arthritis pain; this corresponds to a "small" effect size (10). Devine and Cook (13) reported a mean effect size for psychoeducational surgical pain interventions of .39, corresponding to a "small-to-medium" effect size. Malone and Strube (14) reported generally larger effect sizes in their survey of chronic pain. Their mean effect size for cognitive-behavioral interventions, for example, was .76, corresponding to a "large" treatment effect.

Cohen's (10) designations notwithstanding, a "large" treatment effect of .8 corresponds to only 14% of explained variance; a "medium" effect to 6%; and a "small" effect to 1%. Although these effect sizes are nontrivial, they leave most of the variance unexplained. From the clinician's perspective, it is important to know whether the unexplained variance is due to systematic individual differences in treatment response or to random error. Some treatments have mediocre efficacy with everyone; others work splendidly when the clinician identifies the right patients for them.

Awareness of individual differences in treatment response is also critical for good clinical science. When effect size is small due to individual differences, the study provides a poor basis for generalizing results to new patients who, *a priori,* have a low probability of response. When explained variance is small, the indications for treatment assume primary clinical importance. Malone and Strube (14, p. 237) concluded, "The critical issue at this time is not demonstration of the superiority of one type of treatment over others, but instead the identification of the type of treatment most likely to provide long-term benefit from a specific type of pain for a specific type of pain patient." Suls and Wan (8) stressed the heterogeneity of effect sizes in their review of painful medical procedures, and suggested the importance of individual differences factors as plausible moderators. These considerations support our claims that careful preliminary work on treatment indication, with attention to individual differences in treatment response, is a critical step in evaluation of NP interventions.

SETTING THERAPEUTIC ENDPOINT ACCORDING TO TYPE OF PAIN

Clinicians frequently distinguish three types of clinical pain states: acute, chronic, and mixed forms such as cancer-related pain. Acute pain is that produced by an immediate lesion or pathologic condition; this type of pain disappears as healing progresses. There are two forms of chronic pain. Chronic nonmalignant pain persists after tissue healing or accompanies pathologic conditions that do not heal. It decreases activity and impairs function. The second form is that associated with a disease process that does not heal. Some patients experience acute and either or both of the two forms of chronic pain together. Cancer patients, for example, may have bouts of acute pain or acutely painful procedural pain that is superimposed upon chronic pain. The therapeutic endpoint for NP intervention differs across these types as shown in Table 1.

Meaningful evaluation of an intervention requires that the therapeutic endpoint fit the pain problem treated. Studies of postoperative pain, in its simplest form, need only measure pain intensity following surgery. On the other hand, studies of interventions for chronic nonmalignant pain benefit little from measures of immediate subjective treatment response. For example, if an investigator wishes to study the effect of TENS in patients disabled by chronic low back pain, he or she needs to determine whether the treatment increases patient functional capability over time. It is of limited value to treat patients in clinic and ask them whether the intensity of back pain is relieved during or immediately following

TABLE 1. *Therapeutic endpoints for nonpharmacological intervention*

Type of pain	Therapeutic endpoint(s)
Acute and chronic malignant	Reduced pain Reduced distress
Chronic Nonmalignant	Increased normal function Increased activity
Mixed	Reduced pain Reduced distress Increased normal functioning Increased activity

TENS treatment. If the patient's activity level does not increase over days or weeks because of repeated treatments or ongoing self-treatment (or if it is reduced because the patient feels worse some hours after treatment in the clinic), then the intervention has not had an appropriate clinical effect. Measuring immediate pain report may even be misleading if the investigator interprets transient sensory change as a positive outcome in chronic pain patients. Many of the early studies of acupuncture pain control made this same mistake: investigators scored chronic nonmalignant pain intensity before and immediately after acupuncture treatment but failed to determine whether the treatment had any lasting effect on the patient's activity level or on the chronicity of the pain (5).

Therapeutic benefit does not necessarily equate with analgesia, particularly in chronic nonmalignant pain patients. None of the three endpoints in Table 1 corresponds precisely to analgesia as we traditionally define it in pharmacologic research, that is, modulation of the transmission of impulses signaling tissue injury. Although one can prevent or relieve pain experience by modulating nociceptive transmission, it is also possible to achieve this goal through cognitive modulation. Return to function is a complex process that may or may not involve modulation of nociception. Psychologic therapies that help the patient to live with nociception through control of attentional processes or to understand that the nociception does not demand restricted activity have little relationship to conventional concepts of nociceptive modulation. Therapeutic endpoint, therefore, may or may not correspond to analgesic response as conventionally defined. This is a major difference between pharmacologic therapeutic outcome studies and NP studies.

Because NP interventions are more complex than pharmacologic ones, the multidimensional nature of pain is particularly important. There is now consensus among researchers, if not in the day-to-day clinical reasoning of most practitioners, that pain is not solely a sensory process. It is a complex perceptual and affective state with sensory, emotional, motivational, and cognitive dimensions. Some NP interventions like hypnosis surely involve complex central nervous system processes, but we lack well-defined theory to guide research on such processes.

These considerations show that the therapeutic endpoint for a given NP intervention depends upon the type of pain under study, theory concerning the mechanism of pain relief, and the specific goals of the investigator. There can be no hard-and-fast rules for therapeutic endpoints in pain control studies with NP interventions, but it is important to avoid confusing acute and chronic pain states in such research.

MEASURING TREATMENT EFFECT

Measurement involves the assignment of numbers to phenomena to scale relevant attributes. Key characteristics are determined by theory and research goals. Pain states have attributes such as (a) intensity, (b) duration, (c) frequency of occurrence, (d) probability of occurrence during activity X, (e) aversiveness, and (f) periodicity. One can score these and other characteristics of pain, including certain physiologic correlates.

Pain patients also have characteristics, and when pain is chronic it is often more important to scale the attributes of the patients under treatment than the attributes of the pain itself. This follows from the clinical principle that therapy should endeavor to restore the functional capability of the chronic pain patient and not just relieve a symptom.

Behavior patterns are one type of patient attribute. Keefe and Block (15) identified bracing, rubbing, sighing, and moaning as behavioral manifestations of chronic back pain. They developed a system for coding such behavior patterns from videotapes of patients. The behavioral attributes of other pain states differ, but all behavioral patterns can be quantified by frequency or conditional probability of occurrence once they are identified. General or specific levels of activity are also good patient attribute variables useful for therapeutic outcome studies. Rate or endurance at repetitive work movements (e.g., painting a ceiling, lifting a weight), speed and distance in walking or other locomotion, working to the point of pain, accuracy of work beyond the point of pain, and general up- versus downtime in a 24-hr day can all serve as measures of persons debilitated by pain (16,17). In the right circumstances, such measures can define therapeutic endpoint.

In general, acute pain studies require measures derived from attributes of the pain state. Chronic nonmalignant pain studies require measures derived from attributes of the person in pain and have more to do with the functional capability of the individual than the sensations he reports. Mixed pain states require measures of both sorts. Therapeutic endpoints follow from this breakdown. More than one endpoint can be used in most studies, but the investigator must understand clearly what the different measures mean for the treatment under study.

PRACTICAL PROBLEMS

There are two major problems in research on NP interventions: (a) achieving adequate experimental control, and (b) achieving gradations in treatment (dosing).

Achieving Adequate Experimental Control

Discussions of control are often framed in the language of "placebo" treatments, but control in NP research is a more complicated issue than this. The NP pain researcher typically must introduce an intervention in a context where patients already receive treatments for pain, and he or she must recognize that most pain tends to vary over time according to circadian and ultracadian variation, adventitious environmental events, and with healing. We can see immediately, then, that most studies require controls for "treatment as usual" and perhaps for time as well.

When chronic nonmalignant pain or mixed pain are the targets of a controlled trial of a NP intervention, the investigator will need to account for the possibility that the patients will be treated elsewhere. Cancer patients are likely to receive analgesic medications from their primary care providers, and hospitalized patients are likely to receive pain control medications from house staff. Chronic nonmalignant pain patients tend to be "doctor shoppers," and many will seek relief from physicians outside of the study or from chiropractors, acupuncturists, over-the-counter remedies, biofeedback specialists, or others. Even when outside treatment is objectively ineffectual, it may affect the patient's responses to the study psychologically. In some cases, manipulation treatments, exercise, or other interventions may exacerbate pain in patients under study. There is no standard way to control for these "contaminants," but it is essential to query subjects about concurrent interventions before they go off study.

Psychologic researchers face a further control problem when they teach pain coping skills to patients. Most patients, left to themselves, will cope in their own ways with pain. Some can do very well, and others will do poorly or counterproductively. The intervention introduced by the therapist will therefore interact with these individual differences. Poor copers may benefit maximally. Persons who would otherwise be good copers may benefit little and may even do less well than normal because they are less well suited to the new method than to their normal skills. In the control conditions, good copers will perform well because of psychologic factors, and this will reduce the apparent efficacy of the intervention introduced. Fundamentally, this is a problem of defining treatment indication. Investigators need to determine which patients are suitable candidates before gauging the success of an intervention. New alternatives for measurement of coping skills and better control procedures are likely to emerge in the literature in the near future as researchers become increasingly aware of this problem.

The classical control problem, defined by pharmacologic researchers as double-blind placebo treatment (a procedurally equivalent but ineffectual intervention like an inert tablet) can take on complex dimensions in NP work. In psychological studies of cognitive-behavioral interventions for acute pain, there is no inert treatment: any human contact can have a psychological effect. Therefore, the best control is a single-blind therapist contact condition in which the psychologist meets with control patients for the same amount of time as experimental patients, but conducts no formal intervention.

With TENS for acute pain, one can feign control conditions by using a stimulator without electrical power, telling the patient that the current is too low to detect. However, some patients will not believe this (especially when informed consent procedures introduce the possibility of a false treatment), and careful investigators should determine and record whether the patients believe the control treatment when debriefing them at the end of the study. Control may be best achieved by using combinations of current intensity and pulse frequency that previous studies have shown to be ineffectual.

Control treatments in acupuncture research are an ongoing issue. There is no acupunctural intervention that is known to be wholly ineffectual, so that one risks using an active treatment as a control if one inserts a needle into tissue. Options include placing needles at sites immediately adjacent to, but not at, classically defined acupuncture points, placing needles at irrelevant points, and feigning insertion of the needles. The latter procedure is performed with the patient visually shielded from the treatment field. One can simulate needle insertion by pinching the skin. Alternatively, when acupuncture is performed with a needle in a guide tube with a piston, the investigator can rig a control device that retracts the needle when it appears to insert it. However, as with TENS, patients tend to disbelieve treatments they cannot feel.

In a few cases, control for NP treatments is straightforward. Biofeedback researchers sometimes use false feedback as a control treatment condition. This prevents patients from learning how to control physiological responses and yet they are engaged in the therapeutic activity. Laser treatments offer good options for control as well. Patients cannot feel laser stimulation of acupuncture points. In both of these cases, the researcher can deliver an ineffectual treatment with double-blinding, thus achieving good control.

Achieving Gradations in Treatment (Dosing)

In conventional research, one ought to be able to compare changes from baseline in pain across therapeutic doses by examining means at each dose (pp. 73–78). Pharmacologists derive therapeutic effect from dose-response relationships. Mean values are the standard focal points for their statistical analyses. Repeated measures typically yield log-linear trends in pain reduction over increasing dose. Unfortunately, with NP interventions, manipulation of dose or a related concept eludes us still.

Investigators working with therapies other than drugs face a significant challenge in designing dosing schedules. Indeed, some cannot even define what dosing means for their intervention. Acupuncture is a prime example. There is much speculation but no agreement on how acupuncture works. If, in fact, it does work, then there may be more than one mechanism. Does an acupuncturist use a stronger treatment if he inserts more needles? Or should he stimulate the needles more vigorously upon insertion or perhaps leave the needles in place longer to increase treatment effect? If he believes that he is "releasing his patient's endorphins" by needling, then treatment should become stronger as the therapist elicits greater stress response from the patient. On the other hand, if treatment works by producing sympathetic nervous system inhibition, then treatment strength needs to be gauged some other way.

Does increasing the current on a TENS unit increase dose? Or should the investigator measure treatment duration to gauge strength? Perhaps the length of time the psychotherapist spends with the patient or the time the acupuncture needles are left in the patient is the best indicator of treatment magnitude. The preliminary work to define these fundamental principles has yet to be done.

Schimek et al. (18) attempted to demonstrate a dose-response relationship for electrical acupunctural stimulation in laboratory volunteers undergoing painful electrical tooth pulp stimulation. They varied the intensity of the electrical stimulus and found that analgesic effect occurred with a sufficiently high electrical stimulus intensity (near the subject's level of tolerance), but there were no gradations in response from faint to very strong stimulation. This observation raised the possibility that many NP interventions may be characterized by all-or-nothing relationships between treatment and effect. It may be inappropriate or impossible to demonstrate gradations in treatment response for some of them.

GENERAL METHODS FOR ADDRESSING INDIVIDUAL DIFFERENCES

We advocate examining individual outcomes, but we offer no recipe for how they should be analyzed. Below, we provide a brief general guideline for how one can examine individual treatment response in a data set and note that designs exist for research with single subjects. Approaches to the formal analysis of individual outcomes fall under two principal themes: time series (including single-subject designs) and longitudinal modeling.

Examining Individual Treatment Response

If an investigator hopes to account for important individual differences, he must take care to record all relevant variables when new subjects are entered onto study: age, sex, disease, medication intake, etc. Relevant variables depend upon the nature and immediate circumstances of the study; there is no standard list for what to measure. And there can be no substitute for careful thought. Giving general psychological tests for personality like the Minnesota Multiphasic Personality Inventory, measuring this or that trait, and other casting of broad nets is unlikely to yield anything of value unless the investigator has specific hypotheses in mind. Tests for affective state and coping style are promising for NP work with behavioral interventions because these factors are likely to interact with treatment, but they may be useless for TENS studies in which depressed patients are screened out in advance. A few well thought out variables, chosen with clinical insight, usually will prove more valuable than a plethora of odds and ends.

When sufficient data have been collected, the investigator can examine scatterplots and other graphic depictions of data to explore clusters in treatment response. Do males and females tend to form separate groups in treatment response? Does age correlate with treatment response? When sample size is sufficiently large, multiple regression techniques can identify which variables, if any, predict treatment response along with treatment or interact with treatment in predicting treatment response. Newly developed computer graphics programs allow for three-dimensional and other complex plots that facilitate data exploration, and these can be a great asset in ascertaining individual differences. Data exploration is detective work; it provides clues. These clues require further thinking in light of theory and clinical experience in order to generate hypotheses. Multiple regression and other inferential statistical methods can confirm or disprove individual differences.

Some work on individual differences requires pattern recognition. When the investigator obtains repeated measures of pain and response to intervention, he can profile individual subject data sets and compare the profiles across individuals, looking for relationships between patterns of response and individual difference variables.

Single-Case Design and Analysis

In certain cases, large sample sizes are simply not feasible. There are rare but important single cases that merit scientific report. For example, one might encounter a patient with congenital insensitivity to pain or agenesis of the corpus callosum, but it will never be possible to sample from a population of such patients. Single-subject designs permit an investigator to rigorously assess response to treatment in a single patient. Barlow and Herson (19) have compiled a useful collection of designs and analysis methods for such situations. These methods may prove valuable in determining indications for NP pain therapies. Their potential value remains largely unexplored to date.

Time Series

Some clinical trial designs provide outcome measures at many equally spaced time points. For example, one might track pain patients daily for a month. Given enough time points (more than 30), an investigator could apply time series analyses for the analysis of each individual separately. The auto regressive integrated moving average (ARIMA) model of Box and Jenkins (20) estimates the parameters generating the time series. The investigator can treat these parameter estimates as individual outcomes and incorporate them in conventional analyses.

Longitudinal Modeling

More commonly, clinical trials obtain measures at only a few time points. Rogosa et al. (21) discuss analysis of individual outcomes in the very common two-occasion design. With more than two occasions of measurement, empirical Bayes estimation yields parameters of individual growth curves with optimal mean squared error by incorporating reliability information about the individual trends (22,23). Laird et al. (24) and Laird and Ware (25) offer a random-effects longitudinal model that applies to individual growth curves as well as more general repeated-measures problems.

SUMMARY

Evaluation of NP interventions for pain is complex, because methods differ markedly for acute, chronic nonmalignant, and mixed acute/chronic types of pain. Individual differences in NP treatment response are typically large and further complicate matters. Careful work on treatment indication before study of treatment efficacy can facilitate the process of evaluating these increasingly prominent pain control techniques.

In clinical studies, magnitude of treatment effect is important; it is not sufficient to simply demonstrate that an intervention is significantly different than control conditions. Establishing effective control conditions is challenging with most NP interventions and involves much more than simply introducing a "placebo" control. Whether these treatments permit evaluation of graded treatment-response effects remains at issue; some, like surgical interventions, may have all-or-nothing treatment-response relationships.

REFERENCES

1. Melzack R, Wall PD. Pain mechanisms: a new theory. *Science* 1965;150:971–979.
2. Fordyce WE. *Behavior methods for chronic pain and illness.* St. Louis: CV Mosby, 1976.
3. Miles J. Chemical hypophysectomy. In: Bonica JJ, Ventafridda V, eds. *Advances in pain research and therapy,* vol 2. New York: Raven Press, 1979;373–380.
4. Gianasi G. Neuroadenolysis of the pituitary of moricca: an overview of development mechanisms, technique, and results. In: Benedetti C, Chapman CR, Moricca G, eds. *Advances in pain research and therapy,* vol 7. New York: Raven Press, 1984;647–678.
5. Chapman CR, Gunn C. Acupuncture. In: Bonica JJ, Loeser J, Chapman CR, Fordyce WE, eds. *The management of pain,* 2nd ed. Philadelphia: Lea and Febiger, 1990;1805–1821.
6. Turner JA, Chapman CR. Psychological interventions for chronic pain: a critical review. Part I: relaxation training and biofeedback. *Pain* 1982;12:1–21.
7. Turner JA, Chapman CR. Psychological interventions for chronic pain: a critical review. Part II: operant conditioning, hypnosis, and cognitive-behavioral therapy. *Pain* 1982;12:23–46.
8. Suls J, Wan CK. Effects of sensory and procedural information on coping with stressful medical procedures and pain: a meta-analysis. *J Consult Clin Psychol* 1989;57:372–379.
9. Vincent CA, Chapman CR. Pain measurement and the assessment of acupuncture treatment. *Acupuncture in Medicine VI* 1989;1:14–19.
10. Cohen J. *Statistical power analysis for the behavioral sciences,* 2nd ed. Hillsdale, New Jersey: Lawrence Erlbaum Associates, 1988.
11. Miller RC, Berman JS. The efficacy of cognitive behavior therapies: a quantitative review of the research evidence. *Psychol Bull* 1983;94:39–53.
12. Mullen PD, Laville EA, Biddle AK, Lorig K. Efficacy of psychoeducational interventions on pain, depression, and disability in people with arthritis: a meta-analysis. *J Rheumatol (Suppl 15)* 1987;14:33–39.
13. Devine EC, Cook TD. Clinical and cost-saving effects of psychoeducational interventions with surgical patients: a meta-analysis. *Res Nurs Health* 1986;9:89–105.
14. Malone MD, Strube MJ. Meta-analysis of non-medical treatments for chronic pain. *Pain* 1988;34:231–244.

15. Keefe FJ, Block AR. Development of an observation method for assessing pain behavior in chronic low back pain patients. *Behav Ther* 1982;13:363–375.
16. Sanders SH. Automated vs. self-help monitoring of "up-time" in chronic low back pain patients: a comparative study. *Pain* 1983;15:399–405.
17. Mayer TG, Gatchel RJ, Kishino N, et al. A prospective short-term study of chronic pain patients utilizing objective functional measurement. *Pain* 1986;25:53–68.
18. Schimek F, Chapman CR, Gerlach R, Colpitts YH. Varying electrical acupuncture stimulating intensity: effects of dental pain evoked potentials. *Anesth Analg* 1982;61:499–503.
19. Barlow DH, Herson M. *Single case experimental designs: strategies for studying behavior change.* New York: Pergamon Press, 1984.
20. Box GEP, Jenkins GM. *Time series analysis: forecasting and control,* 2nd ed. San Francisco: Holden-Day, 1970.
21. Rogosa D, Brandt D, Zimowski M. A growth curve approach to the measurement of change. *Psychol Bull* 1982;92:726–748.
22. Bryk AS, Raudenbush SW. Application of hierarchical linear models to assessing change. *Psychol Bull* 1987;101:147–158.
23. Morris CN. Parametric empirical Bayes inference: theory and application. *J Am Stat Assoc* 1983;78:47–65.
24. Laird N, Lange N, Stram D. Maximum likelihood computations with repeated measures: application of the EM algorithm. *J Am Stat Assoc* 1987;82:97–105.
25. Laird NM, Ware JH. Random-effects models for longitudinal data. *Biometrics* 1982;38:963–974.

Subject Index

Neuropathic pain (*contd.*)
  placebos, 208–210, 226–227
  response, 197
  treatment conditions, 197
  treatments, 196–197, 208–210, 226–227
  trial purpose, 195–198, 222–223
crossover design, 210–212, 227–228
drug treatment
  knowledge requirements, 193, 194, 198–200, 223–224
  maximum dose, 198
    response time, 198
    safety, 198
    toxicity, 199
  lorazepam, 199
  McGill Pain Questionnaire, 201–202
  parallel design, 212–213, 227–229
  placebo, 199
  response, 181
  response variability, 180
  visual analogue scale, 201
New chemical entity, 9
No treatment group
  chronic pain, 158
  placebo, 158
Nociceptive pain, cancer pain, 243, 287, 288
Nonnarcotic analgesic, cancer pain, 268–269, 272–273
Nonpharmacological pain treatment, 691–702
  dosing, 699–700
  efficacy, 694–695
  experimental control, 697–699
  individual difference, 700–702
    longitudinal modeling, 701–702
    single-case analysis, 701
    single-case design, 701
    time series, 701
    treatment response, 700–701
  measurement, 696–697
  problems, 697–700
  research goals, 691–695
  therapeutic endpoint, 695–696
    type of pain, 695–696
Nonresponder
  onset, 135
  outcome measures, 135
Nonsteroidal antiinflammatory drug
  cancer pain, 180, 235–236, 268–269
  experimental pain model, 37–38
  low back pain, 292–293
  orofacial pain, 391
  sickel cell disease, 323–325
Normorphine, relative potency study, 78, 80
Norpropoxyphene, plasma concentration-time profiles, 544
Nurse observer, 607–619
  adverse effect, 613
  baseline evaluation, 611–613
  commentary, 621, 627–630
  dropout, 614
  early termination, 614
  entry note, 613–614
    inpatient studies, 613–614
    outpatient studies, 616–617
  exit note, 613–614

  inpatient studies, 613–614
  outpatient studies, 616–617
informed consent, 611
inpatient analgesic studies, 607–614, 621–624
inpatient screening procedures, 627–629
interval evaluation, 611–613
monitoring, 624–625
oral surgery model, 629–630
outpatient analgesic studies, 614
outpatient studies, 624
patient interview, 609, 622–623
record review, 608–609, 622
remediation, 613
selection, 625
training, 617–619, 624–625, 630
  observation, 617
  performance monitoring, 618–619
  reading assignments, 617–618

O

On-demand analgesia computer, 483–484, 508
Onset
  dose, 135
  fine measurements, 135
  meptazinol, 135
  morphine, 135
  nonresponder, 135
  single-dose comparison, 132
  stopwatch measure, 134
Open-label dose administration
  multidose study, 178
  repeated-dose study, 170
Open trial, cancer pain, 255–256
Opiate
  experimental pain model, 37
  pain threshold, 33–34
Opiate adjuvant, cancer pain, 267–279
  clinical trial guidelines, 274–279
  commentary, 283–286
  current use, 268–274
  long-acting drugs, 275–276
  monoamine pathways, 284
  patient selection, 276–278
  short-acting drug, 276
  study endpoints, 278–279
  suggested drugs, 268
  tricyclic antidepressant, 284
Opioid
  adrenocorticotropin, 600
  cancer pain, 237–239
  child, 446
  cortisol, 600
  beta-endorphin, 600
  mechanisms, 49–50
  patient-controlled analgesia, 516–519
    alfentanil, 517
    brain concentration, 516–519
    fentanyl, 517
    morphine, 517
    plasma concentration, 516–519
  pharmacokinetics, 539
  stress hormone, 600–602
Oral surgery pain
  clinical trial, 347–373